A TEXTBOOK

of

OBSTETRICS

by

EDWARD A. SCHUMANN, A.B., M.D., F.A.C.S.

Professor of Obstetrics, School of Medicine, University of Pennsylvania;
Surgeon-in-Chief, Kensington Hospital for Women; Gynecologist and
Obstetrician to Philadelphia General and Memorial Hospitals;
Obstetrician to Chestnut Hill Hospital; Consulting Gynecol-
ogist to Frankford, Jewish, Burlington County and
Rush Hospitals

WITH 581 ILLUSTRATIONS
ON 497 FIGURES

PHILADELPHIA AND LONDON

W. B. SAUNDERS COMPANY, *Publishers*

1936

MADE IN U. S. A.

PRESS OF
W. B. SAUNDERS COMPANY
PHILADELPHIA

TO

JOSEPH BRETTAUER, M. D.

Distinguished physician; trusted
counsellor; true friend.

PREFACE

It is traditional that medical works should be embellished with a preface, and as he who follows tradition gains merit, the writer of this book dares not depart from the rule.

My object in preparing the work has been to present, to students and practitioners of medicine, the art and science of obstetrics as it is regarded at this time. The experience gained as a practitioner and teacher of obstetrics has been drawn upon to present the various phases of this subject in as well balanced a form as possible. The mechanics of childbirth, and its more common complications, have been given great weight, while the more rare conditions are but briefly sketched.

Unproved theories are simply mentioned, but no attempt has been made to avoid controversial topics, it being my belief that both student and physician gain by forming their own opinions after a scrutiny of both sides of a disputed matter.

It is with keen regret that the historical side of obstetrics could not be discussed fully, but the limitations of space in a textbook preclude any full consideration of this fascinating subject, so that it has perforce been eliminated.

I have eliminated the use of proper names as much as possible, in order to clarify the text. Reference to the work of those who have done original work in obstetrics will be found in an appended bibliography.

My very sincere thanks are due to Dr. Adrian W. Voegelin for his unremitting patience and skill in the preparation of photographs, to Miss Olive Stoner and Mr. A. L. Comroe for their painstaking and artistic work upon the illustrations, to Miss Mary Brophy for her long and excellent work upon the manuscript and to Dr. Clayton T. Beecham for his criticism and correction of the material.

Messrs. W. B. Saunders Company by their unfailing courtesy and helpfulness have made the task a pleasant one.

Edward A. Schumann.

1814 Spruce Street,
Philadelphia, Pa.
September, 1936.

CONTENTS

I. INTRODUCTION—GENERAL PRINCIPLES UNDERLYING REPRODUCTION

CHAPTER I

CHAPTER II

CHAPTER III

CHAPTER IV

CHAPTER V

CHAPTER VI

II. PREGNANCY

CHAPTER VII

V. THE PATHOLOGY OF LABOR

CHAPTER XXVIII

CHAPTER XXXV

CHAPTER XXXVI

CHAPTER XXXVII

CHAPTER XXXVIII

CHAPTER XXXIX

CHAPTER XL

VII. OPERATIVE OBSTETRICS

CHAPTER XLI

CHAPTER XLII

CHAPTER XLIII

CHAPTER XLIV

CHAPTER XLV

CHAPTER XLVI

A TEXTBOOK OF OBSTETRICS

I. INTRODUCTION—GENERAL PRINCIPLES UNDERLYING REPRODUCTION

THAT series of events, which, originating in the fertilization of a ripe ovum, culminates in the birth of a mature infant, perfect in all of its mechanisms and prepared to assume at once the physiological activities incident to terrestrial existence, has no parallel, even in the wonder house of natural phenomena.

When the details of the reproductive cycle are surveyed, one must stand in awe of the flawless interrelationship of the biological and chemical principles involved and of the precision with which the same infinitely complicated mechanism is perfectly repeated for countless generations.

Obstetrics is that branch of medicine which deals with the delivery of a woman in childbed, if the term be used in its narrowest sense, the word being derived from the Latin *obstetrix*, a midwife, from *obstare*, to stand before. In its wider meaning, however, obstetrics is concerned with the entire series of phenomena which constitute the reproductive cycle of women, from the development of the sex organs to their senescence, including the ontogeny of the child.

It is apparent that the complicated mechanisms involved, the normal and abnormal physiological processes, the accidents to which mother and fetus are liable, and the tremendous importance to race development of successful production of offspring, render this branch of medicine of the greatest importance.

The maternal mortality during the process of reproduction varies from 0.4 to 0.7 per cent throughout the civilized world and in spite of the improvements in obstetric methods and teaching, these figures have not been lowered appreciably during the past quarter century. Lea well remarks that advances in asepsis and in surgical technic have been nearly balanced by the increased tendency to unwise operative interferences as a result of the confidence inspired by these advances. Just now, there are searching surveys of maternal and infant mortality under way in many countries. In the United States there are a number of such investigations being conducted with great vigor, under the auspices of various medical agencies.

It is hoped that, by careful analysis of the causes of death in the study of large case series, there may ensue a substantial reduction in the mortality rate.

CHAPTER I·

ANATOMY OF THE FEMALE REPRODUCTIVE ORGANS

The female genitalia consist of the intra-abdominal organs, the uterus and its ligaments, the fallopian tubes, and the ovaries; and the extra-abdominal organs, *i. e.*, the vagina, a portion of the cervix uteri, the vulva and the mammary glands.

UTERUS

The uterus is a single, hollow, muscular organ, located in the pelvic cavity, its function being to furnish a place of nidation for the ovum, supply it with pabulum, and expel it when mature.

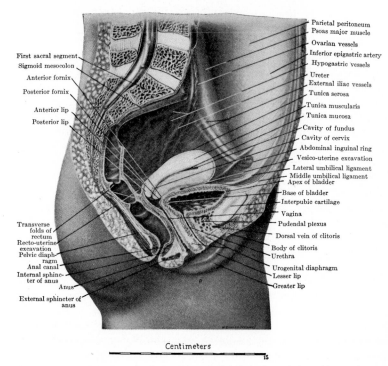

Fig. 1.—Median sagittal section of the female pelvis. (Anson.)

The virgin uterus is shaped much like a small pear, slightly flattened anteroposteriorly and measures on the average 6 cm. in length, 5 cm. in width and 3 cm. in thickness. Its weight is from 40 to 50 Gm., the uterus of the parous women being somewhat larger and heavier.

18

The uterus is divided into two main parts, the *body* or *fundus* and the *neck* or *cervix*. The two are connected by the isthmus, which when considered in an obstetrical sense is termed the *lower uterine segment*. The body of the uterus is much larger than the cervix in adults, particularly in parous women. The fundus uteri lies wholly within the abdominal cavity, whereas the cervix extends downward into the vaginal tube, and is extra-abdominal. The body of the uterus communicates with the fallopian tubes above, and the cervix communicates with the vagina below (Fig. 3).

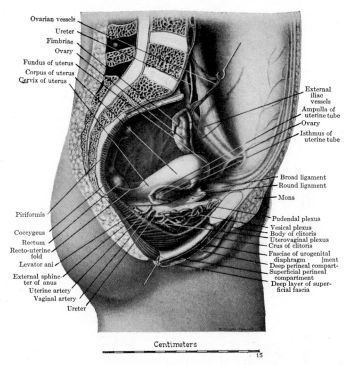

Ovarian vessels
Ureter
Fimbriae
Ovary
Fundus of uterus
Corpus of uterus
Cervix of uterus

External iliac vessels
Ampulla of uterine tube
Ovary
Isthmus of uterine tube

Broad ligament
Round ligament
Mons

Piriformis
Coccygeus
Rectum
Recto-uterine fold
Levator ani
External sphincter of anus
Uterine artery
Vaginal artery
Ureter

Pudendal plexus
Vesical plexus
Body of clitoris
Uterovaginal plexus
Crus of clitoris
Fasciae of urogenital diaphragm   [ment
Deep perineal compart-
Superficial perineal compartment
Deep layer of superficial fascia

Centimeters
15

Fig. 2.—Paramedian section of the female pelvis. The pelvic venous plexuses are shown in relation to the organs. The peritoneum has been cut away to show the ureter and the ovarian vessels. The right ovary is shown in the position which it holds in the living body. (Anson.)

The organ is hollow, being pierced by a cavity which is flattened anteroposteriorly, and broadened out laterally at the fundus, where its lumen becomes continuous with that of the fallopian or uterine tubes.

The cavity is more nearly circular in outline where it traverses the cervix, terminating at a central orifice in this structure termed the *external os*. At the isthmus uteri there is a little constriction of the cavity termed the internal os. The fundus is broad and rounded, and the fallopian tubes are attached to its upper outer aspects which are slightly drawn out to meet the tubes, these angles of the fundus being called the *uterine cornua.* The cervix is almost cylindrical and is divided into a supravaginal and a vaginal portion by the attachment of the vagina to its external surface. The vaginal attachment is

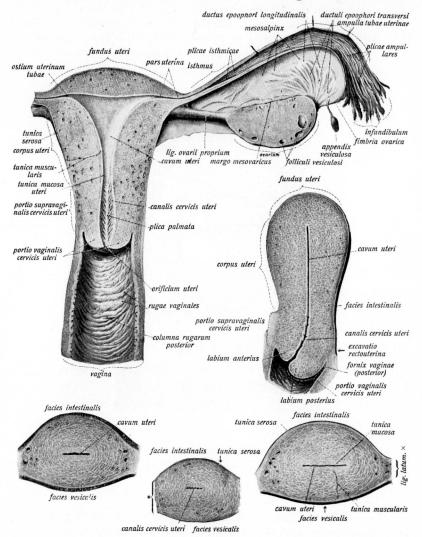

Fig. 3.—Details of the anatomy of the uterus. (Sobotta and McMurrich.)

higher on the posterior aspect of the cervix, about one half of this portion being in the vagina, as opposed to one third of the anterior portion.

The vaginal cervix terminates in a smooth, rounded external orifice, the *external os,* while its uterine end terminates in the internal os which is simply a constriction of the cervical canal at its junction with the cavum uteri.

The urinary bladder is attached to the lower one third of the anterior surface of the uterus.

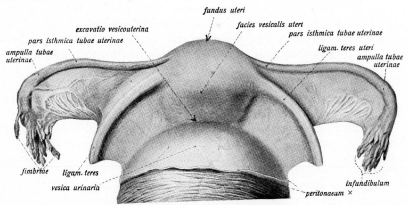

Fig. 4.—The female organs of generation viewed from in front. (Sobotta and McMurrich.)

There is a gentle angle between the cervix and the fundus uteri of from 80 to 100 degrees and the axis of the uterus is therefore a curve, its concavity anterior, the fundus lying in anteversion and with a slight degree of anteflexion on the cervix.

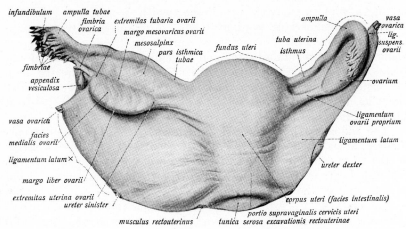

Fig. 5.—The female organs of generation viewed from behind. (Sobotta and McMurrich.)

Ligaments of the Uterus.—The uterus is held in position by a series of ligaments, one pair of which is of muscular tissue, the *round ligaments* or *ligamenta teres*. These structures are of unstriped muscle and connective tissue, and arising from the cornua of the uterus just anterior to the origin of the fallopian tubes, they run diagonally across the pelvis and enter the inguinal canals, where they finally fade into the subcutaneous tissues of the inguinal canals and labia majora. The remaining ligaments consist of three pairs of peritoneal folds, as follows: the *broad ligaments* (ligamenta lata) pass from the lateral aspects of the uterus to the sides of the pelvis, which is divided by them into an anterior and posterior compartment. The broad ligaments enclose within their folds the fallopian tubes, the ovarian vessels and the anastomosing branches of the uterine vessels, with the lymphatics and nerves (Figs. 4 and 5).

The two *uterovesical ligaments* are folds of peritoneum passing from the dorsal surface of the urinary bladder to the cervix uteri.

The two *uterosacral ligaments* are also peritoneal folds passing between the sides of the rectum and the lateral walls of the uterus and forming a space which is known as the pouch or *cul-de-sac of Douglas.*

Structure of the Uterus.—The uterus is composed of three coats; an outer serous, a middle muscular and an inner lining, the mucosa.

The *muscular coat* forms the great bulk of the organ and consists of bundles of nonstriated muscle united by connective tissue and containing considerable elastic tissue. In spite of much study, no definite arrangement of the muscle bundles in the nonpregnant uterus is discernible, but when gestation is present distinct layers of muscle become apparent (*q. v.*).

The *endometrium* is the name given to the lining mucosa of the uterus, a pinkish, velvety membrane, which is perforated by the orifices of innumerable uterine glands. Morphologically the endometrium consists of a covering of surface epithelium, with many glands and interglandular tissue and is richly supplied with blood and lymph. There is no submucosa, the epithelium lying directly upon the surface of the muscularis and its surface is therefore somewhat irregular, as it corresponds to the elevation and depression between the muscle bundles.

The endometrium is covered by a layer of simple columnar epithelium, areas of which are ciliated, and which line the entire cavity of the uterus and the tubes, merging into the peritoneum at the fimbriated extremity of the tubes, and with the vaginal mucosa at the os externum of the cervix.

The epithelium is extended into many simple tubular glands which penetrate to the muscularis and are lined by columnar epithelium, and are surrounded by a rich stroma of cellular areolar tissue. The uterine glands are either tubular or may be bifurcated, and vary greatly in size and tortuosity with the different phases of menstruation. The entire endometrium is from 0.5 to 4 mm. in thickness.

The *cervical mucosa* is thrown into folds on the anterior and posterior surfaces, there being a vertical ridge, with horizontal branches, on both cervical walls. The mucosa is covered by columnar cells, many of them ciliated, which extend usually about two thirds of the length of the cervix, when they begin to become flattened, merging finally with the stratified squamous epithelium which covers the vaginal portion of this structure.

The cervical glands are short, branching or racemose, lined with columnar epithelium and resting upon a basement membrane.

The **fallopian tubes** (**oviducts**) are paired organs springing from the lateral aspects of the uterine cornua, running in a somewhat tortuous course along the upper margin of the broad ligament and enclosed in an extension of its folds (the *mesosalpinx*) toward the side of the pelvis (Fig. 6).

The oviducts are about 10 cm. in length by 5 to 8 mm. in diameter. They terminate in a freely open *abdominal ostium* which lies usually

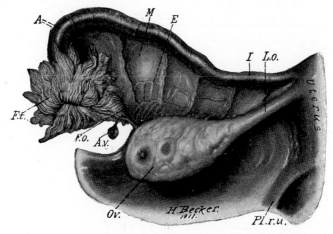

Fig. 6.—*F.t.*, Fimbria; *A*, ampulla; *M*. mesosalpinx; *E*, parovarium; *F.o.*, fimbria ovarica; *A.v.*, hydatid of Morgagni; *Pl.r.u.*, plica recto-uterina; *I*, isthmus tubae. (DeLee.)

on the posterior wall of the broad ligament and is open to the abdominal cavity. At the uterine end, the lumen of the tube is continuous with that of the cavum uteri.

The oviducts are composed of an outer peritoneal covering, loosely connected to the muscular layer of the tube, and sometimes containing vestigial remains of the wolffian tubules.

The muscular coat composes the bulk of the tube wall and is of unstriated muscle fibers, arranged in an outer longitudinal and an inner circular layer, thickest at the uterine end.

The mucosa of the tube is thrown into a number of longitudinal folds, low at the uterine end, growing longer as the ampullae are approached. These *folds* or *rugae* are delicate, branching, papillary processes arching about the lumen of the tube, covered with ciliated columnar epithelium, and they rest upon a slight connective tissue

stroma. The character of the tubal folds changes from the comparatively simple arrangement obtaining at the uterine cornua, to a highly
complex system of finger-like processes found in the ampulla of the

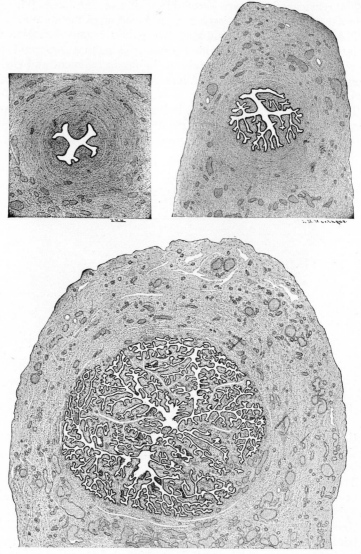

Fig. 7.—Sections through uterine, isthmic and ampullar portions of tube. × 15.
(Williams, "Obstetrics," D. Appleton-Century Co., Publishers.)

tube. For descriptive purposes, the tube may be said to consist of
the *interstitial portion*, which really represents a portion of the uterine
wall at the cornua, which is traversed by the lumen of the tube, end-

ing in a little depression in the upper angle of the cavum uteri. This portion is about 0.2 mm. in diameter. The *isthmus of the tube* is that part which continues from the uterine cornua. It is straight, thin and about 3 to 4 cm. in length, its lumen measuring 5 mm. in diameter (Fig. 7).

The *ampulla* or trumpet-shaped portion of the tube consists of the distal two thirds of the organ, and is wider than the isthmus, usually shows a moderate tortuosity and its lumen is from 2 to 3 mm. in diameter. It ends in a free opening, the abdominal ostium, the end of the tube being expended into the pavilion where it is converted into a series of little fringe-like fingers called *fimbriae*. These fimbriae are covered with ciliated columnar epithelium. The whole tube increases in size gradually, from the uterine end to the abdominal ostium, the outer portion (ampulla) being quite movable and usually somewhat convoluted.

OVARIES

These paired organs lie on either side of the uterus, behind and below the origin of the tubes. They are attached to the posterior

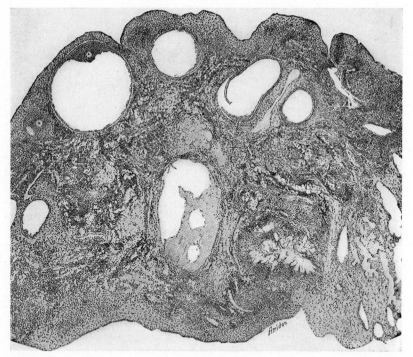

Fig. 8.—Mature ovary. Transverse section. (Dr. Zeit's specimen.) (DeLee.)

surface of the broad ligament by folds of peritoneum, the *mesovarium*. The *ovarian ligaments* are rounded cords of connective tissue with a few unstriated muscle fibers which extend from the inner pole of the ovary to the lateral wall of the uterus, being inserted between the fallopian tube and the round ligament, and lying within the posterior fold of the broad ligament. These ligaments are about 1 cm. in length.

The *infundibulopelvic ligaments* are delicate peritoneal bands running from the distal pole of the ovary to the pelvic wall and are really the lateral terminations of the posterior leaflet of the broad ligaments and contain the blood vessels and lymphatics which supply the ovary.

The ovaries themselves are almond-shaped, silvery white organs measuring on the average 3.5 cm. in length, 1.8 cm. in breadth and 1.2 cm. in thickness. The surface of each ovary is irregular and somewhat nodulated and is covered by a dense connective tissue envelope, the *tunica albuginea*.

On section the gland is found to be made up of a narrow cortex and a much bulkier medulla. The cortex is a compact structure of connective tissue, overlaid by the still more firm tunica albuginea which is covered by columnar epithelium. It contains numerous graafian follicles. The medullary portion consists of loose connective tissue arranged in bundles among which lie the vessels, nerves and lymphatics of the organ (Fig. 8).

THE VAGINA

The vagina is a musculomembranous tube which runs from the cervix above, to terminate at the vulva below. It runs downward and forward, continuing with the axis of the superior strait of the pelvis, and forms an angle of nearly 90 degrees with the anteverted uterus.

The vagina is attached to the margin of the cervix in an oblique direction, the expanded portion just distal to the ring of attachment being termed the *fornix of the vagina*. Obstetricians speak of the anterior, posterior, and lateral fornices. By reason of its oblique attachment to the cervix, the posterior wall of the vagina is longer than the anterior (8.5 cm. and 6.5 cm. respectively).

In nulliparous women the anterior and posterior walls are in contact in the middle portion of the tube, which in section is often compared to the letter H.

The surface of the vagina is thrown into many longitudinal folds called *rugae*, which permit of its enormous distention during parturition.

The bladder and urethra are in contact with the vagina anteriorly, a sheath of loose fibrous tissue connecting the two structures. Posteriorly the vagina rests upon the rectum below and is in contact with the pouch of Douglas above. Structurally the vagina consists of an outer fibrous, a middle muscular and an inner mucous coat.

The outer layer is formed of compact fibrous tissue, with many elastic fibers which make a firm sheath for the tube and connect it with the surrounding fasciae. It contains the vaginal vessels, nerves and lymphatics. The muscular layer is made up of irregularly arranged bundles of unstriated muscle fibers together with much connective tissue. The muscle fibers are arranged in a longitudinal fashion, with some circular bundles, and these fibers intermesh with certain others from the levator ani.

The mucosa is composed of stratified squamous epithelium, resting upon a basement membrane of elastic tissue.

THE EXTERNAL ORGANS OF GENERATION

These organs, grouped under the term *pudendum,* consist of the two labia majora, the labia minora, the clitoris and the orifice of the vagina (Figs. 9, 10).

The pudendum lies as a bulging eminence between the pubes above and the anus posteriorly, and exhibits the opening of the urethra as well as the vagina. The *labia majora* are the homologues of the

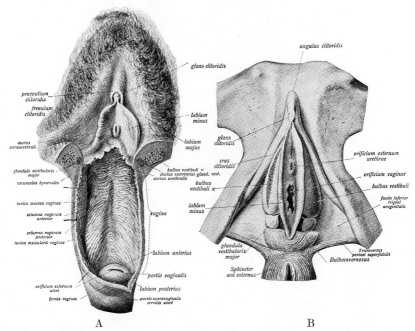

Fig. 9.—A, Superficial anatomy of the external genitalia; B, deep structure of the external genitalia. (Sobotta and McMurrich.)

scrotum in the male. They are folds of skin distended into oval cushion-like eminences, by contained fat and elastic tissue, and vary from plump ovoid forms to flabby and pendulous folds, depending upon the age of the woman. In young adults they measure about 8 by 3 cm. They lie in contact in the midline, and unite above to form the anterior commissure, which develops into a considerable pad of fat known as the mons veneris.

Posteriorly, the labia majora unite anterior to the rectum to form the *posterior commissure.*

The skin surfaces are covered with hair and contain sebaceous glands. On their inner surfaces the skin is smooth and pink. The *labia minora* are folds of skin lying to the inner side of the labia majora, and in young women are concealed by the latter. They are thinner and smaller than the majora to which they lie parallel. The labia minora unite anteriorly, after dividing into two separate folds, a medial one which merges into the clitoris on each side, to form the frenum of the clitoris, and a lateral one which unites with its fellow on the opposite side to form the prepuce of the clitoris.

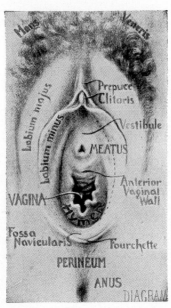

Fig. 10.—Diagram of female external genitalia. (Dickinson.)

Posteriorly, the labia minora fuse with the labia majora to form the posterior commissure. A small transverse fold of skin unites the posterior ends of the lesser lips and is termed the *fourchette.*

Just above and between the fourchette and the vaginal opening is a shallow transverse depression, the *fossa navicularis.*

The **vestibule** (pudendal cleft, urogenital fissure) is the opening of the urogenital canal on the body surface. It is bounded laterally by the labia majora and minora, the clitoris forms its apex, and the posterior commissure is its posterior border.

The urethral orifice opens into the anterior portion of the vestibule, the vagina into the posterior portion.

The **urinary meatus** is the external orifice of the urethra and opens into the vestibule just below the clitoris. It is a slit-shaped space, its mucous membrane somewhat elevated and thrown into small folds. Just beneath the urethral floor are two small glands, Skene's glands, whose ducts open into the posterior wall of the urethra, within the meatus.

The vaginal orifice, in the virgin, is partially closed by a septum of vascular mucous membrane called the *hymen.*

This curious structure appears late in fetal life and is peculiar to the human species and appears to have no particular value. The hymen generally possesses a central aperature though it may be imperforate. Sometimes it is pierced by a number of small orifices (cribriform hymen), sometimes the orifice is semilunar.

The hymen is usually destroyed by coitus, its remains being little tags of mucous membrane (*myrtiform caruncles*) attached to the sides of the vaginal orifice.

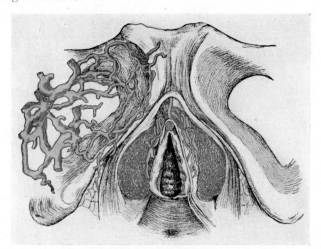

Fig. 11.—Erectile structures of the female genitalia, particularly the highly vascular bulbi vestibuli. (Kobelt.)

The **clitoris** is a small organ, composed of two joined corpora cavernosa, which are the homologues of similar structures in the male. The corpora cavernosa form a cylindrical body about 3 cm. in length the end of which is covered by a glans, which is an extension of the vestibular bulbs.

The clitoris is covered by a *prepuce* in front composed of the joined lateral folds of the labia minora, and has its *frenum* behind, which is also derived from the labia minora.

The **vestibular bulbs** (Fig. 11) are masses of erectile tissue, very vascular, about 5 cm. in length and lying at the sides of the vaginal orifice, just under the labia. Their anterior extremities terminate in the *glans clitoris,* and posteriorly they end as rounded masses, which sometimes extend to the posterior vaginal wall.

The musculature of the pelvic floor will be described in Chapter XI.

THE BLOOD VESSELS OF THE REPRODUCTIVE ORGANS

The pelvic organs derive their chief blood supply from the ovarian and uterine arteries.

The **ovarian arteries** arise from the abdominal aorta, being the homologues of the spermatic in the male. They run downward and laterally lying behind the parietal peritoneum and upon the psoas

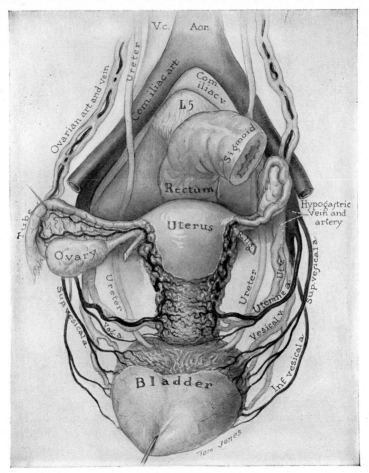

Fig. 12.—The blood supply of the pelvis. (Curtis, "Textbook of Gynecology.")

major muscle, crossing the ureter and the internal iliac artery. At the pelvic brim they enter the infundibulopelvic ligaments, beneath the ovary through the ovarian ligament to anastomose with the uterine of the same side. Branches are given off to the ovary, the tube and the round ligaments.

The **uterine artery** on each side arises from the internal iliac (anterior division of the hypogastric). It lies on the inner wall of the pelvis running toward the midline on the fascia of the levator ani muscle, to the lower border of the broad ligaments, when in the parametrial tissues between the folds of the broad ligament, it crosses over the ureter, about 2 cm. from the uterus. Upon reaching the cervix, at about the level of the internal os, a vaginal branch is given off which courses downward on the lateral vaginal wall. The main vessels run upward along the lateral wall of the uterus, being exceedingly tortuous, and giving off many branches which supply the uterine musculature. At the fundus the vessel separates into branches which supply the ovary and fallopian tube anastomosing freely with the ovarian and the uterine on the opposite side (Fig. 12).

The **vaginal artery,** one on each side, arises from the hypogastric, and runs downward and inward to supply the vagina, and in part, the bladder.

The Internal Pudendal Arteries.—Arise as one of the terminal branches of the internal iliac (ventral portion of the hypogastric). They arise in front of the pyriformis muscle and each one leaves the pelvis through the posterior portion of the great sacrosciatic foramen, crosses the spine of the ischium and again enters the pelvis via the lesser sacrosciatic foramen. The vessel then lies anteriorly on the internal border of the tuberosity of the ischium and finally runs along the side of the descending ramus of the pubis.

The internal pudendal gives off many important branches as follows:

The inferior hemorrhoidal artery, supplying the region of the anus.

The superficial perineal artery, supplying the labia.

The transverse perineal artery, supplying a portion of the pelvic floor.

The artery to the vestibular bulb.

The artery to the clitoris—supplying the corpus cavernosum.

The dorsal artery of the clitoris, supplying the glans and prepuce.

The Middle Hemorrhoidal Arteries.—These paired vessels are branches of the inferior vesical or the internal pudic, and they supply the anal region, anastomosing with the superior and inferior hemorrhoidal vessels.

The Superior and Middle Vesical Arteries.—The superior vesical comes from the hypogastric, the proximal portion of which remains potent after birth. It divides into branches which supply the fundus of the bladder and the sheath of the urethra.

The middle vesical artery is a branch of the superior and supplies the bladder. The inferior vesical artery is a branch of the internal iliac and also supplies the base and trigone of the bladder.

The Veins.—The pelvic veins are peculiar in that, with few exceptions, they have no valves.

They form an extensive network surrounding the pelvic organs, the most important divisions of which are: the pampiniform plexus or the ovarian plexus, lying between the folds of the broad ligament;

the uterine plexus which surrounds the uterus; the vaginal plexus, of which one portion lies in the submucosa, the other external to the muscular sheath; the vesical plexus, and the hemorrhoidal plexus.

These plexuses form terminal veins as the ovarian, uterine, vesical, etc., which accompany their respective arteries in their course.

The *hemorrhoidal plexus* surrounds the lower portion of the rectum, lying under the mucosa. This plexus terminates in the superior, middle and inferior hemorrhoidal veins, the superior hemorrhoidal being of importance, because, emptying into the inferior musculature, it enters the portal system and is the means of communication between this and the general circulatory system.

LYMPHATICS OF THE PELVIS

The lymph glands of the pelvic organs (Fig. 13) are composed of several groups.

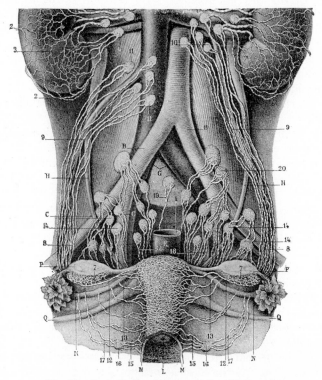

Fig. 13.—Lymphatics of the pelvis. (Sappey.)

The **internal iliac** glands (hypogastric glands) lie between the two divisions of the common iliac artery, and receive the lymphatics from the upper portion of the vagina, the ureter and cervix.

The **cephalic group of inguinal glands** lies under Poupart's ligament lateral to the deep pelvic fascia, and admits the lymphatics from the external genitalia, the labia minora and majora, perineum, vestibule and clitoris.

The **lumbar glands** lie in three well differentiated groups, two lateral and one median. The lateral groups lie under the psoas major muscles and into them empty the lymphatics from the posterior aspect of the abdominal wall.

The median group proximates the common iliac arteries, the vena cava and the lower portion of the aorta. These glands receive the lymphatics from the fundus uteri, ovaries and tubes and from the kidneys. The sacral glands lie on the anterior surface of the sacrum and receive the lymphatics from the rectum and the surrounding bony structures.

The **superficial inguinal glands** run in a long chain under the inguinal ligament and together with the superficial subinguinal glands lying along the upper portion of the long saphenous vein receive the lymphatics from the perineum, vulva and anus, together with those of the lower portions of the abdominal wall.

NERVES OF THE PELVIC VISCERA

The uterus is innervated chiefly by the sympathetic nerve system, to some extent by the spinal nerves, the latter being represented by fibers from the third and fourth sacral nerves. The sympathetic fibers come from the hypogastric plexus, which lies between the common iliac arteries and is continuous with the aortic and renal plexuses.

The hypogastric plexus is further subdivided into the middle hemorrhoidal plexus supplying the rectum, the uterovaginal plexus which runs along the course of the uterine artery and divides to innervate both arteries and posterior surfaces of the uterus.

The vesical plexus accompanies the vesical arteries and supplies the bladder.

The ovaries receive their nerve impulses from the renal and aortic plexuses, the fibers reaching the ovary through its hilum.

The pudendal nerve accompanies the internal pudendal vessels and, with the sacral plexus, innervates the perineum, the skin surface of which also receives fibers from the ilio-inguinal nerve, the perforating cutaneous branches of the second and third sacral nerves, etc.

The nerve supply of the pelvis is most complex, the foregoing description being at best only a brief résumé of the more important nervous elements involved.

3

CHAPTER II

THE PHYSIOLOGY OF THE REPRODUCTIVE ORGANS

Puberty is a term used to define the transition from the immature state of childhood to the maturity of sexual development.

In the girl the changes associated with puberty affect not only the reproductive system but the entire organism, as well as the psyche.

The angular body of the child develops graceful contours with some increase in fat about the hips and shoulders, the hair grows rapidly, especially about the pudendum, the breasts become full and a certain amount of pigmentation appears about the areola, and there may be some nervous instability.

The most noteworthy changes are observed in the genitalia. The labia majora become plump, through the deposition of fat and the labia minora disappear beneath them. The mons veneris grows more prominent and becomes covered with hair (the escutcheon), the vagina lengthens and its mucosa grows more vascular. The uterus and tubes increase markedly in size by a process of hypertrophy, and the ovaries soon present the characteristic adult eminences upon their surfaces which denote the growth of maturing graafian follicles.

The most striking phenomenon of puberty in the female is the advent of menstruation.

Age of Puberty.—Racial differences are marked with regard to the age when puberty arrives. In America and Northern Europe the average age is somewhere between thirteen and fourteen years, 13.9 often being given as the mean for America.

In other races the phenomena appear much earlier, as in India, eleven years, or later, as in Great Britain, fifteen years and so on.

Precocious puberty may occur; many girls, apparently normal in all respects, menstruating at ten years, while in exceptional instances it may occur at eight years of age.

Relation of Puberty to Maturity.—Ovulation and menstruation usually appear some time before maturity as expressed by the capacity for reproduction, most adolescent girls being sterile for from one to three years after the first menstruation.

Cause of Puberty.—Many theories have been advanced to account for the profound systemic changes which mark the transition between girlhood and womanhood, but none have been entirely proved.

It is now generally assumed that the whole impulse is due to endocrine influences, with the pituitary gland as the general activator. It appears that for some reason, as yet not satisfactorily explained, the hypophysis rapidly becomes active and secretes certain hormones which circulate in the blood. Among these are substances which stimulate the ovary and produce maturation of the follicle, and this follicular hormone in turn stimulates the endometrium to activity. Later another hypophyseal hormone is potent in the development of the corpus luteum, which in turn develops an endocrine quality and brings about menstruation. The whole matter is still somewhat in the speculative stage however.

Menstruation is a periodic discharge of blood from the uterus, occurring at regular intervals, lasting for several days, making its initial appearance at the onset of puberty and continuing during the period of sexual maturity, until it disappears with the advent of re-

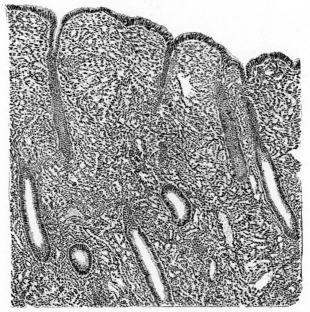

Fig. 14.—The endometrium in the postmenstrual phase (fifth day of cycle). Note especially the straight and narrow glands. (Novak, "Menstruation and Its Disorders," D. Appleton-Century Co., Publishers.)

productive senility, which is called the menopause. The cause of menstruation is not yet clear. It has been held to be due to ovulation and dependent upon it, while other observers hold that the two processes are entirely independent of each other.

Frankel believes that menstruation is governed by the corpus luteum whose hormone (progestin) stimulates the endometrium, and prepares it for the nidation of the ovum and that the death of the latter and consequent regression of the corpus luteum causes menstruation by the withdrawal of the nutrition element in the uterus. Other experimentors, headed by Frank, think that overloading the endometrium with the female sex hormone, followed by the sudden withdrawal of this hormone upon the death of the ovum, produces the bleeding.

Whatever the cause, the phenomenon is beyond doubt controlled by the endocrine system.

Cyclical Changes in the Endometrium.—The great work of Hitschmann and Adler placed the various changes of the uterine mucosa during the menstrual cycle upon a firm basis.

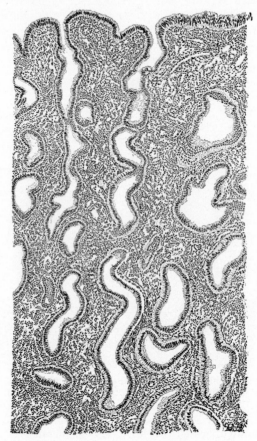

Fig. 15.—The endometrium in the interval phase (fifteenth day). (Novak, "Menstruation and Its Disorders," D. Appleton-Century Co., Publishers.)

It is now definitely known that four major phases occur in the endometrium during the menstrual cycle. These are:

Postmenstrual Phase (Fig. 14).—Immediately following menstruation the endometrium is thin (1 mm.), pale and is covered with a newly regenerated low cuboidal epithelium. The glands are narrow clefts and straight tubules with no convolutions. The epithelium soon grows to assume its usual definitely columnar character. The stroma is dense. This phase lasts about one week after the cessation of bleeding when it passes by a gradual transition into the

Interval or Resting Phase.—In this, which is one of slow hyperplasia, the glands become longer and more tortuous, their orifices widen, the epithelium increases in height and the entire endometrium is much thicker (2–3 mm.). This phase (Fig. 15) lasts about two weeks and then merges into the

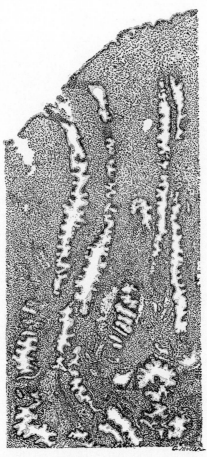

Fig. 16.—The endometrium of the pregravid phase (twenty-fifth day). Note the corkscrew glands, the low, secreting epithelium, and the decidua-like stroma. (Novak, "Menstruation and Its Disorders," D. Appleton-Century Co., Publishers.)

Premenstrual or secretory phase, in which the endometrium is thick (6–8 mm.), velvety and somewhat edematous, while the epithelium lining the glands has become flattened and shows evidence of the secretion of a material rich in glycogen and mucus. The glands are so elongated and so sharply spiraled that they may project above the surface of the endometrium, throwing it into irregularities or eminences. The stroma becomes edematous and its cells may hypertrophy until they resemble decidual cells, the so-called "false" decidual cells (Fig. 16).

The entire stroma becomes infiltrated with leukocytes, and is quite vascular. This phase lasts four to six days and goes into the

Menstruation phase (Figs. 17 and 18), a time of bleeding, during which, as first shown by Schröder, there is a desquamation of the surface epithelium and some of the stroma, the entire upper or com-

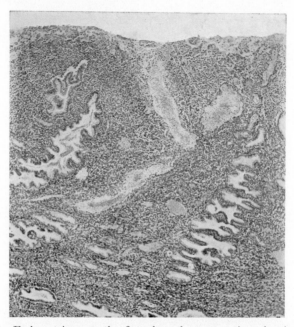

Fig. 17.—Endometrium on the first day of menstruation, showing the compacta, spongiosa, and part of the basalis. The greatly dilated blood vessels, some of which are opening directly on the surface (rhexis), are especially prominent. There is a marked infiltration, especially of the compacta, the upper portion of which is being cast off in small particles. There are considerable individual differences in the degree of this endometrial loss on the first day. (Novak.)

pact layer being cast off, together with considerable of the underlying spongiosa. Novak and Te Linde have shown that the epithelium is cast off in little masses, mostly of necrotic cells and stroma. The bleeding is due to the opening of the blood vessels by the necrotic process. After menstruation, only the stumps of the uterine glands remain, with occasional little islands of tissue and it is from these that regeneration begins, often while menstruation is still in progress (Figs. 17, 18).

The Clinical Aspects of Menstruation.—The usual cycle is one of twenty-eight days but a variation of three to five days is not unusual.

Indeed in my experience the thirty-day type of menstruation is almost as often noted as that of twenty-eight days. In the early years of menstruation irregularity of rhythm is often seen.

The duration of the flow varies in different women, lasting usually from four to six days, though many healthy women menstruate but two to three days.

Amount of Menstrual Blood.—This varies greatly in different women and also in the same woman from time to time. Many investigators have announced average amounts of blood lost, which seem

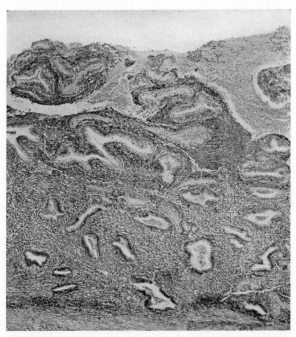

Fig. 18.—Endometrium on second day of menstruation, showing the basalis with only a small part of the spongiosa intact. The compacta and the greater part of the spongiosa have been cast off. (Novak, Nelson's "Loose-Leaf Living Surgery.")

to be somewhere between 4 and 8 ounces. Normal menstrual blood does not coagulate, because of the mucous secretions of the endometrium and because there is no fibrin ferment contained in it.

The onset of the catamenia is often accompanied by mental and physical depression, headache, lassitude, and a sense of heaviness in the pelvis.

These symptoms may persist during the flow or they may disappear when bleeding is well established.

The **menopause,** or **climacteric,** marks the termination of the reproductive period and occurs from the fortieth to the fifty-second year, American women seeming to continue menstruation for a longer period than that given in the various European statistics. Normally the menopause may develop in one of three ways: an abrupt cessaation of the period, with no subsequent return; an irregular but increasing interval between periods, six weeks, two months, four months and so on until presently the flow does not recur; and finally the continuance of regular menstruation, the amount and duration of the flow steadily decreasing until it eventually disappears.

The menopause is associated with many psychic and physical phenomena, descriptions of which have no place in this book.

Cyclical Changes in the Ovary—Ovulation.—There are regularly recurring activities in the ovary which closely parallel those of menstruation and are indeed, in some part, responsible for them (Fig. 19).

The cortex of the ovary of the girl contains many thousands of immature ova surrounded by their follicle cells. With the approach

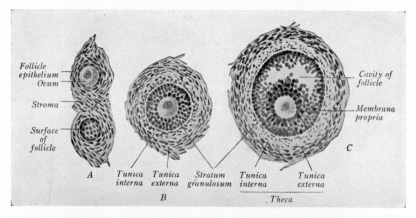

Fig. 19.—Growth and transformation of a human primordial follicle into a vesicular follicle. *A,* Primordial follicles in sectional and surface view. *B,* Enlarged primordial follicle with stratified epithelium. *C,* Young vesicular follicle with fluid-filled cavity. (Bumm.) × about 200.

of puberty certain of these primitive ova begin to enlarge and to approach the surface of the organ. In due time and more or less coincident with the first molimina of menstruation, one of these ovum-containing follicles reaches the surface of the ovary, becomes mature and finally ruptures, permitting the escape of the contained ovum into the peritoneal cavity.

Ovulation.—The rupture of the mature graafian follicle and the discharge of the ovum is termed ovulation and in the human female this begins with puberty and continues at twenty-eight day intervals until the end of the reproductive period (Fig. 20).

Usually only one follicle matures at each period of ovulation, the ovaries roughly alternating, so that each one discharges some 200 ova during the reproductive life of the woman.

Sometimes two or more ova are discharged simultaneously, multiple pregnancy resulting if fertilization follows.

Many thousands of follicles begin to mature and reach various degrees of development before they die, their remains being found in the ovarian cortex as atretic follicles.

The mature follicle is about 10 mm. in diameter and is marked by a rounded eminence upon the surface of the ovary, at the apex of which is an area of great thinness, the stigma.

The mechanism of rupture of the graafian follicle has been the subject of much controversy, whether it be due to increased engorgement of the follicular blood vessels, the constriction of smooth muscle fibers at the theca, or the more popular view that the rupture is due to the erosive action of a ferment developed in the follicular fluid.

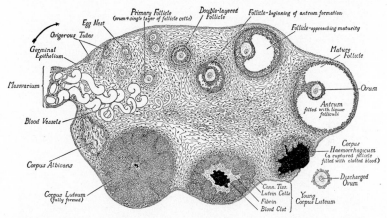

Fig. 20.—Schematic diagram of mammalian ovary showing the sequence of events in the origin, growth, and rupture of the ovarian (graafian) follicle, and the formation and retrogression of the corpus luteum. Follow clockwise around the ovary starting at the arrow. Immediately to the right of the arrow are shown two stages in oogenesis from the germinal epithelium. (From Patten, "Embryology of the Pig," published by P. Blakiston's Son & Co., Inc.)

The rupture is not a sudden bursting, but a gradual opening of the follicle with a slow oozing of the fluid which carries with it the ovum.

The Mature Graafian Follicle.—At maturity the follicle is a cystic, rounded mass 10 mm. or more in diameter. Its walls are derived from the cells of the ovarian stroma and consist of an inner cellular and vascular tunica interna, and an outer fibrous and muscular tunica externa (Fig. 21).

The follicular epithelium proliferates and becomes converted into the membrana granulosa, which is many layers of cells thick, the cells showing many mitotic figures. The granulosa grows out at one point and projects into the cavity of the follicle and its cells surround the ovum, which is embedded into the so-called "discus proligerus." The cells of the granulosa nearest the ovum are arranged in a radiating manner and are called the corona radiata. Within this is a zone of hyaline material called the zona pellucida, and within this space is the ovum, in its perivitelline space. The entire follicle is distended with the clear, slightly yellow liquor folliculi.

The **ovum** is a typical animal cell, about 0.13 mm. in diameter, consisting of a peripheral layer of clear protoplasm which surrounds the germinal vesicle (Fig. 22).

The bulk of the ovum is composed of deutoplasm or yolk protoplasm, made up of coarse and fine granules, of a highly refractile nature.

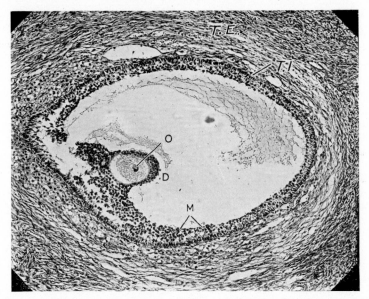

Fig. 21.—Mature graafian follicle. D, Discus proligerus; M, membrana granulosa; *T.E.,* tunica externa; *T.I.,* tunica interna; O, ovum. (Kensington Hospital for Women.)

The eccentrically located nucleus or germinal vesicle is bounded by a nuclear membrane and contains a chromatin network and one or more nucleoli, whose function is unknown.

The Corpus Luteum.—Upon the rupture of the follicle and the discharge of the ovum, the cavity of the follicle remains, lined by the granulosa cells. The cavity at once collapses, leaving a wavy outline and appearing as a flattened vesicle, the outer layer of which is composed of the theca cells which have become large and polygonal and are well vascularized. Within this layer is the rapidly proliferating granulosa layer whose cells become polyhedral, vacuoloated and develop the characteristic yellow color from the presence of lutein, a yellow pigment. The blood vessels of the theca invade the lutein layer, with sometimes considerable bleeding into it.

The mature corpus luteum is a well formed solid yellow body, 1 to 2 cm. in diameter, which lies at the surface of the ovary and sometimes forms a considerable eminence upon it. It is made up of large, clear lutein cells with well marked nuclei. The blood has been mostly resorbed so that the color is a uniform yellow (Fig. 23).

This stage is reached five or six days before menstruation, and shortly before bleeding occurs, the corpus luteum begins to retrogress.

It shrinks in size, becomes fibrotic and loses is yellow color. Fatty degeneration occurs and finally the whole body has been converted into a silvery, fibrous mass called the *corpus albicans*.

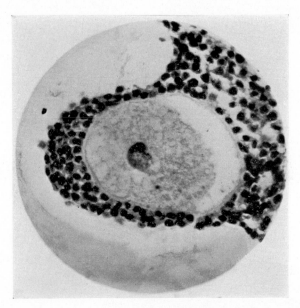

Fig. 22.—The mature ovum surrounded by the discus proligerus. (Kensington Hospital for Women.)

This retrogression occupies some time, but the entire corpus luteum has practically disappeared in three months, and examination of ovaries removed at operation will disclose several of these bodies in various stages of absorption.

The Corpus Luteum Verum (Corpus Luteum of Pregnancy).— Should the ovum become fertilized, the corpus luteum does not retrogress but continues to develop, reaching its maximum growth about the fourth month of pregnancy after which it slowly declines, all trace of it having usually disappeared at the close of the seventh month. The corpus luteum of pregnancy is larger than that of menstruation, contains more fibrous tissue, and contains considerable colloid material and toward the end of its life often contains *calcium*.

The Relation Between Ovulation and Menstruation (Fig. 24).—
Much recent work has apparently established the fact that in the
human female ovulation occurs about midway in the interval be-

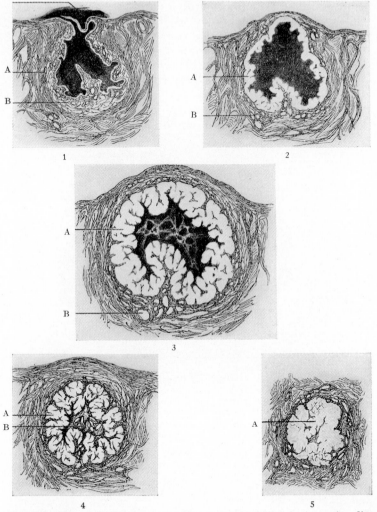

Fig. 23.—The corpus luteum. 1, The ruptured follicle: A, tunica fibrosa;
B, tunica propria. 2, The corpus luteum at twelve days: A, membrana granulosa; B, tunica propria. 3, The corpus luteum at three weeks: A, membrana
granulosa; B, tunica propria. 4, Corpus luteum at five weeks: A, membrana
granulosa; B, vascularized central blood clot. 5, Corpus luteum at eight weeks:
A, corpus albicans.

tween menstrual periods, that is, from the twelfth to the fourteenth
day after the onset of the preceding period. This corresponds to the
interval or resting stage of the endometrium. It is held that many

women can determine the time of ovulation by mild attacks of pelvic pain, located on one side or the other according to the ovary involved, together with the expulsion of a small plug of mucus from the vagina.

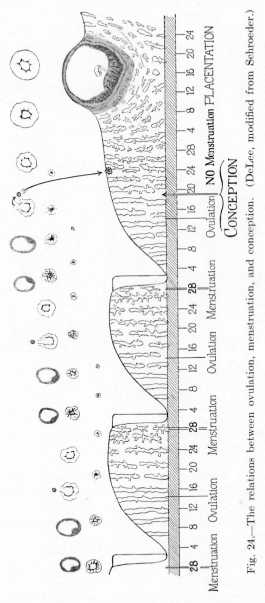

Fig. 24.—The relations between ovulation, menstruation, and conception. (DeLee, modified from Schroeder.)

So generally has this view of ovulation been accepted, that a widely used technic of contraception has been based upon it. Since the life cycle of the ovum has been fixed at three or four days, and the time of ovulation is known, it is only necessary for a couple to refrain from coitus during the period of from the eleventh to the seventeenth day after the onset of the last menstrual period to insure success. This question requires further study before it may be accepted as true. Clinical records of conception occurring after coitus immediately before or after menstruation suggests the possibility that the ovum may remain viable for a longer period than that generally accepted. Also it may be true that rupture of the mature follicle may be induced by intercourse as in certain of the lower animals.

Summary of Current Views Upon the Influence of the Endocrine System Upon the Reproductive Cycle.—Much of modern opinion in this matter is due to the work of Zondek, Frankel, Novak, Frank and many others.

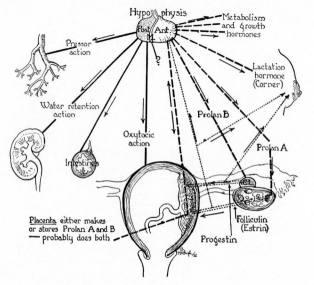

Fig. 25.—Diagram showing the reciprocal relations of the hypophysis with various organs, as of August 1, 1932. (DeLee.)

It is thought that the hypophysis is the motivating agent of the sex cycle although still more recent work hints that there is an underlying factor somewhere in the midbrain (Fig. 25).

The anterior lobe of the hypophysis elaborates four hormones:

1. Growth hormone.
2. Prolan A—follicle ripening—estrin or folliculin.
3. Prolan B—luteinizing hormone—progestin.
4. Metabolism hormone.

Prolan A stimulates the follicle to ripening and the development of its own secondary hormone, estrin or folliculin. This in turn activates the endometrium to regeneration and proliferation.

The follicle having ruptured, the corpus luteum develops, and, stimulated by Prolan B, elaborates its hormone, progestin or lutein, whose function is to prepare the endometrium for the nidation of the ovum and for its nutrition during the early weeks of pregnancy and to inaugurate the secretory phase of the endometrium.

Should fertilization not occur, the ovum dies, the corpus luteum undergoes regression and the sudden withdrawal of its hormonal effect causes menstruation.

If fertilization does occur the corpus luteum continues to grow and maintain the endometrium in its stage of a tissue of nutrition.

The menstrual cycle would then be due to the periodic production of folliculin by the mature graafian follicle and to the effect of progestin upon the growing endometrium, both induced by the hormones of the hypophysis, the final stage of menstrual bleeding being caused by a sudden withdrawal of the ovarian hormone. Further studies may greatly alter this conception and the whole matter must be regarded as still *sub judice*.

CHAPTER III

FERTILIZATION OF THE OVUM—IMPLANTATION

FERTILIZATION or conception implies the union of the male element in generation, the spermatozoon, with the female ovum. In the human species this union takes place in the fallopian tube presumably in its outer third.

The mature ovum escapes from the ruptured follicle and for a time lies free in the peritoneal cavity, in a little space or pocket bounded by the pelvic wall, the broad ligament and the intestinal mass.

The fimbriated extremity of the tube opens into this space, and in some way, as yet not fully understood, the ovum is drawn into it. Possibly the constant waving movement of the cilia, possibly strong tubal peristalsis may be responsible. It has been thought that the movements of the surrounding pelvic viscera play a part, a theory which may explain the curious phenomenon of external migration of the ovum in which this cell, expelled from one ovary, traverses the pelvic cavity, behind the uterus, to enter the tube on the opposite side.

Once in the tube the combined force of the ciliary current and tubal peristalsis slowly force the ovum toward the uterus. The time required for the ovum to reach the uterine cavity after it is received in the fimbriated extremity of the tube has been determined in many of the lower animals but is not definitely known in man, though general opinion states seven days as the requisite time for this transit. The life cycle of the human ovum is likewise unknown, its capability for fertilization after expulsion from the follicle having been estimated at from a few hours (Grosser) to two to three days (Corner).

The spermatozoon reaches the ovum, after it has been deposited in the vaginal vault by coitus, as a result of several types of activity; first by the swimming motion imparted by the undulating tail, and second by the muscular contraction of the uterus.

Upon reaching the tube, the spermatozoa meet the strong ciliary current, against which they cannot propel themselves and they are finally transported to the ovum in a very different manner.

Mucosal folds, compressed by temporary contraction rings in the tube, subdivide its lumen into a series of longitudinal compartments. In each of these, the cilia wave downward along the peripheral walls while a compensatory countercurrent of fluid wells upward centrally. Sperm cells are carried in these currents without regard to their locomotive abilities. By the forming and reforming of such compartments, at various levels, there is an interchange of contents so that

48

the spermatozoa move in an accidental manner both up and down the tube (Arey, Developmental Anatomy). The life cycle of human sperm is not definitely known, but it is probably limited to a few days.

Arey well says that it is highly improbable that the sperm may lie in wait for the egg or the reverse, for any considerable period of time, since the human species is relatively so infertile.

The ovum upon its expulsion from the follicle is mature, but is not capable of being fertilized until the first polar body has been extruded, polar division being completed only after the fertilization has begun. When the spermatazoon meets the egg, which is apparently a more or less accidental process without any definite chemical attraction, the lashing movements of the tail quickly cease and the attached sperm is passively engulfed by the cytoplasm of the egg, the head alone usually entering, although the tail may remain attached. Observations of lower forms has shown that when the sperm has entered the egg there is formed a fertilizive membrane which is impenetrable to additional sperms, and some similar mechanism must be operative in the human species, although not yet demonstrated.

The union of ovum and spermatozoon is followed at once by the profound changes in the nuclei, which result in cell division and multiplication and the development of a new being.

IMPLANTATION

The first stages of cell division and cleavage have not been observed in the human ovum, but following the analogy of lower mammalian types it is probable that after segmentation is complete there results a cluster of cells called the morula mass. There now occurs a rearrangement of blastomeres which results in a capsule of cells called the *trophoblast* at the periphery of the ovum. This trophoblast soon becomes separated from the inner cell mass by the accumulation of fluid, retaining its connection at one point only. The entire ovum is now called the *blastodermic vesicle* of which the trophoblastic covering represents an early growth of ectodermic cells. It is at this stage of development, believed to be reached eight or ten days after fertilization, that the ovum reaches the cavity of the uterus.

The endometrial lining of this organ is at this time under the influence of folliculin and progestin (*q. v.*) and is in the premenstrual stage, in which the mucosa is very thick, edematous, its cells large and hypertrophic and the glands long, convoluted and in a secretory phase and it has been sensitized by the lutein hormone (progestin) to receive the ovum. The fertilized ovum drops from the uterine ostium of the tube and comes to rest on the mucosa, possibly in a little valley between two elevations of the somewhat undulating surface of this tissue, perhaps in the mouth of a uterine gland (Fig. 26).

There follows prompt embedding by the destruction of the surface epithelium as a result of a localized enzymic digestion of the epithelium by the cells of the trophoblast, though there seems to be no

4

real destruction of the subepithelial tissues, the blastocyst only creating a cavity in the epithelium for itself.

This whole process is termed *implantation* and is supposed to consume but one day, the superficial wound in the mucosa being closed over the ovum by the operculum which is a portion of the trophoblast, later replaced by a blood clot.

At this time of implantation the ovum lies in the superficial compact layer of the swollen endometrium, nowhere penetrating the deeper spongiosa (Fig. 27).

Having become embedded, the ovum proceeds to rapid growth, more room being created by additional disintegration of the mucosa by enzyme action, by which also blood spaces are opened, for the required nutrition of the expanding embryo.

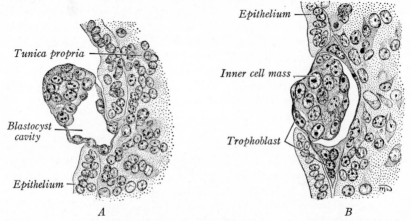

Fig. 26.—Early implantation in the guinea-pig. × 335. *A*, Blastocyst of six days with trophoblast beginning to penetrate the uterine mucosa. *B*, Blastocyst of six days at an advanced stage of penetration. (Arey, after Sansom and Hill.)

All of this activity is due to the trophoblast, which, at first a single layer of ectoderm, rapidly proliferates into a thick strong layer of tissue, which soon becomes transformed into *syncytium*.

The syncytium is composed of an outer strip of protoplasm, without definite cell walls, but containing large, poorly staining, oval nuclei. These ill-defined bodies are called *syncytial cells*, and in certain areas they may be heaped up in irregular masses.

Just under these cells is another layer of low, cuboidal, mononucleated cells, which take the stain much better than the syncytial cells and are called *Langhans' cells*. At term Langhans' cells have almost disappeared.

It is believed (Grosser) that there are two periods in both of which, the outer syncytial trophoblast and the inner, undifferentiated cellular trophoblast, become dominant in turn.

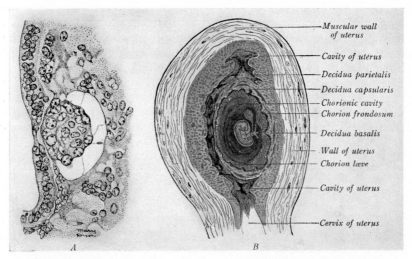

Fig. 27.—Later implantation stages. *A,* Guinea-pig blastocyst, early in the seventh day, with penetration completed (after Sansom and Hill; × 300); the eroded uterine epithelium is being repaired and the trophoblast is suffering partial breakdown. *B,* Section of a gravid human uterus showing implantation relations after several weeks' growth. (Arey, after Thompson.)

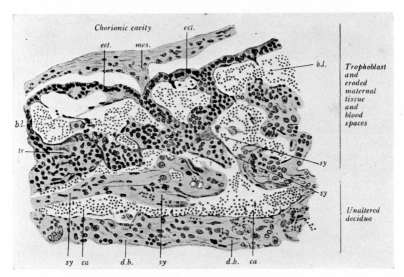

Fig. 28.—Invasion of the human maternal tissues illustrated by a portion of the implanted Peters' ovum. (Arey, after Peters.) × 520. *ect.*, *mes.*, Ectoderm and mesoderm of chorionic wall continued into cellular strands of cytotrophoblast (*tr*) which in turn have produced syncytial plasmothrophoblast (*sy*). Maternal tissue already eroded has given way to blood lacunae (*b.l.*); below, the syncytium is seen tapping a hitherto intact capillary (*ca*) next the unaltered decidua basalis (*d.b.*).

At first both layers are chiefly concerned in the erosive processes leading to embedding, whereas the second generation of cells covers the villi and provides for the absorption of maternal fluids from the newly opened sinuses. The first villi produced are simple strands of trophoblast, while the later ones are complex.

During the first eighteen days after implantation as shown by studies of some of the early human embryos (Miller, Peters, Frassi, Von Spee) the mesoderm begins to send prolongations into the trophoblastic villi to produce secondary or true villi. The trophoblast be-

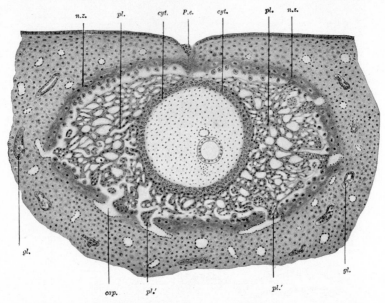

Fig. 29.—Diagram of Teacher-Bryce ovum. (Magnified about 50 diameters.) (T. H. Bryce, Del.); *P. e.*, point of entrance; *cyt.*, cytotrophoblast; *pl.*, plasmoditrophoblast; *n.z.*, necrotic zone of decidua; *gl.*, gland; *cap.*, capillaries; *pl.'*, masses of vacuolating plasmodium invading capillaries. The cavity of the blastocyst is completely filled by mesoblast, and imbedded therein are the amnio-embryonic and entodermic vesicles. The natural proportions of the several parts have been strictly observed. (Bryce and Teacher.)

comes reduced to its two layers, an outer syncytium and an inner cellular layer (Langhans' layer) (Fig. 28).

These maturing villi are composed of the above layers of ectodermic epithelium as a covering and within these layers lies a central core of mesodermal connective tissue, with looped blood vessels, these being the terminals of the umbilical vessels which pass from the embryo through the body stalk to the chorion.

The villi dip into the blood lacunae which have been opened and which coalesce to form the intervillous space in which maternal blood circulates. This phase marks the beginning of placentation (Fig. 29).

CHAPTER IV

THE FETAL MEMBRANES AND THE PLACENTA

FROM the time of implantation the growth of the embryo is parallelled by the elaboration of fetal membranes, which are structures entirely extra-embryonic, but of vital necessity during the period of fetal development. These membranes are the yolk sac, the allantois, the amnion, the chorion and in some sense the umbilical cord, the only

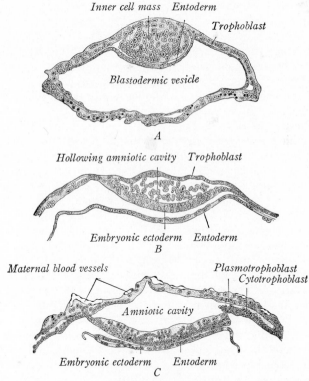

Fig. 30.—Sectioned stages of amnion formation in the bat (Van Beneden). × about 100.

ones of import from the standpoint of the obstetrician being the latter three.

The Amnion.—During early embryonal life a cleft appears in the ectoderm of the germinal area leaving a little cavity which fills with fluid and forces the embryonic plate toward the center of the ovum. The amnion and chorion are concentric, saccular coverings, composed of ectoderm and somatic mesoderm. This double layer is thrown into parallel folds at first just in front of the embryo (Fig. 30, A) and a little later behind it. The ends of the folds presently unite, covering the embryo and when the two layers have fused there remain two enveloping membranes, an inner one lined with ectoderm and covered by mesoderm (the amnion) and an outer one lined by mesoderm and covered by ectoderm (the chorion). The cavity of the amnion is soon filled with fluid and in this sac the embryo hangs suspended (Fig. 30).

The outer portion of this double membrane, the chorion, is the outer covering of the embryo and its ectodermal wall soon becomes thickened and there develop little spaces called lacunae into which maternal blood may enter from the opened blood vessels of the endometrium and which lacunae later become the intervillous spaces. The strands of primary villi soon are thrust out of the chorion later replaced by the mature villi as before described (Fig. 31).

The mature amnion is a silvery white membrane, consisting of its two layers, outer mesodermal and inner ectodermal. The epithelium of the ectoderm is composed of more or less cuboidal cells, which are probably the chief source of the amniotic fluid which distends the sac and in which the fetus is suspended.

The **liquor amnii** is a fluid at first clear, later becoming more opaque, which is secreted by the cells of the amnion in part and probably augmented by accumulation of fetal urine and possibly by transudations from the maternal blood vessels.

The amount of liquor amnii varies greatly in different individuals and in different pregnancies in the same woman. From 500 to 2000 cc. (16 to 66 ounces) is regarded as within the normal limits, more or less than this being pathological.

The amount of fluid increases with considerable regularity until the end of the seventh month when it again decreases until term.

On Analysis.—Liquor amnii is found to be neutral in reaction or faintly alkaline. The specific gravity is from 1.005 to 1.018; it contains albumin, fat and inorganic salts in small amounts and microscopically shows sebaceous matter, exfoliated epithelium from the epidermis of the child, a few leukocytes and some cellular débris.

Function of the Liquor Amnii.—(a) To furnish a fluid cushion, in which the fetus is suspended and by the presence of which the delicate embryo is saved from external injury.

(b) To allow the fetus free motion and prevent adhesions of its body to the surrounding membrane.

(c) To act as a food for the fetus (problematical).

(d) To surround the fetus during the early stages of labor and so save it from undue compression by the contracting uterine muscle.

The Chorion.—The origin of the chorion has been described previously. Once formed its surface rapidly becomes covered by the primitive chorionic villi. These primitive villi are rapidly replaced

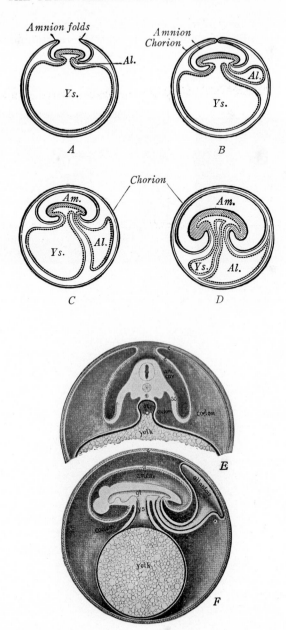

Fig. 31.—Diagrams illustrating the development of the fetal membranes in most amniote vertebrates (*A–D*, in a sagittal plane, after Gegenbauer in McMurrich; *E, F*, stereograms in a transverse and sagittal plane, after Kingsley). In *A–D* ectoderm, mesoderm and entoderm are represented by heavy, light and dotted lines respectively; in *E, F*, ectoderm is hatched, mesoderm gray and entoderm black. *a,* Amnion; *Al.,* allantois; *Am.,* amniotic cavity; *c,* chorion; *gt,* gut; *so,* somatopleure; *Ys.,* yolk stalk and sac. (Arey.)

by the secondary or true villi, each with its loop of blood vessels derived from the allantois and soon to become the umbilical vessels. The entire ovum is covered with villi, which grow out radially and convert the chorion into a shaggy sac, the villi covering the entire surface of the egg (Fig. 32).

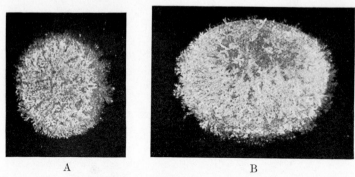

A   B

Fig. 32.—A, The ovum at four weeks; B, the ovum at two months showing the beginning atrophy of the villi on the exposed surface of the chorion. (Bumm.)

By the sixth week of gestation the chorion may be divided into:
The chorion frondosum (placental portion).
The chorion laeve (a smooth, capsular chorion).

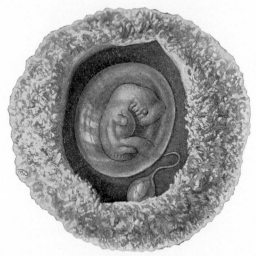

Fig. 33.—Chorionic sac opened to exhibit an 11-mm. human embryo within its unruptured amnion. × 2. (Arey.)

The chorion frondosum represents the fetal portion of the developing placenta, the villi being now compact bush-like tubes with but few branches, and are contained within the open blood sinus (Fig. 33).

That portion of the chorion which is not in contact with the uterine wall rapidly stretches with the growing ovum and its villi become more and more compressed and flat until finally at the third month they lose their shaggy appearance and are reduced to mere flat, opaque plates lying upon the thinned-out chorionic membrane (Fig. 34).

The Decidua.—The endometrium at the time of fertilization has been described as being under the influence of folliculin and progestin and is in its thickened, secretory, premenstrual phase.

At the time of labor the endometrium is cast off, in part with the fetal membranes and placenta, in part during the puerperium. For this reason the endometrium in the pregnant woman is called the decidua (that which falls off). Arey says that its preparation for gestation, the long deferred loss at parturition and the subsequent

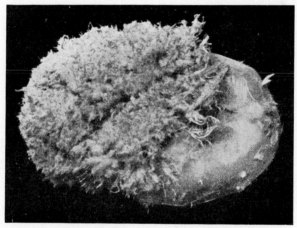

Fig. 34.—The ovum at three months. On the left, the chorion frondosum. On the right the chorion laeve. (Spee.)

repair after childbirth, exaggerate and extend the events of an ordinary menstrual cycle.

The two processes show undoubted fundamental similarities, and the decidual membranes are a direct continuation of the already modified premenstrual mucosa. When the ovum has embedded itself the decidua may be divided into three parts.

The *decidua parietalis* or *vera* which is simply the thickened endometrial lining of the uterus exclusive of the site of the ovum. It reaches its greatest development at the end of the third month, when it reaches 1 cm. in thickness (Figs. 35, 36).

The *decidua capsularis* or *reflexa* which represents the overlapping folds, which fall together over the ovum after the latter has buried itself beneath the surface. This part of the decidua rapidly expands over the growing embryo and finally lies in intimate contact with the decidua vera and with it becomes flattened and thinned out.

The *decidua basalis* or *serotina* which lies next the ovum on the uterine side and becomes developed into the maternal portion of the placenta.

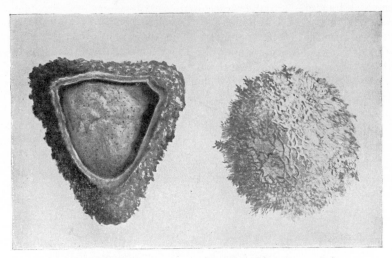

Fig. 35.—The decidua vera and the chorion. (B. C. Hirst.)

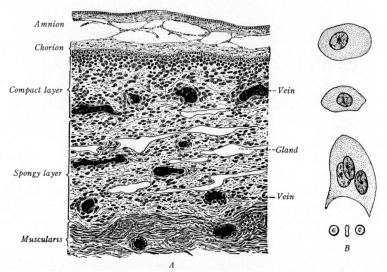

Fig. 36.—Human decidua parietalis. *A,* Vertical section, at about seven months, with the attached fetal membranes *in situ* (Schaper in Lewis and Stöhr; × 30). *B,* Decidual cells at the end of pregnancy (× 450); below are three red blood corpuscles drawn to scale. (Arey.)

All portions of the decidua are composed of two layers: a superficial compact layer containing the straight, nonconvoluted outer ends of the uterine glands and much stroma and a deeper spongiosa layer which presents the branched and tortuous deeper portion of the uterine glands and is richly vascularized.

The deciduae parietalis and capsularis rapidly become thinned out and the glands become thinned out and flattened.

In the basalis both layers continue to hypertrophy and grow into the maternal placenta.

The Placenta.—The earlier stages of placental formation have already been described. The chorionic villi have been shown to develop in great numbers at the area of contact with the uterus, and to dip

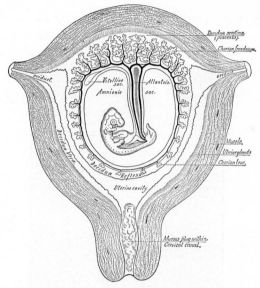

Fig. 37.—Diagram illustrating relations of structures of the human uterus at the end of the seventh week of pregnancy. (B. C. Hirst, modified from Allen Thomson.)

into the large opened blood vessels of the uterine wall which constitute the placental sinus.

By the end of the fourth month the chorionic villi on the free surface of the membrane have all atrophied so that the chorion is bare, while on the uterine surface they have hypertrophied and branched to form the dense network which is the fetal portion of the placenta.

The placenta is a distinctly dual structure—the fetal portion, consisting of the villi and their connective tissue stroma, together with the chorionic membrane itself and the maternal portion, made up of the decidua basalis, or more particularly the altered compact layer of this decidua (Fig. 37).

The Fetal Placenta.—After the fourth month the placental villi are complex, arborescent growths, having branches of varying length, which hang free in the blood sinus. A few of these, the anchoring villi, are still firmly attached to the underlying decidua. While relatively few, there are enough anchoring villi to hold the fetal placenta in intimate contact with the uterine wall.

The individual mature villi consist of a central supportive stem of connective tissue containing the large Hofbauer cells which have presumably a phagocytic power, and there are many lymphocyte-like cells. In this connective tissue core lie the blood vessels, usually two arterioles and two venules, which branch and communicate at the tips of the villa *in a closed circulation*. The villi are covered by the syncytium which in some areas is gathered together into little masses (Fig. 38).

The *chorionic plate* is the capsule covering the placental area, and possesses an outer layer of trophoblast and an inner coat of fibrous

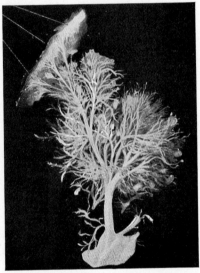

Fig. 38.—Placental villus at five months. Drawn under slight magnification from a specimen floated in water. (Bumm.)

tissue. The fusion of the amnion with the chorion brings the former into contact with the fetal surface of the placenta at the third month of gestation.

The Maternal Placenta.—The maternal portion of the placenta is made up of the stratum compactum of the basilar decidua, together with some fragments of the spongiosa. This tissue is largely a connective tissue stroma, with many decidual cells and some trophoblast derived from the original anchoring villi (Fig. 39).

In the later months of pregnancy the uterine wall grows more rapidly than the fetal placenta and consequently the decidua is thrown into upright folds which penetrate between the masses of villi and form septa which divide the placenta into irregularly quadrilateral lobules called cotyledons. The cotyledons are so developed that each of them (there are usually some twenty) contains a main villus with its branches. The decidua basalis or, as it is now called, the basal plate, forms the medium for the uteroplacental circulation (Fig. 40).

The umbilical arteries and veins pass obliquely through the basal plate and as they do so they lose all of their coats, except one layer of endothelial cells, and they form large sinuses lying between the muscle bundles of the uterus and the decidua. The arteries run in a

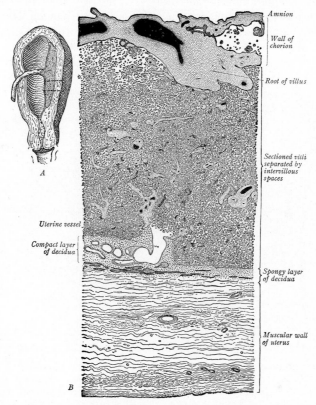

Fig. 39.—Human gravid uterus in section. *A,* Longitudinal section with mature placenta *in situ. B,* Vertical section at seven months (Arey, from Minot; × 5); the area shown corresponds to the rectangle in *A.*

spiral direction while the veins are straight. The growing villi rapidly erode the thin endothelial coat of the veins, until these open directly into the intervillous space, the openings being plugged by the ends of the villi, while there is still some dispute as to whether the arteries ever discharge their blood into the intervillous space. Finally the veins of the compacta are enlarged to form great blood lakes filled with the intermingled branches of the villous tree.

There is a constant circulation of blood in the space, the afferent supply arising from the arteries in the septa while the veins of the cotyledons carry the blood to the venous sinuses. At the periphery is the marginal sinus, an enlarged blood space which never completely encircles the placenta. There is normally no direct intermingling of fetal and maternal blood, the trophoblast covering the villi, the connective-tissue stroma and the capillary endothelium all forming a barrier to direct communication, the interchange being one of diffusion, much as the intestinal villi absorb the fluid contents of the intestine. The pabulum for the fetus, *i. e.*, the proteins, fats and carbohydrates, together with inorganic salts, iron and oxygen, in solution, pass from the maternal blood to the fetus, while the end-products of fetal metabolism are carried in the opposite direction.

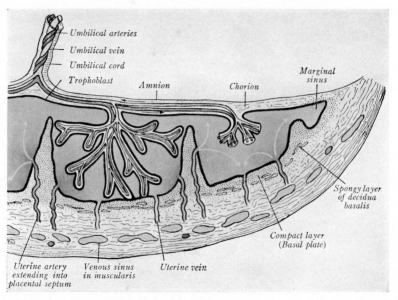

Fig. 40.—Scheme of circulation in the human placenta, as shown in a vertical section. The half of the placenta represented bears one chorionic villus and the stump of another extending into the intervillous spaces of cotyledons. (Arey.)

There is still some question as to whether the placenta acts merely as a dialyzing agent or whether it possesses secretory powers.

The total absorbing surface of the chorion frondosum is calculated at 70 square feet. By comparison, the skin area of an adult is less than one-fourth this amount, but the respiratory area of the lungs of a newborn is some two or three times as great. The smaller absorbing surface and the sluggish "circulation" of the placenta are responsible for the very low oxygen content of fetal blood. This is balanced by the relatively large amount of blood in a fetus, its rapid circulation, and the low oxygen requirements due to bodily quiescence and the non-necessity of a fetus producing its own heat. Among the placental activities, on which there is as yet no complete agreement, should be mentioned the presence and possible local elaboration of hormones and the presence of various enzymes for the splitting of proteins, fats and carbohydrates to be used for fetal nourishment (Arey).

The placenta grows with great rapidity, at first occupying about one fifteenth of the internal surface of the uterus, while at the end of the fourth month it takes up one half of this area and finally at birth the organ covers from one third to one half of the uterus.

The growth is both in thickness, by an elongation of the villi, while the lateral expansion is due to a splitting of the decidua parietalis at the margin of the placenta and an increase in the size of the placental site brought about by the growth of the uterus.

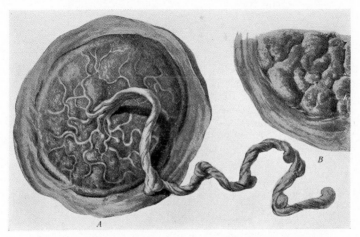

Fig. 41.—Mature human placenta and its adjoining membranes after delivery. × ⅓. *A*, Fetal surface with the umbilical cord exhibiting both false knots and a true knot, and with the yolk-sac remnant near its insertion. *B*, One-quarter of the maternal surface of the same specimen, especially to show cotyledons. (Arey.)

The *mature placenta* (Fig. 41) is a disk-shaped mass of tissue, 7 to 8 inches in diameter and 1½ inches in thickness and weighing usually about one sixth of the weight of the child, or a little over a pound.

It is circular in outline, its margin being fused with a membrane composed of the combined decidua parietalis, the remnants of the capsularis and the chorion laeve.

It is of a deep purplish-gray color and possesses, after detachment and expulsion, a maternal and a fetal surface. The former is divided into cotyledons by the septa from the decidua and presents a velvety surface, irregular and usually studded with blood clots. This portion of the placenta is made up of villi, crowded together, the decidua basalis and the blood vessels and intervillous spaces. On floating bits of the placenta in water the delicate branches and twigs of the villi may be seen clearly (Fig. 42).

The fetal surface of the placenta is covered with grayish, smooth amnion, and its chief characteristic is the mass of large, tortuous blood vessels which stand out from the surface, and are the branches of the two umbilical arteries and the single umbilical vein, which run in the umbilical cord to the child. Hanging from the margins of the placenta are the fetal membranes, which though giving the appearance of a single thickness of tissue may easily be stripped apart disclosing the outer, opaque chorion, still showing remnants of the flat-

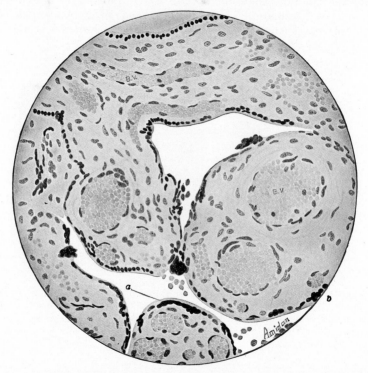

Fig. 42.—Ripe placenta. *a*, Intervillous space; *b*, syncytium. (DeLee.)

tened and atrophic villi, while within this is the smooth, shining transparent amnion. The umbilical cord is inserted into the placenta, usually a little off center, though it may be situated near the margin.

The **umbilical cord** is the structure which connects the fetus with the placenta and, through this, to the uterine wall. Its purpose is to convey the fetal blood to and from the maternal blood sinuses.

The cord is formed at the point of closure of the ventral area of the embryo, where embryonic and extraembryonic tissue meet, which area is called the umbilicus, at the periphery of which the amnion merges into the structure forming the belly wall. The yolk stalk and the body stalk both emerge from the umbilicus and the amnion finally becomes wrapped around these prolongations which also contain the allantois, to form the umbilical cord.

The cord is largely made up of a jelly-like substance (the jelly of Wharton) which is of connective tissue origin.

The mature cord varies from 50 cm. to possibly 100 cm. in length, by about 1 cm. in diameter. It is covered by the glistening amnion with its squamous or low cuboidal epithelium and in substance is made up of the two umbilical arteries and the one umbilical vein, the remains of the allantois, the body stalk and the yolk stalk, the whole connected by the whitish jelly of Wharton.

The cord is usually spiral, twenty to forty turns being commonly seen, but this is subject to great variation. The spiraling is thought to be due to unequal growth of the two arteries, to the movements of the child and the effect of the pulsations of the fetal heart. The arteries and vein are twisted, usually the arteries around the vein, though sometimes they are straight.

5

CHAPTER V

THE GROWTH OF THE FETUS

THE age of the fetus cannot be determined with absolute accuracy, but since it is now generally believed that ovulation occurs from the eleventh to the fourteenth day after the onset of the preceding menstrual period and that the ovum is only capable of being fertilized for about forty-eight hours after ovulation, the time of conception may be fairly accurately determined.

For general purposes one may then calculate the age of an embryo from the twelfth day after the beginning of the last menstruation. This is by no means always accurate, but is true in a sufficient proportion of cases to justify such time as an indication of the probable date of conception.

The length and weight of the embryo at various times in pregnancy have been estimated and a table of averages has been compiled. The length of the embryo may be measured by taking the crown-rump length or sitting height, the crown-heel length or standing height and in early embryos with marked spinal flexion the neck-rump length is often utilized.

The following table from Arey (Developmental Anatomy) gives the statistical averages for human embryos of definite age (Fig. 43).

Age of Embryo	Crown-rump length (mm.)	Crown-heel length (mm.)	Weight in Gm.
Two weeks	0.1	0.1	
Three weeks	1.5	1.5	
Four weeks	2.5	2.5	
Five weeks	5.5	5.5	0.004
Six weeks	11.0	11.0	
Seven weeks	17.0	19.0	
Second lunar month	25.0	30.0	2
Third lunar month	68.0	98.0	24
Fourth lunar month	121.0	180.0	120
Fifth lunar month	167.0	250.0	330
Sixth lunar month	210.0	315.0	600
Seventh lunar month	245.0	370.0	1000
Eighth lunar month	284.0	425.0	1600
Ninth lunar month	316.0	470.0	2400
Full term (269 days)	336.0	500.0	3200

With the age and length of the embryo known, a rule may be evolved to determine the unknown factor in terms of the known.

When the size of the embryo is known, its age may be estimated by:

Crown-heel length in cm. $\times$ 0.2 = age in lunar months.

Crown-rump length in cm. $\times$ 0.3 = age in lunar months.

(For embryos less than 10 cm. long, add one lunar month to the result.)

Conversely when the age of the embryo is known.

Age (in lunar months) ÷ 0.2 = crown-heel length in cm.

Age (in lunar months) ÷ 0.3 = crown-rump length in cm.

(For embryos of the first three months subtract 4 cm. from the result.)

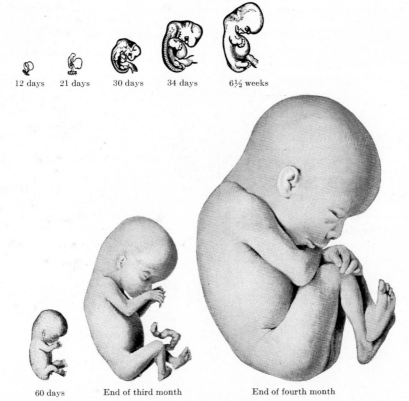

12 days   21 days   30 days   34 days   6½ weeks

60 days   End of third month   End of fourth month

Fig. 43.—The human embryo in natural size, in the first four months of gestation. (Bumm.)

Another practical and commonly used rule is to square the number of months of pregnancy which will give the length of the fetus in centimeters until the fifth month. From this time on, the number of the month is multiplied by 5 to arrive at the length of the fetus.

Reversing this rule gives the age of a fetus of known length.

Summary of the Development of the Ovum and the Change in the Uterus During Pregnancy.—The ovular period occupies the first two weeks after conception, during which time the embryo consists only of the blastocystic vesicle. The embryonic period begins with the third week of gestation.

First Lunar Month.—The embryo is growing rapidly having attained a length of 4 to 5 mm. at the end of this month. Flexion is marked so that the cephalic and caudal extremities are almost in con-

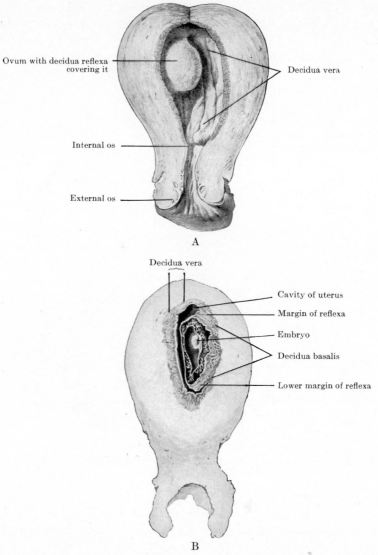

Fig. 44.—Uterus and ovum at four weeks. A, The uterus laid open. B, Mesial section through uterus and embryo. (Bumm.)

tact. The anlage for the various organs have become differentiated. The chorion has begun to develop its shaggy coat, the deciduae are thick, the uterus slightly enlarged and boggy (Fig. 44).

Second Month (End).—The embryo is 30 mm. long, the rudimentary limbs have appeared, the external genitalia appear, the tail process has shrunken, the head assumes a somewhat human appearance (Fig. 45).

Third Lunar Month (End).—The embryo is from 9 to 10 cm. in length, contours of ossification have appeared, fingers and toes are differentiated, and the nails are apparent. The external genitalia become differentiated, the head is still disproportionally large.

The placenta has begun to develop, the chorion beneath the capsularis shows atrophy of its villi.

The decidua capsularis and parietalis are in contact, the uterine cavity almost obliterated.

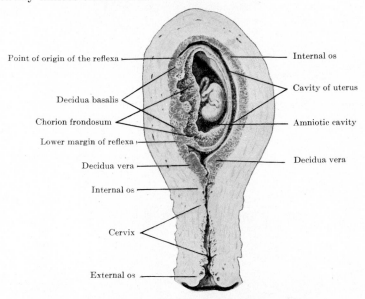

Fig. 45.—Uterus and ovum at the end of the second month of gestation. Sagittal section. (Bumm.)

The entire ovum is about 8 cm. in diameter, the uterus is softened and ovoid and may be palpated just above the symphysis, being about 10 to 12 cm. in length (Figs. 46, 47).

Fourth Month (End).—The fetus is 18 cm. long, sex organs are well differentiated, and centers of ossification are increasing. The skin is red and transparent and meconium is present in the intestine. The fetus is capable of active movement of its well defined limbs.

The placenta is being rapidly formed and is almost complete.

The uterus is soft and somewhat cystic in consistency and is globular in shape, about 15 by 12 cm. in size and easily palpable above the symphysis. The cervix is soft and cyanotic.

Fifth Month (End).—The fetus is 25 cm. long, and weighs about

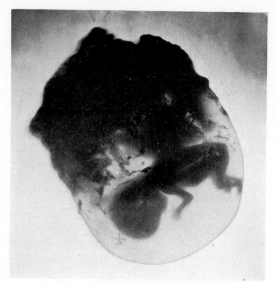

Fig. 46.—Ovum of three months showing fetus lying in the intact amniotic sac, and a few opaque flakes representing the chorion laeve. Placenta is shown as a dense mass. (Kensington Hospital for Women.)

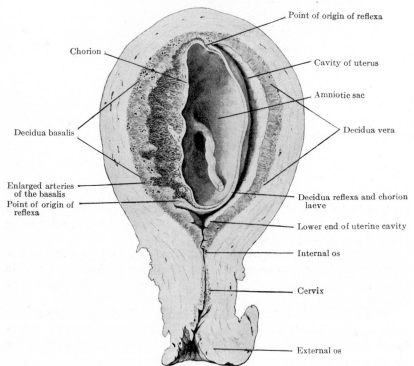

Fig. 47.—Uterus and ovum at end of third month of gestation. Sagittal section. (Bumm.)

350 Gm. (10–11 ounces), the skin is covered with lanugo hair, and true hair appears on the head. The heart beat is visible and may be heard through the maternal abdominal wall. Vernix caseosa is present. The placenta is fully formed, the uterus 18 cm. long and midway to the umbilicus of the mother. Fetal movements have been apparent for about three or four weeks (Fig. 48).

Sixth Month.—The fetus weighs 650 Gm. (22 ounces), is active and viable for a short time after birth. The ovoid uterus reaches the umbilicus, measuring about 22 cm. in length, fetal movements are strongly felt by the mother and the heart tones are easily audible over the abdomen.

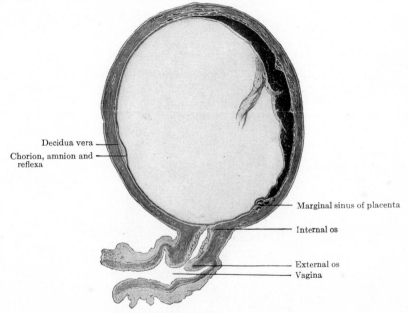

Fig. 48.—Pregnant uterus at five months' gestation. Sagittal section. (Bumm.)

Seventh Month (End).—The fetus weighs about 1000 Gm. (about 2¼ pounds) and is 35–38 cm. long.

The face is wrinkled and the muscles of expression have begun to functionate, the testes have begun to enter the scrotum, and the child may survive if born, although its chances are not promising.

The ovoid uterus measures 27 cm. and the lie of the child can be made out by abdominal palpation, together with the vigorous fetal movements.

Eighth Month (End).—The fetus is 40 to 42 cm. long and weighs about 1600 Gm. (about 3½ pounds). The skin is still red, but much paler than before, and the superficial fat is beginning to appear. The uterus measures 30 cm. in height and is midway between umbilicus and xiphoid.

Ninth Month (End).—The fetus is now 45 to 46 cm. long and weighs about 2500 Gm. (5½ pounds). The nails reach the ends of the fingers and toes, the lanugo disappears, and the face loses its wrinkles and is well plumped out. If delivered at this time the infant has an excellent chance for life. The uterus measures 33 cm. in height and reaches almost to the ensiform cartilage.

Tenth Month (End).—The mature fetus weighs 3200 Gm. (7 to 7½ pounds), is 50 cm. in length and fully developed in all respects.

The uterus measures 36 cm. in length, but by reason of engagement of the head in primiparae, it sinks again in these women to almost midway between umbilicus and xiphoid (Fig. 49).

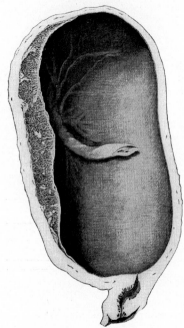

Fig. 49.—Uterus at term, sagittal section. (Bumm.)

The Mature Fetus.—The fetus at term weighs around 3400 Gm. (7 to 7½ pounds) and is about 50 cm. long. The skin is pinkish white, smooth and free from wrinkles. The hair is abundant on the head and may be several centimeters long. The fingernails are firm, and reach to or slightly beyond the tips of the fingers and toes. The cranial sutures are sharply marked, the large anterior fontanel firm, and not depressed below the level of the skull. The body movements are active, the cry strong, the child attempts to suck and the muscles of expression are active.

There is a marked natural variation in the size of the child, heredity playing a large part. Small parents have small children and large ones breed large infants. (The writer is 6 feet, 3 inches tall, his wife 5 feet, 9 inches and their three sons weighed respectively $9\frac{1}{4}$, $9\frac{1}{4}$, and 10 pounds at birth.)

Children of later pregnancies are larger than those of the earlier ones, because of the increased uterine circulation, the tendency toward longer pregnancies in older women and the greater physical development of the mother which comes with maturity.

Intra-uterine disease restricts the growth of infants, and maternal toxemia exerts a profound effect.

CHAPTER VI

THE PHYSIOLOGY OF THE FETUS

Nutrition.—While the fertilized ovum is still in the fallopian tube it is probably nourished by osmosis from the fluids in the tube. In the early days of embedding, the same process is operative but very shortly the chorionic villi dip into the blood sinus so that by the fourth week of pregnancy branches of the umbilical vessels appear in

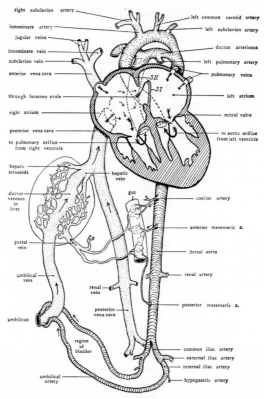

Fig. 50.—General plan of the fetal circulation. (From Patten, "Embryology of Pig," published by P. Blakiston's Son & So.)

the chorionic villi and the direct transmission of nutritive material from mother to infant begins.

The Fetal Circulation (Fig. 50).—Since the lungs of the fetus are inactive, the circulatory system is very different from that required by extra-uterine existence. The blood is oxygenated and receives its nutritive elements from the placenta, whence it is carried to the fetus

74

by the umbilical vein. Entering at the umbilicus this vein rises behind the parietal peritoneum and reaches the liver. At this point the vein divides, one branch unites with the portal vein, circulates through the liver and enters the vena cava via the hepatic vein. The large branch of the umbilical vein is carried through the ductus venosus and empties directly into the vena cava.

The blood in the vena cava comes from the lower limbs of the fetus and is purely venous in character until the fresh arterial stream entering the vessel from the ductus venosus and the hepatic artery causes a mixture of arterial and venous blood in the cava.

The vena cava empties into the right auricle of the heart, where its already somewhat venous stream meets and mingles with the purely venous blood coming from the fetal head and upper extremities and reaching the right auricle through the superior vena cava. The blood in the right auricle is then mixed in quality, and not two separate streams, one venous from the superior vena cava and one mostly arterial from the inferior as has been thought.

Part of this mixed blood now enters the left auricle through the patulous foramen ovale, then goes into the left ventricle and is distributed by the aorta.

Part goes into the right ventricle, and is forced by the systolic contraction into the main trunk of the pulmonary artery, which in the fetus has three divisions, one to each lung and a third which opens into the aorta. This latter division is called the ductus arteriosus and serves to divert a considerable quantity of blood from the functionless lungs. It is probable however, that there is a much greater circulation through the pulmonary arteries and the lungs than was formerly believed. The blood in the aorta supplies the various organs of the fetal body, but eventually most of it reaches the internal iliac and hypogastric arteries and through them enters the umbilical artery to be distributed throughout the placenta for reoxygenation and the absorption of nutritive elements.

Changes in the Circulation after Birth.—The essential differences between the fetal and adult circulation lie in the functionating of the ductus arteriosus, the ductus venosus, the foramen ovale, the hypogastric arteries and the umbilical vessels. After delivery a rapid change takes place in the function of these structures. The infant inspires, the lungs expand, and the pulmonary circulation is fully established almost immediately. Consequently, the bulk of the blood from the right ventricle goes directly into the lungs, the ductus arteriosus gradually closing, until it is completely obliterated by the end of the second week, although it may remain patent for some time longer.

Termination of the cord circulation renders the umbilical vein functionless, and a smaller quantity of blood reaches the right auricle by way of the inferior vena cava.

Hence the pressure in the right auricle is sharply reduced, while the tension increases in the left side of the heart, and thus, the foramen ovale slowly is closed, although it may persist for months and even remain patulous throughout life.

Because of the abolishing of the umbilical circulation, the ductus venosus and the umbilical vein become occluded within the first week after parturition.

Respiration in the fetus does not occur, the lungs being atelectatic. The interchange of oxygen and CO_2 is brought about in the placental circulation by splitting off the oxygen from the maternal erythrocytes by some sort of enzyme activity of the placental cells.

Digestion.—The physiology of the fetal intestinal tract is not yet understood, although it is known that the stomach contains pepsin and rennin at the sixth month, and that bile is secreted by the liver, as shown by the presence of bile salts in the meconium. All fetal nutrition is the result of placental absorption, with the exception of a small amount, perhaps obtained by swallowing liquor amnii.

It must be remembered in considering the physiology of the fetus that its oxygen requirement is low by reason of its restricted movement and the fact that the oxygenation of ingested food is not required. There is no heat loss by reason of the constant temperature of the maternal uterus and the amniotic fluid.

The Physiology of the Placenta.—It has been stated that there is no direct contact between fetal and maternal blood and that the placenta acts as a dialyzing membrane in the osmosis of gases and substances in solution, between mother and fetus.

It is probable that the placenta also has certain glandular activities in its own right.

The passage of water through the placenta in either direction is closely associated with the maintenance of mineral balance between the fetal and maternal fluids.

The transmission of glucose and other carbohydrates seems to be a process of osmosis and depends upon the concentration of the solution, the placenta apparently having no selective action for this substance.

Fat transmission has not been proved and it is probable that the fetus synthetizes its own fats from carbohydrates, chiefly glucose.

Iron is probably taken up in the form of hemoglobin, and the method of transmission of albumin, if any, is not understood.

The question of transmission of bacteria by the placenta has given rise to great controversy, the present opinion being that such passage is quite infrequent, and occurs only if there be some lesion of the villi, with a solution of continuity, or sometimes when there is a supervirulent infection. The tubercle bacillus may sometimes pass the placental filter, but such occurrences are rare, although for some reason the typhoid bacillus appears to enter the fetus rather frequently.

Filtrable viruses do seem to pass, and there are many recorded cases in which the presence of streptococci has been shown in both the maternal and the fetal blood stream.

II. PREGNANCY

CHAPTER VII

THE PHYSIOLOGY OF PREGNANCY

CHANGES IN THE MATERNAL ORGANISM, ASSOCIATED WITH PREGNANCY

THE human female has reached a stage in evolution where pregnancy and childbirth may be said to be an incident in her career, rather than its only purpose. In many of the lower forms of life the females exist only for the performance of the function of reproduction after the completion of which they immediately perish. Indeed, in certain moths, the adults in the reproductive cycle are unprovided with other than a rudimentary digestive apparatus, so that, their eggs being fertilized and deposited, they die of starvation.

In woman, although pregnancy may leave no great permanent impress upon her morphology, still the fact of providing nutrition and tissue-producing element as well, from her own bodily resources with which to serve the developing embryo, necessitates marked changes in all of her organs, notably, of course, those having directly to do with the growth and nidation of the fetus. In general these changes are all hypertrophic in their nature, the increased demands on the entire organism causing compensatory hyperfunction.

The biological relationship of the fetus to the mother is still an unsettled question. Unquestionably the former is in a sense a mass of partly foreign, partly autogenous protein, growing within the body of the mother, but absorbing from her tissues the pabulum necessary for its development and may well be regarded as a separate organism with parasitic tendencies. In short, the child may be likened to a benign tumor developing at its mother's expense but without permanent damage to her body cells. A second group of observers hold that the fetus *in utero* simulates a malignant tumor, not only deriving its nutrition from the mother's tissues but destroying her cells in the meantime.

A third version and the one coming to be most generally accepted is that there is a beneficial physiologic interchange between mother and fetus, the woman developing an increased metabolic rate which more than compensates for the expenditure of tissue elements necessitated by the requirements of the growing embryo.

As put by Paul Bar, when there is a healthy fetus in a healthy mother, pregnancy represents a condition of "symbiose harmonique homogene."

77

This conclusion is in perfect harmony with modern beliefs as to the interchange of growth forces, and is not contradicted by the existence of even such grave disturbance of metabolism as are seen in the toxemias of pregnancy, since the rapid advancement of so complex a relationship as takes place between the embryo and its host must carry with it the great possibility of error in the mechanism of metabolism with the resulting disharmony which we recognize as pathological.

THE MATERNAL CHANGES IN PREGNANCY. LOCAL CHANGES

CHANGES IN THE UTERUS

The uterine alterations in pregnancy may be divided into:
Change in size.
Change in position.
Change in shape.
Change in morphology.
Change in innervation and blood supply.

Changes in Size.—The nonpregnant uterus measures about 7.5 cm. (3 inches) in length, 5 cm. (2 inches) in breadth and 2.5 cm. (1 inch) in thickness, having a cubic capacity of about 1 cubic inch and weighing between 40 and 50 Gm. In women who have borne children, the uterus may be somewhat larger but not markedly so. At term, ten lunar months later, the same organ has been converted into a soft, muscular sac 30 cm. in length, weighing upward of 2 pounds and having a capacity of from 400 cubic inches up.

This tremendous increase in size is brought about by a hypertrophy of all the structures entering into the formation of the uterus, and also by a true hyperplasia. Not only do the tissues increase in size but there is a distinct increase in the number of individual cells. The hyperplasia takes place during the first few months of pregnancy, after which few if any new cells are developed but these present hypertrophy to an amazing extent, some of the muscle fibers measuring ten times as long and five times as broad in the pregnant as in the nonpregnant uterus. There is also a considerable overgrowth of connective tissue (Fig. 51).

Early in pregnancy there is an increased thickness of the uterine wall, but later on the distention of the organ nullifies the increase and at term the wall is about 0.5 cm. in thickness.

The arrangement of the muscle bundles may be studied to some extent in late pregnancy, the work of Hélie in 1864 on this matter remaining unchallenged. Three layers of muscle fibers may be distinguished, an outer thin, a very thick and strong middle layer and a thin inner layer next the mucosa. The outer layer extends from the lower uterine segment to cover the entire fundus and is apparently a continuation of the longitudinal fibers of the tubes (Fig. 52).

The inner layer lies just external to the endometrium. Its fibers encircle the internal os and the orifices of the tubes and pass obliquely upward on both anterior and posterior walls of the uterus.

The thick middle layer forms the bulk of the uterine muscle. It is derived from the circular fibers of the tube and radiating fibers from the uterine ligaments. The muscle bundles run in an interlacing, generally circular direction (Fig. 53).

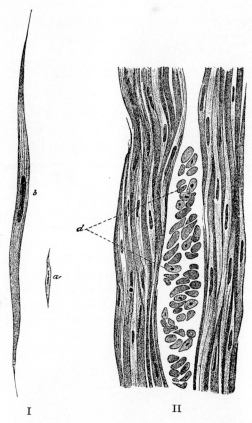

I II

Fig. 51.—The muscle changes in pregnancy. I, (*a*) Muscle cell from non-pregnant uterus, (*b*) muscle cell from a uterus pregnant at term. (After Sarwey.) II, (*d*) Section through the wall of a pregnant uterus. (After Bumm and Rosthorn.)

The combination of these three layers of muscle, each with fibers running in different directions, provides for a lessening of uterine size in all directions, when they contract. Every portion of the uterus is pulled together upon such contraction, this resulting in the powerful expulsive force, responsible for delivery.

The blood vessels of the uterus course between these muscle fibers and are hence twisted and shut off when contraction occurs, which explains the absence of hemorrhage after the child is expelled.

The *cervix* undergoes little change.

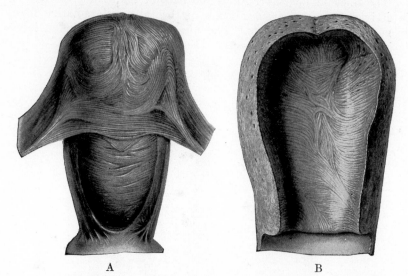

A   B

Fig. 52.—A, External muscular layer of pregnant uterus. B, Internal muscular layer of pregnant uterus. (Hélie.)

Its muscle fibers run generally in a circular direction, with an external layer of oblique and longitudinal fibers which extend through the vesico-uterine ligaments and into the bases of the broad ligaments.

Changes in Position.—The somewhat increased weight of the pregnant uterus causes that organ to sink a little into the pelvis during

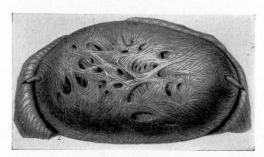

Fig. 53.—Median muscular layer of pregnant uterus. (Hélie.)

the first two months of gestation after which it steadily rises in the abdominal cavity at a fairly constant rate, until the ninth lunar month when it again descends for a short distance, until delivery takes place (Fig. 54). Inasmuch as the uterine enlargement during the first three

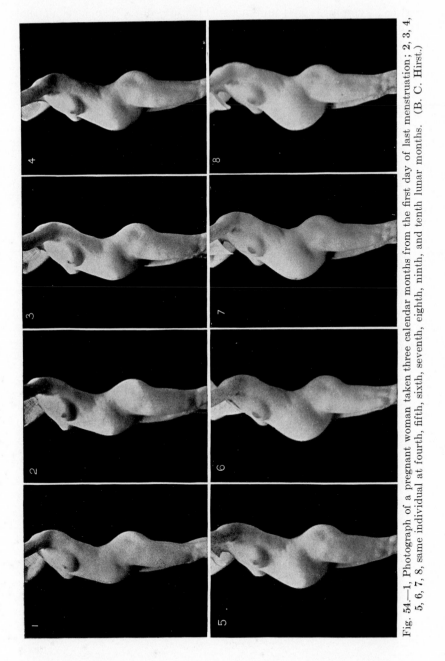

Fig. 54.—1, Photograph of a pregnant woman taken three calendar months from the first day of last menstruation; 2, 3, 4, 5, 6, 7, 8, same individual at fourth, fifth, sixth, seventh, eighth, ninth, and tenth lunar months. (B. C. Hirst.)

months is concerned more closely with an increase in the lateral and anterior posterior diameters the fundus does not rise above the symphysis pubis until the fourth month. At the fifth month it is midway

6

between symphysis and umbilicus (Figs. 55, 56). The level of the latter is reached at the sixth month and at seven months the fundus

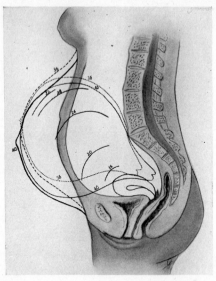

Fig. 55.—Increase in the size of the uterus and alterations in the contours of the abdomen during pregnancy. Lateral view.

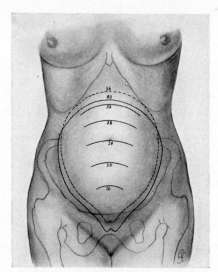

Fig. 56.—Increase in size of the uterus during the several weeks of pregnancy. Front view.

is one third the distance from the umbilicus and the ensiform cartilage, at eight months, two thirds the distance and at eight and one-half calendar months the level of the ensiform is reached. Two weeks before term the uterus and its contents sink to about the eighth month level. This phenomenon is termed lightening, since as the uterus sinks the stomach and diaphragm have more play with greatly increased comfort on the part of the patient (Figs. 57, 58).

There is usually some lateral torsion of the uterus, from left to right, both by reason of the inherent tendency to slight right twisting

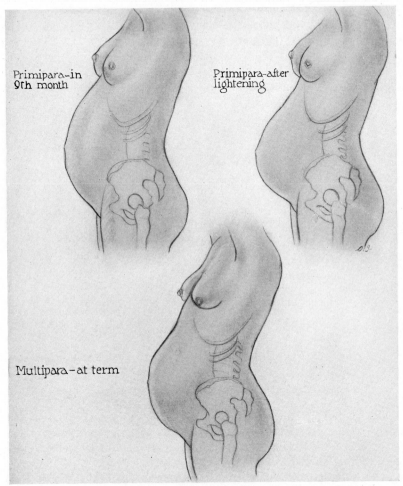

Primipara-in 9th month

Primipara-after lightening

Multipara-at term

Fig. 57.—The contours of the pregnant abdomen. (Redrawn after Tom Jones.)

on the part of the human viscera, as well as to the thrust exerted by the sigmoid and rectum which occupy the left posterior portion of the pelvic cavity. This torsion reaches so marked a degree that not infrequently in an operation for cesarean section, the left ovary, tube and broad ligament will present at the left side of the abdominal incision, while the right adnexa are buried deep in the right flank.

The round ligaments hypertrophy with the uterus and may frequently be palpated as firm tissue cords running obliquely across the abdomen.

The fallopian tubes and ovaries rise with the fundus and it is significant that the areas of pain and tenderness arising from salpingitis complicating pregnancy are higher by far than in the nonpregnant woman and this fact must be taken into consideration when determining a diagnosis.

Changes in Shape.—During the first few weeks of pregnancy the uterus maintains its flattened pyriform shape but at the beginning of the second month, the lower portion of the fundus begins to enlarge very rapidly and the organ becomes globular in shape, the fundus seeming like a sphere resting upon the small, cylindrical cervix.

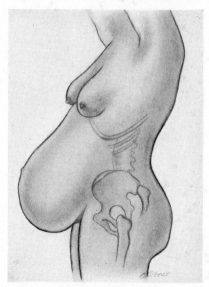

Fig. 58.—Pendulous abdomen. (Redrawn after Tom Jones.)

The globular shape becomes more marked until the end of the fourth month, when the elongation begins to exceed the lateral development, until at term the uterus is more than one and one-half times as long as it is wide.

The anteroposterior diameter of the growing uterus is less than the lateral, because of the limitations placed on expansion in this direction by the spinal column behind and the abdominal wall in front (Fig. 59).

Throughout pregnancy there is a torsion of the fundus upon the cervix toward the right, sometimes reaching above 70 degrees in extent. This is simply an exaggeration of the physiologic slight torsion of the nonpregnant uterus, and is supposedly increased by the push of the gas- and feces-filled sigmoid and rectum to the left.

The area between the cervix and fundus, the lower uterine segment, becomes steadily more compressible and less resistant and upon this fact, coupled with rapid increase in size and weight of the fundus, depends the marked exaggeration of the anteflexion of the uterus in early pregnancy, which, however, gradually disappears after the fourth

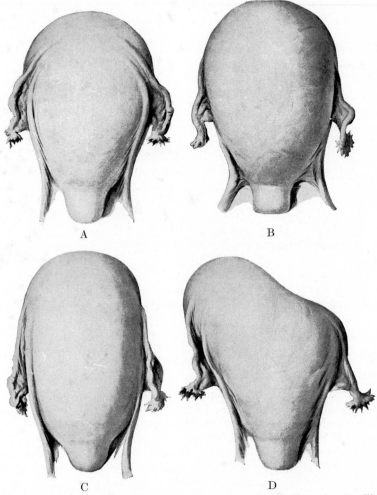

Fig. 59.—Variations in shape of the pregnant uterus. A, Ovoid uterus; B, elliptic uterus; C, cylindrical uterus; D, asymmetric development. (Bumm.)

month, as the fetus elongates and the fundus rises higher and higher in the abdomen.

The **morphology of the uterus** is altered greatly during pregnancy, the first change taking place in the endometrium, which becomes thicker, softer and much more vascular, undergoing the specific changes which result in the formation of the decidua as described in Chapter IV.

The changes in the muscular coat have already been explained.

The serous covering of the uterus shares in the general hypertrophic process and become much thicker during pregnancy, being firmly attached to the fundus, but lying in loose, easily separable folds on the lower uterine segment.

Blood Supply and Innervation.—*The Blood Vessels.*—The arteries increase greatly in diameter, length and tortuosity. At the placental site they empty directly into the dilated uterine veins which are termed sinuses and whence the fetal blood derives its oxygen.

The veins are enormously dilated, and at the area occupied by the placenta they are spread into deep lakes or sinuses, whose thin walls are closely invested with connective tissue, and which lie between the muscle bundles, by whose contraction the sinuses may be occluded. It is by this mechanism that hemorrhage is prevented after the birth of the child and the expulsion of the placenta.

The *lymphatics* share in the general marked development and are found in a great network, at the sides of the uterus under the attachment of the broad ligaments and covering the fundus.

The lymphatics form two layers, one just beneath the peritoneum, the vessels penetrating the muscle bundles and another just beneath the mucosa. The richness of the lymph supply in the pregnant uterus explains the extent and rapidity by which an infection of the endometrium becomes generally distributed.

The Nerves.—The nerves of the pregnant uterus become somewhat thickened and elongated, the neurilemma being the coat most affected. The various nerve ganglia also become somewhat hypertrophied.

CHANGES IN THE CERVIX

The cervix undergoes much less hypertrophy than does the remainder of the uterus, reaching its maximum growth at about the third month when it is 5 cm. long. The most characteristic change in this portion of the uterus is its softening and congestion, the former being available as a diagnostic sign in pregnancy. In older multiparae with much scar tissue about the external os the softening may be very slight; in certain instances almost negligible although the passive congestion is usually present.

Early in pregnancy the cervix assumes a deep violet or purple color as a result of the hyperemia it has undergone and this color persists until involution is completed. The cervical glands are active and secrete a tenacious mucus which shortly accumulates in the cervical canal, being gradually compressed by the increased amount secreted and by the elasticity of the cervical walls, until there is formed a dense, mucous plug, fairly firmly attached to the mucosa of the cervix and remaining in position during pregnancy until dislodged by the uterine contractions of the first stage of labor, when it together with a little blood exudes from the vagina.

The hypersecretion of the cervical glands produces also a fairly abundant white mucous leukorrhea which in healthy women is non-irritating and bathes the vagina during the later months of gestation. The cervical glands become greatly enlarged, at the expense of the interglandular tissue, and finally form a honeycomb or cavernous structure (Fig. 60).

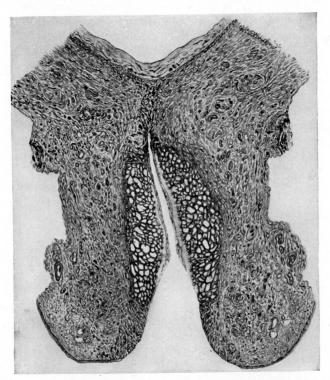

Fig. 60.—Cervix at three months. Note immense development of the mucous glands and the blood vessels. Cervix seems almost like an erectile organ. (DeLee.)

The cervix is not appreciably shortened even at term, when effacement is complete; however, the internal os practically disappears.

The relation of the cervix to the lower uterine segment is still a controversial subject, although it is probable that both uterine body and cervix contribute to make up the distensible, poorly contracted lower uterine segment. There is a sort of no man's land between cervix and corpus called by Aschoff the isthmus, in which the musculature is not so well developed as in the body of the uterus, but more so than in the cervix. It is from this intermediary zone that the distended lower uterine segment develops.

PARAMETRIAL CHANGES

There is some hypertrophy of the dense fibrillar connective tissue of the parametrium, but the most important change is the appearance of many cells of mesenchymal origin which are called clasmatocytes and which, as shown by Hofbauer and others, exert a strong phagocytic action and are powerful factors in the prevention of infection during pregnancy and after labor.

Changes in the Tubes and Ovaries.—The alteration of position of these structures has already been discussed. The morphological changes to which they are subject during pregnancy are largely the result of increased vascularity. Moderate hypertrophy, marked softening and a distinct hyperplasia of the blood vessels are characteristic. Occasionally there develops an abortive and atypical decidua in the tubes, as is so uniformly observed in tubal pregnancy, but this condition is rare and does not give rise to any clinical evidence of its presence.

While true ovulation ceases during pregnancy, the partial ripening of ova seems to continue, the development going on until checked by the internal secretion of the corpus luteum when the growing ova suffer atrophy and finally appear as "the interstitial gland" which is said to possess some of the power of glands of internal secretion but which has not as yet been physiologically accounted for.

Changes in the Vagina.—This organ shares in the general succulence and congestion of the pelvis. Owing to venous engorgement, the vaginal mucosa assumes a violet hue, early in pregnancy, the color deepening as gestation advances until by the fourth month it has become a dark purple. The color is much more marked in brunettes than in blondes, and is so universally present as to be regarded as an important presumptive sign of the existence of pregnancy (see Chadwick's sign).

The mucous secretion which bathes the vagina is also much increased during pregnancy and in some individuals reaches an amount sufficient to cause an annoying leukorrhea. There is also present a considerable hypertrophy of the muscularis and mucosa of the vagina, paralleling the same process in other portions of the birth canal.

The Bladder and Rectum.—Frequency of urination, as will be seen later, is a suggestive sign of early pregnancy, the condition being due to increased congestion at the vesical trigone and to the stretching of the area brought about by the rapid widening of the uterus in the early weeks. This symptom usually disappears after the third month, to reappear during the last four weeks or thereabouts, since at this time the fetus has grown so large that the presenting part exerts a distinct pressure upon the bladder, distorting its cavity and rendering complete evacuation more or less difficult. Varices of the bladder mucosa may be present explaining the occasional hematuria of pregnancy.

The rectum is usually not disturbed during the early portion of

pregnancy but in the last months constipation is a frequent annoyance by reason of pressure. The general increase of blood supply also
predisposes to the development of hemorrhoids at this time.

CHANGES IN THE ABDOMINAL WALLS

Alterations in these tissues are brought about mechanically, by
the overstretching to which they are subjected and to the frequent
excessive deposition of fat which markedly alter the contour of the
woman. The distention of the abdomen is most marked about the
umbilicus, which soon becomes everted, reaching the level of the abdominal wall and may often protrude during the later months. There
may be separation of the recti muscles (diastasis) with a pendulous
abdomen as the result.

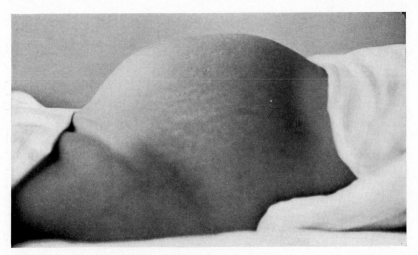

Fig. 61.—The striae of pregnancy.

The **striae of pregnancy** are whitish or silvery, purplish or reddish
lines of varying number and width, which result from the overstretching and disordered arrangement of the connective tissue layer of the
skin (Fig. 61).

They may be radial to the umbilicus, parallel to Poupart's ligament, are irregular in shape, may be confluent, many or few and
sometimes are found on the thighs and breasts. They are more deeply
pigmented in brunettes than in blondes, and remain as little silvery
scars throughout life. A median line of pigmentation is often noted
running from umbilicus to symphysis and called the linea nigra.

GENERAL CHANGES IN PREGNANCY

Heart and Circulatory System.—In late pregnancy the heart becomes displaced upward and assumes a more transverse position, the
area of cardiac dulness being considerably increased. Inasmuch as

the total bulk of the blood is considerably increased during pregnancy and the circulatory demands of the growing fetus plus the enlarging uterus require more rapid circulation, it seems natural that the cardiac output must be amplified. Frey maintains that x-ray studies and the increase in blood volume all indicate cardiac hypertrophy.

Stander found that the cardiac output is increased over one half in late pregnancy and as normal pregnancy is not associated with a fall in blood pressure, it is apparent that normal gestation is accompanied by a marked increase in cardiac work. Stander is unable to say whether the additional heart work is effected by actual hypertrophy of the heart or by calling into function any reserve force of the heart. This increase in cardiac output begins as early as the fourth month and from this time on the demands on the heart steadily become greater.

The cardiac reserve is fully maintained during pregnancy and the electrocardiogram shows no change.

In healthy women the increased demands on the heart are met without difficulty, although there may be some functional disturbance as evidenced by arrhythmia, extrasystole, transient dyspnea and so on.

In patients suffering from cardiac disorder, however, the increased effort required may bring about decompensation and sometimes complete cardiac collapse.

Blood.—It has long been held that there is an increase in total blood volume during pregnancy. This view has been confirmed by the modern, accurate method of investigation and it is true that during pregnancy there is a definite increase in both the plasma and blood volume which disappears during the puerperium. The volume is definitely increased, while the cell and hemoglobin content is relatively but not actually diminished.

The coagulability of the blood is slightly but definitely increased during pregnancy, the readings having a sharp tendency to return to the value found in the nongravid state, during the puerperium (Bland and Goldstein).

There is a distinct "physiological" type of anemia which occurs to some degree in about one half of all pregnant women.

Numerous authors have developed this thesis, the finding of most workers being strongly in accord with each other. Bland, Goldstein and First studied a large series of cases and show that practically one half of all pregnant women show an anemia in various periods of gestation, with red cell counts of 3.5 millions or less.

A distinct hemoglobinemia of 70 per cent or less occurred in three fifths of the patients.

It seems true that this type of anemia grows more severe with the advance of the pregnancy. Recovery during the puerperium is the rule; 92 per cent of Bland's patients exhibiting improvement beginning seven to ten days after labor and being practically complete six months after delivery.

The etiology of physiological anemia of pregnancy is not clear. The older writers felt that it was caused by malnutrition and improper prenatal care, which is possible. However, since the same blood picture is seen in wealthy private patients, this cannot be the sole source of origin. Hofbauer thought the anemia due to a syncytial hemolysin developed in the ectodermal cells of the chorion. With the advance of pregnancy an antihemolysin formed in the mother's blood which prevented further blood destruction. Still other investigators think that the condition is relative, and due to a true hydremia, with increased water of the plasma.

The only definite statement which can be made is that the anemia is due to pregnancy, and in most cases ceases with delivery.

Sedimentation Time During Pregnancy.—The sedimentation rate of the erythrocytes increases progressively with each month of normal pregnancy. Griffin, in the author's clinic at Kensington Hospital for Women, found that the rate in the ninth month is approximately five times that given for the average healthy nonpregnant woman.

There is a return to normal by the fourth week after delivery.

In a group of toxic patients studied at the same time, the sedimentation time was shorter than in normally pregnant women at a corresponding period of gestation. The average readings were from 10 to 15 per cent higher, using the percentage method.

Griffin also found that there is a mild regeneration type of activity in the bone marrow during pregnancy as shown by the Schilling index which presents in the blood a few metamyelocytes and an occasional myelocyte. This tendency does not vary noticeably with the period of gestation.

The blood platelets are not appreciably increased during pregnancy, averaging from 200,000 to 350,000 per cmm.

In most patients there is a rapid gain in platelets after delivery, Bland and his colleagues finding increases of from 50,000 to over 200,000. The cause of this rapid rise in platelets is undetermined, but it has been suggested that their multiplication may be physiologic, a natural response of the body to safeguard against infection.

Leukocytosis.—The physiologic leukocytosis of pregnancy has been known since Virchow. There is a distinct increase of polymorphonuclear cells and of myelocytes. The leukocyte count averages about 15,000 in the later months of pregnancy, rising sharply during labor to 18,000 or 20,000 (DeLee, 34,000), and falls to normal in the six weeks following delivery. The leukocytosis is believed to be in part a measure of the increased activity of the bone marrow engendered by pregnancy and in part to a defense mechanism erected against the toxins of pregnancy.

Knowledge of the existence of the physiological leukocytosis is clinically important since the blood picture, so suggestive of inflammatory reaction, may well confuse the diagnosis in acute abdominal disorders developing in the course of pregnancy.

The blood-making organs are much stimulated by gestation, the spleen and bone marrow undergoing marked congestion and in the case of the former, a considerable increase in weight.

The **blood pressure** varies but little during pregnancy, unless toxemia develops, when its variation from the norm forms one of the most valuable diagnostic signs.

The normal blood pressure in healthy women is 110 to 120 systolic, 75 to 85 diastolic, with individual fluctuation. During the summer months and in women who suffer from fatigue a mild hypotension is the rule. During labor the blood pressure undergoes marked variations, dropping suddenly with the rupture of the membranes, but rapidly rising again thereafter.

Varicosities of the veins involving the lower half of the body are common during pregnancy. Any site may be involved about the vulva, rectum and anus, abdomen and legs, the venous engorgement beginning usually in the upper thigh. The right side is more commonly affected and the superficial veins are first implicated.

Many causes are suggested for the development of varices, among them disturbance of vasomotor balance, obstruction of the great abdominal veins due to the increase of intra-abdominal pressure during pregnancy, etc.

Constipation, cardiac disease, excessive exercise and probably some toxic alteration of the vessel walls may be responsible. The varices may be slight, presenting themselves as little festoons of blue, enlarged veins on the inner aspect of the thighs and calves or there may be great dilatation of the surface veins, sometimes with local rupture and subcutaneous hemorrhage. The vulva may be transformed into a dense mass of engorged veins, greatly distending the labia and sometimes giving rise to massive hematomata during labor, or if external rupture occurs, severe intrapartum hemorrhage.

Respiratory Tract.—The parts of the nasal mucosa described by Fliess long ago as the genital areas undergo some congestion and thickening during pregnancy. These areas are sometimes utilized during labor for the administration of pituitrin, which is rapidly absorbed, when brought in contact with the nasal mucosa on an applicator.

Hofbauer has studied the alterations in the laryngeal mucosa which undergoes hyperemia, edema, and cellular infiltration. The laryngoscopic picture in pregnant women bears a striking resemblance to inflammatory processes, which explains the alteration in the voice of singers during pregnancy.

The lungs undergo hyperemia and edema associated with increased lymph secretion and an aggregation of lymphoid tissue in close proximity to the smaller bronchi. Hofbauer thinks these changes may have some bearing upon the acceleration of pulmonary tuberculosis during and immediately after pregnancy.

The capacity of the lungs is not diminished despite the upward displacement of the diaphragm from the growing uterus. The breathing is more costal than abdominal but the air excursion is increased by greater depth and frequency of the respiration.

Urinary Tract.—The most notable change here is the physiologic dilatation of the ureter and kidney pelves and the hypertrophy of the walls of the former. Much work has been done on this subject and the relation between the morphological alteration in the ureter and the frequency of infections of the urinary tract in pregnancy has been definitely established. Beginning at the fourth month, both ureters are markedly dilated in practically all the women studied. The earlier reports, based upon retrograde pyelography, were inaccurate by reason of the traumatic reaction induced by the passage of the

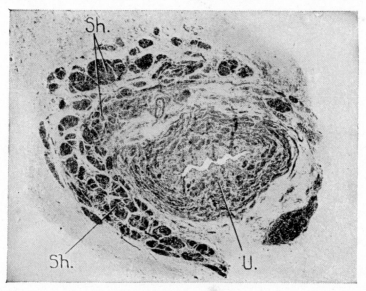

Fig. 62.—Pregnant ureter at term, juxtavesical portion 2 mm. above ureterovesical junction. *Sh.,* Ureteral sheath; *U.,* ureter. (Hofbauer.)

ureteral catheter. The more recent studies based upon intravenous pyelography with skiodan or similar salts bring out the true alteration in the urinary tract. The right ureter is definitely dilated in every pregnant woman, the left one not markedly so in some 10 to 15 per cent of cases. The ureters may reach a diameter of 1.5 cm. or even more. They are also increased in length. The size of the uterus and the position and presentation of the fetus play no part in the production of ureteral dilatation, but it has been thought that these structures undergo a hypertrophy and hyperplasia both in the musculature and in their connective tissue. This hypertrophy as pointed out by Hofbauer is particularly pronounced in the juxtavesical region where the ureter passes through the parametrium and lies in close contact with the bladder and the vaginal vault. This hypertrophy gives to the ureter a certain rigidity sometimes so marked that the whole pelvic course of the structure can often be easily palpated during the later months of pregnancy (Figs. 62, 63).

These changes, together with the decided kinking of the right ureter due to dextrotorsion of the pregnant uterus, brings about a tendency to urinary stasis which underlies the pyelitis so often found to complicate the pregnant state. The ureteral hyperplasia and hypertrophy regresses rapidly after delivery and within twelve weeks the structures have regained their normal morphology (Fig. 64).

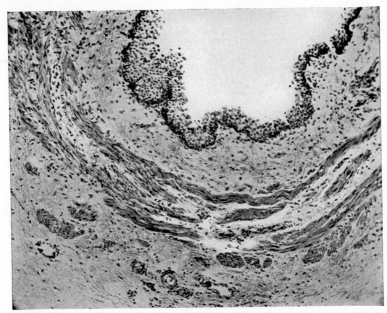

Fig. 63.—Photomicrograph of pregnant ureter 9 cm. above ureterovesical junction (× 84). (Hofbauer.)

Kidney.—There are no decided changes in the kidneys during normal pregnancy although they are most vulnerable to toxic invasion at this time. Cloudy swelling of the epithelium of the convoluted tubules with swelling of the glomerular capillaries may occur, and as a result there may appear in the urine a faint trace of albumin with a very few hyaline casts. This clinical picture has been so often observed that it has been termed "the kidney of pregnancy" and regarded as a regular physiologic change. It would seem, however, that any alteration in kidney structure must be regarded as of pathological origin, probably a very mild expression of toxemia.

The urine is increased in amount, the specific gravity is low and there is no characteristic change in the urinary solids although the chlorides are slightly decreased.

Sugar is often found in the urine of pregnant women and may be a lactosuria originating in the absorption of lactose from the mammary glands and is of no clinical significance. It occurs in from 16 to 20 per cent of all pregnancies. Glycosuria when present is always a sign of some disorder of metabolism although some students speak of a physiologic diabetes of pregnancy, a misnomer.

Acetone and peptone when present in appreciable amounts usually predicate some degree of toxemia, though during the puerperium they may result from the absorption of proteins of the involuting uterus.

Changes in the bladder have been described previously.

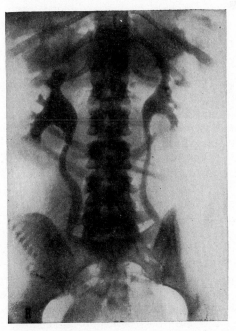

Fig. 64.—Primigravida mens. IX. Fetus in R. O. A. Course of pregnancy asymptomatic. Urine clear. Bilateral ureteral and pelvic dilatation. (Hofbauer.)

Alimentary Tract.—Disturbances of digestion are commonly associated with pregnancy, as noted in the consideration of morning nausea and vomiting (q. v.).

Curious alteration of appetite occurs, the patient experiencing strong craving for special articles of food, sometimes of the most bizarre nature. This is called pica and may become morbid as in DeLee's case of a woman who craved a bite of her husband's arm and actually took it.

The stomach is displaced upward during the later months of pregnancy and sometimes is found with the fundus markedly on the left side against the spleen. There is said to be increase in the secretion of gastric juice which is dilute and watery. The appendix and cecum are displaced upward and to the right, an important point in the diagnosis of acute appendicitis in pregnancy being that the area of localized tenderness is so displaced that confusion is sometimes caused by its nearness to the area of tenderness in cholecystitis.

The liver is displaced upward, backward and to the right. Its function is generally disturbed to greater or less extent, even in normal pregnancy. Tests for liver function are in general use, the bromsulphalein test being one of the best. Five mg. of the drug per kilogram of body weight are injected into the cubital vein, and blood withdrawn from the opposite arm at thirty and forty-five minute intervals. In normal pregnant women the blood serum shows at most a barely appreciable retention of bromsulphalein, forty-five minutes after the injection of the dye. In the toxemia of early pregnancy the retention is far greater, in some instances as high as 20 per cent.

There is generally a distinct diminution in the glycogen content of the cells, only 57 per cent of normal amount being found by Schmidt and his coworkers.

There is also disturbance of the fat metabolism and indeed it seems apparent that pregnancy imposes severe strain upon the liver function, and future study may find in these strains some adequate explanation for the toxemias of pregnancy.

Skin.—The integument undergoes more or less alteration in pigmentation during pregnancy. The areola of the nipple widens, and deepens in color until in brunettes there may be an almost black disk encircling the nipple.

A longitudinal line of pigmentation termed the linea nigra forms on the midline of the abdomen between symphysis and pubis, gradually deepening in tint as pregnancy advances.

On the face there may appear brown patches, the cheeks, forehead and nose being especially favored. When marked the coloring is referred to as the mark of pregnancy and is occasionally very pronounced. The vulva may also be deeply pigmented. Various causes have been assigned for this condition, the most plausible placing the etiology in some imbalance of the adrenal glands. The pigmentation disappears rapidly during the puerperium although in a few women it may persist for a long time.

The sweat and sebaceous glands are stimulated and characteristic skin odors are common.

DeLee says that the subcutaneous fat becomes thicker, the features coarsened.

The **nervous system** reacts to pregnancy in alteration of disposition, many women being depressed and even showing a pronounced tendency to melancholia. Curious perversions of taste with bizarre longings are noted. Neuralgia may develop, especially facial and sciatic, and exaggerated reflexes are often found. Sometimes pregnant women have a tendency to syncope, with short periods of unconsciousness, but unattended by any evidence of cardiac or circulatory disturbance.

The **pelvic articulations** are rendered movable during pregnancy, sometimes to a pathological degree, but even when within the normal limits this increased mobility may be of aid in procuring spontaneous delivery which otherwise would be impossible. x-Ray studies have revealed that there is a constant widening of the symphysis during pregnancy and movement of one pubic bone on the other may be clearly demonstrated. It is probable that these changes are hormonal in character, due to a function of the corpus luteum.

The bones show increased vascularity and there may appear on the inner aspect of the cranial bones thin bony deposits called puerperal osteophytes. Their cause is unknown.

The Hormonal System.—Within the last ten years an enormous literature has grown up around the endocrine glands in pregnancy, but the entire subject is still so vague that little certain knowledge has developed.

Pituitary Body.—Comte and Erdheim have described a definite increase in weight of the pituitary gland during pregnancy which reaches its maximum at the tenth lunar month, the weight further increasing with successive pregnancies until weights of 1.5 Gm. have been reported in multiparae. This increase of size, however, though it may seem to presuppose increased secretory activity does not prove that the pituitary-like substance occurring in the blood and urine during pregnancy is formed by the anterior pituitary since this substance is present in the urine before the pituitary shows any pronounced anatomical changes appearing with the earliest formation of the trophoblast (Philip Smith). Hofbauer describes certain "pregnancy cells" which appear to be modified chromophobe cells, abundant in the anterior lobe. There are also certain alterations of carbohydrate metabolism during pregnancy which seem to be associated with changes in the function of the pituitary, notably the decreased sugar tolerance which is of sufficient importance to have been made the basis of a test for pregnancy rather widely used until it was displaced by the more definite Aschheim-Zondek reaction.

Thyroid.—Correlation between the thyroid and the sex organs has been known for many years. There is a definite increase in the size of the gland during pregnancy, this being due to a true hyperplasia of the adenomatous tissue, together with scattered areas of increased colloid storage. There is an increased iodine content of the blood in pregnant women and the basal metabolism undergoes decided changes.

Parathyroids.—Seitz and others feel that the parathyroids undergo some hypertrophy during pregnancy and they are edematous and more vascular with an increase in their eosinophilic cells.

These changes probably have some bearing upon the increased calcium metabolism, necessary for the growth of the fetus.

7

Adrenals.—Hypertrophy of the cortex is noted in pregnancy and it is possible that increased cellular activity in these glands is responsible for the increased skin pigmentation observed during pregnancy. It may be true that there is an increase of adrenalin in the blood during gestation but this has not been proved.

CHANGES IN THE METABOLISM OF THE MOTHER

The presence of a rapidly growing fetus and its envelopes requires a sudden increase in the requirements as to food and energy imposed upon the maternal organisms.

The extra energy production at the end of pregnancy varies in direct ratio to the weight of the offspring to be delivered. In the human female the energy metabolism expressed in kilograms and hours in the last month of pregnancy is only 4 per cent larger than for a woman in complete sexual rest.

It was formerly held that the energy and food materials necessary for the development of the fetus were derived from the fixed tissues themselves and that the infant flourished at the expense of its mother.

The recent work of Bar has shown that this view is incorrect and that not only is the normally pregnant woman free from pathologic metabolism, but that on the contrary, normal pregnancy is concluded with a metabolic gain on the part of the mother.

The body weight increases during normal pregnancy, the gain being in excess of the weight of the fetus and generative organs, and is due to the bodily inactivity and good dietetic condition during pregnancy and the frequency with which the tissue fluids are increased.

It has been shown that the weight of the fetus remains constant, even when the diet of the mother has been considerably restricted and indeed the infant is reduced in size only when the restriction of food has been severe enough to jeopardize the health of the mother. The amount of weight gained during pregnancy varies with the metabolism of the individual woman, but as abnormalities in appetite are so common, there is generally an excessive gain if the patient be permitted an unrestricted diet. From 20 to 25 pounds' increase is normal if the woman has not been underweight at the beginning of pregnancy. More than this should be regarded as excessive. During the first three months there may be a considerable loss, owing to the nausea and vomiting of the first trimester but this is usually rapidly regained in the succeeding months.

Basal Metabolism in Pregnancy and the Puerperium.—Basal metabolism is the measure of the energy metabolism of a normal subject during complete rest and in the postabsorptive state and is determined by ascertaining the heat production or gaseous interchange in such subject during a certain period. It may be expressed in calories per kilogram of weight of the subject.

Clinically, basal metabolism may be studied by calorimetry, several methods being in use.

The basal metabolic rate in late pregnancy averages from 33 to 35 per cent above the normal for nonpregnant women. During the early weeks the rates obtained showed little or no increase above the normal. Three days after delivery the average basal metabolic rate is 15 per cent above normal and from seven to ten days postpartum it is approximately normal. This delayed return to normal is due to the involution of the uterus and the onset of lactation. Twin pregnancy should show a rate above the average for a single pregnancy, when both twins are well developed. Fetal sex plays no rôle.

The fundamental biochemical alterations during pregnancy have been well summarized by Trumper (Max Trumper, Ph.D., Fundamental Biochemical Factors in Pregnancy) who is freely quoted here:

Protein Metabolism.—The normal adult of constant weight is in a state of nitrogen equilibrium, that is, the nitrogen or protein intake is balanced by the nitrogen output. An insight into the terminal stages of protein metabolism may be gained by examining the nitrogenous constituents of the blood. The most important of these are: urea nitrogen, 12 to 15 mg. per cent; uric acid, 2 to 3.5 mg. per cent; creatinine, 1 to 2 mg. per cent; amino-acids, 5 to 8 mg. per cent; ammonia nitrogen, 0.1 to 0.2 mg. per cent, and other constituents of less importance. In addition there is the undetermined nitrogen fraction which in the opinion of some authorities is of prime importance in certain abnormal conditions. The sum total of these nitrogen compounds comprises what is termed the total nonprotein nitrogen, which ranges normally from 25 to 35 mg. per 100 cc. of blood.

The end-products of nitrogen metabolism are represented by the appearance of these same substances in the urine, but of course in different concentrations.

Protein Requirements in Pregnancy.—The pregnant woman, in contradistinction to the nonpregnant woman, is not in nitrogen equilibrium, her nitrogen output being less than her intake. In other words, she is in a state of positive nitrogen balance. The reason for this is apparent from the fact that the pregnant woman must satisfy the requirements of the growing fetus in addition to those of her growing body. Near the end of pregnancy this positive balance is reduced since the demand for nitrogen by the fetus is diminished.

The intermediate protein metabolism as evidenced by extensive studies of the nitrogenous constituents of the blood is but little altered during pregnancy. There is a slight diminution in urea nitrogen, balanced by a slight increase in amino-acids and ammonia nitrogen. There is also a constant but slight increase in uric acid. A very important variation from the normal is encountered in a study of the plasma proteins. Normally the ratio of albumin to globulin is about 3½ to 1, fibrinogen existing in very small amount. During pregnancy, beginning about the third mouth, there is a diminution in plasma proteins which is due almost entirely to a decrease in the albumin fraction. This results in a relative increase of globulin and fibrinogen, the latter being increased much more than the former.

Urinary findings with regard to protein metabolism in pregnancy differ but slightly from these findings in the nonpregnant state. There is a slight decrease in the output of urea and a corresponding rise in amino-acids and ammonia.

Fat Metabolism.—Alterations in fat metabolism occur during pregnancy but the significance of these changes is difficult to determine. It is definitely established that there is an increase in the concentration of cholesterol and other lipoids as well as of total fat in the blood. Too little is known concerning the metabolism of cholesterol to enable us to interpret these findings to practical advantage. One very important deviation from normal fat metabolism is generally recognized as occurring in pregnancy, namely, a distinct tendency toward a state of mild ketosis. This is evidenced by the excretion of acetone bodies as a result of diets which would not produce this result in the nonpregnant woman. This will be discussed in greater detail in the consideration of acid-base equilibrium.

Carbohydrate Metabolism.—Obviously under the conditions of normal pregnancy, providing as it must for the constant growth of the fetus, a distinct alteration in the carbohydrate requirement must take place. Whether or not there occurs any disturbance of carbohydrate metabolism, it is difficult to say; if it does occur, it is in all likelihood more in the nature of a quantitative than a qualitative change. We do know that in many cases there is an excretion of sugar in the urine. This occurs without any increase in the concentration of glucose in the blood and in the opinion of most investigators is due to a decrease in the renal threshold for glucose rather than to any actual disturbance in carbohydrate metabolism. In other words the permeability of the kidneys is increased, constituting a state analogous to that of renal diabetes. One must remember that not all sugar found in the urine is glucose. Particularly in the later months of pregnancy and during lactation, lactose is apt to be excreted in the urine. Most observers report an increase in the lactic acid content of the blood and urine. This is evidence of some interference with the complete combustion or resynthesis of glycogen in the tissues, but the exact mechanism underlying this increase is debatable.

Acid-base Equilibrium.—There is a definite tendency toward a mild acidosis in pregnancy, beginning in the early months and persisting throughout. This acidosis is in all probability a compensated one, the actual hydrogen ion concentration of the blood changing only in the last weeks of pregnancy. Therefore the statement may be made that normal pregnancy is associated with a state of relative and not actual acidosis. This state is evidenced by the following laboratory findings: a decrease in the alveolar CO_2 tension, decrease in the CO_2 combining power of blood plasma, increase in the excretion of lactic acid and ammonia in the urine and the elimination of acetone bodies. The cause of this acidotic tendency is not definitely known. Most investigators attribute it to a depletion of the alkali reserve incident to the increased production of acetone bodies and lactic acid.

Calcium Metabolism.—It has long been recognized that the pregnant state is associated with some alteration in calcium metabolism. This has been emphasized particularly because of the association of osteomalacia and tetany with pregnancy. This relationship has been exaggerated but it nevertheless is a factor of importance. During the twenty-eighth week the fetus contains only about $5\frac{1}{2}$ Gm. of calcium. At the fortieth week there are 30.51 Gm. of calcium. As pointed out by Hess, the loss of 5 Gm. from the bones of an adult to build up the fetal skeleton could not possibly cause osteomalacia which usually begins before the seventh month of pregnancy. This effect is strongly suggestive of some endocrine action. It is of interest to note that Aub found the calcium balance in early and late pregnancy to be practically identical with that of the nonpregnant state, when maintained on low calcium intake.

The serum calcium tends to diminish as pregnancy progresses, this diminution being very rarely beyond the lower limit of normal. This finding, in the light of modern knowledge, concerning calcium metabolism is strongly suggestive of a condition of hypofunction of the parathyroids, which may be associated with the hyperfunction of the thyroid which exists during pregnancy. The susceptibility to tetany likewise points toward this premise. However, it is believed at present that osteomalacia is more frequently associated with hyperfunction of the parathyroids than with hypofunction. These conflicting facts are difficult to reconcile. One must remember that the subject of calcium metabolism is an extremely intricate one and that the complete story may not be told by the level of serum calcium. The partition of calcium into diffusible and nondiffusible fractions is perhaps of more importance than the absolute level of calcium in the blood, since the ratio between these two fractions affords an insight into the distribution of physiologically active calcium in the tissues. Investigation in this direction is needed to throw more light upon the subject.

Water and Sodium Chloride Balance.—It seems well established that blood volume in the later months of pregnancy is increased. This increase is due to an increase in plasma volume and is associated with a corresponding decrease in specific gravity and in the percentage of hemoglobin and red cells. The serum proteins are likewise diluted in addition to the actual diminution in serum albumin. There is no unanimity of opinion as to the actual volume of blood in pregnancy. Blood studies on sodium chloride have been disappointing and are of no diagnostic value. We do not as yet understand the factors concerning the salt and water balance in pregnancy.

THE DURATION OF PREGNANCY

It is most important that we should know the length of time elapsing between the fertilization of the ovum and the birth of the mature child, but there are so many variable and unknown factors that exact knowledge is still lacking.

From the dawn of history women have reckoned the duration of pregnancy as two hundred and eighty days, ten lunar months, or since the advent of the Gregorian calendar, nine calendar months. This time has been found to be correct by the most detailed modern observation. The length of pregnancy varies slightly among different women, a standard deviation of eleven days either way being regarded as normal. Hard work and insufficient food seem to tend toward earlier delivery and the reverse.

From a medicolegal standpoint, the time elapsing between a presumably fruitful coitus and the birth of a viable child varies in different countries by a wide margin.

In England the legitimacy of a child born three hundred and thirty-one days after the husband went to war was allowed. In France, the law recognizes as legitimate a child born one hundred and eighty days after marriage as well as that of one born three hundred days after the death of the husband. In Germany the limits are one hundred and eighty-one and three hundred and twenty-one days respectively (DeLee). There is no specific statute covering this subject in the United States.

There is but little variation in duration of several pregnancies of the same mother, the normal gestational time for the individual being fairly consistent, age and parity having little or no effect.

It is now thought that ovulation occurs about fourteen days before the next menstrual period, regardless of the length of the cycle and the modern view is that the ovum just extruded from the graafian follicle cannot be impregnated until some hours have elapsed. The time required for the ovum to reach the lumen of the fallopian tube is not known, but since this is due to the combined action of the cilia and the peristalsis of the tube wall, the time is probably several days. Ova probably live in the tubes for a short time (forty-eight hours or thereabout) after which they degenerate and are no longer capable of fertilization.

The spermatozoa have been found in the tubes twenty-four to thirty-six hours after intercourse. It is probable that they reach this objective in much less time, possibly a few hours. The viable period of spermatozoa in the tube is probably two or three days and hence if one adds the life period of the ovum to that of the spermatozoa, it seems likely that the former may become fertilized for an interval of possibly six to seven days after coitus.

As regards implantation of the fertilized ovum, it is significant that an impregnated egg has never been shown in the uterus of a woman who has not missed a menstrual period and therefore it seems true that implantation does not occur before the first day of the supposed menstruation.

CHAPTER VIII

THE DIAGNOSIS OF PREGNANCY

The presence of a living fetus in the womb of its mother would seem to require no especial skill for its determination, but such is by no means the case.

The diagnosis of pregnancy in the earlier months, and indeed, sometimes at term, presents features of uncertainty and obscurity which render mistakes very liable to occur with consequences sometimes ludicrous but more often tragic.

Deliberate or unwitting falsification on the part of the women is common, symptoms being concealed on the one hand by reason of the social obloquy of an illegitimate gestation or the desire of the jaded city dweller to avoid the cares and burdens of a growing family, and on the other hand by the ardent and uncontrollable desire for maternity of the sterile woman whose dreams of the awakening life within her body lead her to unconsciously invent whole trains of suggestive symptoms.

In recent years the development of various hormone tests have made it possible to determine absolutely whether or not pregnancy exists, within a few days after conception. However, these procedures are not as yet in universal use and the recognition of pregnancy still depends in many localities upon the physical findings and the history. Brumm well says that when all available information has been obtained a no more definite opinion should be given than that warranted by the facts. For diagnostic purposes, pregnancy may be divided into two periods according to its duration: (a) a period of doubt including the first sixteen weeks after conception when all signs are presumptive only, and (b) a period of certainty comprising the latter twenty-four weeks.

For convenience in teaching and conducting routine examinations of patient, the period of doubt is further subdivided into the time of presumptive evidence only, and the time of signs the elicitation of which renders a positive diagnosis of pregnancy probable. The former period covering the first ten weeks after conception, the latter the second ten weeks.

DIAGNOSTIC FACTORS

Diagnostic Factors of the Period of Doubt. Prior to the Sixteenth Week

First Group. Subjective Symptoms. Those Noted by the Patient.
Cessation of menstruation.
Morning sickness.
Frequency of urination.

Increased vaginal secretions.

Sensory disturbance of breasts.

Mental and nervous changes.

Second Group.—Objective signs of the first sixteen weeks.

Enlargement of breasts and appearance of colostrum.

Bluish discoloration of vagina and vulva (Chadwick's sign).

Softening of the cervix.

Obliteration of the lower uterine segment (Hegar's sign).

Ladin's sign.

Change in the form, size and consistency of the uterus.

Enlargement of the abdomen.

Increased pigmentation (areola of breast, linea nigra).

Ballottement (Braxton Hicks sign). The intermittent uterine contractions of Braxton Hicks.

Biological tests.

Diagnostic Factors of the Period of Certainty. After the Sixteenth Week

x-Ray discovery of a fetus in utero.

Quickening.

Fetal movements.

The fetal heart beat.

The funic souffle.

The uterine souffle.

Enlargement of the abdomen.

The palpation of the fetal body.

The painless periodic uterine contractions of Braxton Hicks.

THE SUBJECTIVE SYMPTOMS OF PREGNANCY DURING THE PERIOD OF DOUBT

The Cessation of Menstruation.—This phenomenon, usually the first indication of a possible pregnancy noted by the patient is a reliable indicator in most instances. When a woman whose catamenia has been regular and whose health is good, suddenly develops amenorrhea, pregnancy is present as a rule.

As a diagnostic factor, however, the rule is subject to several exceptions.

1. Pregnancy is not the only cause for the sudden occurrence of amenorrhea. Psychic influence, notably the fear of an illegitimate conception in unmarried women, the shock of an assault and so on, may cause an amenorrhea which may persist for several months after which menstruation occurs without any evidence of pregnancy having taken place. In this group belong those not uncommon cases, wherein delicately nurtured and sensitive young women, experiencing sexual excitement for the first time immediately after marriage, develop amenorrhea even sometimes with the associated tingling and irritability of the breasts without later evidence of pregnancy.

Climatic changes, as shown by the histories of young women coming from Europe to the United States, may also be causative, as may sudden exposure to cold, and the occurrence of acute illness, as influenza, scarlet fever, acute rheumatic fever, etc.

In chronic systemic diseases, as the severe anemias, Addison's disease, tuberculosis, diabetes, pituitary and other endocrine disturbances, including hyper- and hypothyroidism this is also true.

Persistent lutein stimulation caused by corpus luteum cysts is sometimes a cause as are certain diseases of the nervous system as dementia praecox, epilepsy or brain tumor.

2. Pregnancy may occur in the presence of a preexisting amenorrhea as before the physiological onset of catamenia. Many cases are recorded where young girls conceive before menstruation. Indeed, among Oriental peoples and in certain savage tribes, marriage at a very early age is the rule. There is no doubt as to the possible fertility of marriages contracted by children. Polak gives examples from Persia and that this is true not only in warm but in cold climates is shown by Rakhmanoff who in Russia attended in childbirth a woman not more than fourteen years of age, of poor constitution and with features still infantile. Menstruation had not yet taken place; the confinement was normal.

During the amenorrhea of lactation pregnancy is usual, and there are many case histories recorded, wherein women become the mothers of large families, without the appearance of a menstrual flow from the first impregnation until the menopause.

After the climacteric, pregnancy may take place as shown by many examples. In some instances one or more years of amenorrhea may be followed by a totally unexpected pregnancy.

Constitutional diseases, the anemias, tuberculosis, local traumas or a curettage, may all be productive of amenorrhea during the course of which pregnancy may occur.

Irregular menstruation, with long intervals, sometimes many months, due to some endocrine imbalance occurs in some women who may conceive at any time during these intervals.

3. Menstruation may continue after conception has occurred.

This fact was known to Hippocrates, who comments on it in his 60th aphorism thus, "If a woman with child have her courses, it is impossible that the child can be healthy."

Inasmuch as the decidua vera and the decidua reflexa do not fuse until some time during the fourth month, it is possible that normal menstruation could continue for that period. Frequently there occurs one scant, abnormal menstruation subsequent to conception, and some women regularly pass through such a postconceptional cycle. There are cases reported in which apparently normal menstruation continues during the entire course of the pregnancy, but most of them are subject to doubt and the bleeding has probably been caused by some form of uterine disease, decidual endometritis, mole pregnancy, etc.

In the rare cases of double uterus, it is conceivable that menstruation from the mucosa of the unimpregnated horn might persist, but here again, the inhibitory action of the corpus luteum of pregnancy theoretically should produce a suppression of the flow.

In general it may be said that sudden amenorrhea, while merely a presumptive symptom is a most important one and taken in conjunction with other evidences and examined with due regard to the possible sources of error as just described, is probably the most reliable of the diagnostic factors.

Nausea and Vomiting: Morning Sickness.—This phenomenon occurs in about 80 per cent of all pregnant women coming under the observation of the writer, the remaining 20 per cent being unconscious of any digestive disturbance. Of those women who do have nausea and vomiting, it is severe and of considerable duration in about 40 per cent and moderate or only slightly annoying in the remaining 60 per cent.

The etiology of this condition is not understood, but the most reasonable explanation is that it is due to a hormone secreted by the syncytium which, when in excess, acts as a toxin. This toxin, developing in a woman of more or less unstable nervous mechanism, produces various grades of reaction. Nausea and vomiting may range from the simple feeling of squeamishness in the morning, to inability of the patient to retain anything in the stomach, with consequent dehydration, starvation and death. This severe development constitutes one of the toxemias of pregnancy and will be described under that heading.

These symptoms rarely develop within a week or two of conception, commonly appear about the fourth to the sixth week and usually disappear during the third month. Occasionally the distress may persist throughout pregnancy, only ceasing after delivery.

In the ordinary case, the patient complains of considerable nausea and possibly slight vomiting, much worse on arising in the morning, greatly aggravated by the odor of food or its preparation, and decreasing during the day, until at evening a meal may be taken or enjoyed. Other women report that they approach a meal with good appetite and no repugnance whatever, only to vomit the entire stomach contents shortly after eating. From this common type, the condition may vary as regards severity.

It need scarcely be said that nausea and vomiting is a purely presumptive symptom of pregnancy, so many other disorders giving rise to the same effect.

Curiously enough there are a few cases recorded where although the wife suffered but little from the morning sickness, the husband was profoundly affected, and while such an event apparently has no basis in fact and would seem to be a mere fabrication, the creditability of the persons involved is so great, there can be no doubt as to this peculiar occurrence. Of course a neurosis is the underlying factor in these cases. Here again the evidence is based wholly upon the statement of the patient and may be entirely false if there is reason to conceal the existence of a pregnancy or to pretend that such condition exists.

Frequent Urination.—Frequency of urination, especially at night, is an important presumptive symptom of early pregnancy, and when it occurs in a healthy woman who has had no previous urinary disorder, and who reports a cessation of menstruation, it is to be regarded as highly suggestive.

The cause of this urinary frequency is probably not a stretching of the trigone or any pressure on the bladder as a result of the enlargement of the uterus; it is caused by the great venous congestion which affects the entire generative tract during pregnancy.

Increased Vaginal Secretion.—Very frequently a patient who suspects pregnancy will report a marked increase in the vaginal secretions, sometimes amounting to a leukorrhea. This is also due, of course, to the congestion and is due to stimulation of the cervical glands and Bartholin's glands, with the production of glairy viscous secretion.

In women who have previously suffered from vaginal discharge, this is almost always appreciably increased during pregnancy.

Symptoms Referable to the Breasts.—Pain and tingling in the breasts is a commonly noted symptom in early pregnancy. About one-third of the patients observed by the author have reported either slight fugitive pains or a distinct sensation of fulness in the breasts coincident with the early months of gestation. The symptoms usually occur about the fourth to sixth week of pregnancy and persist for a month or less. Many patients state that the same sensations have been noted by them just prior to menstruation. They also accompany fibroma uteri, ovarian cysts or breast tumors.

Changes in the Nervous System and Mentality of the Patient.—It has been remarked that pregnant women frequently become irritable and capricious, both as regards their appetite and their social reactions.

Certain women develop marked alteration in their psyche and gay, ebullient natures become quiet and introspective, silent women suddenly turn vivacious, and sometimes well concealed or unsuspected traits of character come to the surface. Such alteration may be trivial or obscure and may pass entirely unnoticed by the patient and her family, but if noticeable and evident the physician should be on his guard lest a more serious and permanent mental change be foreshadowed by the slighter changes noted at this time.

OBJECTIVE, PRESUMPTIVE SIGNS OF PREGNANCY

Bluish Discoloration of the Vagina (Appears Eighth to Twelfth Week).—Usually at about the third month of pregnancy the mucosa of the vulvar outlet, the vestibule of the vagina, becomes deep violet in color, the intensity of the discoloration being more marked in brunettes than in blondes. This is but another evidence of venous congestion, and may be due to anything which increases the venous stasis in the pelvis, as the rapid growth of a tumor, etc., but it is extremely corroborative of pregnancy when taken in connection with other presumptive signs. This phenomenon was first described by Jacquemier in 1836 but was popularized by Chadwick of Boston and hence bears his name. Later in pregnancy the cyanosis extends over the entire vaginal mucosa and the cervix is markedly involved.

This discoloration is more marked in multiparae than in primiparae, especially after some relaxation of the abdominal walls.

Softening of the Cervix (Appears Sixth Week in Primiparae, Later in Multiparae).—This structure in the nonpregnant state is hard and firm in consistency. Very early in pregnancy it becomes soft and velvety, the change being distinctly palpable. Goodell said in his lecture that when the cervix was as hard as one's nose, the woman was probably not pregnant, but if it was as soft as one's lips, gestation was probably in progress. The cervix also increases in size during pregnancy, its muscle cells undergoing hypertrophy and hyperplasia pari passu with those of the uterine fundus.

The cervical mucosa so proliferates that at the end of pregnancy it occupies more than half of the cervix. It assumes a reticulated honeycomb appearance and may easily be mistaken for an adenocarcinoma by microscopic examination.

Hegar's Sign. Obliteration of the Lower Uterine Segment (Appears About Eighth Week in Primiparae, Sixth in Multiparae).—This important and valuable sign is usually best elicited between the sixth and the tenth week of pregnancy, and depends upon the fact that the ovum still occupies only the upper portion of the uterine body, although the lower portion of the uterus is greatly softened; on bimanual examination the upper pole of the uterus is noted as being enlarged, globular and elastic while the cervix is fairly hard and firm. The lower uterine segment may be compressed between the fingers so that the cervix and the rounded uterine body appear to be distinct organs, the lower uterine segment being so soft and compressible as to give the impression of its almost complete obliteration to the touch (Fig. 65).

Hegar's sign depends upon the existence of the above three factors, and when they are found pregnancy is usually present. A common mistake is to consider that Hegar's sign implies only the softening of the lower uterine segment which may occur in the presence of soft myomata of the uterus, subinvolution and so on, but in these instances the globular enlargement of the uterus and the definite separation of the fundus and the cervix do not occur.

Hegar's second sign consists in the elicitation of a definite fold in the anterior uterine wall and may be determined by bimanual examination, an assistant steadying the uterus to prevent its slipping backward away from the examining hand.

Ladin's Sign. Softening of the Anterior Uterine Wall (Sixth Week).—This is an important presumptive sign of pregnancy and may be elicited as early as the sixth week. It depends upon the presence of a soft, fluctuating, elastic area in the anterior wall of the uterus, just above the cervical junction, and is, at the sixth week, about the size of a twenty-five cent piece. This area steadily increases in size until after the third month it is obscured by the general softening of the uterus. Ladin claims that this sign serves to differentiate intra-uterine from extra-uterine pregnancy, and also that the softened area becomes incompressible with the death of the fetus, this being of

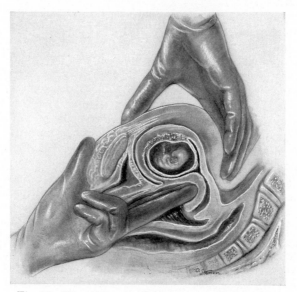

Fig. 65.—The diagnosis of pregnancy. Hegar's sign.

value in the determination as to whether abortion is threatening or inevitable.

Changes in Form, Size and Position of the Uterus.—According to Williams, the existence of an enlarged uterus at any time during child-bearing period should be regarded as presumptive evidence of pregnancy until such a possibility has been clinically eliminated, and this dictum will express the importance of this sign in the diagnosis.

During the first few weeks the uterus does not increase in length but undergoes a considerable thickening from before backward, and to the trained observer may be felt to spread out laterally somewhat further than the nonpregnant state.

At the beginning of the third month the pear-shaped uterine body has become almost globular in form, has increased two or three times in size, and there may be noted a definite accentuation of the normal anteflexion.

During the third month the uterus begins to emerge from the pelvis until at the end of the first trimester it may be clearly felt above the symphysis. The consistency of the organ is definitely altered; the dense, almost fibrous feel of the virgin uterus is rapidly converted into a soft, doughy though elastic consistency, a sensation which may well be compared to that obtained from pressure upon a well inflated child's balloon.

At the third month the fundus uteri may be distinctly asymmetrical in outline, the cornu in the neighborhood of which the ovum is attached, rising and forming a definite unilateral mass until this asymmetry is sometimes so marked as to lead the examiner to the

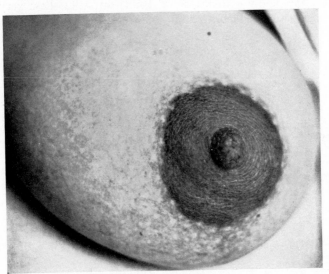

Fig. 66.—Pigmentation of areola and hypertrophy of Montgomery's glands in pregnancy.

belief that a cornual pregnancy may exist. As pregnancy advances and the ovum increases in size, this asymmetry disappears, the uterus becoming regularly increased in size (Piskacek's sign).

Enlargement of the Abdomen.—Enlargement of the abdomen is not a particularly important sign, since it does not take place until the diagnosis has been rendered positive by accumulation of evidence. As pregnancy proceeds, the uterus rises in the abdomen until at the sixth month it reaches the umbilicus which now, rather than being inverted, becomes either level with the abdominal wall or distinctly protrudes.

Pigmentation and Changes in the Breasts.—Enlargement of the breasts and more particularly an increase in the density of the mammary tissues may be noted as early as the second month. There is usually some increase in the pigmentation about the nipple, the so-called "areola," and some distention of the superficial veins in the areola. There also develop small, papular, sebaceous glands, which have been termed "The Glands of Montgomery," and on pressure upon the nipple there may be expressed a thin serous fluid known as colostrum which is a transudate composed for the most part of serum albumin and contains numerous brown bodies called colostrum corpuscles, which represent cast-off epithelial cells that have undergone fatty degeneration (Fig. 66).

With regard to the value of breast changes as a diagnostic factor, the author is inclined to believe that the increase in the size and consistency usually predicate some form of uterine congestion. The pigmentation, however, is not in any way regular in its distribution, and there are many patients, even brunettes, who show very little if any increase in pigmentation at this time. The same holds true in

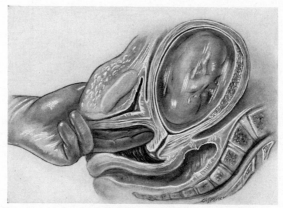

Fig. 67.—The diagnosis of pregnancy. Ballottement or Braxton Hicks sign.

the pigmented line on the abdomen, running from the xiphoid to the symphysis, and known as the linea nigra. This discoloration, so important in the eyes of older obstetricians, is extremely unreliable as a means of diagnosis, and while its presence may suggest pregnancy, its absence by no means precludes such a possibility.

Ballottement or Repercussion (Fig. 67).—This maneuver, popularized by Braxton Hicks whose name it bears, depends upon the fact that the fetus during the earlier months of pregnancy is far smaller than the cavity of the ovum and that it is floating free in the liquor amnii for the first five months at least. The sign is best elicited during a bimanual examination, when the vaginal fingers give the cervix or lower uterine segment a quick but gentle thrust upward; the fetal body may be felt lightly impinging upon the abdominal hand, or if this is not so by reason of fat abdominal walls, the rebound of the fetus will be shortly transmitted to the vaginal fingers as a light tap.

Ballottement is a very satisfactory aid in making a diagnosis of pregnancy from the sixteenth to the thirty-second week. Before this time the fetus is too light to be felt and as pregnancy advances it fills the uterine cavity and is too large to be floated away from the fingers. The sign may be impossible to elicit in cases of placenta praevia when this organ is interposed between the fetus and the vaginal hand and it may be simulated by a movement of the entire uterus especially if it be the seat of a small fibroid tumor in the presence of ascitic fluid.

Pigmentation of the Skin.—The linea nigra, a dark brown line running down the midline of the abdomen from umbilicus to symphysis and sometimes extending upward to the ensiform, has long been regarded as indicative of pregnancy.

This discoloration is not usual during the first few months and frequently is never seen. It is, of course, most marked in brunettes, and with other skin discolorations, is probably due to some dysfunction of the adrenals.

DIAGNOSTIC FACTORS IN THE PERIOD OF CERTAINTY

The Roentgen Diagnosis of Pregnancy.—It is the consensus of opinion of roentgenologists that a definite diagnosis of pregnancy by x-ray is impossible before the fourteenth week, although isolated cases are reported in which fetal centers of ossification were demonstrated as early as the ninth week. Case concludes that the roentgen method by the demonstration of fetal bones does not yet determine with any consistency the presence of pregnancy until three to six weeks before the appearance of definite clinical signs of fetal life.

After the fourteenth week, obesity or the coexistence of a tumor does not invalidate the correct diagnosis of pregnancy. All of the fetal bones are not usually visible at this time, but a few vertebrae, ribs, bones of the extremities and (uncommonly) the cranial bones may be noted (Fig. 68).

Pneumoperitoneum by the transabdominal route and the injection of small quantities of iodized oil into the uterine cavity have both been recommended for the earlier x-ray diagnosis of pregnancy, but since both procedures carry with them a certain danger, they have been almost completely superseded by one of the accurate and safe biological tests.

Quickening is the term applied to the first sensation experienced by a mother of the movements of the fetus in utero. The use of the word is archaic, it being a survival of the Roman law that the child was not endowed with life until its motions had been felt by the mother and hence its destruction before this time was a minor felony but if the offence were committed after quickening it was murder and punishable by death.

The sensation of quickening has been described as a gentle flutter, like a bubble bursting in the abdomen. The first motions are usu-

8

ally not recognized by a mother bearing her first child for several days or a week after they have been first noticed, but as the fetus grows more active, certainty soon replaces doubt in her mind.

Sometimes in women of stolid temperament the motion is not observed for weeks and even months after the active fetal movements may easily be palpated by the physician.

The phenomenon may be noted as early as the tenth week, but experience has shown that the greatest number of instances occur be-

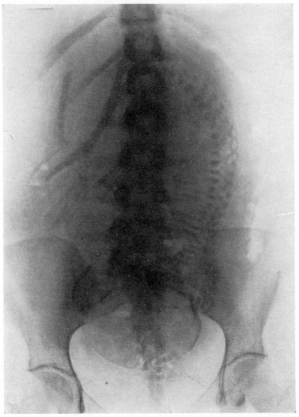

Fig. 68.—Roentgenological diagnosis of pregnancy. Normal pregnancy at eighth month. L. O. A. (Kensington Hospital for Women.)

tween the end of the twelfth and sixteenth weeks after conception or better between the fourteenth and eighteenth weeks after the last menstruation.

Multiparae perceive the motions of the fetus earlier than primiparae, previous experience having taught them what to expect. The movements vary greatly in degree from day to day being excessive when the mother is fatigued, cold or ill with a febrile disease. They are lessened by warmth and rest. Ballantyne has pointed out that the fetus sleeps and that there is a periodicity of active motion and passivity which corresponds to the phases to somnolence and wakefulness in the child.

It has also been observed that exposure to the roentgen rays as when determining a diagnosis of pregnancy by this means will throw the fetus into violent, almost spasmodic movement.

Quickening is a useful corroborative evidence of pregnancy but is of little value in a doubtful case, since as long ago stated by Hamilton "No woman ever yet fancied herself pregnant without also persuading herself that she felt the motions of the child."

Among women of intelligence the date of quickening may be utilized roughly to foretell the probable duration of pregnancy, De-Lee's suggestion being to count twenty-two weeks ahead in primiparae to find the probable date of confinement and twenty-four weeks in multiparae.

Fetal Movements.—When capable of being appreciated by the obstetrician, fetal movements constitute an absolute diagnosis of pregnancy. There is nothing comparable in the whole domain of physical diagnosis to the sensation transmitted to the palpating hand by the motion of fetal extremities.

The movements may be felt, seen and heard, although palpation is by far the most accurate method of diagnosis. Two types of movement are generally recognized—a slow, heaving, twisting motion as the broad back of the fetus rises against the uterus, and a multiple, irregular, tapping and sliding movement as the extremities are flexed or extended and glide along the uterine wall.

The motions of the fetus are at first palpable about the fourteenth to the sixteenth week, sometimes earlier, but before the twentieth week they are so faint and doubtful that diagnosis prior to this time is somewhat dubious. As pregnancy advances the movements become more definite, until in the later months they may be so violent as to cause considerable annoyance to the mother and to be visible even through the clothes.

The fetal activities may also be determined by auscultation, a little tap transmitted to the ear being significant of a fetal extremity striking against the uterine wall.

These movements as have been said constitute an absolute diagnosis of pregnancy although they may be simulated to some extent by active peristalsis and by voluntary contraction of the abdominal muscles especially among sterile women who have become obsessed by their intense desire for maternity until the wish becomes translated into a delusion that pregnancy exists. In these cases the self-deception as well as the false information given to the physician is often amazing in its accuracy of detail. (See Pseudocyesis.)

The Fetal Heart Sounds.—Of all the signs of pregnancy, auscultation of the fetal heart is the most positive and when these sounds are definitely audible there can be no doubt as to the condition.

Curiously enough it was not until 1818 that Mayer of Geneva announced the fact that the fetal heart tones could be heard by applying the ear to the abdomen of the mother, the phenomenon being independently discovered by Kergaradec of Paris in 1822.

Some observers have noted the heart sounds as early as the eleventh week, but they are not usually audible until the twentieth week and even then they are so faint as to be heard only under the most favorable circumstances.

The sounds may be developed by the employment of any form of stethoscope or by applying the unaided ear to the abdomen which has been covered by a towel or napkin.

These sounds have been aptly compared to the ticking of a watch under a pillow or as they were termed by the older obstetricians "tictocs." The rate varies from 120 to 160 beats per minute and while marked variation, especially an increase, may occur without cause, persistent considerable variation in the heart rate predicates some fetal pathology and where such condition obtains the fetal heart should be auscultated with great frequency with the thought in mind that either some anomaly of the fetal circulation exists, which may render the infant incapable of an extra-uterine life or that some mechanical agency is responsible for interference with the placento-fetal blood interchange and that induction of premature labor may be necessary to preserve the life of the child.

For a time it was thought that variations in the fetal heart rate could be utilized as a means of determining the sex of the child, a rate of well over 145 beats per minute indicating a female and well under 145 a male.

Inasmuch, however, as the average rapidity is about 144 it is clear that the rule is so indefinite as to be of but little practical value. When the rate drops sharply the fetus is usually undergoing dangerous pressure; either compression of the skull or pressure upon the cord.

The heart tones may be confused with the maternal pulse, but except in cases of thyroid toxemia with tachycardia, or where the mother's heart is dilated and undergoing compensatory hypertrophy as in those cases of extremely acute nephritis beginning sometimes late in pregnancy, the difference in rate will serve to clear up the confusion.

The technic of auscultation of the pregnant abdomen is simple, but only repeated practice will enable the student to detect the faint pulsation.

The room must be absolutely quiet, the patient relaxed and not nervous, and the abdomen exposed.

For the direct method, the ear is placed firmly but not heavily on the abdominal wall, first at a point to the left of and below the umbilicus and thence moved about until the sounds are heard with their maximum intensity. The abdomen should be covered by a thin napkin or gauze.

In using the stethoscope, the model to which the observer is accustomed will probably give the best results; and care must be taken that the bell of the instrument does not move on the skin of the abdomen with the respiratory excursion and with a resulting friction sound which may completely obliterate the heart tones. When this interference does occur, a little lubricant applied to the abdomen will usually obviate it. If the child be small, and the pregnancy not far advanced, the stethoscope should be placed in the median line just above the symphysis, and it is advisable to fix the body of the child against the anterior wall by manual pressure on the sides of the abdomen, to secure the best transmission of the heart sounds.

The Funic Souffle.—Synchronous with the fetal heart rate is a sharp, high-pitched, whistling sound heard in about 10 to 15 per cent of all cases, its point of greatest intensity being almost anywhere on the abdomen.

It was first described by Kennedy who rightfully attributed it to some interference with the current of blood flowing through the umbilical cord. The souffle can sometimes be made out on deep pressure with the ball of the stethoscope over the cord in these women.

In cases where the funic souffle is heard during labor, the fetal heart being at the same time retarded in rate, the prognosis is bad for the child, since some intra-uterine asphyxia is evidently in progress.

The uterine souffle, first described by Kergaradec as the placental souffle, is a low-pitched blowing sound caused by the rush of blood through the uterine sinuses and is most marked in the region of the uterine artery, low down in the pelvis. This sound is, of course, synchronous with the maternal pulse and may be noted in cases of soft myomata, etc., being but an indifferent aid in the diagnosis of pregnancy.

Enlargement of the Abdomen.—The abdominal enlargement is not visible until the end of the fourth month, at five months the uterus is midway between symphysis and umbilicus, at six months it reaches the umbilicus which begins to protrude and it then continues to rise at a rate of about 4 cm. per month until it almost reaches the xiphoid at the end of the ninth lunar month.

Lightening.—About three weeks before term, the fetus sinks into the brim of the pelvis and the presenting part engages, the patient experiencing the sensation of lightening, the fundus dropping to about its level of the eighth month. This descent of the fundus is more marked and definite in primiparae than in multiparae, occurring in the former about three weeks before the maturity of the fetus and in the latter about a week or ten days before term. In the writer's observation many multiparous women do not seem to experience lightening at all.

The Intermittent Uterine Contractions of Braxton Hicks.—Beginning early in pregnancy, sometimes during the third month, the uterus will be found to undergo a periodic contraction, its walls becoming firm and hard but without any sensations being noted by the mother. As pregnancy advances these contractions increase in vigor until at the seventh or eighth month they may be very easily felt by laying the hand on the abdomen when in a few moments the soft, cystic uterus will begin to grow hard and firm and the fundus to rise against the abdominal wall. These contractions may be known to the patient who will call the attention of the obstetrician to their presence. The contractions usually occur ten or fifteen minutes apart, although an interval of several hours may intervene. They are of moderate corroborative value as diagnostic factors, but may be present in cases of submucous fibroid tumor and hematometra.

The Signs and Symptoms of Pregnancy Arranged in the Order of Appearance:

First four weeks:
Amenorrhea, pain and tingling in breasts, frequency of urination, increase in vaginal secretions. (Biological tests positive.)

Second four weeks:
Amenorrhea, breast signs, frequency of urination, increase in vaginal secretion, Hegar's sign, Ladin's sign. Softening of the cervix.

Third four weeks:
Amenorrhea, morning sickness, uterus may be palpated above symphysis, softening of the cervix, cyanosis of the vaginal mucosa (Chadwick's sign), colostrum—increased pigmentation in breasts.

Fourth four weeks:
Morning sickness grows less, uterus well above symphysis, ballottement, uterine souffle, x-ray positive (?), quickening.

Fifth four weeks:
The above signs. *The fetal heart sounds.* Uterus reaches umbilicus. Marked areolae of nipples.

Sixth four weeks:
Continuation of the signs enumerated plus fetal movements felt by physician, striae develop in the abdominal skin, uterus reaches to and grows above umbilicus.

Seventh four weeks:
All signs more marked. Uterus rises to one third the distance between the xiphoid and the umbilicus.

Eighth four weeks:
Uterus reaches almost to the xiphoid, all signs highly definite.

Ninth four weeks:
Uterus reaches xiphoid.

Tenth four weeks:
Lightening, uterus sinks to its eighth month position.

BIOLOGICAL PREGNANCY TESTS

The Aschheim-Zondek Test.—In 1928 Aschheim and Zondek contributed the greatest advance in obstetric diagnosis since Mayer of Geneva demonstrated the fetal heart tones in 1818.

This test together with a few important modifications has been subjected to an intense and critical scrutiny in the eight years which have elapsed since its appearance and in that time it has superseded all other devices for determining the presence of pregnancy in the early weeks. It is correct in over 99 per cent of cases and is simple of performance, requiring no special training. With its best modification, the Friedman test, it may be employed in connection with an office practice, independent of elaborate laboratory facilities.

The Aschheim-Zondek test is based on the fact, first, that large amounts of the hormone of the anterior pituitary body are excreted in the urine during pregnancy, and second, that when urine containing this hormone is injected into immature female mice, ovulation occurs. The original technic involves the use of six immature female mice weighing from 6 to 8 Gm. each. It has since been shown that when available it is better to use animals of a known age, twenty-one to twenty-four days.

The six twenty-one to twenty-four-day-old mice are injected subcutaneously with urine, three times daily for a period of forty-eight hours as follows:

Mouse 1. 6×0.2 cc. urine.
Mouse 2. 6×0.25 cc. urine.
Mouse 3. 6×0.3 cc. urine.
Mouse 4. 6×0.35 cc. urine.
Mouse 5. 6×0.4 cc. urine.
Mouse 6. Control (not injected).

The urine is a fresh morning voided or catheterized specimen, filtered and, if alkaline, weakly acidified with acetic acid.

One hundred hours after the first injection the animals are killed and autopsied and the ovaries examined microscopically and macroscopically.

The reactions observed are called anterior pituitary reactions (A.P.R.).

A.P.R. I consists of the stimulation of the ovary to follicle maturation and is not suggestive of pregnancy.

A.P.R. II consists in the development of corpora haemorrhagica showing as one or more minute purplish black spots in the ovaries.

A.P.R. III consists in the formation of corpora lutea, grayish yellow elevations resulting from the luteinization of unruptured follicles.

A.P.R. III can be demonstrated by covering the ovaries with a drop of glycerin and crushing them between a glass slide and a stout coverglass. The luteinized follicles can then be distinguished from primordial or maturing graafian follicles by their more opaque and granular appearance, when examined under the low power of the microscope.

Robert Frank points out that this difference in opacity disappears in about fifteen minutes as the glycerin clears the tissues. It may be necessary, sometimes, to cut serial sections of the ovaries, if the former method proves ineffectual.

A.P.R. II and A.P.R. III are diagnostic of pregnancy.

Accuracy of the Test.—In a report of 1000 cases Aschheim demonstrated 98.2 per cent accuracy and stated that in the cases in which accurate results were not obtained in the first test, subsequent tests gave results which were later substantiated.

Frank in 321 cases reported 96.9 per cent accurate, all of the errors being in the direction of negative results in the presence of pregnancy. In no case was the test positive in the absence of pregnancy.

Other observers concur in this high percentage of accuracy, so that it may be said that for all practical purposes, the Aschheim-Zondek test is positive as a diagnosis of early pregnancy.

Duration of Pregnancy When Test is First Positive.—Aschheim and Zondek reported cases in which the test was positive five days after the first missed menstrual period. It is almost always positive within the first month of pregnancy, so that it may be said that the test is applicable when no other method of diagnosis is of any value.

Objections to the Test.—The time required, one hundred hours, the number of immature female mice needed, with the consequent necessity of having a large number of breeding females always at hand and the number of injections requiring very close attention, combine to make this otherwise most valuable test somewhat cumbersome.

These objections are well overcome by two modifications which have achieved much popularity, *i. e.*, the Friedman and the Mazer-Hoffman tests.

The Friedman Test.—In his work upon ovulation in the rabbit, Friedman demonstrated that intravenous injections of 5 cc. of urine from a pregnant woman into a female rabbit provokes ovulation in the same manner as in the mouse, the advantage being that ovulation occurs within twenty-four hours, either because of the injection of a single large amount directly into the blood stream, or because of the sexual peculiarities of the rabbit. Based upon these facts, Friedman and Lapham developed their test which is based upon these fundamental facts.

1. The ovaries of an isolated, immature female rabbit contain neither corpora lutea nor corpora haemorrhagica, inasmuch as the rabbit does not ovulate spontaneously, but only after coitus.

2. The urine of pregnant women contains some substance, or sub-

stances, which simulate in their biologic effects the anterior lobe of the pituitary.

3. The ovary of the rabbit quickly responds to the injection of these substances by the formation of corpora lutea or corpora haemorrhagica.

The Friedman test was continued and developed by Schneider who used a rabbit twelve to fourteen weeks of age, injected intravenously 5 to 7 cc. of urine and performed autopsy twenty-four to thirty hours after injection (Fig. 69).

This test has been further developed by Mathieu, Palmer and Holman, whose technic is followed by the author in his work and is as follows:

A rabbit at any age greater than three months may be used, but if older than about four and a half months, care must be taken to isolate the animal from the male for thirty days before it is used. The gestation period in a rabbit being thirty-one days, it is easy to determine in about three or four weeks' time by palpation whether the female has or has not been exposed to the male. If the animal has been continuously isolated from three months of age, this precaution is not necessary.

The specimen of urine is collected at any time during the day, preferably in the morning, acidified with 10 per cent acetic acid and treated with toluol (one drop to 50 cc. of urine). The urine specimens are then collected by the technician, usually about 7.00 P. M., and injections are made at that time.

Depending upon the apparent concentration of the urine, 10 to 17 cc. are injected into the marginal ear vein of the rabbit. If the specimen is amber colored, it is probably concentrated and 10 cc. is sufficient. When the specimen is pale and has the appearance of water, the larger dose is used. This method is empiric. From three to five minutes' time is taken to make the injection, so as to prevent intravascular clotting.

The rabbits are killed at 7.00 A. M., thirty-six hours after the injections of the urine, and each ovary is examined. A positive reaction is determined by the presence of corpora haemorrhagica which may be dark red in color, or if rupture has occurred recently, may be bright cherry red, and almost pin point in size. Corpora lutea may also be present, and if the animal is a virgin and has not been used for a previous test, are further evidence of a positive reaction. The changes in the rabbit's uterus are not significant. Occasionally the uterus in both positive and negative reactions is seen to be enlarged five times its normal size. (This is probably due to an increase in the amount of the ovarian hormone contained in the injected urine.)

Accuracy of the Test.—Friedman and Lapham in their series showed 100 per cent correct.

Schneider also reports complete accuracy but warns against the use of immature rabbits, which may cause error in that these young animals do not ovulate even under stimulation.

This is probably the simplest and most certain biological test yet devised.

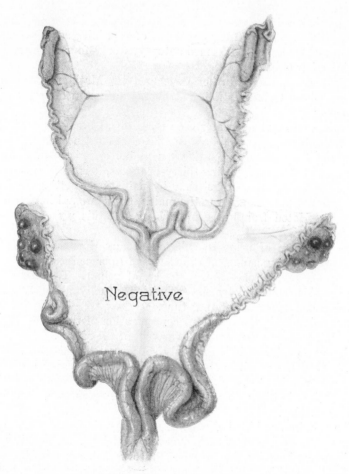

Fig. 69.—The Friedman pregnancy test. Note the hemorrhagic follicles and the swelling and congestion of the uterus in the positive test. (Mathieu, Palmer, and Holman, Northwest Medicine, May, 1932.)

Duration of the Pregnancy When Test is Positive.—Always within the first two weeks after conception, sometimes within a few days after fruitful coitus.

There are no objections except the unimportant one of the cost of the animals, but as this is usually cheerfully borne by the patient, it is of no significance. Some technicians prefer not to sacrifice the rabbits but to examine the ovaries *in vivo* via laparotomy, in which case the same rabbit can be used many times, sufficient interval being allowed to permit regression of the corpora lutea.

The Estrin Pregnancy Test (Mazer-Hoffman).—This test depends upon the vaginal smear method and the artificial induction of estrus in the castrated mouse by the estrin content of the urine. This test was originated by Mazer whose work is here quoted.

Technic of the Estrin Test for Pregnancy.—Three to five mature female mice, ranging in weight from 20 to 25 Gm., are used for this test, since old or immature animals are often less responsive to the effects of estrin treatment. They are examined daily for the occurrence of estrous cycles and, if found to be normal in this respect, are castrated in the following manner:

The animal is placed in a jar filled with ether vapor and fully anesthetized. It is then stretched upon a board, ventral surface down, and held fast thus by means of pins stuck through the extremities. A low, dorsal skin incision is made along the spine, and the flaps of the incision retracted and likewise held fast with pins. The ovaries are then removed through small wounds made with the tips of pointed forceps in the overlying muscles, the peritoneal folds running from the ovaries to the renal regions serving as guides. The removed ovaries and tissue are then pressed between two slides and examined under the microscope or through an ordinary hand lens in order to make sure that the ovaries are included in the excised tissue. The muscle wounds heal readily; it is not necessary to close them. The skin flaps are sutured with linen thread. A technician can perform the castration within three to five minutes, with practically no operative mortality.

Vaginal smears from the castrated animals are then taken daily for two weeks and microscopically examined for evidence of estrus in order to exclude the possibility of regeneration of an overlooked fragment of ovarian tissue or the presence of an accessory ovary. If the castrated test animals show no evidence of estrus at the end of this period they are then treated thus: 15 cc. of morning urine of the tested patient are injected subcutaneously in six divided doses into each of 3 or 5 castrated animals used for this test, in the course of two days. The specimen of urine employed should be kept in a refrigerator to prevent bacterial growth to which the animals are sensitive.

Smears of the vaginal secretions of the injected mice are examined once a day until the third day when evidence of cellular activity in the form of nucleated epithelial cells may be noted. This does not, however, constitute a positive reaction, since a slight increase in estrin excretion, characteristic of some amenorrheic and menopausal women, may occasionally produce such a reaction in the vagina of the test animal. If such activity is noted, it is necessary to examine the vaginal secretions twice or thrice daily in order not to overlook a frank estrous reaction of several hours' duration.

Much depends on the correct interpretation of the vaginal smear. A mild reaction, such as described above, must be disregarded because urine of nonpregnant women contains minute quantities of estrin and may produce such a reaction. A preponderance of non-nucleated epithelial cells and the absence of leukocytes and mucus constitute a positive pregnancy reaction. This is usually obtained on the fourth day after the first injection. One may be inclined to disregard the significance of the presence of some leukocytes and mucus in the smear. In our opinion, it is erroneous to interpret such a smear as a positive reaction for pregnancy. It is better to repeat the test, under these circumstances, before deciding upon the positiveness or negativeness of the findings.

The platinum loop employed in securing the vaginal secretion for the smear, if faultily handled, may carry some nucleated, squamous epithelial cells from the vulva, and convey the impression that the cells are derived from the vagina. An abrupt transition from diestrus in one of the test animals should therefore be viewed with suspicion and be corroborated by another smear. A delayed reaction (six to seven days of the first injection) is equally unreliable. Vaginal smears obtained from moribund animals, too, are misleading because of the dehydration of the vaginal mucosa current in pathologic conditions. The urine of women who have recently received estrin therapy may—one should also remember—render false positive reactions.

Advantages of the Mazer Test.—It is inexpensive, the mice can be repeatedly utilized for test purpose, the mortality incident to the injection of urine being about 10 per cent.

Accuracy.—This test is not so sensitive in early pregnancy as the others, but it is more accurate when positive.

Summary.—The three biological tests for pregnancy are astonishingly accurate and have rendered this diagnosis one of the most certain in medicine.

Occasional errors due to the presence of hyperthyroidism, approach of the menopause, ovarian cysts and primary ovarian failure, may occur, but these are so infrequent as to constitute only a small percentage of the whole and are no deterrent to the performance of these valuable diagnostic aids.

THE DIAGNOSIS OF LIFE OR DEATH OF THE FETUS

The decision as to whether the child in utero is living or dead is a most important one in many instances, and unfortunately cannot be reached with any degree of certainty until one or two weeks have elapsed since the death of the fetus. The matter is usually brought to the attention of the obstetrician by the mother, who has noticed a cessation of fetal movements and is greatly alarmed thereby. Far more often than otherwise, this stillness is more apparent than not, and the patient being reassured that all is well with her and her child, the movements recur within a day or two.

So long as positive evidence that the fetus has perished is lacking, it should be considered as living and no measures to institute delivery should be attempted.

The diagnosis of fetal death is based upon cessation of fetal movements after they have been felt. Absence of fetal heart sounds after they have been heard. The cessation of growth of the uterus and its contents as shown by measurements of the height of the fundus. This sign is only available after comparative measurements have been made over a period of days and weeks. The sharp increase in the intensity of the painless uterine contractions, which according to Shears is the most significant of all symptoms. The contractions suddenly increase greatly in force and on palpation of the uterus it would seem that labor must be in progress, although the patient is not cognizant of the contraction. Polyuria and frequency of urination are inconstant signs but a valuable affirmative if present. The vaginal discharge of bloody or grumous liquor amnii, which, however, may also be significant of some decidual endometritis or a slight partial separation of the placenta. The palpation of the loose, movable, macerated cranial bones, the scalp hanging like an edematous bag and the bones being easily made to overlap one another, sometimes with a crackling. A feeling of malaise, undefinable illness and weight in the abdomen on the part of the patient. Tumefaction and congestion of the breasts with possibly a slight secretion of milk followed rapidly by a loss of tone with marked relaxation and diminution in size of these organs. In the early months a sudden relief from annoying nausea and vomiting.

The history of the case is of importance since the same accident may have befallen the patient in previous pregnancies.

Taken singly none of these signs are absolutely indicative, but when a number of them are to be detected, particularly the palpation of the softened and macerated fetal skull, the probability of fetal deaths is strongly suggestive and the parents should be prepared for this eventuality.

During late pregnancy, the death of the fetus may be detected in a woman otherwise normal, by a drop in the basal metabolic rate as compared with the average. The increased basal metabolic rate in late pregnancy is due to the growing demands of the fetal organism and placenta.

Then according to Baer, the basal metabolic rate in normal cases tested during late pregnancy, averaged from 33 to 35 per cent above the normal for nonpregnant women of a surface area equal to that of the pregnant women. When the rate in a pregnant woman drops approximately to that normal in the nonpregnant state, death of the fetus may be predicted.

ROENTGENOLOGIC EVIDENCE OF FETAL DEATH

Several criteria of fetal death, demonstrable in the *x*-ray plate, have been described but so far none give any absolutely reliable information.

Overlapping of the cranial bones with asymmetry of the head is one such type of evidence, but this may be confused with the moulding of approaching labor.

Angulation of the caudal half of the fetal spine has also been observed in dead infants, but this also is unreliable. Faint visualization of the fetal skeleton due to decalcification has been suggested as positive evidence of fetal death, but as many technical factors affect the density of the skeletal shadows, this is also indefinite.

Anthropometric data published by Scammon and Calkins allow a reasonably accurate opinion as to the age of a fetus if its occipito-frontal diameter is known. Even with very coarse roentgenographic measurements of this diameter, roentgen estimates of fetal age have agreed surprisingly well with the actual age (as estimated from menstrual or delivery dates) in a considerable number of cases. Disproportion between ages thus calculated and the supposed duration of gestation constitutes a valuable criterion of fetal death and accurate fetometry by stereoroentgenographic methods ought to improve the validity of the diagnosis.

This subject has been carefully worked out by Schnitker and his associates, whose article contains a complete bibliography and who point out that absence of any one or all of the criteria does not exclude the possibility that a fetus is dead because they all depend upon the degree of maceration. It seems worth while, therefore, to point out that the roentgenographic diagnosis of movement of a fetal part occurring during the roentgen examination constitutes conclusive evidence of fetal life.

Treatment.—Noninterference is the rule, since infection or putrefaction of the dead fetus *in utero* is extremely uncommon and spontaneous delivery of the softened and macerated body usually takes place within a few days or possibly weeks after death has occurred. Repeated examinations are contraindicated as is the use of douches, local treatment, sexual congress or indeed anything which might carry infective matter into the uterine cavity. Only in those rare cases of missed abortion or missed labor (q. v.) is any interference justified.

THE ESTIMATION OF THE DURATION OF PREGNANCY AND THE DETERMINATION OF THE PROBABLE DATE OF CONFINEMENT

The welfare of the patient and her necessary economic arrangements, securing hospital accommodations, the engagement of the nurse, the preparation of the lying-in room all demand reasonable certainty as to the probable time of labor. Unfortunately, this cannot be absolutely predicted since many sources of error exist which may render all calculation useless and in addition as has been seen in the discussion as to the duration of normal pregnancy, this period varies with the individual and indeed may vary within considerable limits in the same woman during different pregnancies.

Two general sources of information are at the command of the obstetrician—certain data given by the patient, and the estimation of the size of the uterus and of the fetus or both as determined by mensuration.

Information given by the patient.

1. **The Fruitful Coitus.**—Many women aver that they experience certain indefinable but none the less positive sensations within a few hours after impregnation. While this seems somewhat fantastic and is not to be relied upon, it may have some basis in truth and should be taken into consideration at least. When, however, a single intercourse is followed by separation of husband and wife or in cases of assault or rape, the date is fixed and may safely be utilized in arriving at a conclusion. The accepted rule is to count two hundred and seventy-three days from coitus to arrive at the date of confinement. In a majority of instances this rule will be accurate within ten days.

2. **Calculation Based Upon the Time of Appearance of the Last Menstrual Period.**—This is the most accurate and widely used method of determining the probable date of confinement at our command. It is known that conception occurs usually just subsequent to a menstrual period and for this reason the date is fairly accurately fixed by the last previous catamenia.

Naegele's rule, the one in general use, is to count back three months from the first day of the last menstruation and add seven days to obtain the approximate date of labor. For seven months of the year this rule is correct, but in April and September six days, in December and January five days and in February four days should be added to obtain a date two hundred and eighty days after the first day of the last menstruation. Thus, if a pregnant woman last noted the appearances of her menses on March 15th, labor should take place on December 22nd.

It must be remembered that inasmuch as the date of impregnation is an unknown factor, and the normal term of gestation varies in different women, no rule for determining the time of delivery can be accurate, but the method just stated will be found to be correct within seven days in the vast majority of instances.

3. **Quickening.**—Perception of the life of the fetus by the mother has been stated to occur during the sixteenth week in multiparae and the eighteenth week in primiparae and the time of labor may be therefore predicted by counting ahead twenty-four weeks in the former and twenty-two in the latter group of patients. Since quickening depends so much upon the individual characteristics of the mother as to the time of its onset, this sign is an unreliable one and is only of value as corroborative evidence.

Information Gained from an Estimate of the Size of the Fetus, in Whole or in Part (of special value when the onset of the last menstruation period is unknown).—1. *Ahlfeld's Rule.*—The size of the fetus varies in direct ratio with its age, Ahlfeld's rule being to divide the fetal length by five during the last five months of pregnancy to determine its age, and to extract the square root of the fetal length to obtain the age prior to the fifth month.

Length of fetus		Age
50 cm.		10 months
45 cm.		9 "
40 cm.		8 "
35 cm.		7 "
30 cm.		6 "
25 cm.		5 "
16 cm.		4 "
9 cm.		3 "
4 cm.		2 "
1 cm.		1 month

The practical application of this formula lies in an estimation of the length of the fetal ellipse (from buttock to vertex) by direct measurement.

In primiparae, because of the early engagement of the fetus, one arm of a previously sterilized pelvimeter is placed against the presenting part in the anterior vaginal vault, while the other part is placed on the abdomen in firm contact with the opposite pole of the fetus. The length obtained is equal to one half the length of the child, when straightened out, plus the thickness of the abdominal wall, and therefore, when doubled and 2 cm. subtracted to allow for the abdominal wall, the fetal length is obtained (Fig. 70).

Distance between fetal poles minus 2 multiplied by 2, equals length of fetus from which the age can readily be calculated from the table given above.

2. *MacDonald's Rule.*—The height of the fundus uteri, measured with a tape from the top of the symphysis to the top of the fundus, the tape applied to the midline of the abdomen. This formula was devised by MacDonald and bears his name (Fig. 71).

The rule states that the distance from the symphysis to the top of the fundus uteri, measured in centimeters over the curve of the abdomen, if divided by the constant factor 3.5 will give the duration of the pregnancy in lunar months. It is only applicable after the sixth month. Thus when the fundus is 35 cm. from the symphysis, the duration of the pregnancy is ten lunar months or term. At eight lunar months the height of the fundus is 28 cm., at seven months 24 plus cm., and so on.

This method of computation is reasonably accurate, with a factor of error of about two weeks.

3. *Mensuration of the Fetal Cranium.—Perret's Maneuver.*—The

position of the fetal head is carefully determined (always before engagement) with reference to the pelvic brim and then the occipitofrontal diameter is directly measured with the pelvimeter as it lies

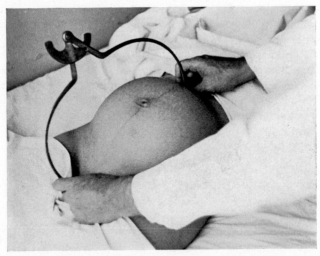

Fig. 70.—Measuring the length of the fetus by Ahlfeld's rule.

more or less transversely across the inlet, without making any allowance for the thickness of the abdominal wall.

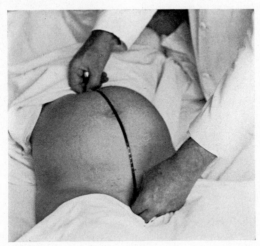

Fig. 71.—Measuring the length of the fetus by MacDonald's rule.

From this figure the biparietal diameter is estimated by calculation, according to a table originated by Perret and elaborated by MacDonald.

The height to which the fundus uteri rises during pregnancy is a

9

wide though fairly accurate index of the duration of gestation. At the fourth month the top of the fundus is usually distinctly felt above the symphysis pubis; at the fifth month midway between the symphysis and the umbilicus; at the sixth month on a level with the umbilicus; at the seventh month about four fingers' breadth above the umbilicus; at the eight month two thirds of the distance between the umbilicus and the ensiform cartilage; and early in the ninth month it reaches almost to the ensiform. At this time lightening occurs and the fundus descends to about the level it occupied during the eighth month. The factors of error in this method of computation are: multiple pregnancy, variations in the anatomical position of the umbilicus in different persons, marked relaxation of the abdominal wall, obesity and hydramnios.

THE DIAGNOSIS OF PREVIOUS GESTATION

Occasionally it becomes necessary that the obstetrician ascertain whether or not a woman has previously been delivered of a child, the information usually being required in medicolegal cases.

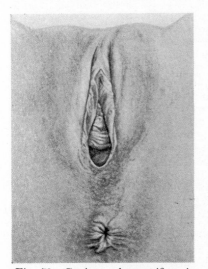

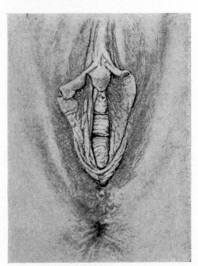

Fig. 72.—Gaping vulvar orifice, injury of urogenital trigonum muscle, and prolapse of lower anterior vaginal wall. (B. C. Hirst.)

Fig. 73.—Gaping vulvar orifice with rectocele and cystocele from a former labor. (B. C. Hirst.)

Ordinarily this diagnosis is simple, but when a considerable interval of time has elapsed since the last pregnancy some difficulty may be encountered.

The history is naturally of no avail since the patient has denied any previous pregnancies.

The facts upon which the diagnosis rests are:

Striae and scars upon the abdominal wall.

Relaxation and laceration of the perineum as shown by a bulging of the posterior wall of the vagina when patient strains (Figs. **72, 73**).

Deep tears of the hymen with the formation of irregular masses of tissue at the lower lateral orifice of the vulva—the myrtiform caruncles (Fig. **74**).

Deep tears and scars in the cervix.

Pendulous and flabby breasts with striae and deeply pigmented areolae.

Pendulous and relaxed abdominal walls.

If all of these conditions are present a fairly definite diagnosis of previous pregnancy may be made, but it must be remembered that

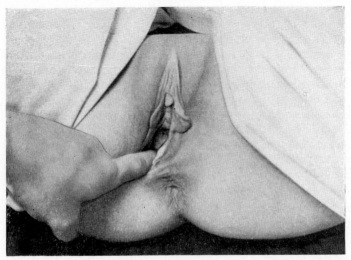

Fig. 74.—Testing the levator ani muscle in the right posterior vaginal sulcus. In this case there was a deep tear. (B. C. Hirst.)

each of them may be due to some cause entirely unrelated to pregnancy.

Striae on the abdomen—these irregular wavelike scars, silvery white when the pregnancy has occurred years before, pinkish or purplish in a recent case, may be the result of a sudden loss of weight in an obese woman, they may accompany abdominal tumors, may be seen sometimes in adolescent girls and are said to accompany typhoid fever. In addition there is a considerable number of individuals among whom striae never appear regardless of the number of pregnancies.

Relaxation and laceration of the perineum may be the result of traumatism, operations or aberrant sexual practices. However, the characteristic bilateral laceration of the perineum, with large or small v-shaped rectoceles in the middle is a most important sign, and one rarely found except after the delivery of a child.

Deep tears of the cervix are also quite characteristic but may have other origins as the congenitally split cervix or as a result of severe endocervicitis.

In rendering an opinion as to the existence of a previous pregnancy, the physician should take all of the factors entering into the question into careful consideration and when doubt exists, the patient should always be given its benefit.

THE DIFFERENTIAL DIAGNOSIS OF PREGNANCY

Theoretically, there should be no confusion between pregnancy and other abdominal conditions, but in fact, the greatest difficulty is sometimes experienced in arriving at a definite conclusion by examination alone. The biological tests for pregnancy, however, usually render this diagnosis simple.

The conditions most commonly rendering a diagnosis uncertain in their order of frequency and difficulty of determination are:

Spurious pregnancy or pseudocyesis.

Fibroid tumor of the uterus.

Hematometra.

Ovarian cystomata.

Other abdominal tumors.

Pseudocyesis is a state of affairs where a woman either ardently desiring offspring, or in deadly fear of the consequences of an illegitimate connection, becomes convinced that she is pregnant and makes every effort, conscious and unconscious, to convince her medical attendant that such is the case. A certain number of these cases are purely psychic, "delusion of desire," but such are not difficult of diagnosis, the physical findings being ample to exclude pregnancy.

Another and larger group, however, are sufferers from hypopituitarism with its attendant phenomena of rapid and marked obesity, atrophy of the sex organs with amenorrhea, somnolence and increased sugar tolerance, in short, the dystrophia adiposogenitalis or Fröhlich's syndrome as it is commonly called (Fig. 75).

In these cases the woman has usually menstruated regularly, has been married for some years with constantly increasing desire for children. Suddenly menstruation becomes scant, and in a few months ceases altogether, weight is gained very rapidly, the abdomen especially increasing in size and the patient becomes convinced she is pregnant. All preparations for the reception of the expected arrival are joyously made, the nurse is engaged and the woman applies to her physician not for a diagnosis of pregnancy, since in her own mind this is established as a certainty, but to recount her symptoms and to bespeak his services for the impending delivery. Ludicrous, not to say pathetic, errors have been made in the treatment of these women because the physician has accepted the statements of the patient without verifying them by painstaking physical examination.

The subjective symptoms of pregnancy are of no value in the diagnosis of pseudocyesis, except in so far as a lack of knowledge on the part of the patient may cause her to place an important happening, such as quickening, so far back in her history as to make the continuance of pregnancy impossible at the time of the examination. Morning sickness, etc., all may be reported in the utmost detail.

The physical findings are definite.

The small, hard, uterus and the more or less atrophied condition of the external genitalia, the hard cervix and the soft and flabby breasts are usually sufficient to base a positive diagnosis upon them.

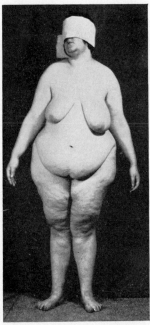

Fig. 75.—Case of hypopituitarism with pseudocyesis.   (Philadelphia General Hospital.)

It must be remembered that as these women are usually extremely obese, examination is sometimes attended by the greatest difficulty and sometimes may only be completed satisfactorily by the aid of an anesthetic.   The writer has no hesitation in advising this procedure when an attempted bimanual examination is unsatisfactory and when the circumstances of the case lead him to suspect pseudocyesis.

Fibroid Tumor of the Uterus.—In the presence of single, large, soft fibromata or myomata a differentiation from pregnancy is sometimes difficult especially if the patient, preferring hysterectomy to the birth of an illegitimate child, falsifies the history, with the denial of the symptoms of early pregnancy.

The diagnosis depends upon those factors of certainty before alluded to—the fetal heart tones, the fetal movements and the presence of a fetal skeleton as demonstrated by the x-ray. The marked softening of the cervix, Hegar's sign and ballottement are usually absent, although in certain types of rapidly growing, soft, submucous tumors they may be closely simulated.

It is astonishing how closely a smooth, regular myoma may simulate the pregnant uterus as is borne out by the many instances when a gynecologist, proposing a hysterectomy for the removal of such a tumor, finds to his chagrin, the uterus the seat of a normal pregnancy. With the development of the x-ray such mistakes are inexcusable since with its aid any doubtful case can be absolutely cleared up as to the presence of a fetus.

The diagnosis of pregnancy complicating a previously present fibroid tumor, sometimes offers difficulty, but time will usually determine the matter, the fetal heart tones and movement becoming apparent after the twentieth week.

The greatest uncertainty arises when the sudden enlargement of a fibroid tumor known to be present, with amenorrhea replacing the usual metrorrhagia, and with the associated symptoms of bladder irritability and pelvic pain, render it necessary to decide whether the tumor is undergoing inflammatory change or some rapid variety of degeneration, or whether pregnancy has supervened. Here the subjective signs are of great importance and the patient's statements as to morning sickness and the onset of amenorrhea must be carefully regarded. A true conclusion cannot be reached before the advent of fetal heart tones and movements, the perception of which may be considerably delayed by reason of the size of the underlying tumor. Here again the x-ray is of value. Biological tests will at once determine the diagnosis.

Ovarian Tumor.—Differentiation of pregnancy from these growths should offer no great difficulty, since careful bimanual examination will always disclose the small, hard uterus, not connected with the tumor mass, while the uterine signs of pregnancy are always absent.

Hematometra resulting from traumatic occlusion of the cervix, the result of operation or inflammatory disease, sometimes may be mistaken for pregnancy. Amenorrhea, progressive globular enlargement of the uterus, softening of the cervix and cyanosis of the vaginal mucosa may be present and on occasions the differentiation of these conditions from early pregnancy is impossible. Time will clear up the matter since no fetal heart tones or movements develop, and the x-ray is persistently negative for a fetal skeleton.

Most abdominal tumors can be distinguished from pregnancy at a glance but when such is not the case, repeated examinations are to be made, under anesthesia if necessary, and the physician should be careful to express no definite opinion until all doubts are settled in his own mind and he is prepared to defend his diagnosis under any circumstances.

CHAPTER IX

THE MANAGEMENT OF PREGNANCY

PRENATAL CARE

PRENATAL care is the supervision, care and instruction given to pregnant women.

By careful and frequent observation and examination the incidence of the toxemias of pregnancy as well as other progressive illnesses of the pregnant woman can be reduced to a minimum and many competent observers hold that with complete prenatal care, eclampsia, that death-dealing complication of late pregnancy, may be completely eliminated.

Prenatal care also provides for the accurate determination of the relative size of fetus and pelvis, the type of presentation and position whether normal or abnormal, and by this means the probable nature of the labor may be forecast, and a planned delivery arranged, which will insure to mother and child maximum safety against the accidents of parturition.

In the present day of general obstetrical information and education the pregnant woman seeks medical advice at a very early date—usually within three months, and the duties of the medical attendant are very definite.

First Visit:

1. Obtain a short, concise past history.
    a. Occurrence of familial diseases and malignancy.
    b. Scarlet fever and diphtheria, because of their sequelae—weakened kidneys and myocarditis.
    c. Complete menstrual history.
    d. Operations.
2. History of previous pregnancies—dates, illness during, nature of labor, etc.
3. Physical examination. To be routinely carried out in the presence of a nurse, or at the home in the presence of the husband, at the very earliest date.

    Details: a. Throat (tonsils), and teeth. Have all cavities filled at once.
    b. Thyroid and associated signs of thyroid disease.
    c. Routine examination of heart and lungs.
    d. Breasts: inverted or erect nipples. Condition of tissues.

135

e. Abdomen: Tone of wall.
              Height of uterus.
              Presence of hernias.
              Rashes.
f. Pelvis: With gloved hands, to determine the
             size of uterus, size of pelvic outlet,
             and lacerations.
       Take G.C. smear routinely.
Misc.:   a. Measure pelvis with pelvimeter.
         b. Blood pressure.
         c. Urinalysis.
         d. Wassermann.
         e. Blood count.

Subsequent Visits.—The patient should be instructed to return to her physician at intervals of three weeks, during the first seven months of pregnancy, and of two weeks thereafter.

At these visits she is instructed to bring a 4-ounce bottle of urine, which need not be a morning specimen, but should have been voided on the day of the examination. Each time the woman should be questioned as to her well being, effective sleep, etc., and any required advice given. Special inquiry should be directed toward the existence of headaches, edema, or marked constipation. Weight should always be recorded and made a subject of major discussion with the patient. Too great weight increase is the rule in pregnancy and unless the patient be well advised she will approach her labor obese, nonresistant to infection and toxemia and faced with the difficult task of reducing after the puerperium, in order to regain her usual figure.

Most authorities give the permissible weight gain in pregnancy as from 20 to 25 pounds but in the experience of the writer it is apt to average nearer 30, one reason being that the initial visit to the obstetrician is commonly made early in pregnancy when the nausea and vomiting so characteristic of this period have brought about a reduction from the normal weight average.

If the gain be more than 3 pounds per month, the patient should be instructed to reduce the amount of food taken. Fats, cream, starches and an excess of sugar should be curtailed. The usual principles of weight control are applied as in any other condition requiring its practice.

Maintenance of a balanced diet is requisite and pregnant women should not be permitted to reduce arbitrarily during this time. The blood pressure, both systolic and diastolic should regularly be taken and recorded at each visit. Hypotension is encountered in a large number of patients, systolic readings of 100 mm. or even less being very common. Lynch, Newell, and Williams have all noted the frequency of hypotension during pregnancy and regard it as of little significance. It does, however, seem to tend to languor and fatigue and possibly to some increase in the duration of labor.

Hypertension is one of the great warning signals of impending toxemia. Especially is this so when a pressure, normal during the first few months, steadily rises as pregnancy proceeds until it reaches a level 10 or 20 points above the initial reading.

Even more alarming is a sudden sharp elevation of 20 points or more. In either case, the patient with increasing tension must be regarded as potentially toxic and closely watched. Should the hypertension continue or increase after saline purgation, rest and a sharp restriction of diet, the patient should be considered definitely toxic and treated in accordance with the principles set forth in the section on management of toxemia.

The urine should be examined with the utmost care, the development of pronounced albuminuria, or the presence of a number of casts denoting the onset of toxemia.

At the seventh month, the patient should be completely reexamined, the position and presentation of the fetus being determined at this time. Again, at the ninth month a careful obstetrical examination should be made to recheck the type of delivery anticipated and to prepare to meet any difficulties which may be expected to occur

THE HYGIENE OF PREGNANCY

In the human species pregnancy is a normal, physiological process which of itself should cause no disturbance of the well being of the expectant mother. Inasmuch, however, as there is developing within the woman's body a new being whose functions of growth, nourishment and the excretion of waste products are all dependent upon extra efforts on the part of the maternal organism, it follows that pregnancy predicates a severe strain upon the mother which may readily lead to disabling damage or even may result in her death. The management of pregnancy, therefore, implies the reduction of the maternal strains and stresses to a minimum and the prompt recognition and immediate treatment of failure of any organ or system of organs.

Dress.—The dress of the pregnant woman should, in general, follow her inclinations in this regard. When pregnancy advances to the point where abdominal enlargement is apparent, she should be encouraged to wear garments which, while accommodating her changed figure, still retain lines of grace and beauty. Patterns for such garments or the ready-made dresses themselves are now readily obtainable and the morale of the patient is greatly increased if she is confident that her appearance is such that it will not excite unfavorable comment. The usual corset may be worn until about the fifth month when it should be discarded and one of the many excellent maternity corsets now made by almost all manufacturers of these articles should be substituted. It is not wise to permit a pregnant woman to go about uncorseted since the protruding abdomen needs some measure of support.

The shoes should not be changed unless swelling of the feet necessitates the use of a larger size. The woman who has been accustomed to wearing high heels should continue to do so during pregnancy and vice versa, a sudden change in this regard being often responsible for backache of unexplained origin.

Exercise.—The usual activities of the woman may be continued throughout her pregnancy with the exception of arduous physical labor and of such athletic exercise as may result in accident or heavy falls. Horseback riding and tennis are interdicted not by reason of the sports themselves, but on account of the danger of falls. Dancing, golf, walking, are advised.

Ordinary household duties are beneficial as the mind of the patient is kept occupied and the work provides necessary exercise. Heavy lifting and arduous labor should not be permitted, however, by reason of the danger of abortion in the earlier months or of premature separation of the normally implanted placenta later in pregnancy. Abundance of sunshine and moderate exercise in the fresh air are essential.

Bathing.—Full use should be made of the skin as an organ of elimination during pregnancy. A daily bath, preferably a shower, is an important part of the regimen of this period. The bath should be neither hot nor cold, but pleasantly warm, and should be followed by a brisk rub.

There are several cases on record of severe abdominal injury sustained by women who, heavy with child, slip and fall while entering or leaving the bathtub. Accordingly patients are to be apprised of this danger and instructed to use bath mats of rubber in the tub to prevent slipping.

Normally pregnant women in whom there is no tendency to kidney insufficiency may enjoy sea bathing in locations where there is no surf, the danger of injury from buffeting by waves prohibiting surf bathing. Swimming in quiet waters may be moderately practiced, but no diving is permissible. Outdoor bathing of any sort should be restricted to short periods in water not too cold; 68° F. is about as low a temperature as the pregnant woman can well withstand and in days when the water temperature drops below this figure the bath should be dispensed with.

Automobiling.—The advent of the motor car has rendered the study of the effect of motoring upon pregnant woman a matter of some importance. It has been found that the strain of resisting road shocks, sudden starting and stopping and rapid turns, is quite exhausting and too frequently results in debilitating fatigue. Also there is some nerve strain dependent upon steady and long-continued exposure to the wind created by a rapidly moving vehicle which may prove injurious. For these reasons, long severe tours are prohibited during pregnancy. On the other hand, the relaxation, change of scene and fresh air to be obtained through moderate uses of the motor car are of inestimable benefit, and patients should be encouraged to go out every day if possible. For the first six months a woman chauffeur may drive her own car, using reasonable care as to speed and accident.

Diet.—The food of the pregnant woman forms the basis of a large literature both lay and medical and as is usual in such cases has been vastly overestimated as to its importance. The nutritional problems arising during gestation may be stated as follows:

The frequency of abnormal appetite causing pregnant women to overeat, with a consequent excessive gain in fat and greater strain upon the already laboring excretory organs.

The tendency to overingestion of proteins and urea rich foods, with the attendant danger of kidney failure.

The various methods by which food intake may be made to regulate the size and weight of the fetus.

With regard to the quantity of food eaten, it is generally true that pregnant women overeat. An undernourished patient has a better chance of withstanding the stresses of labor and of avoiding toxemia than one who is excessively overfed. The diet should be mixed, with an abundance of green vegetables and fruits and overindulgence as to quantity is to be forbidden.

Because of the attendant strain upon the renal system, meat, fats, and eggs should be restricted. It is well to insist that not more than 4 ounces of meat, fish or eggs be eaten per day and during the last two months of pregnancy meats should be taken only on alternate days.

Sweets in moderation are advised, it having been shown that the ingestion of glucose and other sugars in moderate amounts tends to prevent the hepatic variety of toxemia.

Free use of fluids is to be encouraged, especially milk, buttermilk, and water. Tea and coffee may be taken in accordance with the previous habits of the patient, although the excessive drinking of tea as practiced by some women should be strongly discountenanced. An adequate amount of water should be taken, and this insisted upon by the physician.

Alcoholic drinks are in general harmful, although an occasional glass of wine or a small cocktail may agreeably stimulate a depressed woman with good effect.

Dietary Methods of Reducing the Weight of the Child.—It seems reasonable that if the food intake of the mother be restricted, the child will be reduced in size and weight and deliver, therefore, easier. Observation, however, proves this view erroneous, since the child being a true parasitic growth, develops at the expense of the maternal tissues no matter how marked the degree of underfeeding.

Regulation of the Bowels.—Constipation is the rule during pregnancy, though some women undergo no changes in their functions, while a very few suffer from diarrhea.

Evacuation of the bowels should occur daily, and if constipation supervenes, it is to be met by the use of gentle laxatives, as the mineral oils in doses of 1 to 3 ounces at bedtime, phenolphthalein in one of its many combinations or cascara sagrada. When hyperacidity complicates, sodium phosphate in drachm doses daily before breakfast is very satisfactory. An occasional irrigation of the colon with warm tap water, preceded by a cleansing enema of soap and water, is a practice to be recommended.

Attention to the bowels should be emphasized to the patient as many women grow careless in this respect. When diarrhea occurs, unless as the result of some transient dietary indiscretion, it is usually due to lack of intestinal tone—the lienteric diarrhea of the older observers. Tincture of nux vomica with small doses of paregoric will usually arrest the condition. If refractory diarrhea is present careful study of the feces for amebae or other parasites must be instituted, and the proper treatment administered.

Maternal Impressions.—That mental shocks and strains can produce direct effects upon the body of the fetus in utero has been a popular belief since recorded time. To such a wide extent has this view been held that every instance of malformation of an infant, from the most insignificant nevus to the most bizarre monstrosity, is readily explained by the lay members of the family by reference to some incident occurring to the mother during her pregnancy. This notion is not only of great antiquity but is also of world-wide distribution, Ploss having noted its existence among the primitive people of India, China, South America, Western Asia and East Africa.

It is interesting to note that the power of mental impression had many adherents in the United States, Fordyce Barker strongly supporting it before the American Gynecological Society in 1887, his views being shared to greater or less extent by Goodell and others.

Scientific opinion of the present day denies the possibility of the direct transmission of a maternal impression upon the fetus.

The physician should be very definite regarding this matter. The strongest emphasis should be laid upon the fact that the fetus is fully formed at the end of the sixth week and that no mental image created in the mother's mind can have any effect whatsoever upon the child.

On the other hand, since it seems true that profound anxiety and worry can and does influence the health and development of the fetus, it is most essential that pregnancy be regulated with regard to a quiet, well ordered mind, as free as may be from nervous shock and strain.

Preservation of the Figure.—It is the duty of the obstetrician to so advise his patients that they may guard against the relaxed, pendulous abdomens which are so often a source of annoyance and sometimes are responsible for serious illness after pregnancy is over.

Here, as in most medical problems, prophylaxis is of the greatest importance. The swimming, tennis-playing girl of today runs but little risk of losing the tone of her abdominal muscles as compared with her languishing sister of a generation ago.

Vigorous exercise during adolescence and young womanhood and the entering upon marriage in a state of physical fitness are essential.

After impregnation has taken place, there is no longer time to strengthen the abdominal muscles, so they must be afforded adequate support. The wearing of corsets should be advised, a simple girdle during the first few months and a sturdy, elastic sided maternity corset, which supports, without compressing the abdomen and which fits snugly over the sacrum during the later period.

The support of the abdomen is even more important in relaxed multiparae, in whom the abdomen may become so pendulous that mal-presentation not infrequently results. Some of these patients cannot stand the pressure of a corset and the necessary support must be given by means of a scultetus bandage or some variety of elastic surgical belt.

Particular injunction against too great compression of the gravid uterus should be given especially when the patient as a result of vanity or the necessity of concealing her condition might be apt to adopt such plan.

During the puerperium, gentle massage of the abdominal walls will serve to maintain their tone and immediately upon getting up from child-bed the patient is advised to wear a firm binder or to reapply her maternity corset, coming back to her regular garment as soon as possible.

Coitus.—Marital relationship may be indulged in cautiously during pregnancy, care being taken to avoid the period of usual menstruation for the first three months. After the seventh month intercourse is prohibited as not a few cases of puerperal infection can be traced to active coitus very shortly before labor. In addition there is always a slight but distinct danger of a traumatic premature separation of the placenta being brought about by such practice.

The author has personal knowledge of two fatal cases (both occurring in the experience of Professor Barton Cooke Hirst) in one of which the uterus at term was ruptured as the result of intercourse with a heavy husband while, in the other, the intra-abdominal pressure had been so forcibly increased from this same cause that the cecum was ruptured, a fatal peritonitis following.

Care of the Teeth.—The old adage "for every child a tooth" is known to every woman, although the recent work of Bill seems to show that the influence of pregnancy in producing dental caries is much exaggerated. By way of prophylaxis, calcium is indicated since the whole problem is one of decalcification of the mother, that the growing fetus may be abundantly supplied for its great needs.

Calcium chloride in 5-grain capsules is valuable as is the syrup of calcium lactophosphate in doses of 2 drachms after meals. Abundant milk in the diet is probably the simplest and best method of administering calcium.

Should caries develop, prompt dental attention should be advised. The analgesic technic of modern dentistry permits any necessary procedure to be carried out, without the slightest danger of terminating the pregnancy or of any untoward result. The old idea that dentistry may cause premature termination of pregnancy is no longer true since the agony and nerve shock which formerly accompanied such procedures are no longer present.

Sleep.—The strain and stress to which women are exposed during gestation, render it imperative that they secure abundant sleep to restore the nervous tone.

A minimum of eight and preferably ten hours at night with a rest of an hour in midafternoon is sufficient. The afternoon rest is peculiarly beneficial and should be taken whenever circumstances permit.

Care of the Breasts.—Most women desire to nurse their offspring and to the end that the function of lactation may proceed without difficulty it is well to prepare the breasts during the latter months of pregnancy.

There is little that may be done to insure lactation, but the nipples should receive attention in order that any abnormalities may be corrected, if possible, long before the birth of the child.

Nipples which are flat, inverted or infantile are to be treated by massage, chiefly traction.

The patient should be instructed to anoint the nipples twice daily with cocoa butter and then gently make traction upon them, pulling them and releasing them with a sort of milking motion, in order to stimulate the erectile tissue and to increase nipple length.

If the nipples are soft and painful they may be bathed daily with alcohol 30 per cent, to bring about a hardening of the surface epithelium.

Despite this treatment true inversion of the nipples cannot be corrected and women suffering from this deformity are rarely able to nurse their infants.

Morning Sickness.—This annoying symptom causes great uneasiness to many women, although not severe enough to warrant formal treatment as is advised in the more marked cases. The patient, if possible, should remain in bed during the morning, and is to avoid contact with food and its preparation early in the day, if such arrangement can be made. At luncheon time a meal may be taken, the nature of the food being immaterial. By evening the symptoms have generally disappeared and the woman is able to prepare and enjoy dinner.

In some patients a dry diet of cereal, toast, crackers, etc., is much esteemed, whereas others require liquids only to combat the nausea. Drugs are of but little avail, although a standard prescription of soda bicarbonate, aromatic spirits of ammonia and peppermint water, taken before eating is sometimes beneficial.

For the management of the more advanced cases, the reader is referred to the section upon toxemia of early pregnancy.

Nervous System.—Insomnia, restlessness and anxiety are common accompaniments of what is otherwise a normal pregnancy. A tranquil life, abundant rest and moderate daily exercise in the open air do much to dispel these unpleasant manifestations. For insomnia, the bromides may be used freely, doses of 10 grains of sodium or potassium bromide at bedtime being quite useful. When insomnia is more aggravated, the barbiturates may be used, with caution, but opium should on no account be exhibited.

Backache and Pains in the Legs.—Sometimes give rise to distress. Backache is due to the change in posture produced by the weight of the pregnant uterus in front, and possibly to some sacro-iliac strain, the result of faulty position. A well-fitting abdominal belt is of the greatest value as is the daily rest, with the application of dry heat to the back. Pain down the course of the sciatic nerve, due to pressure of the presenting part, is often annoying and very difficult to manage. The knee-chest position, which permits the uterus to rise in the abdomen and so relieve the pressure, is sometimes of avail, heat sometimes helps and the occasional use of acetylsalicylic acid in 5-grain doses, orally, does relieve the distress for a time. Sciatic pain disappears with delivery.

Tingling and numbness of the hands and feet seem to be an expression of calcium deficiency and are almost always promptly improved by the addition of this mineral to the diet.

Milk is probably the best agency to securing calcium and patients suffering from deficiency should drink approximately a quart per day. Calcium itself may be administered or calcium phosphate in doses of 10 grains three times daily, calcium lactate 20 grains or calcium gluconate in similar dosage. The combination of cod liver oil or viosterol with calcium is often advantageous and many elegant preparations of these drugs are now supplied by pharmaceutical houses.

Determination of Sex.—Despite a huge literature which has accumulated upon this interesting subject, the matter is still entirely in the realm of conjecture and the wise physician will not commit himself to an opinion.

Selection of Nurse.—The patient should be instructed to secure the services of the best type of nurse permitted by her financial budget, and to engage her as early as possible so that she may be certain of attendance when labor sets in. Most specialists in obstetrics have lists of nurses who understand their methods and who are usually very acceptable to patients.

Surgical Operations During Pregnancy.—Surgery is to be avoided during the course of pregnancy if this be possible.

Acute lesions, as appendicitis, ovarian cysts causing symptoms, etc., must be treated by operative intervention, it being borne in mind that pregnant women bear anesthesia badly, and that there is the ever present danger of abortion or premature labor.

CHAPTER X

THE FETUS IN UTERO. POSITION AND PRESENTATION

THE posture of the fetus in utero is of the greatest import as
to the conclusion of labor, since if the smallest and most conical fetal
diameter lies in contact with the cervix, the uterine contractions will
speedily force this wedge into the cervical canal and bring about
normal dilatation, while if a broad and impassable fetal diameter
impinges upon the cervix, spontaneous labor will be rendered impossible no matter how forcible the uterine contraction.

During the early months of pregnancy, the fetus is so small that
it floats about quite freely in the liquor amnii, but by the fifth month
it has grown large enough to fairly well fill the uterine cavity and
it then assumes a definite relationship with respect to the long axis of
the uterus.

Before discussing this relationship, certain obstetric terms which
are used in this connection must be defined.

Lie.—By this term is meant the relationship of the long axis of the
fetus to that of the mother. Thus when the two spinal columns are
parallel, the lie is said to be *longitudinal,* when they are at right
angles (approximately) the lie is said to be *transverse,* and when the
long axis of the fetus is oblique to that of the mother, the lie is
termed *oblique,* a term rarely used.

Reasons for the Lie of the Fetus.—It has been said that in the
latter half of pregnancy the fetus fills the uterus and by simple accommodation its long diameter tends to occupy the long diameter of
the uterine cavity. If for any reason this relationship should become
disturbed and the fetus turn to an oblique or transverse lie, the reflex
muscular contraction of the uterus and the voluntary movements of
the child's limbs will tend to restore the normal parallelism. Combined
statistics show that longitudinal lie occurs in about 99.5 per cent of
all cases.

Attitude or Habitus.—This term refers to the relation of the fetal
parts to each other, without regard to any external influence. Thus in
normal attitude the spinal column is slightly curved, the concavities
forward, the head flexed, with the chin in contact with the sternum,
the arms flexed and crossed on the chest, the thighs flexed on the
abdomen, the legs on the thighs and the feet on the lower legs.

The whole body forms a rough ovoid called the fetal ellipse,
which closely conforms to the contour of the uterine cavity. The
fetal ellipse is bipolar, the occiput forming one pole, the breech the
other. A line passing from one pole to the opposite one, and form-

ing a chord to the curve of the spinal column is called the longitudinal axis of the fetus.

This attitude of general flexion is not fixed since the fetus moves its limbs freely about in this uterine cavity, but it always comes to rest in the flexed posture. Warnekros has shown in his roentgenological studies that rather general movements take place, the spine straightening, the extremities extending and the head undergoing marked variation in deflection.

Presentation refers to that part of the fetal body which presents itself in the center of the plane of the pelvic brim. Thus in a longitudinal lie—there may be cephalic or breech (caudal) presentation; in transverse lie, back, umbilical, shoulder or buttock presentation.

Cephalic and breech presentation are further subdivided with respect to the degree of flexion present.

Cephalic Presentation
{
Vertex, when flexion is complete and the occiput is the most dependent part.
Sincipital, when the head is midway between flexion and extension.
Brow, when extension is beginning.
Face, when extension is complete.
Parietal bone, when there is no anteroposterior flexion, but a sharp lateral flexion of the head.
}

Breech (Caudal)
{
Sacrum, or frank breech when flexion of the lower extremities is complete.
Footling, when one or both feet present.
Knee (single or double).
}

FREQUENCY OF THE VARIOUS PRESENTATIONS

A summary of the last 3200 deliveries at Kensington Hospital for Women discloses a ratio of the several positions and presentations almost identical with the large series already reported.

Cephalic presentations numbered	3162 or 95.6	per cent
Breech presentations numbered	133 or 4.15	per cent
Transverse presentations numbered	5 or 0.156	per cent

Of the cephalic presentations, the vertex presented in 3140 or 99.3 per cent. The remainder being made up of transverse arrest with the head midway between flexion and extension, face (8 cases) and brow (2 cases).

Reasons for the Frequency of Cephalic Presentation.—Cephalic presentations occur with such frequency that this is regarded by many writers as the only physiological presentation, combined statistics showing that about 96 per cent of all cases terminate in this position. The explanation of this phenomenon is somewhat obscure. It would seem obvious to anyone observing a newborn infant, that the larger, heavy cephalic extremity would sink by gravity into the lower uterine segment, but upon experiment it has been found that the specific gravity of the infant is in such balance that the body floats evenly when suspended in fluid, the head sinking very slowly and to a but slightly lower level than the buttocks.

Veit and Matthews Duncan recently suspended a dead fetus in a fluid of approximately the same specific gravity as the body (1050–1055) and found that the head and right side sank immediately. This was correctly thought to be due to the weight of the head and liver respectively. Later, however, the classical work of Schatz proved that when a fetus is suspended in a fluid medium of approximately identical specific gravity with the liquor amnii (1008–1009) the buttocks had a greater tendency to sink than the head. These experiments were later confirmed by Williams of Johns Hopkins.

The most probable explanation lies in the application of Pajot's theory of accommodation which states that when an ovoid body lies free in an ovoid container, the two long axes tend to become parallel, which is especially true if the container has contractile power; as has the uterus (DeLee).

Late in pregnancy the uterine cavity is of a perfect oval contour laterally and having a marked depression on its posterior aspect due to the impingment of the lumbar spine which thrusts sharply forward against the uterus as this compressible organ lies in contact with it.

The assumption of an almost perfect ovoidal form, by the fetal body, the cephalic extremity being the small end of the ovoid has already been shown, and it follows that if the law of accommodation be true, the small portion of the fetal ovoid will conform to the small end of the uterine cavity, which is the lower uterine segment.

In about 97 per cent of all cephalic presentations, the fetus presents by the vertex, i. e., the occiput lies in the middle of the plane of the pelvic inlet.

The explanation of the marked preponderance of vertex presentation is quite simple. The fetal head articulates with the spinal column at the occipital condyles, which lie on the posterior aspect of the skull, about two thirds of the head being anterior to this articulation as against one third lying posterior to it. If the head be in the usual "military" position with respect to the trunk it is obvious that when uterine contractions begin to exert their force upon the fetal trunk, this force is transmitted to the head, which is thrust downward into the pelvic brim. As soon as the head meets with resistance of the bony pelvis and the soft parts lining the inlet, it begins to flex, since the anterior end, being much the longer end of the lever, yields to the pressure sooner than does the short posterior end of the same lever arm. As a consequence, complete flexion occurs fairly rapidly and the head passes the pelvic inlet with the chin in contact with the chest, the vertex first.

Variation in the mechanical factors just described may bring about the small proportion of positions other than anterior vertex. These will be taken up in the discussion of labor in the various abnormal presentations.

Position is a term meaning the relation of an arbitrarily designated point on the presenting part to an arbitrarily determined portion of

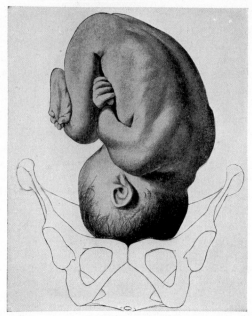

Fig. 76.—Vertex presentation. Occiput left anterior. (Bumm.)

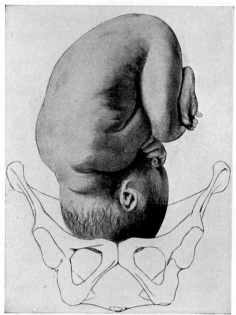

Fig. 77.—Vertex presentation. Occiput right anterior. (Bumm.)

the maternal pelvis. For this purpose the pelvis is divided into left and right anterior and posterior quadrants.

A point of direction is chosen on each presenting part, which point is primarily directed toward one or another of the pelvic quadrants,

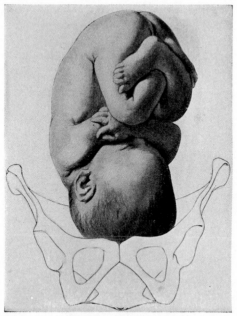

Fig. 78.—Vertex presentation. Occiput right posterior. (Bumm.)

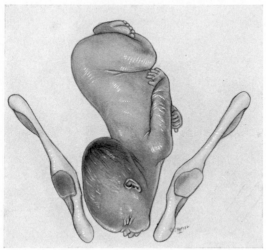

Fig. 79.—The deflexion attitudes. Complete extension resulting in face presentation.

and which during the mechanism of labor should ultimately come to rest under the pubic arch (Figs. 76 and 77).

The point of direction in vertex presentations is the occiput, in brow the large fontanel, in face the chin, in breech the sacrum, in oblique the scapula and in true transverse lie the umbilicus or back.

Each presentation of the fetus, then, is susceptible of six major positions, left anterior, posterior or transverse and right anterior, posterior or transverse.

The various positions with their Latin names and the abbreviations as approved by the International Medical Congress, Washington, D. C., 1887, are as follows:

CEPHALIC PRESENTATIONS

1. Vertex—occiput, the point of direction (Fig. 78).

Occipito-laeva anterior .... O.L.A.
    "   laeva transversa .... O.L.T.
    "   laeva posterior .... O.L.P.
    "   dextra anterior .... O.D.A.
    "   dextra transversa .... O.D.T.
    "   dextra posterior .... O.D.P.

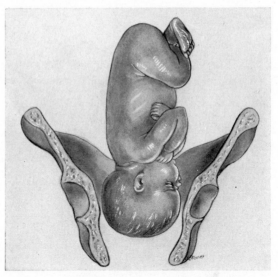

Fig. 80.—The deflexion attitudes. Incomplete flexion resulting in median vertex presentation.

2. Face—chin, the point of direction (Fig. 79).

Mento-laeva anterior .... M.L.A.
    "   laeva transversa .... M.L.T.
    "   laeva posterior .... M.L.P.
    "   dextra anterior .... M.D.A.
    "   dextra transversa .... M.D.T.
    "   dextra posterior .... M.D.P.

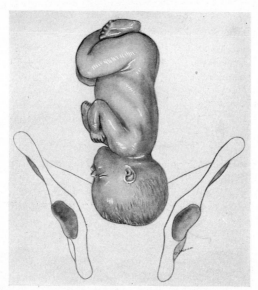

Fig. 81.—The deflexion attitudes. Moderate extension resulting in bregma presentation.

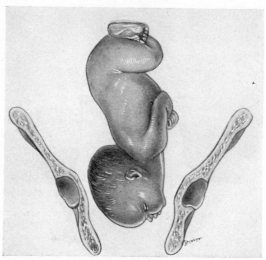

Fig. 82.—The deflexion attitudes. Partial extension resulting in brow presentation.

3. Brow—the brow, the point of direction (Figs. 80, 81, 82).

Fronto-laeva anterior .... F.L.A.
   "   laeva transversa .... F.L.T.
   "   laeva posterior .... F.L.P.
   "   dextra anterior .... F.D.A.
   "   dextra transversa .... F.D.T.
   "   dextra posterior .... F.D.P.

PELVIC OR BREECH PRESENTATIONS

1. The sacrum, the point of direction (Fig. 83).

Sacro-laeva anterior .... S.L.A.
" laeva transversa .... S.L.T.
" laeva posterior .... S.L.P.
" dextra anterior .... S.D.A.
" dextra transversa .... S.D.T.
" dextra posterior .... S.D.P.

TRANSVERSE PRESENTATIONS

1. Shoulder—the scapula, the point of direction (Fig. 84).

Scapulo-laeva anterior .... Sc.L.A. Back anterior
" dextra anterior .... Sc.D.A.   positions
" dextra posterior .... Sc.D.P. Back posterior
" laeva posterior .... Sc.L.P.   positions

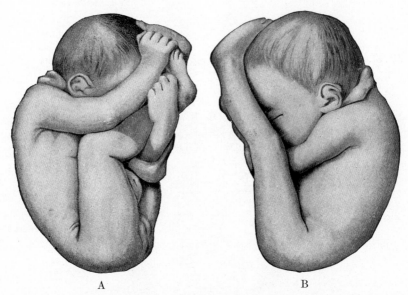

A   B

Fig. 83.—A, Simple breech presentation. B, Frank breech presentation. (From Edgar's "Practice of Obstetrics," published by P. Blakiston's Son & Co., Inc.)

The most common position of the fetal head is O. L. A., occiput to the left and anterior, next in order is O. D. A. the occiput to the right and anterior, third is O. D. P. occiput to the right and posterior and finally O. L. P. occiput to the left and posterior.

The fetal back lies anteriorly by reason of another manifestation of the law of accommodation. The maternal lumbar spine presents its convex inner surface toward the uterus and the flexed fetal spine is even more convex on its outer aspect. Naturally, two convex surfaces have but a small point of contact, so that the fetal back slips laterally to the maternal spine, and tends to slide forward, permitting the fully movable limbs to adapt themselves to the forward bulge of the maternal spine.

With the mother in the erect position and moving about, the fetal back naturally tends to occupy the roomy anterior position of the uterine cavity, especially if the abdominal walls be slightly relaxed.

The reasons for the high proportion of cases in which the fetal back lies to the left of the midline are: first, the physiologic dextro-lateral torsion of the uterus, which throws the larger area of its cavity to the left and anterior, and second, the thrusting forward of the rectum and sigmoid into the pelvic cavity, which tends to decrease

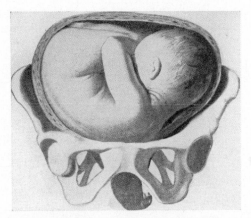

Fig. 84.—Shoulder presentation. (B. C. Hirst.)

the left oblique diameter of the brim and also to push the left side of the uterus forward, carrying with it the fetal back and head. The position of the back is, of course, that of the head, there being normally no unequal tension of the neck muscles, so that the occiput most usually enters the pelvis anteriorly and to the left, O. L. A.

DIAGNOSIS OF POSITION AND PRESENTATION

The Obstetrical Examination.—Satisfactory diagnosis of the relation of fetus to uterus and pelvis is possible only after the sixth month of pregnancy, since before this time the child is so small that its contour cannot be felt clearly. The methods used in the obstetrical examination are inspection, abdominal palpation and auscultation, vaginal examination and, if necessary, roentgenography.

The patient should lie on her back on a table or bed, the abdomen exposed. By inspection the general size and shape of the abdomen are disclosed, the amount of pigmentation is noted, the position of the umbilicus, whether inverted, flat or protruding, is observed as are any evidences of herniae.

The height of the fundus is measured in fingerbreadths or centimeters in relation to the level of the umbilicus, this point giving some hint of the size of the fetus and hence of the duration of pregnancy.

The normally pregnant uterus is ovoid in contour, symmetrical and broader above than below. The moving fetal parts may be seen as irregular, shifting protuberances appearing at different points in the upper uterine segment as the fetus moves its limbs about.

Multiple pregnancy or hydramnios is suggested by a more globular outline of the greatly distended uterus.

Abdominal palpation discloses the true lie and presentation of the fetus. The method of abdominal palpation is as follows:

The Four Maneuvers of Leopold.—Standing beside the table or couch, one of the examiner's hands is placed about over the center

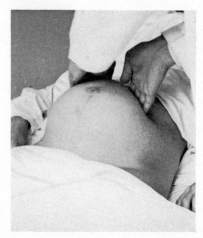

Fig. 85.—The diagnosis of fetal position. First maneuver. Determining what is in the fundus.

of the uterus and after a little manipulation the fingers may be easily depressed into the area in front of the child's abdomen and between the abdomen and the extremities (Fig. 85); with the hand in this position, the fetal body will be found to be fairly well fixed in the abdomen and the examiner's other hand may palpate the broad, smooth, rounded fetal back on one side or the other (usually the left) of the median line, while the irregular extremities may be felt on the opposite side of the abdomen. At this time the extent and vigor of the fetal movements may be likewise determined (Figs. 86 and 87).

The position of the fetal back with relation to the long axis of the mother having been established, presentation is next sought; for this purpose the examiner stands facing the feet of the patient, and with hands at right angles to the abdominal wall, makes gentle but firm pressure with the finger tips backward just above Poupart's ligaments on either side. In the event of a cephalic presentation, the rounded, globular, fetal head will present itself, lying across the pelvic brim (Fig. 88). Should a painstaking palpation of this lower pole of

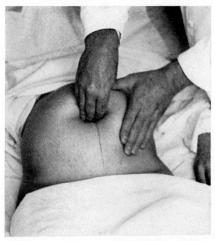

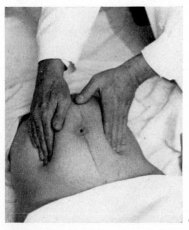

Fig. 86.—Diagnosis of fetal position. With one hand pressing firmly in the region of the umbilicus, the other differentiates the body of the fetus from the extremities.

Fig. 87.—The diagnosis of fetal presentation. Second maneuver. Locating the back.

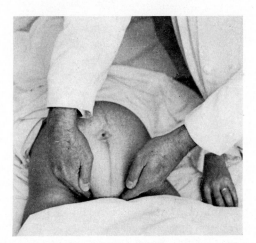

Fig. 88.—The diagnosis of fetal position. Third maneuver. Determining what is in the lower uterine segment.

the uterus fail to disclose the presence of a fetal head, this structure must be sought for elsewhere, and the examiner again palpates the upper portion of the uterus, finally locating a smooth, globular, movable mass high in the fundus, making certain a diagnosis of breech presentation. If the fetal head does not occupy either the fundus or the lower uterine segment, the presentation must necessarily be a transverse or oblique form, and the head in such event will be found either in one or the other flank of the patient, or lying laterally at about the middle of the uterine enlargement (Fig. 89).

Another method of palpating the head is the unimanual which consists in lightly grasping this structure between the extended thumb and forefinger of one hand, the examiner facing the patient's head and his elbow pointed toward her feet. In this manner the unengaged head may be easily grasped and moved about. During the last weeks of pregnancy, the fetal head will be found flexed and fixed firmly into the pelvic brim, in primiparae the phenomenon termed "engagement." In multiparae the head usually lies high in the pelvis, well above the brim even during the early portion of the first stage of labor.

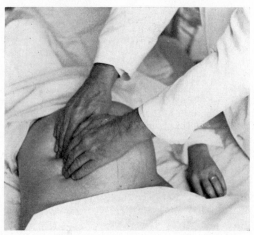

Fig. 89.—The diagnosis of fetal position. Ascertaining whether the fetal back is anterior or posterior.

The fetal skull possesses a characteristic smoothness and density which to the experienced hand is positive evidence of its presence. After the beginning of the eighth month if the patient be well relaxed, the head may be firmly but gently grasped and pushed into the pelvic brim. If it sinks fairly easily into the pelvic cavity, the obstetrician may rest assured that no marked disproportion exists and that labor should prove spontaneous. If, on the other hand, the head at this time will not enter the pelvis but resists a fairly firm pressure, it is probably true that some degree of disproportion is present, and that labor will prove long and difficult, probably requiring operative measures to secure delivery.

Shears lays great stress upon the recognition and location of the shoulder which lies in the average size infant 7 cm. from the biparietal diameter of the flexed head.

The shoulder may be found in a cephalic presentation, either by carrying the fingers downward over the fetal back until a sharp depression is reached. This is the neck, and the small knoblike projection just above it is the shoulder. Another method is first to identify the head and then slide the fingers upward until the shoulder is reached. In fat abdomens or where hydramnios is present, this maneuver is difficult of execution but in the majority of cases it is fairly simple. If the distance from the symphysis to the shoulder be well above 7 cm. the head is not engaged but lies above the brim of the pelvis, while if this distance be less than 7 cm. the head is in all probability engaged.

The shoulder lies about twice as far lateral to the median line in occiput posterior presentation as it does when the occiput is anterior.

By careful systematic palpation of the abdomen, the obstetrician

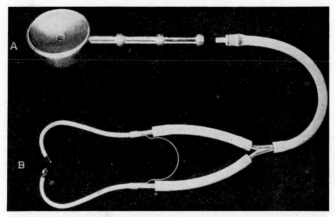

Fig. 90.—Fetal heart stethoscope; A, bell; B, binaurals. (Leff, in Amer. Jour. of Obstet. and Gynec., vol. 20, 1930. C. V. Mosby Co., Publishers.)

has ascertained the size of the fetus, its position and presentation, the presence of abnormalities as hydramnios or tumor of the uterus, multiple pregnancy and the activity of the child as manifested by its movements.

Extension of the head as in face presentation may easily be recognized by abdominal palpation. The very prominent occiput lies just behind the symphysis pubis, with a deep cleft marking the juncture of the extended head with the fetal back. Such finding is almost certainly indicative either of face presentation or of the presence of a tumor occupying the lower anterior portion of the uterus.

Abdominal auscultation: the fetal heart tones may be heard, theoretically at the twentieth week of pregnancy but for practical purposes they are not definite until the twenty-fourth week at least. Either the unaided ear or a stethoscope may be utilized, the heavy, huge instrument devised by Leff (Fig. 90) being an admirable one for this purpose. The bell of the instrument is moved about the abdomen and the area of greatest intensity of the fetal heart tones is sought and marked. When this area lies below the umbilicus, the fetus is in cephalic presentation, when above it, in breech (Fig. 91).

When heard loudest in one of the lower quadrants, the evidence suggests that the fetal back is anterior and to the side of greatest intensity, but sometimes in face presentations the chest of the infant lies close to the abdominal wall of the mother and the directly transmitted heart tones are heard with great intensity near the midline.

When the back is posterior, the heart sounds may best be heard far in the flank.

Auscultation of the fetal heart, then, offers presumptive or corroborative information as to position of presentation, but is by no

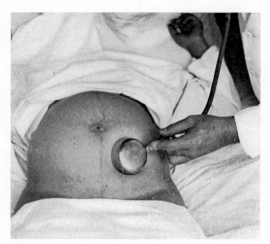

Fig. 91.—Auscultation of the fetal heart sounds.

means an absolute method of diagnosis. The rate and rhythm of the heart beat gives valuable information as to the well being of the baby.

Very thick abdominal walls and hydramnios may render the location of the fetal body obscure and cause the heart tones to be inaudible. Under such circumstances x-ray examination may be necessary to clear up the diagnosis.

Vaginal Examination.—Next in order is the vaginal examination. For this purpose the patient's feet should be placed in stirrups and the buttocks drawn to the edge of the examining table. The vaginal outlet is lightly sponged with a 2 per cent lysol solution, and two fingers of the examiner's hand, covered with a sterile glove, are introduced into the vagina. The information to be obtained from this examination is—first, the nature of the pelvic floor, whether or not its fibers have been torn or relaxed by previous pregnancies; second, the presence or absence of vaginal secretion and its characteristics, if present; third, the condition of the cervix, whether normal, lacerated from previous pregnancy or, unhappily, the seat of a malignant tumor; fourth, the length of the diagonal conjugate of the pelvis, and the determination of any bony deformities which may exist within the pelvic cavity.

If the pregnancy be well advanced, pushing the head into the pelvic brim with the abdominal hand, while the vaginal fingers estimate the relative size of passage and passenger, will often give information of the utmost importance concerning the nature of the labor. If the pregnancy be early there may be elicited upon vaginal examination the softness of the cervix, the cyanosis of the vaginal mucous membrane, Hegar's sign, ballottement and all the local evidences which have been described in the chapter devoted to the diagnosis of pregnancy.

Vaginal palpation is of but little aid in the exact diagnosis of fetal position unless the head be firmly engaged, and the cervix effaced and to some extent dilated, which conditions are only present very late in pregnancy or at the onset of labor.

III. LABOR

CHAPTER XI

THE ANATOMY AND PHYSIOLOGY OF LABOR

Synonyms.—Parturition, delivery, accouchement, confinement, travail, childbirth.

Labor may be defined as the process by which the mature ovum, *i. e.*, the fetus, its placenta and enveloping membranes, is expelled from the uterus, through the vagina and into the outside world.

Among the higher animals reproduction has become an almost purely physiological mechanism, an incident in the life of the mother, and labor has come to be regarded as a function theoretically purely physiological, but the entire phenomenon is so complicated and in mankind the boundary between the pathologic and physiologic is so nebulous that very often the processes of labor become converted into a series of lesions, either mechanical or inflammatory or both, in their nature.

The expulsion of the ovum is brought about by a primary force, the intermittent contractions of the muscles constituting the upper segment of the uterus, assisted by a secondary force, the voluntary contractions of the musculature of the abdominal wall.

These forces in turn are opposed by the passive resistance offered the descending fetus by the undilated cervix uteri, and the pressure exerted upon the presenting part by the bony and soft tissues comprising the pelvic girdle. According to the degree of preponderance of one or the other of these antagonistic force groups, the labor is easy and nontraumatic or difficult and associated with more or less injury first to the maternal soft tissues and to some degree to the presenting, descending fetal body.

CAUSES OF LABOR

The search for the factors underlying the onset of labor has so far been unsatisfactory in that no one determining cause can be ascertained. It is common opinion among obstetricians that several agents acting in conjunction bring about the uterine contraction at the correct time—that is when the fetus is mature. It is unknown whether the fetus itself exercises any influence upon the induction of labor, or whether the provocative factors all lie within the maternal economy.

If one reasons by analogy, there must be some fetal influence, since the eggs of birds all hatch upon a definite date corresponding with the maturity of the fledgling and without any maternal control whatsoever. It is true that the mature avian embryo chips at the eggshell in order to obtain its freedom, a voluntary effort not noted among mammalian fetuses, but there must be some chemical change in the shell, a desiccation of the lining membrane, which permits the feeble efforts of the chick to become effective. In the human uterus, it would seem that some ferment or toxin elaborated by the metabolism of the mature infant and acting upon the innervation of the uterus, is instrumental in originating the periodic contractions.

The theories developed on this subject throughout the centuries are legion and form in themselves a fascinating review of the development of medical thought.

1. The ancients thought that the infant literally struggled to attain a terrestrial existence and attained its end by its own unaided efforts.

2. Galen and his followers held that the progress of the descending head stimulated the nerves of the cervix and the great ganglion groups which encircle the lower uterine segment and their view has by no means been abandoned as witness the present day method for induction of labor; packing the cervical canal, moderate dilatation of the cervix instrumentally or manually, etc.

3. Overdistention of the uterus with its consequent contraction of necessity has been advanced as a cause of labor but this is incorrect since the uterus at term in a normal pregnancy is not overdistended as may readily be observed during the performance of cesarean section, while on the other hand in the presence of hydramnios or multiple pregnancy, the organ may be enormously stretched without any appreciable tendency on its part to fall into contractions.

4. Changes in the decidua; fatty degeneration, thinning of the septa bounding the glandular spaces of the decidua and thus making separations more easy are considered as a cause of labor but the regular occurrence of such change remains unproved.

5. The presence of an excessive amount of carbon dioxide in the blood leads to excessive uterine contractions as shown by Brown-Séquard in 1854 and confirmed by subsequent investigation. It has not been proved, however, that such increase of blood CO_2 occurs just prior to labor, and a definite conclusion as to its mechanism has not been reached.

6. The influence of the menstrual cycle has been advanced as a cause for the onset of labor, it being a fact that at the time of the menstrual period, pregnant women are prone to experience symptoms as a return or increase in the nausea and vomiting, sacro-iliac pain, a feeling of heaviness and weight in the pelvis, all tending to show that some obscure influence is being exerted at this time. Why labor should develop at a certain menstrual period, however, is not known and therefore this hypothesis must be regarded as purely speculation.

7. Toxins or end-products of the metabolism of the fetus discharged into and accumulating in the blood of the mother in constantly increasing amounts as the fetus becomes more mature, may at a given

11

moment of saturation stimulate the uterine muscle to contraction and so bring about labor. While this theory has not been proved it seems to conform more to the known facts than any of the others. It is generally conceded that there exists in the medulla a center governing uterine contractions and if this be true, such center would be much more easily stimulated by toxins circulating in the blood than by any local uterine change.

8. Most writers emphasize the importance of accident, as sudden violence, jarring in a motor car, coitus, profound or sudden emotional stress, etc., as a cause of labor, if such accident should occur when the parts are ready, the cervix softened, the uterus irritable and the fetus mature. Accidents, however, while instrumental in bringing on delivery, should not properly be classified as one of the essential causes of labor.

9. Since the discovery of the various gonadal hormones in the female, it has been suggested that the interaction between estrin and the pituitrin gland is inhibited during pregnancy by the presence of the active corpus luteum. Toward term, the latter undergoes retrogressive changes, and the estrin may again exert its influence upon the posterior lobe of the pituitary which is activated to a point sufficient to stimulate the uterus to contraction.

The whole fascinating subject remains shrouded in obscurity although it seems there is a growing possibility that the researches of physiological chemists may shortly solve the problem.

THE FORCES OF LABOR
THE FORCES OF EXPULSION

1. **The Uterine Contractions.**—The primary and essential factor in childbirth is the power exerted by the contracting musculature of the uterine fundus, a purely involuntary function but one which may be affected by the emotions as in the sudden cessation of contractions upon the appearance of the physician or the reverse. During the later months of pregnancy there have developed the painless but evident intermittent uterine contractions which increase in intensity as the ovum becomes ripe. At the onset of labor these contractions suddenly change their nature and become painful. Why the contractions of an organ composed of unstriped muscle should cause pain (the only instance in the body) has given rise to much discussion and various agencies have been described as causative, i. e., pressure upon the nerve endings caught between the muscle fibers, etc. No explanation is entirely satisfactory but it seems to me that the traction upward upon the lower uterine segment as the contraction of the upper segment lessens the area of the uterine cavity and the lower segment is pulled upward against the presenting part must bear some relation. Furthermore, one often observes in cesarean section the immense engorgement of the veins of the broad ligaments and the vessels on the

posterior uterine wall and it is more than possible that these rapidly alternating and violent local disturbances of veins may have some influence.

The Force Exerted by the Labor Pains.—Various more or less crude experimental technics have been developed to ascertain the force of the uterine contractions with, naturally, a wide divergence in the final estimate. The methods used range from the estimation of the force required to rupture the membranes outside the body (Duncan, Ribemont, etc.) which was found to vary from 4 to 37.58 pounds with an average of 16.7 pounds. Obviously this is an inaccurate and meaningless experiment since the force of expulsion must

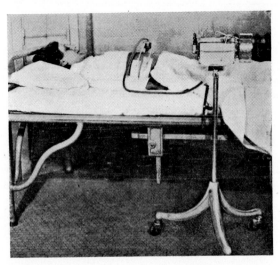

Fig. 92.—The hysterograph applied to the abdomen of a patient in labor. The recording apparatus is also set up. (Dodek, in Surg., Gynec., and Obstet., vol. 55, 1932.)

necessarily be greater than that required merely to rupture the membrane.

Schatz in 1876 introduced into the uterus a rubber bag connected with a manometer. His work is classic and must be regarded as truly representing the state of affairs inside the uterine cavity except insofar as the normal contractions may be altered by the presence of a foreign body.

Schatz found the intra-uterine pressure during a resting period to be 20 mm. of mercury while during the height of a contraction the mercury rose from 80 to 250 mm. which corresponds to a force of from 8½ to 27½ pounds, and which may be regarded as representing the state of our knowledge of the subject.

Other plans of determining the expulsive powers have been attempted such as calculation of the traction exerted during forceps delivery, the force of which sometimes reaches a maximum of 100 pounds. These methods are so obviously erroneous in principle that they require no further consideration.

Dodek has recently devised an external apparatus for graphically recording the uterine contractions, which is based upon the principle that during each contraction the anteroposterior diameter of the

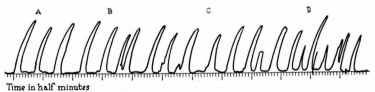

Time in half minutes

Fig. 93.—Normal first-stage tracings in primipara showing double contractions and fetal movements; left occipitoposterior position, three fingers' dilatation. A, No analgesia or anesthesia; B, contractions painful, patient comfortable between pains; C, patient more uncomfortable between pains and complaining during contraction; D, patient very uncomfortable and complaining. (Dodek, in Surg., Gynec., and Obstet., vol. 55, 1932.)

uterus and the abdomen is increased, the more severe the contraction, the greater the increase. The apparatus (Fig. 92) consists of a closed air system, the plunger and diaphragm of which are fastened to the abdomen so that each contraction causes a compression of the air which in turn affects a sensitive rubber tambour supporting a writing point.

Using this device, Dodek reached several definite conclusions concerning the labor pains, which are well shown in the accompanying diagrams (Figs. 93, 94).

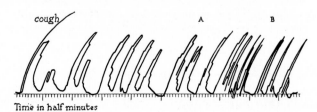

Time in half minutes

Fig. 94.—Transitions from first to second stage. Note the superimposed tracings caused by increased pressure or "bearing down" at B. Patient was a primipara; vertex presentation; no anesthesia or analgesia. (Dodek, in Surg., Gynec., and Obstet., vol. 55, 1932.)

The Nature of the Uterine Contractions.—The musculature of the uterus, as has been said, is of an extremely complex arrangement and has not yet been accurately described, though painstaking efforts have been made to determine the exact distribution of the muscle bundles. For obstetrical classification, the uterus is divided into the upper contractile portion or *upper uterine segment* and a passive portion which must undergo thinning and dilatation to permit the expulsion of the fetal body and which is termed the *lower uterine segment*, the division point between the two segments being the internal os.

Upon the onset of labor the upper uterine segment contracts in all its diameters, but it also retracts or is shortened from fundus to internal os. The exact mechanism of the shortening is not clear but during the contractions the muscle fibers are rearranged, those which were end-to-end during quiescence being side-to-side during the onset of pain. By this means the thickness of the uterine wall is greatly increased and the intra-uterine area considerably diminished.

At the level of the internal os the muscle fibers are mainly arranged in a circular manner, running horizontally around the organ, and into these circular bands are inserted the longitudinal and oblique fibers of the upper segment. These latter exert an upward and outward action upon the lower segment, pulling it against the resistance of the fetal head, and since this lower segment is of comparatively poor musculature and is rendered periodically ischemic by pressure against the head, it gradually thins out, stretches and is slowly pulled upward over the fetal presenting part which is at the same time being thrust downward by the contraction of the upper uterine segment. A proper understanding of this mechanism is most important.

The plane of demarcation between the thickened and active upper segment and the passive, thinned out lower one is termed the contraction ring or the ring of Bandl, in honor of him who first described it. In certain cases of obstructed labor, where the powerfully contracting fundus is unable to force the fetus through a contracted pelvis, the lower uterine segment becomes very thin and the contraction ring rises, with each pain higher in the abdomen until in extreme cases the lower segment is stretched to the tearing point and rupture of the uterus occurs at the point of junction of the two segments.

The Labor Pains.—Each contraction wave must be regarded as a distinct entity consisting of three phases, increment, acme, and subsidence, the whole movement occupying a space of time varying from five to ten seconds in early labor with progressive increase in duration until at the height of the first stage they may persist for a minute and a half. The period of increment is longer than the other two. During the second stage the pain again becomes somewhat shorter, thirty to fifty seconds being the average and at this time each full contraction may be subdivided into two or more shorter waves.

The pains are not equal in duration of intensity, a very long and severe one being frequently followed by two or three relatively insignificant contractions, or there may occur two or three very marked efforts in succession. The whole phenomenon may be likened to the surf on a sandy beach during a rising tide; a steadily progressive advance, but with clearly apparent variation between the height and length of the individual waves.

The uterine contractions are always accompanied by pain, although the intensity of the suffering varies with the type of the individual and the nature of the labor.

Absolutely painless labor does not occur except in the presence of grave disease of the spinal cord when the essential motor innervation of the uterus is not disturbed but the sensory centers in the cord are cut off. Under such circumstances labor may take place without sensation of any sort on the part of the patient.

The degree of suffering naturally varies with the psychology of the individual and the nature of the labor.

At the onset of labor the pains recur at intervals of from twenty to thirty minutes usually and gradually become more frequent and intense until at the height of the second stage they may be one minute or even less apart.

There is considerable variation in the contractile force of individual uteri as well as in the intensity with which they respond to the stimulus provoking labor.

Thus in one woman the pains will be augmented at a regular and even rate, the interval between them increasing in direct ratio as their intensity increases.

In other patients there seems to exist some disorder in the uterine innervation or musculature as a result of which the contractions are irregular as to time and intensity, pains of moderate degree and at long intervals often persisting for several days without definite increase in severity. This condition, known as inertia uteri, will be more fully described elsewhere.

2. The Force Exerted by the Abdominal Walls.—The voluntary contraction of the abdominal muscles plays a large part in expediting the expulsion of the child after the dilatation of the cervix is complete and there remains the resistance of the pelvic tissues to overcome. During the first stage of labor, before dilatation is complete, the abdominal muscles are of no service and indeed, if they are put into play by the patient, considerable harm may result as the entire uterus with its contents may be forced down into the pelvis with damaging stretching of the ligamentary supports of the organ.

As the expulsive period of labor approaches the contractions of the abdominal walls which have been purely voluntary become almost involuntary, the patient bracing herself, closing the glottis and fixing the diaphragm and making violent straining efforts with the abdominal muscles. There results some direct pressure on the uterus but the effect is mainly brought about by the decrease in the intra-abdominal area and the great increase in pressure. In normal labors these auxiliary forces are of great importance although expulsion may occur independently of them as shown by cases in which paraplegia existed with complete paralysis of the abdominal wall, and where labor progressed to an uneventful termination.

THE FORCES OF RESISTANCE

The obstacles to the birth of an infant are the tissues which must be dilated to permit the passage of the fetal body—the lower uterine segment, the cervix, vagina, structures of the pelvic floor and the vulva. The bony pelvis in a normal case offers just enough resistance to give

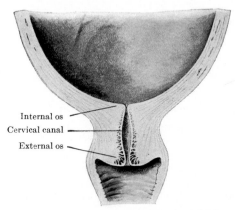

Fig. 95.—Cervix of a primipara at the beginning of labor. (Bumm.)

the soft parts time for dilatation and only in cases of disproportion between mother and child does it occasion difficulty. The body of the child is the third factor in the forces of resistance.

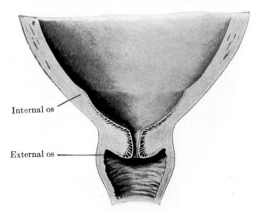

Fig. 96.—Cervix of a primipara during the first stage of labor. Partial obliteration of canal. (Bumm.)

1. **The Cervix and Lower Uterine Segment.**—The mechanism of the obliteration of the cervix and the mode of formation of the lower uterine segment have given rise to endless controversy (Fig. 95).

The *cervix*, in the later months of pregnancy, gives an impression of being greatly shortened in addition to the broadening from side to side and the marked succulence and softening. The shortening, however, is apparent and not real, since on palpation through the patulous cervical canal, its length is found to be from 2.5 to 3 cm. from external to internal os. This apparent shortening is brought about by the anteflexion of the uterus near term and the dilatation of the upper portion of the cervical canal during the terminal weeks (Fig. 96).

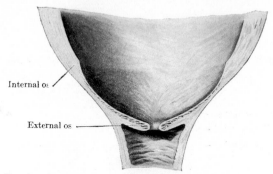

Internal os

External os

Fig. 97.—Cervix of a primipara during first stage of labor. Canal almost completely obliterated. (Bumm.)

The lower uterine segment is that portion of the uterine wall below the fundus and just above the internal os, *the isthmus of Aschoff* (Fig. 97). This definition is not universally accepted, some observers holding that the lower uterine segment is in part derived from the cervix, while others deny the existence of an isthmus.

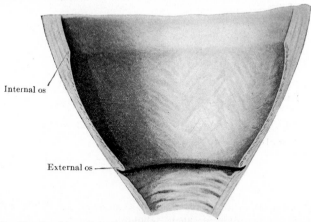

Internal os

External os

Fig. 98.—Cervix of a primipara during second stage of labor. Obliteration of canal and dilatation of external os completed. (Bumm.)

The contraction ring of Bandl is a circular band of dense muscle which forms after uterine contractions have been present for some while, at the junction of the upper and lower uterine segments. Above the ring is the thick, retracting upper uterine segment while below it is the thinned-out lower uterine segment and the cervix (Fig. 98).

The dilatation of the cervix is compassed by the combination of three factors:

1. The engorgement and softening of the tissues of the cervix by serum and lymph forced into them by the contracting fundus.

2. The pull of the fundus upon the musculature of the cervix tending to drag it upward over the presenting part.

3. The hydrostatic dilatation produced by the pouch of membranes below the presenting part being forced into the cervical canal in the form of an elastic, conical wedge.

The first factor is simple of explanation. As the upper uterine segment contracts it becomes ischemic and forces the blood and lymph down into the relaxed lower uterine segment whose tissues become engorged and softened by the pressure of the excessive vascular supply (Fig. 99).

The second factor acts by reason of the fact that the upper uterine segment tends to contract equally in all directions, which pull would

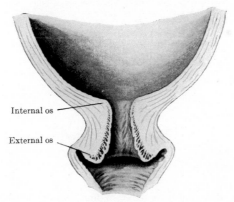

Internal os

External os

Fig. 99.—Cervix of a multipara during the first stage of labor. Beginning of dilatation. (Bumm.)

soon nullify itself were there no focal point on which it could concentrate. The internal os constitutes a break in the continuity of the uterine muscles and in consequence all contraction waves end at its borders and their entire intensity is transmitted to the fibers surrounding the os, which is strongly and steadily pulled open as a result.

The third factor, and a very important one, is the hydrostatic dilatation resulting from the protrusion of a pouch of membranes filled with liquor amnii, into the cervical canal. It is obvious that were the force not reduced in some way the powerful uterine contractions would at once rupture the membranes as they protrude from the external os, but the head of the fetus, dividing the uterine cavity into an upper and larger compartment and a lower and smaller area acts as a ball valve to shut off the lower uterine segment during a contraction, to prevent the distention of the pouch of membranes to a bursting point, and to absorb a considerable portion of the force of the contractions. The bag of waters is the name given variously to the presenting pouch or to the entire amniotic sac, the latter definition being preferable (Fig. 100).

At the onset of labor the amnion lies over the internal os, becoming slightly convex as the uterus contracts and gradually bulging into the opening os. From this point the action of the bag of water is vigorous, the pouch filling the cervical canal and being distended with fluid from above at each labor pain, it acts as a dilator and also as a reflex excitant for renewed and increased uterine contractions.

As the cervix dilates more and more, the pouch of membranes becomes larger and the strain upon the delicate amnion and chorion is greatly increased, until it bursts when dilatation is complete in normal cases. This phenomenon termed the "rupture of the membranes" usually indicates that the second stage of labor is well under way.

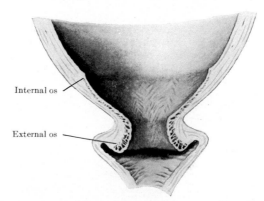

Internal os

External os

Fig. 100.—Cervix of a multipara later in first stage dilatation and effacement proceeding. (Bumm.)

Recent experience with the course of labor, after its induction by rupture of the membranes, leads to the conclusion that our views with regard to the functions of the membranes in aiding dilatation must be revised.

When the membranes are ruptured, dilatation proceeds with slightly greater rapidity than when the sac is intact, nor is there a greater tendency toward laceration of the cervix. It seems that the membranes act rather as a brake upon too rapid dilatation, rather than an aid to it; and that their use is in bringing about a slow equable stretching rather than the rapid one induced by the presence of the head alone.

It is probable that the pull of the retracting upper uterine segment is the principal factor in this process (Fig. 101).

Effacement.—Before actual opening of the external os takes place, the internal os is stretched and the cervical canal becomes thinned out and flattened until its walls decrease from a centimeter in thickness to about a millimeter. The length of the cervical canal diminishes from 2.5 to 3 cm. to almost nothing (Fig. 102).

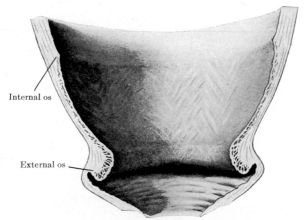

Fig. 101.—Cervix of a multipara at the end of the second stage of labor. Dilatation is complete and effacement practically so. (Bumm.)

This thinning of the cervix is variously termed obliteration or effacement and true dilatation does not begin until effacement is complete. Effacement begins, in primiparae, during the last week of pregnancy and is often almost complete before the onset of labor.

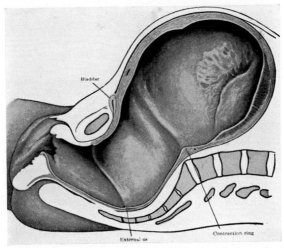

Fig. 102.—Braune's frozen section. The head has passed through the cervix and come to rest on the pelvic floor. (DeLee.)

In multiparae, the external os has been stretched and torn by previous labor until it no longer offers any resistance so that the internal os is the only barrier to dilatation (Fig. 103).

2. The Pelvic Floor and Perineum.—When the cervix has been completely dilated, the chief resistance to the expulsion of the child is that offered by the muscles of the pelvic floor, notably the levator ani.

This great muscular diaphragm forms the bottom of the abdomino-pelvic cavity and in addition to providing for the support of the pelvic organs it is pierced by fenestra for the openings of the rectum and vagina and acts in great measure as a sphincter for both these canals, or better, furnishes anchorage for the special muscle bundles constituting these sphincters (Fig. 104).

The levator ani muscle arises from the posterior surface of the body of the pelvis, the spine of the ischium, and from the white line or lower border of the pelvic fascia in the interval formed by the

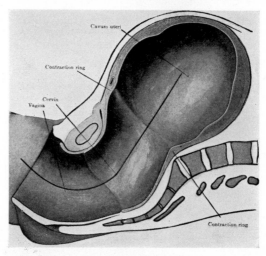

Fig. 103.—The completed parturient canal. Black line indicates the axis of canal. Note sharp bend at narrow pelvic plane. (DeLee.)

divergence of the rectovesical and obturator fasciae. The fibers of the muscle may be divided into three sets. The anterior fibers pass along the side of the vagina and meet their fellows of the opposite side in the interval between the rectum and vagina, where they are inserted into the central tendon of the perineum; the middle fibers blend with the longitudinal ones of the rectum and the external sphincter ani; the posterior fibers are divided into those which join with corresponding fibers of the opposite levator ani muscle to form the median rectococcygeal fibrous raphe and those that are inserted into the tip of the coccyx (Deaver).

According to Dickinson whose work on the levator is most illuminating, the muscle rather resembles a horseshoe or a sling attached to the pubes in front, its sweep reaching horizontally backward to circle, like a collar, the rectum and vagina (Fig. 105).

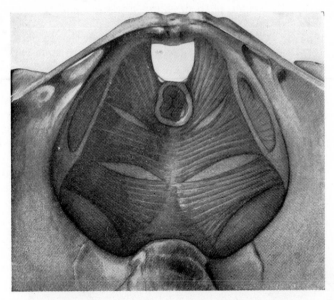

Fig. 104.—Diaphragma pelvis. Levator ani viewed from above. Same dissection
as Fig. 105. (DeLee.)

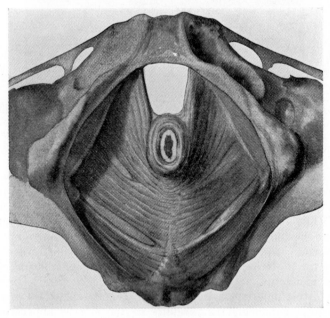

Fig. 105.—Levator ani from below. (DeLee, drawn from a dissection made by
E. Calhoun and E. Potter, N. W. Univ. Med. School.)

Its action in women is to drag the lower ends of the vagina and rectum forward, level to the symphysis.

Luschka says of the composition of the levator that in many women it is so thin as to be almost membranous. Its flat bundles are loosely bound together, and even open up here and there into fissures filled with connective tissue and fat.

In addition to the levator ani, there are as active components of the pelvic floor: *a. The coccygeus*, which muscle arises from the ischial spine and spreads its fibers like a fan from the tip of the coccyx up the sides of the two lower sacral vertebrae, filling the space left open behind the levator.

b. The Bulbocavernosus.—As the coccygeus completes the muscular diaphragm behind the levator, so a thin, weak muscle helps to close

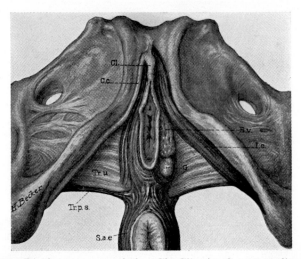

Fig. 106.—Diaphragma urogenitale. Cl., Clitoris; C.c., crus clitoridis; Tr.u., trigonum urogenitale (triangular ligament); B.v., bulbus vestibuli; G., glandula vestibularis major (Bartholini); Tr.p.s., musculus transversus perinei superficialis; S.a.e., musculus sphincter ani externus; I.c., musculus ischiocavernosus. (DeLee.)

the opening between the shanks of the horseshoe—the bulbocavernosus or constrictor cunni. Each muscle starts posteriorly from the perineal fascia at a point nearly midway between the sphincter ani and the fascia while a small bundle only is connected with the sphincter itself. In front the convergent ends separate into three portions: one passes to the under surface of the corpus cavernosum of the clitoris, a second goes to the posterior portion of the bulb and a third blends with the mucous membrane between the clitoris and the urethral orifice. The action of this muscle consists chiefly in compressing the veins of the clitoris thus enhancing the turgidity of the erectile apparatus (Fig. 106).

c. The Pelvic Fascia.—In common with all other muscles the levator ani is supported by powerful sheets of fascial investiture to support and control its contractions. The pelvic outlet may be divided into two triangles, one having its apex at the symphysis pubis, the other one pointing to the sacrococcygeal joint. The common base line is one drawn transversely just in front of the tuberosities of the ischia. In the anterior triangle are located the orifices of the urethra and vagina, while the rectum occupies the posterior.

The levator fasciae result from the cleavage of the iliac fascia into three layers, one covering the interior surface of the obturator internus, a second and very dense sheet lines the levator ani on its under surface and is known as the levator fascia, while the third division covers the levator on its inner or upper surface and is the rectovaginal fascia.

The Action of the Levator Ani.—Contraction of this muscle draws the anus and the posterior wall of the vagina toward the symphysis and it is capable of so firmly closing the lower end of the vagina that coitus and digital examination are impossible. It is in exaggerated cases of levator ani spasm beginning during orgasm that the reported cases of penis captivus have occurred.

The Levator Ani as a Force of Resistance.—When this muscle is inordinately powerful as is not infrequently the case, it may be a potent agent in the production of dystocia. On such occasions the head descends and rotates normally until the pelvic floor is reached when progress ceases, even though the uterine contractions remain active and the pelvic floor seems elastic. Under anesthesia, forceps delivery is usually easy, the spastic contraction of the muscle during a pain being overcome by the anesthesia and the slight pull required to overdistend the spastic fibers.

Rarely serious dystocia with even impossible delivery may occur as a result of extreme contraction of this muscle with permanent thickening and shortening (Budin).

3. The Pelvis.—The relationship of the pelvis to the infant traversing its cavity was long a subject of violent medical dispute.

The ancients held that birth was accomplished by the separation of the pelvic bones, though whether their conclusion was based upon a study of labor in the guinea-pig, in which this phenomenon actually does occur, is not known. Even so distinguished a physician as Ambroïse Paré adhered strongly to this doctrine and maintained it in his writings.

Vesalius in 1543 first accurately described pelvic anatomy, and among obstetricians Van Deventer in 1701, Wm. Smellie in 1752, Levret of France and Stein in Germany, began to present an accurate knowledge of pelvic form. In this country Hugh L. Hodge studied the planes of the pelvis and his classic work remains unchallenged.

The pelvic girdle is formed of four bones, the sacrum, the coccyx, and the right and left innominate bones, each of which is further subdivided into an ilium, ischium and pubis. The coccyx is made up of four fused segments, but is usually independent of the sacrum with which it articulates. The ilia are firmly united to the sacrum by the sacro-iliac synchondroses, which articulations are important from the obstetrical standpoint. The two pubes are fused anteriorly. For anatomical details the reader is referred to the appropriate textbooks.

The Pelvis Obstetrically Considered.—The pelvis is divided into two parts by a bony ridge, the linea terminalis, into the upper or false pelvis and the true pelvis. The former is made up of the flaring basin of the ilia, and the last lumbar vertebra, shaped like a flat funnel and of no obstetric interest save that it forms a support for the uterus and child during pregnancy and directs the latter into the true pelvis at the proper time.

The false pelvis is also of obstetric importance in that its bony prominences present certain landmarks which by their position in relation to one another give the obstetrician definite information re-

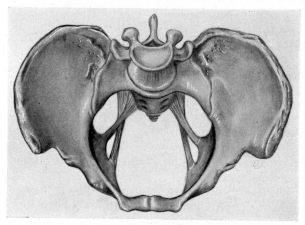

Fig. 107.—The pelvis viewed from above.

garding the size and contour of the deeply situated true pelvis. The true pelvis is all that portion of the basin situated below the brim. Its cavity is a little wider in every direction than the brim itself, while the false pelvis is a great deal wider; the brim is therefore a somewhat narrowed bony ring or aperture between these two, hence the term "strait" is given it.

From the obstetrical standpoint then, the study of pelvic anatomy may be confined to the true pelvis, its shape, size, position and direction. The cavity of the true pelvis is in shape a cylinder, with a slightly curved angle at its lower end. The upper portion or brim and the lower portion or outlet are smaller than the middle portion and are hence called the superior and inferior strait respectively. The large middle portion is called the cavity or excavation (Fig. 107).

The pelvic canal is long posteriorly, 12½ cm., and quite short anteriorly, 4½ cm. The shape of the true pelvis is not possible of description if the canal be taken as a whole. But inasmuch as the pelvic canal is of different form at different levels, and the relationship of the fetal shape to its surrounding bony walls varies at these different levels, it becomes necessary to study the outline of the canal at such various planes.

The first of these levels or planes has been fixed at the pelvic inlet or brim or superior strait and is bounded by the promontory of the sacrum, the iliopectineal lines, the crests of the pubis and the upper edge of the symphysis. It is cordiform in shape and in the bays on either side of the promontory rest the large nerve trunks and blood vessels of the pelvis, so situated as to be free from the pressure of the fetal head.

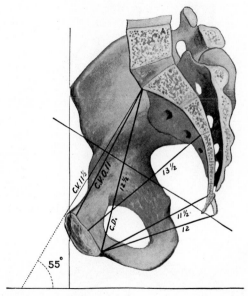

Fig. 108.—Sagittal section of pelvis showing diameters (Hodge). C.V., Anatomical conjugate; C.V.O., obstetrical conjugate; C.D., diagonal conjugate.

In studying the pelvic canal from above downward it appears that it expands below the pelvic inlet and then contracts again as it approaches the outlet. It is convenient, therefore, to lay off a plane at the level of greatest expansion and another at the level of greatest contraction which are called, respectively, the plane of pelvic expansion and the plane of pelvic contraction (the pelvic planes of Hodge). The shape of the pelvic canal at the plane of pelvic expansion, passing through the middle of the symphysis, the top of the acetabula and the sacrum between the second and third vertebrae is almost exactly circular, being only a trifle larger in its anteroposterior than in its transverse diameter (Fig. 108).

The shape of the pelvic canal at the plane of pelvic contraction
12

which passes through the tip of the sacrum, the spines of the ischia and the lower surface of the symphysis is distinctly elliptical, being a centimeter longer anteroposteriorly than it is transversely (Fig. 109).

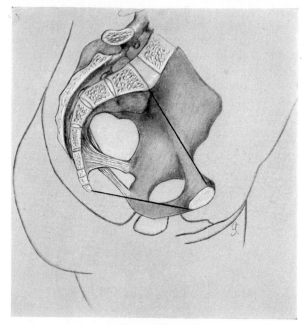

Fig. 109.—The boundaries of the true pelvis. Lateral view.

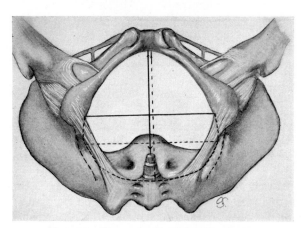

Fig. 110.—The normal pelvis from below.

Finally the shape of the pelvic outlet or inferior strait is cordiform from the projection forward of the tip of the sacrum and the coccyx (Fig. 110).

Pelvic Size.—In determining the size of an irregularly shaped canal like that of the pelvis it is necessary again to resort to certain typical planes on different levels and to measure typical diameters in these planes.

Beginning with the cordiform pelvic inlet the dimensions may best be estimated by a measurement of the following diameters:

An anteroposterior diameter measured from the middle of the promontory of the sacrum to the symphysis pubis about ⅛ inch below its upper edge. This measurement averages in well developed caucasian women 11 cm., is called the conjugata vera or true conjugate and is the most important single diameter in the pelvis.

Next a transverse diameter which is the longest distance from side to side of the pelvic inlet, measuring on the average 13.5 cm., and two oblique diameters measured, the right one from the right sacro-iliac synchondrosis to the opposite iliopectineal eminence, the left from the left sacro-iliac juncture to the opposite iliopectineal eminence, and averaging 12.75 cm. the right usually a trifle longer than the left by reason of the right-footedness of most persons as has been explained.

At the nearly circular plane of pelvic expansion it is possible to measure but two diameters, an anteroposterior averaging 12.75 cm. and a transverse averaging 12.50 cm.

At the plane of pelvic contraction, the anteroposterior diameter measured from the tip of the sacrum to the lower border of the symphysis pubis is 11.5 cm., while the transverse measured between the spines of the ischia is 10.5 cm.

At the inferior strait, the anteroposterior diameter measured from the tip of the coccyx to the lower border of the symphysis is 9.5 cm., but this is not a fixed measurement as the coccyx is normally movable and in labor is displaced backward.

The transverse diameter measured between the tuberosities of the ischia is 11 cm.

Pelvic Position.—By pelvic position is meant the angle or inclination of the pelvis to the trunk and to the horizon. The inclination of the plane of the superior strait to the horizon when the individual is in the erect posture is 55 degrees, and of the inferior strait 10 degrees. This inclination changes greatly however with change of position of the individual. It disappears in a squatting or sitting position, and is increased by leaning backward. The greater the inclination of the superior strait, the greater the divergence of the axis of the superior straight from the long axis of the uterus and consequently the greater must be the divergence in direction of the presenting part from that of the rest of the fetal body when the former engages in the strait.

This may be entirely overcome, however, by placing the woman on her side and flexing the thighs on the abdomen and is therefore of but little obstetric importance.

Pelvic Direction.—By this term is meant the direction of the pelvic canal, and this depends almost entirely upon the curvature of the sacrum and therefore varies in almost every individual pelvis. The sacral curve varies from an almost straight line to the arc of a small

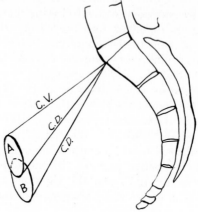

Fig. 111.—The effect upon the conjugate diameters of variations in the height of the symphysis and the inclination of the plane of the pelvic brim.

circle. It may be said that the pelvic direction is a line parallel with the sacral curve and equally distant at all points from the pelvic walls.

Variations in the Conjugata Vera Caused by Different Types of Symphysis.—The angle of inclination of the pelvic brim may be con-

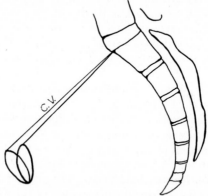

Fig. 112.—Shows the effect upon the true conjugate of variations in the obliquity of the symphysis pubis.

siderably altered by the length of the symphysis, without any difference in the diagonal conjugate.

Thus, as shown in Fig. 111 the true conjugate may vary by fully a centimeter while the diagonal remains the same. Also the inclination of the symphysis is of considerable import. A straight symphysis decreasing the comparative length of the conjugata vera as compared with the diagonal while a markedly inclined one increases the comparative length. Hence it is always important to estimate the length, thickness and inclination of the symphysis, which may easily be done with the pelvimeter (Fig. 112).

4. **The Fetus as a Resistant Force.**—The fetus itself is an important passive agent among the forces of resistance, the pressure and friction caused by its passage absorbing much of the power of expulsion. The fetal head by reason of its bulk, hardness and the fact that it is the presenting part in so large a majority of labors is the most vital portion of the child in this connection (Figs. 113, 114).

The head is of an irregular ovoid form and may be divided into a rigid and immovable area (the face) and an elastic and yielding

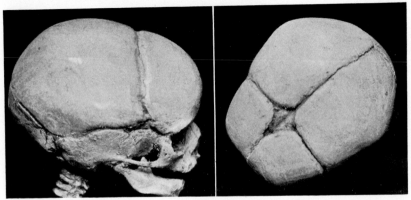

Fig. 113.   Fig. 114.

Fig. 113.—Lateral view of fetal skull showing coronal, occipital and lambdoid sutures.

Fig. 114.—The fetal skull from above, showing the anterior and posterior fontanel and the sagittal sutures.

portion, the cranium. The face in the fetus at term is small, the great mass of the head being made up of the cranial vault, which is composed of the two parietal, the occipital and the frontal bones, all of them elastic and movable, their edges soft and separated by spaces, later to unite as the sutures. The bones are held together by their chondrocranium.

The Sutures.—The sutures of obstetric interest are:

The sagittal: running in the midline anteroposteriorly, between the parietal bones.

The frontal: running between the two as yet ununited halves of the frontal bones.

The coronal: between the frontal and parietal bones on each side.

The lambdoid: between the occipital bone and the two parietals.

The junctions of these sutures are marked by certain spaces, which result from the rounding of the corners of the cranial bones, the defects being covered with the membranous chondrocranium. These spaces are termed *fontanels* and are of great obstetric interest in that they furnish location points from which the examiner can determine the position of the head in relation to the pelvis.

Anatomically there are six fontanels, the anterior, the posterior, and the laterals, two on each side known as the pterion and the asterion. The anterior fontanel is a diamond-shaped space, situated at the juncture of the frontal and parietal bones, with four sutures indicated from its four angles, the sagittal behind, the frontal in front and the two coronary, one on each side. In the fetus at term this space is about a centimeter in length, it is soft, the membrane covering it being loose and impressionable and no matter how extreme the molding of the head, this fontanel is never closed. Situated as it is, at the anterior end of the cranial vault, the large fontanel is a most important diagnostic point, since easily palpated, its position determines at once the location of the anterior position of the fetal head in the pelvic diameter and at the same time it indicates the degree of flexion as more or less of the cranial vault must be passed by the examining finger until the fontanel is reached.

The small or posterior fontanel is a small triangular space, situated at the juncture of the sagittal suture with the lambdoid, and bounded by the posterior margin of the parietal bones and the anterior border of the occipital. This suture is obliterated during labor by the overlapping of the bones.

Two sutures which have not been described because they are of no obstetric significance are the lateral, or temporal suture, which divides the parietal from the temporal bones at the sides of the head.

At the juncture of these sutures with the coronal anteriorly and the lambdoid posteriorly are the four lateral fontanels which may be mistaken for the greater and lesser fontanels. The anterior ones are close to the posterior border of the orbit, and the laterals adjoin the ears, which orientation should serve the obstetrician to avoid error.

In some 4 per cent of fetal skulls there is a so-called "false" fontanel or, as termed by Arnold Lea, a sagittal fontanel which is really the result of faulty ossification of the parietal bones and is a lozenge-shaped space lying in the sagittal suture about midway between the anterior and posterior fontanels.

To avoid error from this source it is well always to follow the sagittal suture to its posterior and anterior terminations.

Certain diameters and circumferences have been chosen to indicate the size and shape of the fetal head.

The Diameters (Fig. 115).—The diameters in general use are:

Fronto-occipital—from the root of the nose to the most prominent aspect of the occiput.

Biparietal—the widest transverse diameter of the head, extending from one parietal base to the other.

Bitemporal—the shortest transverse diameter running between the temporal bones.

Occipitomental—running from the chin to the most prominent portion of the occiput.

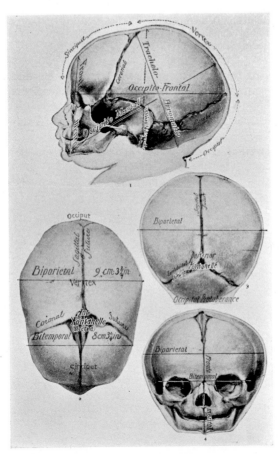

Fig. 115.—Fetal skull seen (1) from the side; (2) from above; (3) from behind, and (4) from in front, showing sutures, fontanels, and diameters (Dickinson).

Suboccipitobregmatic—which corresponds to a line drawn from the anterior angle of the great or anterior fontanel to the lower surface of the occiput, below the occipital tubercle.

The circumferences commonly used are the largest, which corresponds to the plane of the occipitofrontal diameter measure 34.5 cm.

The smallest, corresponding to the plane of the suboccipitobregmatic diameter measuring 32 cm. in the average.

All of these diameters are to some considerable extent modified and reduced by molding during labor.

Boy babies are usually larger than girls and consequently have larger heads, and there is also some racial variation, negroes having smaller craniums than caucasians.

Biparietal diameter	B.P.	9.5 cm.
Bitemporal diameter	B.T.	8.0 cm.
Suboccipitobregmatic diameter	S.O.B.	9.5 cm.
Occipitofrontal diameter	O.F.	11.0 cm.
Occipitomental diameter	O.M.	13.0 cm.

The trunk of the child is somewhat compressible and hence offers less resistance than the head although it is somewhat larger.

The shoulders vary greatly in width and if excessively broad as in a large, postmature male child, they may give rise to serious dystocia.

The bisacromial diameter is 11 cm., the circumference at the shoulder 34 cm. The bisiliac diameter is 9 cm.

CHAPTER XII

THE MECHANISM OF LABOR

The mechanism of labor comprises that series of forces and resistance by whose action a hard, somewhat compressible and fairly flexible body, the fetus, is thrust into, through and finally out of an irregularly circular canal, sharply curved in its lower third, the maternal pelvis. The process is a complicated one, much more so in human beings than in the lower mammals, and its details are not yet clearly understood, although the general principles were clearly stated by such writers as Baudelocque and Smellie and were closely described by Nägele in his essay of 1819. This whole complicated process has been much studied, generally by repeated digital examination of the parturient woman, lately by repeated roentgen photography during labor, and in some instances by the immediate inspection of the parts in women who have perished intrapartum.

Factors Concerned.—The factors concerned in the mechanism of labor may be defined as:

1. The fetus, which is in effect an irregular and moderately elastic cylinder to which is attached at one extremity a slightly elastic ovoid, the fetal head. The connection between the two is made by the freely moving universal joint, the craniovertebral articulation.

2. The pelvis, which may be defined as a short inelastic cylindrical canal, sharply curved at its lower end and having its posterior length several times greater than its anterior length.

3. Certain forces of expulsion, *i. e.*, the involuntary contraction of the uterine muscle, plus the voluntary contraction of the abdominal muscles, the combined effects of these forces being to cause the descent of the fetus through the pelvic canal.

4. Certain forces of resistance, being the bony pelvis, the cervix uteri and the muscles and fasciae of the pelvic floor, which tend to obstruct and delay expulsion and which exert a powerful influence in determining the direction in which the fetal body shall traverse the pelvic canal and in causing such molding of its more elastic portions as shall permit such passage and subsequent egress with a minimum of obstruction.

Phases.—The mechanism of labor may be divided into three phases. *Flexion and engagement* during which the fetal presenting part is molded, compressed, and forced into the pelvic inlet; second, *rotation and descent,* during which the presenting part is made to conform to the varying shape of the pelvic cavity, and to pass through it, together with the dilation of the soft portions of the birth canal; third,

185

disengagement or extrusion during which the fetus finally passes through the pelvic outlet and over the distended perineum to be born.

It has already been shown that some **96** per cent of all presentations are cephalic, and the commonest of these, L. O. A., will be taken as a typical example in mechanism.

The steps in the mechanism in a vertex presentation are as follows:

1. Flexion, engagement, and molding.
2. Descent and dilation of the cervix.
3. Internal rotation.
4. Birth of the head by extension.
5. Restitution.
6. External rotation.
7. Birth of the shoulders.
8. Birth of the body of the fetus.

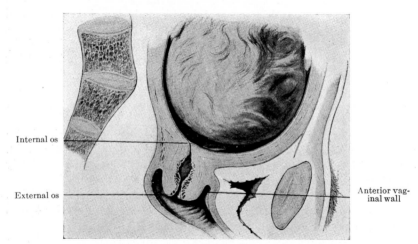

Internal os

External os

Anterior vaginal wall

Fig. 116.—The unengaged head at the end of the seventh month of pregnancy. (Bumm.)

It must be clearly understood that these steps do not occur separately but that one blends into the other so that the entire downward movement of the child is a continued and progressive one, each phase of the process merging gradually into the succeeding one.

Flexion and Engagement.—*Engagement* is a term used to express the entrance of the presenting part into the pelvis and is said to have occurred when the widest diameter of the flexed fetal head, namely, the biparietal, has entered the superior strait. A head is not engaged when its greatest transverse diameter is still above the plane of the superior strait, and if at this time it be freely movable, it is said to be *floating* (Fig. 116).

The phenomenon of engagement usually occurs about three weeks prior to term in primiparae, but only appears in multiparae at the onset of labor. The reason for this variation is not quite clear, but it is probably due to the greater tonicity of the abdominal muscles in primiparae, as well as to the greater frequency and intensity of the

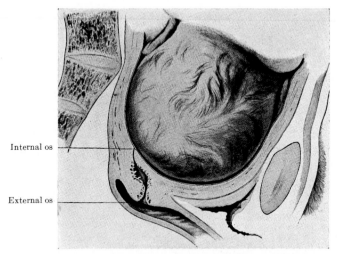

Internal os

External os

Fig. 117.—Vertex presentation at term. The head engaging. (Bumm.)

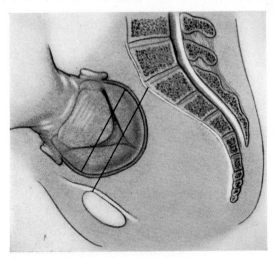

Fig. 118.—The head at the pelvic brim prior to engagement. The sagittal suture occupies the middle of the plane of the superior strait. There is no lateral flexion of the fetal spinal column. Synclitism.

painless uterine contractions of Braxton Hicks, during the later months of a first pregnancy (Fig. 117).

At the beginning of engagement, the child lies with its spine well curved, occupying one side of the uterus and at a considerable angle to the plane of the inlet, while the occipitofrontal diameter of the head lies at a right angle to the cervical portion of the spine, and the latter being markedly curved forward, the head is flexed in respect to the body.

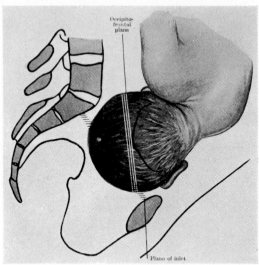

Fig. 119.—Anterior asynclitism (Nägele's obliquity, from DeLee).

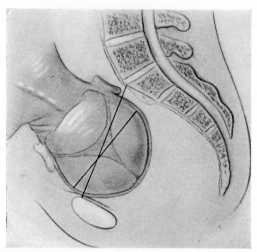

Fig. 120.—The head engaging. Beginning lateral flexion of the head on the body. The anterior parietal bone impinging upon the symphysis. Beginning posterior asynclitism.

Synclitism is defined as the condition when the fetal head lies fairly straight on the neck, perhaps inclined a trifle laterally toward either shoulder, with sagittal suture lying midway between promontory and pubes (Fig. 118).

Anterior *asynclitism* occurs when the anterior parietal bone first descends into the pelvic brim, the sagittal suture moving toward the promontory and lateral flexion of the head increasing. Posterior asyn-

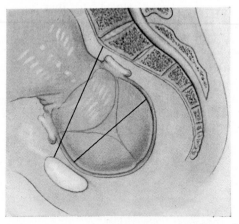

Fig. 121.—Engagement continues, posterior asynclitism increasing.

clitism is the reverse of this, the posterior parietal bone first descending and the sagittal suture moving toward the symphysis (Figs. 119, 120).

The sagittal suture lies usually in the transverse diameter of the brim but may be in one or the other oblique (Fig. 121).

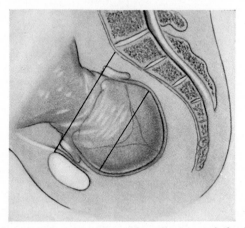

Fig. 122.—Complete engagement. The widest diameter of the head has passed beyond the true conjugate and synclitism is restored.

During engagement the posterior parietal eminence drops into the inlet, coming to rest beneath the promontory while the anterior parietal eminence is still above the symphysis, the sagittal suture lying well forward of the midtransverse diameter of the brim, and quite near the symphysis. This mechanism, called posterior asynclitism or Litzmann's obliquity (Fig. 122) is the common one as disclosed by the roentgenologic studies of Caldwell and Moloy, as directly opposed to the view held by Nägele in 1838, and since generally accepted, namely, that the sagittal suture normally is directed toward the promontory, with the anterior parietal bone first descending into the pelvis giving rise to anterior asynclitism or "the obliquity of Nägele." The writer is in accord with Caldwell and Moloy that the latter mechanism is uncommon and occurs only when a pendulous abdomen might direct the fetal head toward the posterior wall of the pelvis thereby permitting the anterior parietal bone to drop into the inlet (Fig. 123).

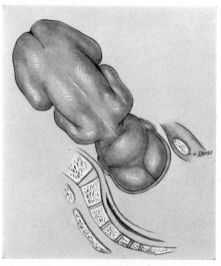

Fig. 123.—Normal engagement. Owing to the inclination of the pelvic brim, the posterior parietal bone of the fetus slips under the promontory and there comes to rest, while the anterior parietal bone is still above the symphysis.

As engagement proceeds, the obliquity of the plane of the pelvic brim to the long axis of the fetus becomes even more evident, so that in order to enter the brim the fetal head must descend below the promontory before it lies in contact with the inner aspect of the symphysis pubis. At this stage the posterior parietal bone remains at rest beneath or at the level of the promontory, while the anterior parietal bone descends behind the symphysis, the sagittal suture now being directed more nearly in the midtransverse of the pelvis, synclitism being restored and engagement completed.

Flexion.—In order to traverse the pelvic canal easily, it is necessary that the head present in extreme flexion, although complete extension may also permit its passage.

The purpose of flexion is obvious, there being presented to the birth canal a suboccipitobregmatic diameter of 9 cm. with a circumference of 31 cm., as opposed to an occipitofrontal diameter of 11 cm., with a circumference of 35 cm.

The fetal head before engagement lies usually in the transverse diameter of the pelvic brim, the occiput often slightly anterior to the brow. The head is midway between flexion and extension. It has already been shown that when the force of the uterine contractions force down both sinciput and occiput, the greater length of the former, in relation to its point of articulation with the spine, tends to greater resistance against the pelvic walls, and it is hence detained while the shorter occiput descends.

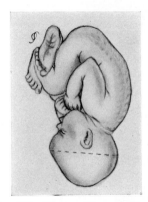

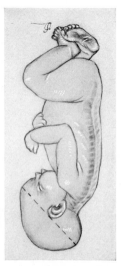

Fig. 124.—The position of the child before engagement. Note the curvature of the spine and the deflexed position of the head.

Fig. 125.—Showing the effect of uterine pressure with the consequent straightening of the fetal spine and its influence upon the production of flexion and anterior rotation.

Furthermore, the child lies at the brim with the spine markedly curved. When uterine contractions occur, the lateral pressure on the fetal body straightens the spine thus lengthening it, the resulting force being exerted upon the craniovertebral articulation, and forcing the occiput downward and forward. This mechanism is well shown in Figs. 124 and 125.

Molding.—The head of the fetus, just before term, is rounded, the vertex of the cranium of an almost spherical form, obviously not well fitted to be thrust through a curved and resistant canal. The constantly recurring force of the uterine contractions slowly driving the vertex into the pelvis causes the cranial vault to yield to the pressure of the surrounding uterine and pelvic walls, with the result that the bones comprising the vault override each other sometimes to a marked extent. This is possible because ossification of the cranial sutures is incomplete, the connection between the bones being very loose, and the fascial covering quite elastic. In vertex presentations the face and forehead are flattened, and the frontal bones and the occipitals are overlapped by the two parietals which in turn overlap, that one which is first subjected to the pressure of the sacral promontory being depressed under the other. As a result of these processes, the head assumes a long, bluntly conical ovoid form, the occipitofrontal diameter much increased, the biparietal and suboccipitobregmatic correspondingly decreased. This is called molding and is

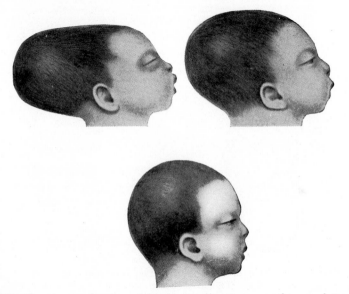

Fig. 126.—Caput succedaneum at birth; its disappearance three and ten days later. (Williams, "Obstetrics," D. Appleton-Century Co., Publishers.)

essential to spontaneous delivery in cases where the fetus is of full size and growth and the pelvis normal in contour. When it does not occur, either by reason of postmaturity of the fetus with the attendant advance in cranial ossification, or as a result of pathologic presentation—brow, face, etc.—dystocia generally results. A sequel of molding is the occurrence of numerous minute hemorrhages in the dura and in the periosteum, these bleedings being traumatic, but rarely giving rise to symptoms unless the hemorrhage be excessive.

That portion of the presenting vertex which is in contact with the soft or dilated cervix and is therefore most free from pressure develops a localized, boggy, edematous swelling of the soft tissue overlying the cranial bones. This swelling is called a caput succedaneum and is located upon the most dependent portion of the head, usually the inner surface of the parietal and the anterior part of the occipital bones. The swelling is due to an infiltration of the subcutaneous connective tissue and of the tissues beneath the galea, with a serosanguineous transudate, accompanied by ecchymoses in the skin and hematomas of varying size in all layers of the scalp. It is now generally assumed that the caput is the expression of the difference between the atmospheric and the intra-uterine pressure, greatly increased during each uterine contraction (Fig. 126). The location of the caput is naturally directly dependent upon the position and presentation of the child during labor and can therefore be utilized immediately after birth to determine what variety of mechanism of labor was operative.

Following flexion, molding and engagement, the head, impelled by the force of the uterine contraction acting upon the fetal spinal column, begins to descend in the pelvis. In primiparae, if the vertex has entered the pelvic brim several weeks before the onset of labor, the head lies much lower in the pelvis than among multiparae in whom engagement rarely occurs before the first stage of labor begins. In either event, descent once begun continues in association with the other movements of the presenting part, to be described, until delivery occurs.

Descent and Rotation.—*Descent.*—Engagement being completed, the increasing force of the uterine contractions bring about descent.

Since the uterus contracts equally in all directions the force is equally distributed through the bag of waters, but there is a noncontractile area, the lower uterine segment, with an opening at its inferior point, the cervical canal. Hence the force of the contraction tends to impel the contents of the uterus, first into the nonresistant portion and finally into the opening, which dilates to receive them as a result of the pressure from above.

The fetal body is elastic, and one of the first effects of pressure exerted upon it from all directions except from below is to straighten the curved spine, before alluded to, and to convert the body into as nearly a straight cylinder as possible. This straightening, which is very apparent on *x*-ray examination, is opposed by the direct pressure of the fundus uteri upon the buttocks of the child.

The uterine contractions naturally force the fluid contained within the membranes into the spaces and crevices about the neck of the child, leaving little or no fluid in the fundus, which naturally comes into contact with the buttocks and forces them downward, thus tending in some measure to again bend the spine since the pressure of the slowly yielding cervix opposes the rapid descent of the head.

By the power of the uterine muscles, then, the head is steadily forced into the opening of the gradually dilating cervix and out into the cavity of the pelvis. Synchronously with this descent, there begins another phase of the mechanism, namely, internal rotation.

13

Summary of Descent.—Descent is the inevitable resultant of four sets of forces:

1. The intra-uterine fluid pressure of the liquor amnii.
2. Direct pressure of the contracting fundus upon the buttocks of the child.
3. The voluntary contraction of the abdominal muscles.
4. The straightening and extension of the fetal spine.

As descent proceeds, flexion becomes more marked, the force of the uterine contractions acting to thrust down both sinciput and occiput into equal resistance, the longer lever arm of the sinciput being detained while the occiput descends.

Internal rotation is the turning of the head from the oblique into the anteroposterior diameter of the pelvis, and represents the most marked difference between the mechanism of labor in man and the lower animals. In the latter the long, wedge-shaped head of the fetus, without frontal prominence, and the extreme inclination of the pelvis permit the head to slide through the long anteroposterior diameter without twisting or rotation. In man the development of the forebrain with its high frontal bulge and the reduction of the obliquity of the pelvis renders it necessary that the head should enter in one diameter—the oblique, and leave in another—the anteroposterior. Internal rotation begins when the most dependent portion of the head meets the resistance of the pelvic floor and the cause of the movement has caused great debate among obstetricians. The older view was that the shape of the pelvis alone determined the turning, inasmuch as the superior strait presents a long, transverse diameter and the inferior strait a long anteroposterior one. However, when the coccyx is displaced backward in labor, the outlet develops a nearly circular outline and therefore rotation would not be necessary to secure delivery.

The first impulse toward internal rotation is probably due to the fact that the convex maternal lumbar spine tends to thrust the body of the fetus forward and as the vertebral column of the child is straightened as before described, it exerts pressure upon the occipital condyles, tending to force the occiput forward (Fig. 127). This movement is aided by the bulge of the rectum in the left bay of the sacrum which tends still further to force the occiput anteriorly. As descent continues, the flexed occiput comes into contact with the musculofascial slings of the pelvic floor and with the spine of the ischium upon which it further turns forward.

The upper portion of the pelvic floor represents a curved plane running forward, downward, and inward. These directions, therefore, are imposed upon any movable body impinging upon the pelvic floor and impelled by a force from above.

In addition to these inclined planes of the pelvic muscles and fasciae, there is the contour of the bony pelvis which practically follows the same direction. The spine of the ischia projects sharply into the lumen of the pelvis and anterior to the spine, the sides of the pelvis curve gently downward, forward and inward, thus forming a part of the lateral inclined planes.

The pelvic floor, or that portion of it composed of the levator ani muscle, forms a sort of trough or sling down which the occiput slips until it is directed under the pubes, the long axis of the fetal head adapting itself to the long axis of the trough in which it lies, *i. e.*, anteroposteriorly. It has been shown that the occiput is generally lower than the sinciput, owing to the flexion of the head, and therefore it is the first portion of the fetal ellipse to meet the resistance of

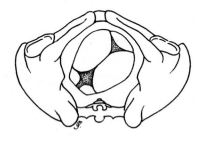

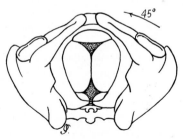

Fig. 127.—The mechanism of labor in L. O. A. Internal, anterior rotation of the occiput as palpated through the vagina.

the pelvic floor and to be impelled along the lines of the pelvic planes until it has rotated through one eighth of a circle and the sagittal suture lies directly anteroposteriorly. Sellheim's careful studies led him to develop another theory of internal rotation, which unquestionably plays some part in the production of this complicated phenomenon.

Sellheim regarded the fetal body as a compressed cylinder, flexible in certain limited directions. The trunk cannot move freely anteroposteriorly because of the morphology of the spinal column and the lateral pressure of the arms and legs, but it bends easily from side to side. The head bends freely on the neck from before backward by extension, and it also has a slight lateral elasticity. It will be seen that the lateral bending of the trunk and the anteroposterior bending of the head form two lines of direction which cross each other at right angles.

Now if the cylindrical fetus is to pass through the sharply curved birth canal it must rotate on its long axis so as to bring the portion in which bending can most easily occur into line with the axis of the pelvic canal, or until the nape of the neck is adapted to the knee of the canal. Or as Colonel Buchanan puts it, "The secret of success is whether you get the pivotal points together." Descent continues during internal rotation, the whole movement being a spiral thrust of the fetus through the pelvic canal (Fig. 128).

Disengagement, Extension and Birth of the Head.—Internal rotation being completed, the sharply flexed head reaches the vulva and

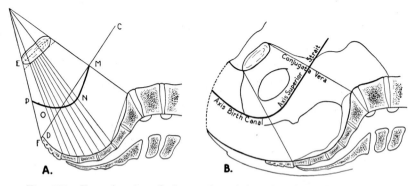

Fig. 128.—Two theories of the static pelvic axis. (A) "Curve of Carus" (redrawn from Bedford, 1861) representing the midpoint of planes from symphysis; CD, axis of superior strait; EF, plane of inferior strait; MNP, central curved line. Earlier obstetricians assumed that the width of the symphysis formed the anterior boundary of the true pelvis rather than the entire depth of the fore pelvis. (B) Straight axis perpendicular to inlet to level of spines. (Redrawn from Williams, 1930.) This theory does not regard the relationship to the inclination of the sacrum. Other authorities have pointed out this fact, but failed to define the axis clearly from the anatomical standpoint. (Caldwell, Moloy and D'Esopo, Amer. Jour. of Obstet. and Gynec., Dec., 1935, C. V. Mosby Co., Publishers.)

then undergoes another essential movement, that of extension. At this time the occiput is under and beyond the pubis, the nape of the neck lying under the arch of the pubis and the forehead has passed beyond the coccyx. Now the resultant of two forces, the pressure of the uterine contraction from above and the elastic resistances of the musculofascial sling forming the pelvic floor from below, begins to act, and the parietal eminences being held firmly by pressure of the lateral fibers of the levator ani near the pubis, the chin leaves the chest, the occiput appears in front of the pubis, the brow greatly distends the outer portion of the perineum and is born by continued extension, the bregma, forehead, nose, mouth, and finally the chin escaping over the greatly stretched anterior aspect of the perineum. Immediately

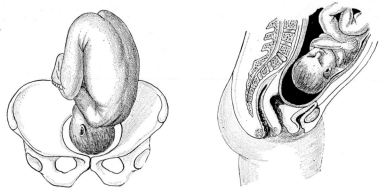

Fig. 129.—The mechanism of labor in L. O. A. The head above the brim, before engagement.

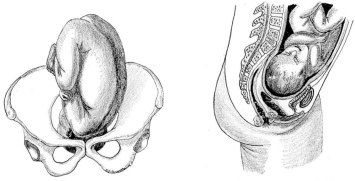

Fig. 130.—The mechanism of labor in L. O. A. The head engaged in the inlet.

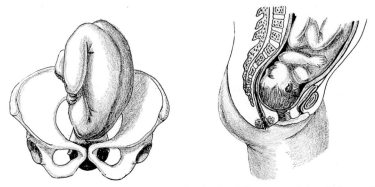

Fig. 131.—The mechanism of labor in L. O. A. The engaged head descending. Internal rotation going on. Flexion complete.

after birth the head falls forward, the chin coming into contact with the anal region (Figs. 129, 130, 131).

Restitution.—As soon as the head is born in a L. O. A. the chin rotates slightly to the mother's right, the sagittal suture resuming the oblique position in which it lay before internal rotation occurred. This movement is simply an untwisting of the neck and a return to the normal tonicity of the two sternocleidomastoid muscles, the left

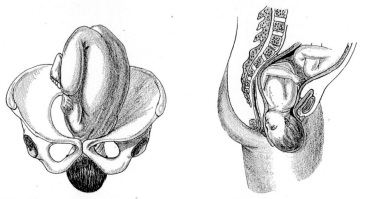

Fig. 132.—The mechanism of labor in L. O. A.   The head delivered by extension.

side of the neck having been placed in considerable tension during internal rotation (Figs. 132 and 133).

External Rotation.—This is the movement imparted to the head by the internal rotation of the shoulders, which does not occur synchronously with that of the head.   The shoulders lie in the pelvis in

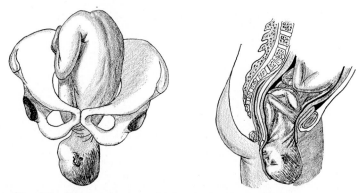

Fig. 133.—The mechanism of labor in L. O. A.   External rotation.

the opposite oblique to that occupied by the sagittal suture.   The anterior or right shoulder, being lower than the posterior or left, strikes the pelvic floor first, and in obedience to the same law of rotation that governed the head, the shoulder moves forward, downward and inward, until the bisacromial diameter lies in the anterior-posterior axis of the pelvis. The shoulder, moving from right to left, naturally transmits its line of movement to the head, the sagittal suture being always at right angles to the bisacromial line. The head, therefore, turns further toward the mother's right until the face points directly to the right thigh.

Restitution and external rotation frequently take place in such rapid sequence that they are practically one continuous movement and are quite commonly so described (Fig. 134).

Birth of the Shoulders.—Complete rotation of the shoulders having occurred, descent continues with the uterine contractions until the right or anterior shoulder stems under the symphysis and is there delayed. The downward force continuing, the posterior or left shoulder sweeps over the perineum by a process of lateral flexion of the spine, to be delivered, following which the anterior shoulder slips from under the symphysis and is rapidly extruded.

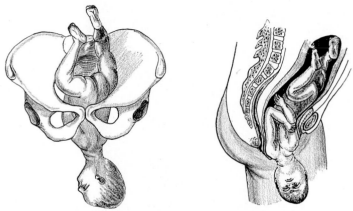

Fig. 134.—The mechanism of labor in L. O. A. Delivery of the shoulders.

Birth of the Body.—After expulsion of the shoulders, the fetal body undergoes a marked lateral flexion and rapidly sweeps through the cavity, its concave side above, the convex below, thus conforming to the curve of the pelvic basin, and is easily and rapidly delivered. The mechanism of right occiput anterior position is identical with that of the left, the words "right" and "left" being simply interchanged.

The Mechanism of the Third Stage of Labor.—The birth of the placenta and membranes comprises two distinct mechanisms, separation of the placenta from the uterine wall, and extrusion of the organ (Fig. 135). Separation does not begin until after the birth of the child, the placenta remaining firmly fixed in situ until after this event, the intra-uterine pressure being an important factor in maintaining this relationship. During labor there is a slight decrease in the area of the cavity of the uterus due to its contraction, and the placenta, accommodating itself to this smaller site of attachment, becomes thicker, its margins rounded. At this time there is probably a slight separation of the central portion of the placenta from the uterine wall with rupture of the vessels in the spongiosa and a small hematoma behind the center of the organ. When the child has been delivered the uterus is greatly decreased in size, and the placenta, being contracted parallel with its uterine attachment, has become almost twice as thick as at the onset of labor.

According to the studies of Frankel there is at this time a sharp rush of blood into the placental site, which, acting like a hydraulic

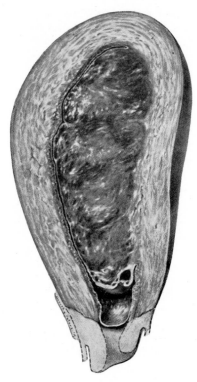

Fig. 135.—Vertical section through uterus removed by supravaginal hysterectomy following cesarean section ($\times$ $^2/_3$). Note thickness of muscle walls, increase in thickness of placenta, and decrease in area of its attachment. (Williams, "Obstetrics," D. Appleton-Century Co., Publishers.)

wedge, serves to separate further the placenta from the uterine wall. Intra-uterine pressure being relieved, there is nothing to hold the placenta in contact with the uterine wall and separation continues with considerable rapidity. Eventually the placenta becomes so thick and contracted that it can no longer follow the steadily diminishing uterine site, and is peeled off from the uterine wall, the separation being greatly aided by the pressure of the growing retroplacental hematoma. The line of division of the placenta from the uterus is in the spongiosa of the decidua serotina. In the meantime the membranes have been pulled from the decidua by the diminution in size of the contracting and retracting uterus, and are thrown into many folds in what remains of the uterine cavity (Figs. 136 and 137).

Expulsion of the placenta occurs when separation is complete, or nearly so, and is caused by additional uterine contractions forcing this organ against the internal os and then through the cervical canal, which is already beginning to reform, until the placenta lies in the

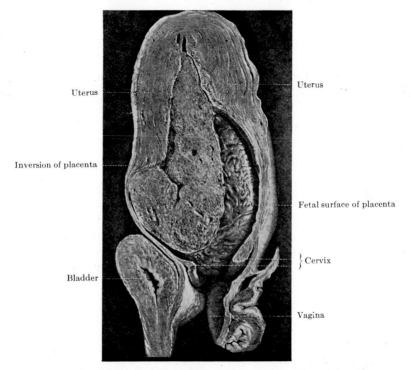

Uterus

Uterus

Inversion of placenta

Fetal surface of placenta

} Cervix

Bladder

Vagina

Fig. 136.—Third stage of labor. Right half of uterus. Placenta partly separated and inverted, with fetal surface presenting at os. Unequal contraction of fundus indicates placental separation by muscular contraction with absence of the traditional retroplacental hematoma. (Titus and Andrews, Amer. Jour. of Obstet. and Gynec., vol. 7, 1924, C. V. Mosby Co., Publishers.)

lower portion of the cervix and the vagina. Now the abdominal muscles contract voluntarily and the placenta escapes from the vulva, the membranes trailing after it, sometimes still adherent to the uterine wall.

Two mechanisms have been described for the expulsion of the placenta. The first is that of Schultze, in which the placenta turns inside out, umbrellawise, the cord and the fetal surface appearing at the cervix and the placental cone, closely apposed to the circumference of the cervix being pushed through the external os, the membranes following (Fig. 138). The second mechanism of expulsion is that described by Matthews Duncan, in which the separated placenta slides down the uterine wall, its relation remaining unchanged, until the lower edge appears at the external os, from which it is extruded, followed by the rest of the organ (Fig. 139). The placenta usually

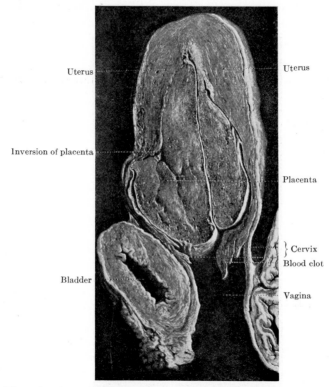

Fig. 137.—Third stage of labor. Mesial section through uterus. Placenta rolled on itself and sectioned in such a way as to show a membranous septum, with fetal surface presenting at external os. Marked muscular contraction of upper portion of uterus, lower segment still thinned out. (Titus and Andrews, Amer. Jour. of Obstet. and Gynec., vol. 7, 1924, C. V. Mosby Co., Publishers.)

escapes from the vulva by the Schultze mechanism, but the statements of Warnekros and Weibel are rather convincing as to the method of separation of the organ from the uterine wall. These writers cut the cord immediately after the birth of the child and injected the placenta with a fluid opaque to the x-ray. Immediate roentgenograms showed that the placenta always passed through the lower uterine segment edge first, that separation occurred early, after a very few uterine contractions, and that there was but little evidence of the retro-placental blood clot. They maintained that the placenta always leaves

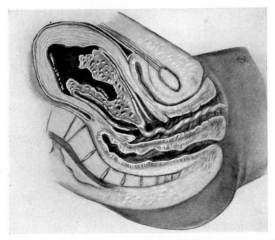

Fig. 138.—Mechanism of the third stage of labor. Schultze's method of expulsion of the placenta.

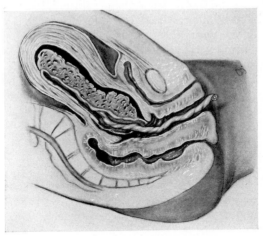

Fig. 139.—Mechanism of the third stage of labor. Duncan method of expulsion of the placenta.

the uterus in this way, and that the mechanisms of Schultze and Duncan only develop in the vagina.

CHAPTER XIII

THE CLINICAL COURSE OF LABOR

Labor has been defined as the resultant of certain forces of expulsion in opposition to other forces of resistance.

Clinically the advent of labor is foreshadowed in primiparae by the occurrence of *lightening*, when the presenting part sinks into the pelvic brim. This takes place from two to three weeks before term and is noticed by the patient in that certain discomforts to which she has grown accustomed are relieved while new ones replace them. Thus the crowding upward of the diaphragm, with its dyspnea, epigastric fulness and digestive disturbances is much ameliorated. On the other hand, pressure of the descending head upon the bladder causes urinary distress and the same pressure exerted upon the nerves of the pelvis produces sciatic pain and a sense of bearing down. Lightening is not particularly noted by multiparae, nor does the figure change in those women as it does in primiparae, when the descent of the fetus occasions a definite change in the abdominal contours.

In both primi- and multiparous women the painless uterine contractions which have been present during the late months of pregnancy become more or less noticeable in the week or ten days preceding term and in many instances they become severe enough to be termed false labor. The only differentiation between these premonitory pains and actual labor is the fact that they are usually irregular, and cease spontaneously after several hours. True labor is ushered in by (*a*) uterine contractions, recurrent in type, painful, and steadily increasing in severity and decreasing as to the intervals between them; (*b*) the escape of a small amount of blood-tinged mucus from the vagina; (*c*) dilatation of the cervix.

Stages of Labor.—Clinically, labor is divided into three stages, the first, from the onset until the cervix is completely dilated and effaced. The second, from the complete dilation of the cervix to the expulsion of the child and, third, from the delivery of the child until the placenta has been ejected.

The *length of labor* varies in different individuals and during different pregnancies from a few minutes to several days, a rough average duration being eighteen hours in primiparae and twelve hours in multiparae. Of this time, the first stage in primiparae average sixteen hours, the second one and three-quarter hours and the third one-quarter hour, while in multiparae the ratios are eleven hours, three-quarter hour and one-quarter hour, respectively.

It is obvious that so many variables enter into the mechanism of labor that the time factor must remain indefinite. The nature of the uterine muscles, whether irritable and active or sluggish, the state of the cervix, whether soft and pliable or dense and resistant; the proportion between fetus and pelvis; the presentation and position; the degree of molding attained by the head; the form and elasticity of the muscles and fasciae of the pelvic floor; all of these factors tend to vary the length of labor. Heredity, race and age also enter into the problem as witness Pharaoh's midwives, who gave as their excuse for not destroying the men children of the Hebrews the fact that "the Hebrew women are not as the Egyptian women, for they are lively and are delivered ere the midwives come in unto them."

The First Stage.—(a) The pains are at first worst in the back, gradually involving the entire uterine area and extending upward toward the umbilicus. They occur at first at irregular intervals—ten to twenty minutes, steadily growing closer until they are separated by three or four minutes. At this time the woman may be moving about, or resting, apparently undisturbed until a pain comes on, when she contracts her facial muscles sets her teeth, the eyes become suffused and she may bend over to compress the abdomen, often emitting a slight groan at the height of the pain. If the abdomen be palpated at this moment, the uterus will be felt as a hard, firm globular mass, relaxing as soon as the contraction has ceased.

(b) During pregnancy the cervical canal is closed by a plug of tenacious mucus. With the beginning of cervical dilatation and effacement small blood vessels are torn and the mucus plug, now blood stained, is loosened from its attachment to the cervical mucosa and escapes from the vagina as a bloody, gelatinous mass, known to the laity as the "show" and rightly regarded as a valuable sign of beginning labor. Sometimes the mucus is detached and expelled by the premonitory pain, so that its discovery is not absolute evidence of true labor.

(c) Dilatation of the cervical canal and effacement of the cervix, when clearly demonstrable are the most reliable signs of beginning labor, although here again, cases are recorded whenever the cervix dilated up to several centimeters, but has later retracted and remained undilated for some days.

The first stage of labor being thus established, the pains steadily become more severe and of longer duration, the woman crying or moaning in distress. On palpation the uterus during a pain, is felt as a globular mass almost boardlike in its hardness, the contractions beginning before pain is experienced and lasting a few moments after the pain has passed.

The patient is anxious and restless and often desires to pace the room, stepping to lean over the footboard of the bed in an effort to relieve her agony. If lying down she rolls about on the bed, turning on her side with legs flexed on the abdomen during the uterine contractions. After some hours of increasing discomfort, the clinical picture changes.

The Second Stage.—The patient, feeling a pain coming on, braces herself, seeks for something upon which she may pull and with a moan, contracts her abdominal muscles in an endeavor to expel the foreign body in her pelvis. The face is flushed, the eyes suffused, the brow beaded with perspiration, the veins of the forehead and neck stand out and the whole picture is that of violent effort. The diaphragm is fixed, the teeth clenched, and the breath held while the expulsive straining goes on. Suddenly the air is expelled from the lungs with a characteristic grunting sound, the diaphragm and the abdominal muscles are again relaxed, while a full breath is taken, when the straining again begins until the uterine contraction has ceased. At this time, if left to herself, the patient is apt to assume a squatting position on the floor or bed, in an instinctive attempt to increase the diameter of the pelvic outlet and to enable the abdominal muscles to exert their

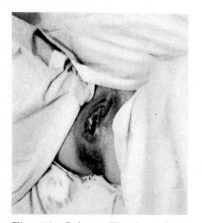

Fig. 140.—Labor. The head beginning to separate the pillars of the vulva. Note the dilatation of the anus.

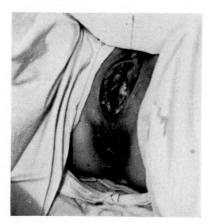

Fig. 141.—Labor. The head being born by extension.

utmost contractile force. At this time the membranes usually rupture, with a gush of liquor amnii. Vaginal examination at this stage of labor will disclose the cervix completely dilated and slipped back over the child's head, which now fills the cavity of the pelvis making strong pressure on the perineal floor, pushing the rectum backward and the bladder forward.

Inspection shows the perineum flattened and bulging, the rectum everted; usually with a crown of distended hemorrhoids surrounding the anus. The vulvar outlet gapes a little and is bathed with bloody mucus while small amounts of feces may be squeezed out of the anus (Fig. 140).

As the pains come on, the vulva dilates and the wrinkled scalp of the child comes into view. At each contraction more of the head appears, distending the vulvar outlet, only to disappear in the interval between contractions, as the elastic tissues of the perineum push it back (Fig. 141). This process may continue for from twenty minutes to an hour, the slow stretching and alternate relaxation of the perineum being Nature's prophylaxis against laceration. Presently the widest, biparietal diameter of the head passes the outlet, the occiput emerges from under the symphysis, the forehead, brow and face slip over the perineum as the head extends and with a shriek of agony from the patient, the head is born (Fig. 142).

Then follows a short cessation of uterine contraction, while the patient lies quietly recuperating her forces for the completion of the delivery. The livid, cyanotic head protrudes from the vagina, the face turning toward one or the other thigh of the mother, the phenomenon termed restitution.

The child during this period is in no danger, its placental circulation being intact. In a few minutes the labor pains recur, and as the

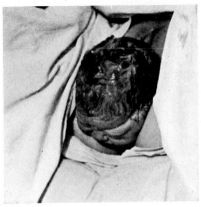

Fig. 142.—Labor. The head delivered. Note the contraction of the fetal facial muscles.

shoulders within the pelvis undergo rotation, the head is observed to turn further and further to the side until it lies practically transverse. Then, the expulsive force continuing, the anterior shoulder appears under the symphysis pubis; the posterior shoulder distends the perineum and finally slips over it and emerges. The anterior shoulder then escapes and is rapidly followed by the body of the child, which is too small to offer further resistance. The birth is announced by a gasping respiration or two, followed by a lusty cry and a rapid disappearance of the cyanosis.

As soon as the child is born, the woman becomes quiet and relaxed and may have a chill, which is probably nervous in origin.

The relief from intense suffering is so great and the rest from extreme muscular effort so grateful, that the patient rests happily, serene in the knowledge that she has passed through her travail, and that for the present at least, the world holds no further terrors for her.

The Third Stage.—After fifteen or twenty minutes have passed, during which the muscle bundles of the uterus are being rearranged, the third stage of labor begins. There is another onset of labor pains, not so severe however. The uterus which has lain flat in the abdomen now rises and appears as a dense round mass about the level of the umbilicus. This is the fundus now engaged in expressing the placenta which has become detached. This structure now escapes from the vulva either in the form of an inverted umbrella, the cord in the center, the method of Schultze, or it emerges sideways, one edge appearing first, as described by Matthews Duncan. The membranes are dragged out with the placenta as a sort of train.

With the expulsion of the placenta, labor is over and the puerperium begins. Examination of the patient at this time reveals a woman lying exhausted and relaxed, but content. The pulse may be rapid from the recent exertion. The temperature is slightly elevated from the same cause.

The abdomen is flat and soft, the uterus a hard globe, reaching almost to the umbilicus and easily movable from side to side.

The vulva is slightly swollen, with a slight trickle of blood, mixed with liquor amnii.

The general impression is that of a patient who is recuperating from very exhausting physical strain.

CHAPTER XIV

THE CONDUCT OF LABOR

DUTIES OF THE PATIENT—PREPARATION FOR DELIVERY IN THE HOME

Engagement of the Nurse.—The expectant mother should engage the services of a nurse, as early in pregnancy as possible, the nurse to be of the best training and experience consonant with the social condition and financial standing of the family.

Many women prefer that the obstetrician select for them a nurse of his choice and it is well for him to have a list of skilled and competent women, trained nurses if possible, with some so-called "practical nurses" to care for the less affluent women under his care.

Articles Required for Home Delivery.—Long before the calculated date of confinement, the patient should have gathered the materials for the conduct of labor under aseptic conditions. These articles are as follows:

2 white enameled basins
1 two-quart enameled pitcher
½ pound surgical absorbent cotton
1 box vaginal pads
1 pair white stockings
4 ounces saturated solution boric acid
1 bucket for waste
1 square rubber sheeting, 36-inch
6 squares
6 towels (may be old)
1 sheet (may be old)
2 ounce lysol
1 douche pan

The sheet, towels and stockings are to be wrapped separately in muslin, in neat packages and baked in the oven for one-half hour on three consecutive days. This will satisfactorily cleanse the linen, which, however, is not to be considered as sterile.

At the time of delivery abundant boiled water, both hot and cold, should be in readiness.

The Lying-in Room.—This should be the sunniest and best ventilated bedroom available, though in summer a cooler room is preferable. Excess furniture and heavy hangings should be removed although it is not necessary to dismantle the chamber to simulate the actual bareness of a hospital operating room.

At the time of delivery, the carpet should be protected by a thick layer of newspaper and care should be taken to protect furniture against the scars of chemicals or utensils containing hot water.

At the very onset of labor, the patient should be instructed to have the genitals shaved. This may be done by the nurse or by a member of the family. After shaving a simple soap-suds enema is taken, unless the pains are strong and tumultuous, and labor seems imminent.

Under such condition, it is far better to have the bed soiled with formed feces than to permit liquid matter to flow about the pudendal region, with possible vaginal infection.

Next in order is a bath, *not in the tub,* but a warm shower if available, otherwise a general washing with soap and water in which the patient is assisted by the nurse or attendant. If the membranes are ruptured the bath is omitted. After the bath the woman is clothed in a clean nightgown and repairs to the delivery room, in which the bed has been moved into a convenient position, with a board inserted under the mattress to keep the springs from sagging during the efforts of labor.

PREPARATIONS OF THE PHYSICIAN

The Obstetric Satchel.—In remote districts the obstetrician must carry with him sufficient instruments and supplies to enable him to cope with any obstetric emergency. This is doubly true of the specialist who may be called into consultation in cases of dystocia.

However, the greater part of the United States is now abundantly supplied with hospitals and the universal spread of excellent highways makes transportation of patients entirely practicable, so that it is far better not to attempt formidable operative procedures in the home, when convenient hospital facilities are available.

The supplies needed for the general practice of home obstetrics are as follows:

FOR ASEPSIS

Two sterile hand brushes.
One surgeon's gown and cap.
One white duck suit.
Four pairs sterile rubber gloves.
Four ounces lysol.
Three jars sterile gauze and cotton sponges.
Four ounces 90 per cent alcohol.

MEDICINES

One quart of ether.
One ounce of fluidextract of ergot.
Six ampules of ergot
Three of pituitrin.
Three of sterile camphorated oil.
Two ampules 1 per cent $AgNO_3$.
A working hypodermic syringe with tablets of morphine and scopolamine

SUNDRIES

Linen bobbin (sterile) for cord.
Six tubes twenty-day catgut No. 2.
One wide-mouth jar with sterile silk gut.
One nickeled copper pan.
History sheets and cards for physician and nurse.
Birth certificates.
One sterile version sling.

INSTRUMENTS

One pair Simpson forceps.
Two scissors, long and short.
Four artery forceps, long and short.
One tissue forceps.
Two vulsella.
One long uterine packing forceps.
One broad retractor.
One box needles.
One needle-holder.
One head stethoscope.
One silver catheter.
One rubber catheter.
Two tracheal catheters.
One baby scale and tape measure.
One anesthetic mask.
One pelvimeter.
One Kelly pad.
One Arnold aspirator.

FOR POSTPARTUM HEMORRHAGE

One douche can and tube.
One salt solution needle.
Three 2-drachm bottles sterilized salt.
One package or tube 2-inch gauze packing.
One pack 4-inch gauze packing

All of the supplies may be carried in one large bag, although it is simple to convey the instruments and medicines, suture material, etc., in one small obstetric bag, while the linen, Kelly pad, packing and so on are contained in a small suitcase.

The Answer to the Call.—The patient, who in most instances should have enjoyed painstaking prenatal care by the physician for some months, is instructed to notify him immediately upon the occurrence of recurring abdominal pain, the expulsion of bloody mucus, or the rupture of the membranes, which frequently occurs independently of other signs of labor.

Immediate response to the call is an absolute obligation, since many of the intrapartum accidents to mother and child may be averted if the physician is present to observe the early course of labor. Having satisfied himself that no abnormalities have presented themselves and that a competent nurse is in attendance, the physician may leave, if in his opinion delivery will be long deferred, but his whereabouts should be known to the family so that he may be summoned at once when needed.

GENERAL PRINCIPLES CONCERNING THE CONDUCT OF LABOR

1. Labor being a process associated with traumatism and with the laceration of tissues, must be regarded as a surgical condition and must be conducted throughout in accordance with the details of absolute aseptic technic.

2. Every effort should be made to eliminate or minimize the suffering incident to childbirth.

3. Labor should be allowed to proceed and terminate spontaneously in every case wherein there is no definite indication for some variety of operative interference. [The wise statement that the first essential for a good obstetrician is to have fat buttocks and know how to sit on them, is attributed to Newell of Boston.]

4. When an indication for interference arises, that form of delivery should be selected which offers the least danger of mutilation or mortality of mother or child.

5. Operative interference should never be undertaken to serve the convenience of the accoucheur or to satisfy the demands of a patient or her family.

On the other hand in the presence of complications which render spontaneous delivery doubtful or impossible, bold interference should be practiced, before the resistance of the patient is lowered by exhaustion.

THE MANAGEMENT OF THE FIRST STAGE OF LABOR

Upon the arrival of the obstetrician, he should first reassure the anxious woman as to the successful outcome of her travail, and should then obtain an idea of her general physical condition. Pulse rate, blood pressure and temperature should be noted, the duration, character and spacing of the uterine contractions observed, after which the position and presentation of the child is rechecked by abdominal palpation and auscultation as described in Chapter X. Especial attention is paid to the rate and rhythm of the fetal heart tones. If the pelvis is known to be normal, from previous mensuration, and the head is firmly engaged, no vaginal examination is necessary at this time, although a single, careful examination will determine the degree of effacement and dilatation of the cervix, the state of the membranes and the exact position of the presenting part, together with the detection of any abnormality such as prolapse of the cord.

In late years rectal examination has gained many advocates, it being held that the probability of infection is greatly lessened by this maneuver and that equal or nearly equal information may be obtained.

With this view the author is not in accord, believing that a single vaginal examination well carried out is productive of more accurate knowledge of the pelvis and its contents than any number of rectal investigations. Furthermore, since the lower one third of the vagina has been shown to harbor pathologic bacteria, it seems reasonable that to rub the contaminated vaginal mucosa about the cervical orifice is possibly more likely to further infection than a properly conducted vaginal examination.

It is true that repeated palpation via the vagina is unwise and serves no useful purpose.

It is the practice of the writer to make one thorough vaginal examination early in labor and then content himself with a minimum number of rectal investigations, very gently carried out, and in most cases omitted entirely.

Technic of the Vaginal Examination.—The patient is draped with the knees flexed, and if very corpulent, is drawn across the bed, the buttocks at its edge, and the legs held by attendants who sit on either side of the woman.

The physician then rolls up his cuffs and scrubs with brush, soap and running water as for an operation. The hands are dried on a sterile towel, a sterile gown is donned and sterile gloves drawn on. The entire perineal area is then carefully scrubbed with soap and water and sterile cotton sponges, care being taken not to enter the vulvar orifice. The labia and the pudenda are then painted with an antiseptic—diluted tincture iodine, 4 per cent mercurochrome, metaphen or whatever solution best suits the individual practitioner. The gloves are now changed and with the finger of one hand separating the labia, the first and second fingers of the examining hand are introduced into the vagina, under the eye, and if possible not touching the external surfaces. By sweeping the finger about the pelvic cavity, its capacity may be ascertained, the resistence of the pelvic floor estimated, the amount of cervical effacement and dilatation discovered; whether or not the membranes have ruptured, the status of the head, the position of the fontanels and of the sagittal and other sutures. Should a labor pain come on while the fingers are in the vagina, the movement of the head may be learned as well as the progress of molding.

It is emphasized that one careful vaginal examination is sufficient in all cases, except when the development of dystocia renders further investigation imperative.

Technic of the Rectal Examination.—The patient being draped as above and the physician having scrubbed, a glove, preferably, but not necessarily sterile, is drawn on, anointed with petroleum or other lubricating jelly and one finger gently introduced into the rectum. With practice one can determine the effacement and dilation of the cervix, the position of the head, with its sutures and the station of the presenting part. The presence or absence of intact membranes is difficult to determine by this method, and the capacity of the pelvic cavity cannot be estimated.

Should labor be unexpectedly prolonged, rectal examination may be repeated to ascertain the cause of the dystocia.

The Information to be Gained by Vaginal Examination.—1. The shape and capacity of the pelvic cavity should be estimated, and checked against previous findings, q. v.

2. The degree of dilatation and effacement of the cervix is determined, it being well to estimate the diameter of the os in centimeters, rather than by "fingers."

3. The pouch of membranes is sought to learn whether or not

rupture has occurred. There is usually a little liquor amnii between the head and the membranes, which may be felt if they are intact. If ruptured, the rough hairy scalp will present itself to the examining finger.

4. The position and presentation is determined by palpating the sagittal suture and the fontanel or fontanels, this being only practicable when the cervix is sufficiently dilated to admit the finger. If this be the case, the sagittal suture may be felt as a ridge, curving over the fetal skull, but with a flat arc, as contrasted with the coronal or lambdoid sutures which are sharply curved.

The relation of the sagittal sutures to the promontory or to the symphysis, will determine the degree and nature of asynclitism if such be present.

The small fontanel is **Y** shaped and often is palpable as a little irregular elevation at one end of the sagittal suture. The anterior or greater fontanel is diamond shaped and much larger.

5. The station of the head is to be noted in relation to the spines of the ischia, the left one being usually selected. The presence or absence of engagement is a matter of great importance in primiparae. When the head lies free above the pelvic brim it is said to be floating. It is fixed when it is firmly lodged in the inlet and engaged when the widest biparietal diameter has passed the pelvic brim. At this time the lowest portion of the head has reached the spines of the ischia.

The head is in midplane when the vault of the cranium has reached the level of the tuberosities of the ischia and is at the outlet when the biparietal diameter has passed these bony prominences.

6. Abnormalities in presentation and position are carefully studied with the examining finger, and noted.

7. The passage of meconium mixed with liquor amnii in a head presentation is a danger sign of impending fetal asphyxia. In a breech presentation meconium merely indicates pressure upon the abdomen of the child and is much less significant.

8. The condition of the pelvic floor, whether rigid and resistant or soft and elastic, is observed.

The examination being completed, the obstetrician should again assure the patient that all is well and that the labor is pursuing its normal course. Any evidence of presumable complication should be reported to the family, out of the hearing of the woman, and the suggestion made that possibly consultation will be necessary should this eventuality be considered probable by the physician.

The husband and relatives are usually much concerned about the duration of labor and the physician must tactfully explain that while this cannot be accurately determined in hours and minutes, so long as the pains continue with increasing force, that delivery will not be long delayed, whereas should they diminish in frequency and intensity, considerable time may be required. It is never wise to commit oneself to a specific time limit in so variable a process.

The first stage of labor is managed by watchful expectancy on the part of the physician, with frequent abdominal palpation to determine progress and regular half-hourly auscultation of the fetal heart tones. This precaution is of great importance, since the condition of the child may be accurately followed by the rate and rhythm of the heart sounds. Irregularity and wide variation in rate should predicate imminent danger to fetal life and call for delivery as soon as practicable.

The bladder should be emptied every four hours, by catheter, if need be, since a distended bladder is a common cause for delay in the second stage as well as errors in rotation or flexion.

If the labor is a long one, simple soap-suds enemata, every twelve hours, will serve to keep the rectum empty and prevent obstruction from this cause.

Abundant fluid intake is advisable, water, milk and sweetened drinks, maintaining the water balance and anticipating acidosis.

Light food should be given at regular intervals, to keep up the woman's strength and to prevent the profound exhaustion and relaxation which so often follow a long and difficult delivery.

As soon as the pains become strong and the woman begins to complain some form of analgesia should be instituted. Relief from pain is every mother's right and the recognition of this fact by the medical profession and the development of so many successful methods for achieving it is one of the signal advances of modern obstetrics. Barnes has well said that during labor one should not study how much a woman can endure, but what she can accomplish.

So important is this matter of analgesia and anesthesia that the whole subject has been considered in detail in Chapter XV to which attention is directed.

Many women seek to shorten labor by bearing down efforts during the first stage of labor, and nurses are apt to encourage this practice. The patient is to be instructed not to bear down at all until she feels the urge to do so, since premature expulsive effort leads to early exhaustion of the abdominal muscles which are then incapable of exertion when their added force is needed in the second stage. Also, forcing down a fetus against an undilated cervix tends to stretch the uterine ligaments and may facilitate the occurrence of prolapse later in life.

CONDUCT OF THE SECOND STAGE

At this time in a properly managed labor, the patient will be under the influence of an analgesic, lying quietly in bed, tossing and moving at the height of a pain. The uterine contractions are strong and succeed each other with great rapidity until presently the wrinkled scalp comes into view. The woman meanwhile has been contracting the abdominal muscles and bearing down with her pain, an effort which goes on even through the dulled senses of narcotized patients.

If left to her own devices, the woman, if not narcotized, would now probably instinctively seek a squatting position to widen the pelvic outlet and to increase the force of the abdominal muscles by flexing the thighs against the abdomen as a brace. The squatting position may be simulated to some extent in bed, by an exaggerated lithotomy position, the legs held in place by attendants.

As the scalp parts the labia and progresses further and further with each uterine contraction only to recede in the interval, the obstetrician should "stand and wait," as manipulations at this time are of no avail. Feces appearing at the anus may be wiped away by a backward sweep of a cotton sponge, care being taken not to soil the gloved

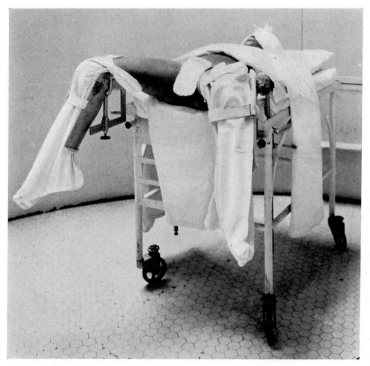

Fig. 143.—Patient prepared for delivery before draping. Piper leg holders.

hand. The perineal region may now be recleansed with soap and water, followed by painting with 4 per cent mercurochrome, 5 per cent tincture of iodine or other antiseptic solution, after which sterile drapes are applied (Fig. 144). Presently the broadest part of the fetal head, the biparietal diameter, appears at the vulva. Now the obstetrician makes firm pressure on the head, pushing the occiput upward against the symphysis, in order to relieve the distended perineum from pressure (Fig. 145). If the woman is sufficiently conscious to obey instructions she should be instructed not to bear down, but to relax and breathe through her mouth. As the pelvic floor distends and delivery becomes imminent, the perineum should be protected by the free hand of the obstetrician, who places the thumb on one side of the perineum and the first and second fingers on the opposite side, making two

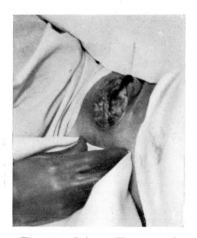

Fig. 144.—Labor. The protection of the perineum with thumb and forefinger. For illustrative purposes, the perineum is shown undraped.

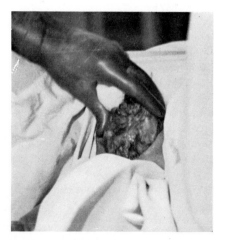

Fig. 145.—Too rapid delivery of the head being retarded by pressure upon the occiput.

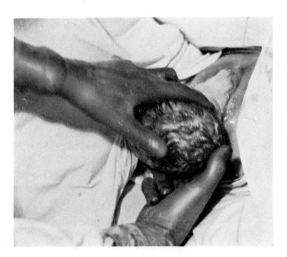

Fig. 146.—Labor. The anterior shoulder stemming under the symphysis.

points against which the fetal head may impinge and be forced forward, thus taking the strain off the perineum itself. At this time episiotomy may be done if thought advisable (Fig. 146).

Episiotomy.—In 1742 Fielding Ould proposed to cut the perineum to facilitate delivery and ever since this practice has been followed more or less. In 1918 Pomeroy of Brooklyn suggested its routine performance in primiparae and his plan has received wide support (Fig. 147).

Episiotomy is a valuable measure in that it replaces a ragged and irregular laceration by a sharp-edged, incised wound which may be placed where it will do the least harm, even if its limits be extended by the passage of an overly large or badly flexed head.

It is by no means necessary to cut the perineum in all patients. Many multiparae possess such relaxed and elastic vaginal outlets that no lacerations occur and in a considerable number of primiparae, particularly younger women, the tissues are sufficiently distensible to permit delivery without injury or at worst with so small a laceration in the fourchette as to require but little effort for its repair. How-

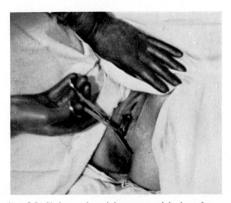

Fig. 147.—Mediolateral episiotomy with bandage scissors.

ever, in many cases episiotomy is of great value in preserving the integrity of the pelvic floor.

Time of Performance.—Episiotomy should not be done until the head is crowning, so that the elasticity of the perineum may be observed and the relative size of the head made known.

If mid or high forceps operation or version is planned, it is well to incise the pelvic floor before introducing the instruments or the hand, as laceration frequently occurs at this time.

There are three sites for the episiotomy:

    a. Median—from the introitus directly backward in the midline, to within 1 cm. of the anal margin.

    b. Mediolateral—from slightly to one side or the other of the midline and carried obliquely outward for 3 or 4 cm. to end well outside of the anal ring (Fig. 148).

    c. Lateral—directly transverse to the vagina, beginning at the commissure.

Episiotomy should be performed whenever there is beginning laceration of the perineum, or when the skin surface becomes blanched during a pain and gives the impression that it has reached its elastic limit.

The median incision is best, when the head is fairly small, the perineum broad, with considerable space between the vaginal and rectal orifices, and when but little additional room seems required.

Mediolateral episiotomy is preferred when the expulsion of the child offers difficulty, the head being large and the perineum narrow and rigid. The lateral episiotomy is an unsatisfactory operation and is not advised.

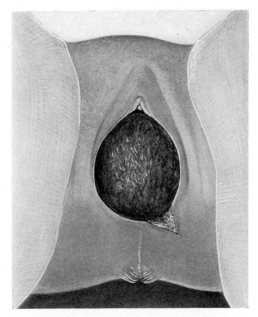

Fig. 148.—Mediolateral episiotomy tending toward lateral.

The incision may be made with scissors, preferably not too sharp pointed, or with a scalpel and care should be taken not to perforate the rectovaginal septum with the scissors point, a too common accident. The wound should be as long as required, and no longer.

In the mediolateral type there may be free bleeding from branches of the inferior hemorrhoidal and internal pudic arteries, which sometimes must be controlled by ligature.

The repair of episiotomy incision is simple, if median; more difficult in mediolateral and its steps are clearly shown in Fig. 149.

In a short time the parietal bones slip past the rami of the pubis and the face emerges over the perineum and the head is born. The cord should immediately be sought for and if found around the child's neck it may be slipped over the head or pushed backward so that the shoulder may be delivered through the enlarged loop. Rarely it may be necessary to cut the cord between ligatures, after which delivery must be completed at once.

The face of the baby becomes intensely cyanosed, but the child is in no danger because the placental circulation is still intact and respiration has not been established.

The Delivery of the Shoulder.—There is a great temptation to complete delivery as soon as the head is delivered by making im-

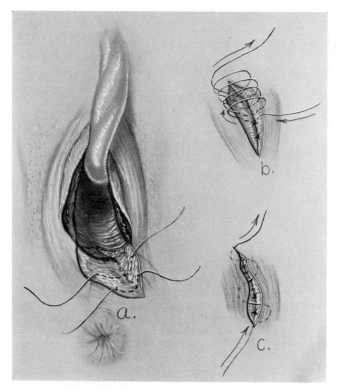

Fig. 149.—Repair of episiotomy wound.

mediate traction upon it. Such procedure results in dragging the unrotated shoulders through the perineum with the probability of extending any present laceration or indeed inaugurating such accident, as well as possibly causing irreparable injury to the child by rupture of a portion of the brachial plexus (Fig. 150).

After the birth of the head there is an appreciable pause in the forces of labor, after which the contractions recur. The rotation of the shoulder may be followed by observing the head, which turns slowly until the face looks directly at one or the other of the mother's thighs—the phenomenon of external rotation. When the shoulders are completely rotated and lie in the anteroposterior plane their delivery may be facilitated by making traction on the head, in a direction directly backward, until the anterior shoulder stems under the symphysis, when by elevating the head sharply but gently, the posterior shoulder slips over the perineum, which has been buttressed against injury by the thumb and finger as in the delivery of the head.

When the shoulders are delivered the rest of the body of the child is rapidly born without effort (Figs. 151, 152).

As soon as the child is delivered the woman should receive a hypodermic injection of 1 cc. obstetrical pituitrin and an intramuscular injection of 1 cc. of any standard preparation of ergot.

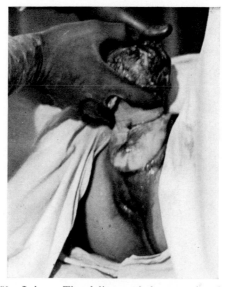

Fig. 150.—Labor. The delivery of the posterior shoulder.

It is held that the administration of oxytocics before the expulsion of the placenta may tend to incarcerate this organ behind a contracting cervix and lower uterine segment, but this does not occur in practice. The pituitrin acts immediately to favor uterine contraction and placental separation, while the ergot, acting much more slowly, maintains contraction after the placenta is expelled. There is usually an interval of from five to twenty minutes between the birth of the child and the expulsion of the placenta.

Attention to the New-born Child.—The child should receive attention immediately upon delivery, the infant being usually placed on the mother's abdomen, lying on its right side to favor closure of the foramen ovale.

If the delivery has taken place in a hospital, the question of identification of the infant is of importance from a medicolegal stand-point, many embarrassing situations having arisen by reason of the claims of parents that babies have been interchanged.

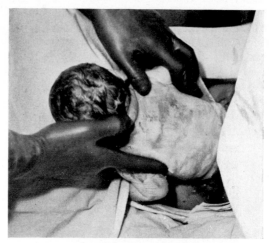

Fig. 151.—Labor. Delivery of the body, the cord being held out of the way.

Many elaborate apparatus are in use for this purpose, but the necklace or bracelet of lettered beads, forming the name of the mother and fastened by a compressed, pierced shot, so that it is

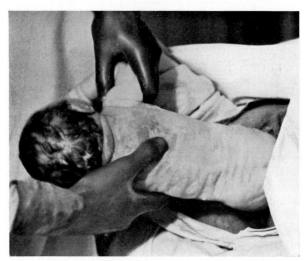

Fig. 152.—Labor. The delivery about to be completed.

not removable, has proved absolutely satisfactory in the institutions served by the writer. *The necklace should always be applied to the child before it is separated from the mother.* This is easily accomplished by having the necklace, shot and shot compressor sterilized with the instruments, the application being made by the nurse before the cord is cut. If the nurse, obstetrician and probably the anesthetist can bear witness that this procedure was carried out, substitution will be difficult to prove in a court of law.

In the home, of course, measures for identification are not necessary. There is a law existing in several States making it obligatory for footprints of the child and fingerprints of the mother to be recorded on the same sheet of paper, immediately after delivery. This is a spectacular but dubious method of identification.

Ligature and Care of the Cord.—The cord should not be ligated until pulsation has ceased or become very faint. A ligature of sterile narrow tape should then be tied very firmly about ½ inch from the skin margin, taking care not to include any skin in the ligature. A hemostat is then placed on the placental side of the ligature and the cord cut, a stump 1 inch or more being left for the possibly necessary religature.

The cut end of the cord is painted with tincture of iodine or alcohol and the stump dressed by covering with a square of sterile gauze, which is held in place by an abdominal bandage, wound for a few turns about the abdomen, the end tucked in.

There are more or less elaborate apparatus for cord compression, the Zeigler clamp and others, and in some clinics it is the plan to apply a hemostat close to the skin margin, leave it *in situ* for six hours and then remove it. All of these are unnecessary refinements, nothing being more satisfactory than a well-placed ligature.

Attention to the Child.—Promptly upon being born the infant, after a few irregular gasps, begins to breathe regularly and usually cries. Since there is danger of the respiration of mucus, blood and liquor amnii, which fluids may have collected in the nasopharynx during labor, it is well to remove them first by gently milking the trachea from below upward with a stroking motion of the finger and then by aspirating the nose and pharynx with an Arnold aspirator, which should form a part of every obstetric kit.

The mouth may be wiped free of mucus with a small pledget of cotton wrapped about the finger. Gauze should not be used as its rough mesh may injure the delicate mucosa and offer a portal for the entrance of thrush or other infective organisms.

All of these measures should be carried out, even before the cord is tied and cut.

Prophylaxis Against Gonorrheal Ophthalmia.—As soon as practicable (immediately upon the birth of head and while waiting for the shoulders to rotate, if possible, is the author's practice), a prophylactic instillation of silver into the eyes of the child and into the vulva, if it be a girl, must be made. This precaution may never be neglected as ophthalmia, with possible resulting blindness, may develop among people in whom the existence of gonorrhea is not even suspected.

The lids being retracted by the nurse's fingers, or better by small retractors designed for the purpose, one drop of a 1 per cent freshly prepared solution of silver nitrate is to be instilled into each eye, without preliminary irrigation. The 1 per cent silver solution need not be neutralized by normal saline as is necessary to prevent irritation if the 2 per cent solution as originally proposed by Credé be employed. Twenty-five per cent argyrol is also a satisfactory prophylactic agent.

Two essentials of the prophylaxis are that one must be certain that the silver solution reaches the conjunctiva and is not spilled on the lids, and second that the instillation must be carried out promptly.

Introduction of the silver into the vulvar outlet may inhibit the development of gonococci at this site and so guard against gonorrheal vaginitis.

The child is then wrapped in a warm blanket and laid aside in a warm place; its basket or crib in the home; the usual heated bassinet in the hospital delivery room; abundant warmth being one of the necessities for the new-born child. The head should be on a lower level than the body and the infant must be inspected frequently during its first hours of extra-uterine life to insure proper respiration and to guard against possible hemorrhage from the cord stump.

THE MANAGEMENT OF THE THIRD STAGE

The mechanism of the third stage of labor consists of two points: separation of the placenta from its uterine attachment and expulsion

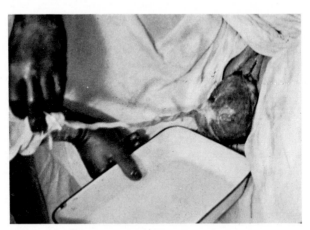

Fig. 153.—Labor. The third stage; the placenta is being extruded by voluntary contraction of the abdominal muscles.

of the organ from the birth canal. The separation is brought about by a gradual diminution of the placental site by uterine contraction until the placenta is literally squeezed off from its attachment to the uterine muscle (see Mechanism of Labor) (Fig. 153).

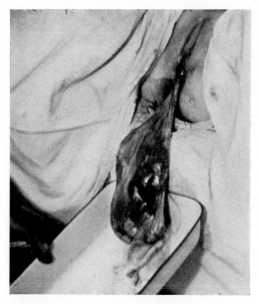

Fig. 154.—The placenta being received into a sterile basin. Note the train of membranes.

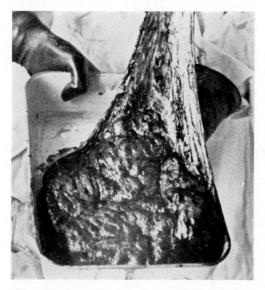

Fig. 155.—Inspection of the expelled placenta.

Clinically, the separation of the placenta can be determined by the behavior of the uterus. The fundus, which was flat and a little below the level of the umbilicus, now becomes globular and rises above the

15

umbilicus where it appears as a distinct tumor under the abdominal wall. The lower uterine segment just above the symphysis which was flat and unnoticeable now fills out. Also the cord descends for from 10 to 15 cm. coincidently with placental separations (Figs. 154, 155).

While the uterus is retracting and separation is going on, there is little or no pain experienced by the patient, but when the detached placenta lies in the lower uterine segment labor pains recommence, though not so severe as before. After several strong contractions, aided by the abdominal muscles, the placenta appears at the vulva and is extruded, with the membranes trailing behind together with the escape of a considerable blood clot: the retroplacental clot.

This mechanism should be completed in from five to thirty minutes after the birth of the child, but very commonly extrusion of the placenta does not occur spontaneously, the pains ceasing when the structure lies partly in the vagina and partly in the cervical ring whence its removal must be completed manually.

The management of this third stage is of the greatest importance, since by the neglect of certain simple precautions, severe hemorrhage or puerperal sepsis may result. In 1853 Credé announced his method of placental expression by vigorous compression of the uterus through the relaxed abdominal wall immediately after delivery. Some years later Credé modified his technic, allowing spontaneous separation and expulsion to take place, waiting thirty minutes and only then compressing the uterus.

The modern plan of administering pituitary extract as soon as the child is born facilitates separation, stimulates the uterus to contraction and generally brings about delivery of the placenta within ten minutes. The cord should be laid on the abdomen of the woman to prevent contamination from feces and any fringes of membrane hanging from the vulva should be cut off and laid aside so that the envelope of the ovum may be later reconstructed to insure complete evacuation of the uterus.

The time-honored custom of massaging the uterus after delivery as well as the less harmful plan of holding the fundus are mentioned but to be condemned. Nothing is gained by their practice and much harm from unnecessary traumatism may result. The postnatal uterus should be watched, however, and may be gently palpated from time to time to make sure that it is not relaxing and filling with blood. After a few minutes the uterine contractions will recur, and the placenta be forced into the vagina. If it be not promptly expelled, the uterus may be lightly held and used as a plunger to force the placenta to the vulvar opening, when the removal may be completed with the finger (simple expression of the placenta, Fig. 156). The following membranes should be slowly and gently withdrawn and in case they are torn in the process and shreds remain, all those which are outside the vulva are grasped with a hemostat and carefully withdrawn. Any bits which lie in the vagina are left to come away with the lochia as indiscriminate internal manipulation may lead to infection. Most of the bleeding after delivery occurs between the separation of the placenta and its expulsion and in practice it is wise to hasten the latter process as described above as soon as one is certain that separation has occurred.

Should the placenta not separate after thirty minutes, the Credé expression may be utilized. This consists in firmly grasping the uterine fundus and steadily compressing it, to squeeze the placenta

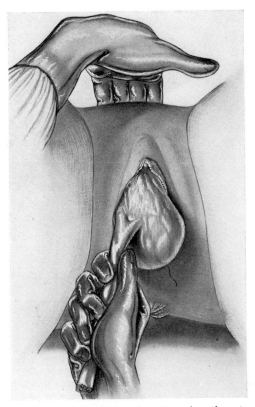

Fig. 156.—Simple expression of the placenta using the uterus as a piston. The hand holding the cord makes little or no traction but guides the descent of the placenta.

from its attachment. Care must be taken not to thrust the uterus downward into the pelvis, which tends to overstretch its ligamentous attachments. If, in spite of vigorous Credé manipulation the placenta remains adherent, the cord may be clamped at the vulvar orifice and cut off, and the case left to nature for as long as twenty-four hours. It is better, however, to perform manual removal, after an interval of two hours, or if hemorrhage or any other indication arises (Fig. 157).

Manual Removal of the Placenta.—For this purpose the patient must be rescrubbed, redraped and reanesthetized. The obstetrician likewise again cleanses his hands, changing gown and gloves. The labia are separated and the hand enters the vagina, following the cord until the placenta is reached, and the other hand on the abdomen holds the uterus steady. The fingers then seek the edge of the placenta, gently insinuate themselves between it and the uterine wall and begin the separation with a sort of peeling motion, following the plane

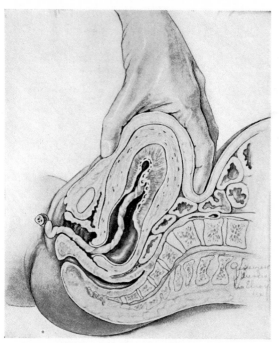

Fig. 157.—Credé method. The placenta is not yet separated. The firmly contracted uterus is compressed, not pushed downward, in order to squeeze the retained placenta out of the corpus cavity. When this is accomplished the placenta is then delivered by a downward push as described for "simple expression." (Baer.)

of cleavage. The separation is usually accomplished without difficulty and the placenta may be withdrawn intact.

If the placenta does not separate easily all attempts to remove it must be abandoned at once, because one is then dealing with placenta accreta (*q. v.*) which cannot be removed manually. In such cases possible attempts at removal may lead to fatal hemorrhage, perforation of the uterine wall or sepsis, and the placenta must be left *in situ,* the uterus packed, if bleeding, while arrangements are carried forward for the performance of hysterectomy, the only safe plan of treatment. Under no circumstances should traction be made upon the cord, as this leads to inversion of the uterus or improper separation of the placenta.

Inspection of the Placenta.—The placenta is placed in a flat dish, or held, maternal surface upward, in the hand of the obstetrician, the membranes folded back and the surface wiped dry with a gauze sponge. The organ is then carefully inspected to make certain that no cotyledons remain in the uterus, and also that there are no torn blood vessels at the edge of the membranes, to betoken the detachment of an accessory lobe or placenta succenturiata.

As Baer well says, it is a great comfort in the puerperium if fever and evidences of pelvic infection develop to be able to say positively that the uterus was left empty.

The Repair of Birth Injuries.—In hospital practice it is a good plan to inspect the cervix before the expulsion of the placenta, so that one may perform any necessary repair after that organ has been extruded. For this purpose a Sims speculum is inserted into the vagina, and with a hand steadying the cervix by lightly holding the cord, the former is exposed to view and after sponging with a gauze sponge held in ring forceps, any deep laceration is noted and the necessity for its repair determined.

Small, clean cervical lacerations require no attention, but those extending deeply into the body of the organ as well as multiple or stellate lacerations should be repaired forthwith.

Immediately after the placenta has been extruded and inspected repair of all recent birth injuries should be performed. This is described elsewhere (Chapter XXXV).

With the repair of birth injuries, the conduct of labor is completed and that of the puerperium begins.

The Amount of Blood Loss in Normal Labor.—Bleeding during the third stage of labor arises from the placental site, from laceration of the cervix and of the perineum and anterior vaginal wall.

The amount varies with the size and weight of the patient, the size of the placenta, the length and character of the labor and obviously upon the degree of laceration of the birth canal. The normal limits are from 100 to 300 cc., a hemorrhage of 500 cc. being an excessive normal and more than this amount of blood loss should be regarded as a pathological postpartum hemorrhage (*q. v.*).

CHAPTER XV

ANALGESIA AND ANESTHESIA IN OBSTETRICS

ALLEVIATION of the pangs of childbirth, seemingly so natural an event in obstetrical practice, has in the past met with decided opposition in part from the medical profession, but more especially from the church. There are records of trials for witchcraft during the sixteenth century, the charges being that the accused attempted to abolish the pain of labor by charms and other means. Indeed, the history of the introduction of chloroform and ether by Sir James Y. Simpson presents a picture of the conflict between science and ecclesiastical authority at once amusing and depressing to contemplate. The Scotch clergy especially were vehement in their attack upon the morality of obstetric analgesia, basing their contention upon an old Scottish belief. In 1591, for example, a lady of rank, one Eufame Macalyane, was charged with seeking the assistance of Agnes Sampson for the relief of pain at the time of birth of her two sons and was accordingly burned alive on the Castle Hill of Edinburgh.

Simpson's use of chloroform was generally denounced from the pulpit as impious and only after a long struggle in which the Queen of England took an active part by permitting herself to be anesthetized at the birth of her son (Edward VII) was relief from the agonies of childbirth considered as comporting with the Christian faith (see Dun's Life of Sir James Y. Simpson).

In America there was considerable clerical opposition to the employment of anesthesia in obstetrics but the attacks were sporadic and did not long continue.

During the past half century there has been a steady development of knowledge regarding the factors necessary for a successful eutocia until, at this time, relief from the pain of labor is demanded by every woman of intelligence and the demand is met by most obstetricians—even the general practitioners following the obstetrics specialist in learning the best methods and drugs to be employed.

General Principles.—The general principles involved in the induction of eutocia may be stated as follows:

All parturient women should be spared as much of the suffering incident to labor as may be, with due regard to the subsequent welfare of mother and child.

Analgesia or the rendering of the patient insensible to pain should be employed in all cases wherein operative delivery is not contemplated.

Anesthesia to the surgical degree should be induced in all cases involving operative procedures.

Indications and Contraindications.—Obstetric analgesia is indicated whenever the pains of labor begin to overcome the moral resistance of the patient so that she loses the ability to cooperate, or when she presents signs of exhaustion by the nervous and physical strains of delivery.

The contraindications to the induction of analgesia are those labors in phlegmatic women in whom there is but little reaction to the suffering of childbirth, and cases in which fetal life is threatened as evidenced by feeble irregular heart sounds. When this occurs, the patients should preferably be deeply anesthetized as soon as operative delivery is practicable.

Associated or coincidental illness of the patient, as cardiac disease, toxemia, acute infections, etc., are not contraindications to the use of analgesic measures. On the contrary, by minimizing shock and relieving the mental distress, analgesia is an important adjuvant to the successful delivery of these women.

In general it may be said that analgesia should be induced in the vast majority of obstetric cases. Properly practiced, the danger is almost negligible, and the relief of pain and suffering so gratifying, not only to the patient herself but to her relatives and those in attendance upon her, that the employment of measures to secure this end is always justified. Nothing tends to disorganize an obstetric technic more than the shrieks of a frightened and suffering woman, supplemented by the tears of her female relatives and the anxiety and distress of her husband.

METHODS OF SECURING OBSTETRIC ANALGESIA DURING THE FIRST STAGE OF LABOR

There are seven types of analgesia and anesthesia in common use, and by selection of the agent indicated in a given case, either singly or in combination with another, satisfactory relief from pain may be secured in practically every instance.

The methods and drugs are:

    a. Morphine or an analogous opium derivative in combination with scopolamine hydrobromide.

    b. The barbiturates, nembutal, pentobarbital, sodium amytal, etc.

    c. Ether and oil per rectum (Gwathmey technic).

    d. Local anesthesia secured by infiltration with some cocaine preparation.

    e. Nitrous oxide-oxygen.

    f. Ether, chloroform or ethylene.

    g. Spinal anesthesia.

The first three are particularly effective in the first stage of labor. At this time the apprehension of the patient regarding her forthcoming delivery is usually at its height and as the backache and steadily increasing pain of the uterine contractions continue, the woman ordinarily becomes highly nervous and complains bitterly. As soon as labor is definitely well begun and the pains begin to grow sharp, analgesia should be considered, regardless of the degree of cervical dilatation, except that morphine should never be given when delivery is probable within two hours, by reason of the danger of a narcotized infant in which respiration may fail to be established.

Morphine and Scopolamine Analgesia.—The morphine-hyoscine combination was first advocated in obstetrics by Steinbuchel in 1902 and was much lauded by Gauss in 1906, who elaborated the technic of its use and coined the happy term "Dämmerschlaf" or twilight sleep. Unfortunately, the lay press took up the matter of relief of pain during labor about this time and exaggerated accounts of its successes were published in magazines and newspaper articles throughout this country. This in itself was sufficient to prejudice the profession against it and when the reports of narcotized babies and women thrown into maniacal excitement by the drugs began to accumulate the method fell into further disrepute.

The original doses were undoubtedly too large in the attempt to secure absolute amnesia persisting throughout labor.

The writer, however, is persuaded that, taken by and large, morphine and scopolamine with a modification of the original conduct of twilight sleep gives more uniformly satisfactory results than any form of analgesic agent of which he has knowledge.

The indication for its use is the first stage of any labor, which probably will go on for two hours or more before delivery.

The contraindications are: First, an idiosyncrasy to scopolamine, possessed by certain persons, which becomes apparent shortly after the first injection by active excitement and restlessness when, of course, the treatment is discontinued.

Second, in presumably short labors, lasting two hours or less, there is said to be some danger of stillbirth or at least difficulty in inducing the baby to breathe. Inasmuch as the patient must be closely watched by a skilled observer, the method is not practicable in home deliveries unless the physician is prepared to remain in the house throughout the labor, although the same objection may be properly made to any of the analgesias in common use.

From one to six hours after delivery the women wake up, with a very variable remembrance of what has occurred. If memory be stimulated by a recital of the incidents of labor, almost complete recollection may be possible, but if all reference to the details are omitted, the accouchement usually remains a blank in the mind of the patient.

Technic.—When the first stage is well begun, the relatives of the patient are informed that she is to be given medication for the relief of pain and they are requested to avoid her room, and keep the house as silent as possible. The delivery room is then darkened, and after explanation as to the proposed treatment, the patient's ears are lightly plugged with cotton.

An initial subcutaneous injection of morphine sulphate, $\frac{1}{6}$ grain, and scopolamine hydrobromide, $\frac{1}{150}$ grain, is then given. Fifteen or twenty minutes after the exhibition of the drug, the patient becomes drowsy and presently falls asleep, to partly rouse herself during a pain, and straightway doze off again. After one or two hours, the intervals of wakefulness increase and the woman again begins to complain. Scopolamine hydrobromide, $\frac{1}{200}$ grain, is now given hypodermically and the dose may be repeated at two- to three-hour intervals until as many as six injections have been given. The morphine is not repeated.

By this plan most patients can be carried through a long first stage of labor and most of the second stage in quiet, without complaint and with subsequent practically complete amnesia concerning the events of labor. The bladder must be emptied by catheter at six-hour intervals, if the patient fails to respond to the ordinary stimulation of distention by voiding. As the second stage progresses, the patient must be carefully watched, since it is the experience of those using this analgesia that babies are often born in bed, without noticeable reaction on the part of the mother. Ordinarily, however, the distention of the perineum overcomes the inhibition of the drugs and the pains of delivery must be relieved by the supplemental use of nitrous oxide, or other inhalation anesthetic.

Low muttering delirium is common after scopolamine, the face is flushed, the pulse rate decidedly increased and the skin hot and dry.

After many years' intensive employment of morphine and scopolamine analgesia, the writer has not often met with respiratory difficulty in the babies and is convinced that this untoward sequel to its use is very infrequent.

The Barbiturates.—Various derivatives of barbituric acid have been used with success as analgesic agents. Nembutal in 6 to 9 grain doses by mouth, sodium amytal 6 to 12 grains by mouth, or 6 grains intravenously, pentobarbital in 4- to 6-grain doses, all of these with or without scopolamine, $\frac{1}{150}$ to $\frac{1}{200}$ grain. These drugs are given when the first stage has well begun and repeated in about one half the original quantity, in three or four hours.

In a careful study of various analgesic agents, Irving and his coworkers reached the conclusion that a combination of pentobarbital and scopolamine is the most effective of any of the methods employed, resulting in 86 per cent of absolute loss of memory of labor, 14 per cent of incomplete amnesia and no failures. Its sole objection is the fairly high percentage of restlessness which these investigators control by the supplementary instillation of rectal ether.

Nembutal in doses of from 6 to 9 grains produces complete amnesia, and is becoming very popular among women who report that they have no recollection whatsoever of any of the events of their delivery after this drug has been administered.

The restlessness which it induces is, in my opinion, a direct contraindication to its use in long labors with the prospect of a difficult forceps delivery after many hours. This because of the exhaustion which follows. Restlessness is so marked that beds having high sides are found in hospitals where nembutal analgesia is routine, and the patient throws herself about and struggles almost continually in many instances. It is said that a small dose of morphine ($\frac{1}{12}$ grain hypodermically) will control the restlessness. In other cases the action of nembutal is ideal, especially when combined with scopolamine as above explained.

Ether in Oil by Rectum.—Some years ago Dr. J. J. Gwathmey developed at the New York Lying-in Hospital a method of analgesia which he termed "synergistic," because it combines the narcotic and analgesic action of several drugs, morphine, ether, magnesium sulphate and alcohol. To these he added quinine sulphate to counteract the depressive effect of the drugs upon the uterine contractions.

The morphine and magnesium sulphate are administered hypodermically, the ether, quinine and alcohol by rectum. The method in our experience has given very variable results, which apparently cannot be forecast. In some women there is practically complete relief from pain, they resting and sleeping quietly, although the uterine contractions continue unabated. In some the relief is so slight and of such short duration that other analgesics must be added to achieve success.

Lately the technic has been modified by the substitution of pentobarbital for the magnesium sulphate, and the use of a 5 to 10 per cent solution of sodium bicarbonate as an enema instead of the usual soapsuds.

The following details are quoted from the recent article of Gwathmey and McCormick:

ETHER-OIL MIXTURE.—The formula for the rectal mixture, as now used, is ether, 2½ ounces (75 oc.), quinine alkaloid 20 grains (1.3 Gm.), alcohol 45 minims (3 cc.), paraldehyde 2 drachms (8 cc.) and liquid petrolatum or olive oil enough to make 4 ounces (120 cc.).

These agents are mixed in the following order: (1) Quinine and alcohol, (2) paraldehyde, (3) ether, (4) oil. The mixture is then stirred, strained through cotton, bottled and corked.

Preliminary Procedure.—The patient, having had a cleansing enema and a bath, and having been placed in bed, is addressed by the obstetrician as follows: "We are desirous of making your labor as painless as possible. Therefore, when your pains become uncomfortably severe, let the nurse know and she will give you a couple of capsules to relieve you. When the pains again become uncomfortable notify her as before and she will give you another capsule and perhaps a hypodermic. Later when this medicine begins to lose its effect, she will inject a solution into your rectum."

The following routine is then employed: the patient is given orally 3 grains and 1½ grains (0.2 and 0.1 Gm.) respectively of pentobarbital sodium. One-sixth or ¼ grain of morphine is usually given hypodermically with the second instead of with the first dose of pentobarbital if the patient is a primipara and labor is active. On the other hand, if the labor is not uncomfortably active, or if it is of the prolonged type, the second dose of pentobarbital may be repeated once or oftener before the morphine is given (not more than 10 to 12 grains [0.6 to 0.7 Gm.] in twenty-four hours). When the effects of the morphine begin to wear off, the ether-oil-quinine solution is administered by rectum and repeated as often as required, except that the quinine is omitted after the second instillation. Usually one instillation suffices. Morphine is omitted if delivery is anticipated within four hours and is rarely necessary if the patient is a multipara. If delivery is anticipated within four hours, the oral administration of pentobarbital and the rectal ether-oil instillation are promptly given simultaneously. After the pentobarbital is administered, the patient should be kept quiet. She is given only the necessary attention. The environment should be such as to favor her falling asleep. If she is in a ward, the bed is screened; if in a room, the shades are lowered and the light is excluded; the door is closed. The patient must be watched while asleep, as she may turn from side to side during contractions and fall out of bed.

Rectal Instillation.—The patient is placed on her left side, with the buttocks at the side of the bed. Seaweed, or tragacanth lubricating jelly (not petrolatum), is liberally applied about the anus. A well-lubricated 22 F. catheter is inserted from 6 to 8 inches into the rectum. It is important that the catheter pass the presenting part. It is held in place with the left hand. With the right hand the bulb is compressed at the conclusion of a pain not more than twenty or thirty times a minute. The mixture may be poured in a funnel. During the administration of ether mixture the patient is told to breathe deeply, with her mouth open, and to draw up with the anal sphincter, as if she were trying to avoid expelling gas; this will induce reverse peristalsis and permit the fluid to run in more rapidly. After all the ether mixture is passed out of the catheter, the catheter is clamped to prevent air being drawn into the return. The catheter is then gently withdrawn. Pressure is made with a towel over the anus during three or four contractions after the catheter is withdrawn. The patient may now be on her back or whatever position is most comfortable. The quiet appearance of the patient should not be misleading: she may be having strong contractions and should be watched carefully. The rectal instillation may be given at intervals of two and one-half hours if necessary. At actual delivery, ethylene, nitrous oxide or ether is given by inhalation, but not chloroform. When the baby is born, if a gas-oxygen apparatus is used, all anesthetic is cut off, and 5 per cent carbon dioxide and oxygen, under pressure, is given before the cord is cut.

The advantages of this method are its safety, there being practically no maternal or infant mortality attributed to its use. There are no contraindications. It does not unduly prolong labor, and it may be used with ether or nitrous oxide if subsequent anesthesia becomes necessary.

Paraldehyde.—This drug has been becoming quite popular within the past few years and has considerable value. It is administered by rectal injection in doses of from 6 to 8 drachms, thoroughly mixed with an equal quantity of olive oil.

The bladder and bowels being empty, the injection is made with a soft rectal tube and syringe, between pains. It is important to wait until pains are well established and regular at about five-minute intervals, and the cervix should be well effaced and dilated to 2 to 3 cm. before administration. If before this time the pains are too annoying they may be allayed with one of the barbiturates in multiparae, or by morphine $\frac{1}{6}$ grain and scopolamine hydrobromide $\frac{1}{150}$ grain in primiparae.

A burning sensation in the rectum, and possibly hiccups may follow the injection and have no significance.

Within fifteen minutes the patient usually is drowsy and soon falls asleep, moving about during pains but rarely restless, and should this occur toward the end of the second stage, light ether analgesia or nitrous oxide during delivery will facilitate this process. With the use of paraldehyde, complete amnesia may be secured in a majority of the cases, nor does there seem to be any untoward effect upon mother or fetus.

SECOND STAGE ANALGESIA

Local Anesthesia.—Late in the first or early in the second stage, infiltration of the cervix or perineum with $\frac{1}{2}$ per cent solution of novocain sometimes gives excellent results. This plan has been advocated by Gellhorn of St. Louis and others and forms a valuable addition to the obstetric armamentarium.

The vagina and perineal region being scrubbed as for an operation, the cervix is exposed with a bivalve speculum. A 10-cc. syringe armed with a long and fairly heavy injection needle is filled with $\frac{1}{2}$ per cent novocain solution and about 1 cc. of the solution is injected deep into the four quadrants of the cervix. Care should be taken that the cervical wall be not transfixed and the solution merely passed into the vagina, or unhappily, the needle permitted to enter the fetal head. The speculum is then withdrawn and the needle reintroduced into the mucocutaneous border at the fourchette. By repeated radial lines of injection the entire perineum may be reached, with complete analgesia lasting for an hour or sometimes more. This valuable procedure is not more popular, perhaps, because its performance is somewhat irksome and requires considerable preparation.

The Inhalation Anesthetics.—*Nitrous oxide and oxygen* seem to have been first suggested for obstetric use by Klikowitch of Leningrad.

In America, Lynch and Webster introduced the method to the United States in 1913.

For anesthetic purposes the usual surgical technic is employed, which requires no comment here.

As an analgesic, nitrous oxide and oxygen is usually administered in an 80:20 mixture. At the onset of a pain as noted by the patient, three or four deep breaths of gas are given after which the inhaler is removed and the procedure repeated with each pain. If the analgesia be not permitted to lapse into anesthesia, the uterine contractions are not inhibited and delivery is not delayed.

Unconsciousness, cyanosis and severe headache indicate that too much nitrous oxide has been given and the amount should be reduced.

There are many light, portable, nitrous oxide apparatus on the market, the use of any of them rendering the administration simple and efficient. The method is expensive and should not be practiced in the home without the presence of one skilled in anesthesia.

Ethylene (CH_2CH_2) is a gas obtainable in cylinders, like nitrous oxide, and all modern machines for administering the latter may also be used for ethylene. It is given with oxygen in various proportions, depending on the patient and the operation to be performed. A concentration of 80 to 90 per cent of ethylene is usually necessary to induce anesthesia.

It is preferable to nitrous oxide in cases of hepatic and renal disease, in cardiopathies and in hypertension, because of its nontoxic properties and because it is not a depressant to the circulatory system.

The infant usually breathes freely, without signs of asphyxia. The gas is administered in a similar manner to nitrous oxide.

The chief contraindication to the use of ethylene is its highly explosive quality, but this may be practically eliminated by having the operating room well humidified, and by seeing to it that exposed flame, cautery, or leaking electrical switch which may spark upon contact and any sources of fire are eliminated from the operating room.

Chloroform.—This agent usually regarded as the most dangerous of the anesthetics may be used as an analgesic during labor, with great satisfaction and a minimum of risk. Certain principles must be observed in its administration however.

First, it must be remembered that chloroform is known as the most dangerous of the drugs commonly used as an anesthetic, Gwathmey placing chloroform and oxygen as eighth in the list of anesthetics and chloroform and air as last, as regards safety to life. This sequence is based upon deep surgical anesthesia, however, and does not apply to the use of this agent as an analgesic in which capacity it is here considered.

Second, the remote deleterious effects of chloroform—liver degeneration, etc., are not seen after its use as an analgesic, in the extreme dilution which is the keynote to its successful employment in this field.

During chloroform analgesia the patient's head must be on a line with the body. Administration in the upright position is absolutely interdicted.

There must be no constricting clothing to interfere with respiration.

The drug should be dropped upon folded gauze or a handkerchief, 5 drops being usually a maximum to control each labor pain, and the gauze should be held at least 1 inch from the nostrils to insure free dilution with air.

As soon as the pain has ceased the chloroform should be withdrawn, not to be replaced until required for further analgesia.

The patient should never be permitted to lose consciousness.

One hour is about the limit of safety for the duration of a chloroform analgesia. The skin and mucous membrane of the mouth and nose should be protected from irritation by a thorough application of an oily film, petrolatum or cold cream before chloroform is administered.

The author has had no experience with chloroform as an anesthetic in obstetrical operations, but believes its use to be fraught with danger, and that ether is by far preferable for this practice.

Ether.—As an analgesic ether is not usually indicated, since its irritating effect on the respiratory system, its unpleasant odor, and the fact that a considerable quantity of the drug is required before insensibility to pain results, makes it an agent of but little value. Occasionally, however, ether may be used with success in this capacity.

Absolute Anesthesia.—When any operative interference is contemplated, analgesia should be abandoned, and deep surgical anesthesia substituted. It is important to remember that the success of obstetric operations varies almost directly with the depth of the anesthesia. It is imperative that the uterine musculature and that of the vagina and pelvic floor be completely relaxed in order that the danger of uterine rupture and serious injuries to the birth canal may be avoided.

For this purpose, ether and oxygen or ether and air are the anesthetics in general use and of the greatest convenience and safety. The principles of ether administration need no comment here, the usual surgical method of induction and maintenance of anesthesia being employed.

One point is of importance and that is that the longer and deeper the anesthesia, the more persistent the uterine relaxation, and the greater the tendency to postpartum hemorrhage, which accident should always be feared and guarded against in such cases.

Objections to Analgesia and Anesthesia.—There is obviously some danger of poisoning by the anesthetic used and while it seems true that the woman in labor is less liable to the accidents of anesthesia than other patients, enough accidents have been recorded to make a formidable list.

Again analgesia may, in some instances, lead to a high state of excitement and delirium on the part of the patient and indeed, it may become necessary in this type of case to substitute anesthesia for analgesia and to terminate labor by forceps or version to save the patient from the exhaustion of her drug excitement.

Such cases are unusual, however, and should not prevent the employment of analgesia.

The duration of labor is usually somewhat lengthened in consequence of analgesia, uterine contraction being lessened in vigor, and the intervals between them increased. This delay is more than compensated for by the increased comfort of the patient and should not be regarded as in any sense a contraindication to analgesic measures.

Precautions to be Taken During Obstetric Analgesia.—The fetal heart must be auscultated at frequent intervals, five minutes during the end of the first stage and even less time elapsing between auscultation as the head passes over the perineum. Irregularity or a marked variation in rate of the fetal cardiac impulses should be a signal to immediately terminate the labor in the interests of the child.

Spinal anesthesia has been used in obstetrics, but aside from its employment in connection with cesarean section, I cannot see any reason for its use in this connection.

In the event of any operation becoming necessary, ether anesthesia to the surgical degree is employed, and here it is absolutely necessary that the services of a skilled anesthetist be employed. Nothing is more conducive to calamity or, at best, to imperfectly performed obstetric operation, than for the obstetrician himself to attempt the anesthetization of the patient, or to entrust this most important feature of the technic to a lay relative or to an inexperienced nurse.

It is the right of the parturient woman and her child to enjoy alleviation of the sufferings of the former, and the immunity from the perils of birth of the latter and it is correspondingly the duty of the medical attendant to arrange for a systematic and scientific management of this important feature of the conduct of labor.

CHAPTER XVI

THE PUERPERIUM

THE puerperium (puer, a child, parere, to bring forth) may be defined as the period between the end of the third stage of labor, and the restoration of the pelvic organs as well as the entire biologic processes of the body to their pregravid state.

This definition is somewhat faulty as such return never completely occurs, the relaxation of the pelvic floor, the distortion of the cervical canal, the abdominal striae and alteration in the form of the breasts being permanent effects of gestation. It is estimated that from eight to ten weeks are required to complete the process of involution and repair, but the time is naturally influenced by the nature of the pregnancy and the type of the labor, whether or not infection has inhibited the process or whether possibly the resistance and tissue-building ability of the patient have been lowered by massive hemorrhage.

THE PUERPERIUM IS A COMBINATION OF GENERAL AND LOCAL CHANGES

GENERAL CHANGES

During the course of labor the patient presents the picture of violent and sustained exertion. The pulse is accelerated, the temperature slightly elevated, leukocytosis is at its height, and all metabolic activities are on a higher plane. Immediately upon the completion of the third stage, the picture changes to one of fatigue, rest and the rehabilitation of the drained physical and mental forces.

The patient lies quietly in bed, the pulse rather slower than normal, often dropping to 60 beats per minute, although in modern obstetric technic anesthetics are so generally used that the pulse rate may be maintained at a much higher level for some hours, as a result of these drugs.

Also in prolonged and difficult labor with excessive blood loss there may be evidence of mild shock often persisting for twenty-four hours or more.

The Temperature.—During labor the temperature rises slightly to fall to subnormal when the process is complete. After an hour or two the temperature again rises and commonly reaches 99.5° or even 100° F. during the first twenty-four hours postpartum. This rise may be due to the absorption of septic products from the puerperal wounds, but is more likely a reaction from effort plus the effects of anesthesia and trauma.

Should the temperature remain elevated for more than the first twenty-four hours, foci of septic absorption must be sought. In about one tenth of cases, there occurs a chill of moderate severity, but unaccompanied by temperature rise, immediately after the delivery of the child. DeLee believes that the chill represents infection during labor, but as it is generally so transitory, follows so closely upon delivery and is not marked by fever, the cause probably, as thought by most observers, lies in a combination of exposure of the skin, nervousness, fatigue and possibly blood loss. When these factors are reduced to a minimum as in the modern lying-in room and when terror has been banished by analgesia, the chill is seldom encountered.

The Respiration.—There is but little alteration of respiration, although the inspiration becomes deeper by reason of the free movement of the diaphragm, when the size of the uterus is reduced. Rapid shallow respiration after labor is a danger sign betokening shock from some cause.

The Blood.—During labor there is normally a fairly high leukocytosis, counts of from 20,000 to 30,000 being common. The white cells rapidly fall to normal after delivery, until they reach normal in from two to three days.

There is said to be a decrease in the total amount of the blood, varying, of course, with the amount of hemorrhage during delivery.

The erythrocytes vary from 3,500,000 to 5,000,000 in the normal, being proportionally reduced in the many women who have had some anemia during pregnancy.

Intra-uterine death of the fetus and multiple pregnancies may be associated with a moderate eosinophilia.

The Skin.—Sweating after labor is free from an increased function of the sweat glands. This normal sweating must not be confused with the cold leaking skin of hemorrhage or shock, from which it is easily distinguishable by the general condition of the patient.

The Urinary Tract.—During the first three days postpartum, there is polyuria as a result of decreased intra-abdominal pressure. Trauma to the bladder and urethra during labor frequently cause urinary retention for the first twenty-four to forty-eight hours, catheterization at this time being required to empty the bladder.

The bladder walls are edematous and may disclose petechial hemorrhage as a result of prolonged pressure by the descending head.

The **urine** at first contains hyaline casts, many white cells and a few reds, together with a trace of albumin and a little lactose as a result of mammary-gland activity.

Peptone is present due to the absorption of the tissues of the involuting uterus. The specific gravity is unchanged from 1008 to 1025, the urea is slightly increased, and the inorganic content is practically unchanged.

The Intestinal Tract.—Moderate tympany due to slight ileus as a result of relaxed abdominal muscles and the trauma of labor is common for the first few days. Constipation is the rule, enemata and laxatives being generally required.

16

Body Weight.—There is always considerable loss of weight after labor, beyond that of the fetus, liquor amnii and placenta.

This is due to the fluid loss, from milk secretion, lochia, urine and sweating and varies from 6 to 8 per cent of the total body weight.

LOCAL CHANGES

Involution of the Uterus.—At the end of labor the uterus is a compact bulk of muscle, 15 to 20 cm. in length, possibly 12 cm. in width and weighing from 1200 to 1500 Gm. In one week the weight is reduced about one half, in two weeks two thirds, and at the close of the puerperium, eight weeks after delivery, the organ has been reduced almost to its pregravid size, weighing from 40 to 50 Gm.

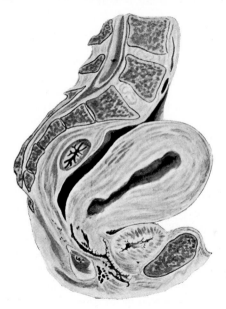

Fig. 158.—Sagittal section of pelvic organs, to illustrate direction of axis of uterus shortly after delivery. (Sellheim.)

At the completion of the third stage of labor the uterus may be palpated, as a hard rounded mass, with variations in its consistency as contraction or periods of relaxation occur (Fig. 158).

Its upper border lies about two fingerbreadths below the umbilicus, usually a little to the right of the midline. The uterus is larger laterally than in its anteroposterior diameter, lies in sharp anteflexion, and is extremely movable, with an excursion of several inches.

On the first day postpartum, the fundus rises higher in the abdomen, as a result of the accumulation of urine and feces in the bladder and rectum.

From this time, its bulk rapidly grows less, so that five days after delivery the fundus lies about 4 or 5 fingerbreadths above the pubis and by the twelfth day it has disappeared behind the symphysis and can no longer be felt.

This remarkable phenomenon is called involution and is brought about by several factors:

The muscle cells are not reduced in number, but each individual cell undergoes a diminution in size from 171 μ in length by 11½ μ in width, to a length of 17½ μ and a width of 4½ μ (Sanger).

This process is brought about by fatty degeneration of the muscle tissue, and by an autolysis in which the protein content of the cells breaks down into simple compounds which are resorbed and later excreted by the urine. It has been shown that an increase in nitrogen in the urine occurs simultaneously with the reduction in the size of the uterus, and decreases as the puerperium proceeds, until a normal output is reached at the end of the puerperium. Slemons made the interesting observation that, in a woman in whom the uterus had been removed at cesarean section, the characteristic increase in the nitrogen output was lacking, and that the difference practically corresponded to the quantity of urea contained in the uterus.

The biochemistry of this process is not yet clear, but it is thought to be aided by the marked anemia of the uterus after labor.

Involution and Regeneration of the Endometrium.—Upon the completion of labor the interior of the uterus is covered with a somewhat ragged coat of decidua and at the placental site there remains the spongiosa layer, the placenta having separated in the cleavage plane between this and the compacta. The line is very irregular, so that in places a thick layer of decidua is retained, in others only a few layers of cells remain while in others the muscularis is practically bare.

Under the remnants of decidua lie the stumps of the uterine glands from whose mucosa the regenerated endometrium is to emerge. Outside the placental site, the endometrium is practically completely restored within three weeks after delivery. During the first two or three days the decidua vera is blood stained and from 1 to 3 mm. in thickness. After seven days the superficial layer is infiltrated with blood, the cells have become hyaline or necrotic and are thickly interspersed with leukocytes. In a few days more this dead tissue is exfoliated and discharged with the lochia and there is exposed an underlying layer of uterine glands separated by a stroma made up of maternal cells only. Shortly the epithelium spreads over the raw surfaces and the normal uterine lining is restored.

Changes in the Placental Site.—The placental site, as clearly shown by Williams in his last paper, is at first flat and difficult to differentiate from the remainder of the uterine cavity, but with eight or ten hours, the uterus becomes less firmly contracted, blood enters the sinuses of the placental site which now appears as a rounded, elevated area with a rough, ragged surface. This area consists for the most part of distended vessels, some arteries undergoing obliteration, some veins filled with blood which is becoming fibrinized and organized. By the twentieth day, the placental site is a hyaline mass which almost fills the now small uterine cavity and impinges upon the regenerated mucosa of the opposite side. New endometrial tissue underlies this site and grows rapidly into the fibrinized area, gradually undermining it and causing its ultimate exfoliation and complete disappearance by the eighth week, postpartum. For details of this process the reader is referred to the splendid paper of Williams, above referred to.

Involution of the Cervix.—Since the cervix does not share in the formation of decidua, no exfoliation or regeneration need occur.

Immediately after labor, the cervical canal is represented by a soft, flabby collar of tissue, which rapidly contracts and elongates until a week after delivery the canal is from 3 to 5 cm. long, the circular muscle wall contracted, the cavity about 1 cm. in diameter. In three weeks the cervix has regained its normal length and muscular tone, but in most instances reveals laceration of varying extent, the two surfaces uniting, or if extensive, remaining as gaping areas covered with granulations.

There may have been hemorrhage into and between the cervical muscle bundles which is slowly resorbed.

The virginal circular contour of the os externus is almost invariably altered by labor, the opening becoming oval, possibly irregular in outline as a result of the uneven healing of lacerations.

The Vagina.—After the completion of labor, the vagina is a relaxed, stretched tube, frequently lacerated in several areas and markedly hyperemic.

In a few days the tissues begin to regain their tone, the congestion disappears and the vaginal walls lie in contact with each other. The introitus gapes and remains open for a variable period, depending upon the degree of stretching it has undergone and the extent of laceration. After six or eight weeks the vagina has fully regained its former elasticity, the rugae have reappeared, and the vulvar outlet is again closed, although there is inevitably some relaxation, mainly of the anterior wall, with gaping upon straining. The remnants of the hymen remain as little tags of mucosa on either side of the outlet, known as carunculae myrtiformes.

The Abdominal Walls.—At first the abdominal walls are greatly relaxed and loose. The recti muscles may be widely separated, the examining hand dropping into a deep sulcus between their internal margins, which separation may present, with a bulging between the recti when these muscles are contracted, called diastasis recti.

The deeply purple striae slowly lose their color and contract although they remain permanently as silvery white, linear scars.

The abdominal walls regain nearly their pregestational form and tone after the completion of the puerperium and especially if the patient has taken appropriate exercise, but some relaxation is usually permanent.

The Lochia.—Discharge from the uterus lasts for from four to eight weeks after delivery. For the first three or four days the discharge is almost pure blood, with some small clots—the lochia rubra or lochia cruenta. On the second day there may be one large clot expelled as the uterine cavity rapidly diminishes in size. Persistent bleeding with many clots is pathological and should arouse suspicion of a retained placental cotyledon, bleeding from a cervical laceration or imperfect involution of the uterus.

After the third or fourth day the lochia becomes of a brownish color and a smooth creamy consistency, possessing a peculiar sweetish and quite characteristic odor—the lochia sanguinolenta.

The color gradually fades until on about the twelfth day the discharge has become yellowish, contains many leukocytes and is called lochia alba.

This gradually decreases in amount and consistency until it appears as a mucoserous discharge, which has completely disappeared upon the completion of involution.

The amount of the lochia varies greatly and may be from 300 to 1400 Gm. *Microscopically* the fluid contains red and white blood cells, fragments of deciduae, in various stages of degeneration, fat, mucus, cholesterin and bacteria. Many observations have been made upon the bacteriology of the puerperal birth canal, it being found that the cavity of the uterus is generally bacteria free, just after labor, while the vagina contains a number of organisms, including the streptococcus.

In a day or two the upper cervix contains bacteria which shortly invade the uterine cavity itself. There is then an ascending infection from the vagina, but by the time the organisms reach the uterus, involution is well established, the puerperal wounds are healing and the invaders find but little soil upon which to propagate.

Furthermore it is probable that the usual bacterial flora is non-virulent to the tissue of the host.

Changes in the Breasts; Lactation.—Unlike the other mammals, in which milk appears in the breasts coincidently with labor and often comes before, the human female does not begin to secrete milk until the second day postpartum in multiparae and the third in primiparae. The secretion occurs not only after full-time labors, but also after abortions from the fourth month and I have noted it following ectopic pregnancy.

The cause of lactation remains obscure, but it has been observed that hypodermic injection of theelin and progestin followed by extract of the anterior lobe of the hypophysis will stimulate the process, but that each of these agents is inactive without the other.

The *breasts* are paired, superficial organs composed of masses of glandular tissue traversed and supported by strands of fibrous tissue and covered by a thick layer of fat. The glandular tissue forms a somewhat conical mass, the apex of which corresponds to the position of the nipple, the base loosely connected to the fascia of the pectoralis major and serratus anterior muscles.

The glandular tissue (Fig. 159) is made up of compressed racemose glands divided into 15 or 20 lobes, each lobe further subdivided into lobules and these in turn into numerous acini. The lobes are bound together and supported by a considerable amount of fibro-areolar

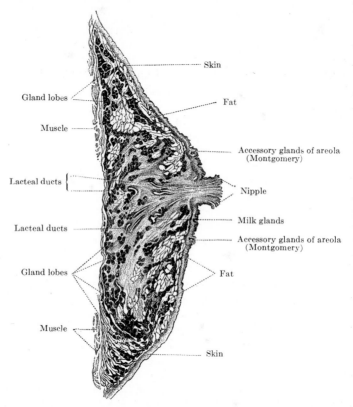

Fig. 159.—Section through the mammary gland, three weeks postpartum. (Bumm.)

tissue, the stroma of the gland. This whole pinkish-white mass is overlaid by a layer of fat, which dips into and fills up the inequality of the irregular surface of the gland tissue. Springing from the lobes are the lactiferous ducts which pass upward toward the nipple and open on its summit without intercommunication. The nipple is a wart-like eminence, containing some erectile tissue and situated on the apex of the breast. It is surrounded by an areola of more or less deeply pigmented skin, which is thrown into wrinkles and presents a series of little globular projections known as the glands of Montgomery and supposedly due to the presence of underlying cutaneous glands. At the summit of the nipples are the openings of the lactiferous ducts.

Physiology of Lactation.—At first there is marked swelling of the cells lining the glands, and great lymphatic engorgement. Within forty-eight hours the gland cells break down into fat globules, the plasma of the milk is furnished by the lymphatics and secretion is established.

Clinical Course.—For some weeks prior to labor and for from two to three days after it the breasts, though enlarged, remain soft. There may be expressed from the nipple a few drops of a yellowish sticky material called colostrum, composed of lymph, a few fat globules and some ovate or round cells, possessing several nuclei and first fat globules, called colostrum cells.

In two or three days the breasts become much swollen, turgid, sometimes painful and tender. This is known as simple engorgement and has no pathological significance being due to a lymph stasis. Within a few hours milk may be stripped from the nipple, and after one or two nursings, the engorgement subsides and a regular rate of secretion is established. In many multiparae and some primiparae, this engorgement is absent, lactation coming on quickly and smoothly. In some others, the function begins with great abruptness, the patients stating that they feel the milk "rushing in" with great rapidity. Once established, the milk supply is regular, the breasts filling in sequence. Careful training of the child and the establishment of regular habits of nursing are essential to normal secretion.

Lactation may be continuous for three or four years, but usually ceases in about one year. In the United States most urban mothers wean their children at nine months, while in rural districts nursing is, as a rule, carried on for some time longer.

Amount of Milk.—This is extremely variable but the average is probably from 30 to 40 ounces in twenty-four hours.

Heavy, fat and pendulous breasts usually secrete poorly, especially if they are the organs of fat, large women.

Small, slim women, with fairly firm, conical breasts having an abundance of gland tissue, usually show a large capacity for milk secretion.

Once the secretion is established, the breasts must be emptied at regular intervals or the function ceases. If for any reason the child may not nurse for a day or two, the breasts should be emptied at four-hour intervals by stripping or by some form of breast pump, to insure maintenance of lactation.

The Composition of Human Milk.—Human milk is a sweet, yellowish-white fluid composed of a thin serum containing innumerable fat droplets.

Chemically the milk varies in different women, at different intervals and even from day to day but its general composition is:

Water .... 86.5 per cent
Solids .... 12.5 per cent which are made up of
Milk sugar .... 6.25 per cent
Fat .... 3.75 per cent
Protein .... 2.25 per cent
Salts .... 0.75 per cent

Milk contains enzymes, antibodies to infection and many vitamins.

The Management of Lactation.—In order to secure a regular and abundant milk supply, the patient must be of tranquil mind, have a full-balanced diet, and establish regular habits of nursing. In the twenty-four hours after birth the infant should be placed to the breast at six-hour intervals, with the object of stimulating the gland epithelium to secretion, and second to utilize the mechanism by which traction on the nipple induces uterine contractions.

After the first twenty-four hours the nursing intervals may be either three or four hours, most obstetricians favoring the former period and most pediatrists the latter. The standard time for nursing is ten minutes at the beginning, gradually lengthening to twenty minutes. The child should nurse but one breast at each feeding except under exceptional circumstances.

The training of mother and child to regular nursing habits is most important and a painstaking nurse is invaluable in aiding in this. Before each nursing the nipple should be washed with a sterile solution (boric acid is traditional) and after the feeding, the cleansing should be repeated and the breast dried, after which the nipple is protected by a small square of gauze or clean muslin, or a lead nipple shield.

The importance of breast feeding cannot be overestimated and where the mother seems disinclined to trouble herself with the duty, it is the office of the physician to explain that the ratio of infant death during the first year of life is as one in a breast-fed baby to five who are bottle fed. Furthermore involution of the uterus is much stimulated by nursing and the psychological effect upon the mother cannot be overlooked.

The quality of milk naturally varies with different women and at different times in the same woman, but only rarely is a mother's milk unsuitable for her baby. A fresh pregnancy diminishes both quantity and quality of the secretion and in such event, the child should be weaned at once.

The food of the mother, if well digested, does not alter the character of the milk, whereas many drugs pass into it, and maternal illness is often reflected in the reaction of the infant to its food supply.

THE MANAGEMENT OF THE PUERPERIUM

Four essentials control the conduct of the period immediately after labor:

1. Rest.
2. Avoidance of infection.

3. Nourishment of mother and child.

4. Maintenance of normal bodily functions to insure involution.

After the fatigue and mental strain of labor, the patient should be allowed forty-eight hours of complete rest, in a quiet room, not too brightly lighted. She should be encouraged to sleep as much as possible and to roll from side to side at her convenience. Many women rejoice in the ability to sleep upon their abdomen, which pregnancy has prevented. Husband, mother and father should be the only permitted visitors and the presence of a room full of chattering relatives more or less laden with the virus of the common cold or worse disease, is evidence of a badly conducted puerperium. When lactation is well established, visitors are welcome but always in moderation. Insomnia and restlessness are combated by the administration of bromides at night or the very occasional use of a barbiturate hypnotic as sodium amytal, 3 to 6 grains.

Careful study of a series of cases at Kensington Hospital has convinced the staff that the routine use of ergot in the first ten days of the puerperium minimizes subinvolution of the uterus, promotes better drainage and shortens the period of lochial discharge. Accordingly, unless contraindicated for some reason, puerperae are given 20 minims of fluidextract of ergot three times daily for the first ten days postpartum.

C. T. Beecham working in this clinic noted the following facts:

1. Lochia rubra was more persistent in patients receiving no form of ergot during the puerperium.

2. Subinvolution occurred in much higher percentage (41.4 per cent in nonergot cases than in fluidextract cases (13.2 per cent), and was completely absent in the ergoklonin series.

3. A satisfactory puerperium was observed in 58 per cent of cases receiving no oxytocic drug, in 87.8 per cent of cases receiving fluidextract of ergot, U.S.P. There was less striking difference in the morbidity percentages in the three groups than in the figures showing degree of bleeding and subinvolution.

4. From a study of a series of 551 cases ergot appears to be a useful and necessary aid to a normal puerperium, preferably in the form of a preparation of known ergonovine content.

After-pains.—Few primiparae and most multiparae suffer from intermittent painful uterine contractions, which may be very severe and may last for three or four days postpartum. Relief may be obtained by the administration of

Paregoric	1 ʒ
Acid. acetylsalicylic.	5 gr.
Fl. ext. ergot	20 ♏

at four-hour intervals until relieved. Pituitrin, 0.5 cc. hypodermically, is also valuable in this condition.

The use of a firm abdominal binder, snugly fitted from costal margin to pelvic brim, affords great comfort, promotes involution of the abdominal parietes and assists in maintaining the figure. After the third day, the use of the binder should be discontinued and the patient encouraged to exercise. The movements for the first day or two are limited to the head and arms. Raising the head from the pillow, elevating the arm to a vertical position and then extending them to right angles with the body and the reverse.

Two days later (unless there has been extensive perineal repair) the legs are flexed and drawn up to the abdomen alternately, in addition to the arm motion; in another two days the patient lies on her side and performs walking motion with her legs and finally after ten days she may assume the knee-chest position in bed for twenty minutes morning and evening. Many other gentle movements may be suggested, the foregoing being merely an outline.

Diet.—For the first day after labor the diet should be light—an egg, tea and toast, milk, orange juice and broth are sufficient. On the third day and thereafter a generous balanced ration is welcome, only very highly seasoned and indigestible dishes being forbidden.

The Emunctories.—If unable to void the parturient woman is to be catheterized at ten-hour intervals. It is a great mistake to insist upon voiding until the woman is clearly able to do so, as unfortunate urinary retention often follows such practice.

A simple soapsuds enema is given the day after delivery and thereafter a gentle laxative as milk of magnesia, small doses of cascara sagrada (30 minims of the fluidextract), etc., is administered "pro re nata."

The Avoidance of Infection.—In a well managed hospital, the patient may be placed in bed after delivery without any vulvar protection but draining upon a pad of sterile gauze.

Generally this plan is not feasible, however, and the vulvar outlet should be protected with a sterile pad, to be changed when saturated. After every urination and defecation, the vulva should be irrigated with a warm antiseptic solution (lysol, 1 per cent, metaphen 1:1000, etc.), poured over the vulva from a pitcher, the patient being upon a douche pan. If stitches have been placed, blood and mucus which may have accumulated upon them are to be removed by gentle wiping with a cotton ball held in forceps. No vaginal douche is permissible nor should the pledget of cotton be permitted to enter the vulva. Nonabsorbable sutures are removed on the tenth day.

It is a tradition that parturient women should be out of bed on the tenth day and this is the usual practice in normal cases. At first the patient simply sits up, with her feet hanging out of bed for a few minutes in the morning. In the afternoon she is permitted to be up in a chair for from one-half to one hour. Following this, the sitting up period is steadily lengthened and the woman allowed to walk a little. By the fourteenth day the woman may leave the hospital, or if at home may move about freely on one floor. In three weeks she may continuously use the stairs.

By the sixth week all usual activities may be resumed, but heavy toil should be delayed for two more weeks if possible.

Shower baths may be taken after the woman is up and about, but no tub baths are allowed until the cessation of lochial discharge.

Retroversion of the Uterus.—Almost one in four women present retroversion during the puerperium. A vaginal examination just previous to leaving the hospital or at the close of the bed period will disclose the condition and if present the patient is asked to assume the knee-chest position twice daily for twenty minutes each time. Polak was very fond of the "kangaroo walk" in which the woman walks about her room on hands and feet, the knees and elbows being held straight. The use of a pessary at this time is not generally advisable, since the perineum is apt to be still weak from the repair of lacerations.

At the end of six weeks a detailed vaginal examination is made, the cervix exposed with a speculum and any granulating areas cauterized with the electric cautery, a nasal tip being utilized and the linear cauterizations made radially to the os, $\frac{1}{8}$ inch apart and not more than $\frac{1}{16}$ inch in depth. At this time, if retroversion persists with symptoms of subinvolution or backache, a Hodge or Smith-Hodge pessary is applied, to hold the organ forward, otherwise the condition may be ignored. The pessary should be removed, the parts inspected and the cleansed pessary reintroduced at monthly intervals until the retroversion is corrected.

Care of the Breasts.—The management of normal lactation has already been described. For the treatment of breast lesions the reader is referred to Chapter XXXVIII.

The Reappearance of Menstruation.—The old view that amenorrhea continues during lactation is in error. Several studies of extensive series have been made and it appears that about one half of all lactating women menstruate within three months after delivery, four fifths menstruate before the cessation of lactation, this number being still higher in primiparae.

Lactation amenorrhea does not protect against pregnancy, but conception is less likely than usual because ovulation does not occur so frequently.

THE NEWBORN CHILD

Immediately after birth manifold alteration takes place in the physiology of the child. The changes in the circulation have already been described.

Respiration is initiated by the increase in the carbon dioxide content of the blood, as a result of the reduction in placental circulation during labor and its complete cessation after delivery.

Efforts at respiration usually begin in a few moments after birth, the first breathing being abdominal, but soon the thoracic muscles are involved and regular respiration is inaugurated. At first the movements are spasmodic and irregular, but soon they develop a regular rhythm. The infant at birth is somewhat cyanotic, but shortly becomes pink and rosy. With the first respiration there is usually crying, which should be vigorous and loud. Delay in respiratory activities may result from partial asphyxia, narcosis or intracranial birth injury, all of which possibilities should be investigated and appropriately treated as found.

Temperature.—An initial drop in body temperature of from 1° to 2° F. is usual, but as the heat-regulating mechanism in the medulla and the vasomotor system becomes operative, the temperature returns to normal within a few hours.

The Kidneys.—The bladder of the newborn contains urine and often a male baby will urinate spontaneously and rather copiously while the cord is being tied and cut. The exact time for the onset of kidney function in intra-uterine life has not been determined. Anuria in an infant may be due to phimosis, some congenital defect in the urinary passages, or to an absence of or defective kidneys. The urine may be albuminous for a few days.

Digestive Tract.—Digestion is accomplished by the digestive juices except the ferments of the pancreas and the salivary glands which appear a little later. For the first two or three days following birth the stools are composed of meconium, a greenish black, tarry, viscid substance, having no odor and which may be found in the fetal intestines from the fourth month of pregnancy.

Within a few days, the stools become lighter in color, nonliquid and contain little lumps of fat and casein, eventually becoming the smooth, yellow, normal fecal material. The normal frequency of defecation in the newborn is from three to four times in the twenty-four hours. The mechanism of sucking is present at birth and its absence should lead to a search for possible intracranial injury.

The Blood.—The hemoglobin in the newborn reaches 105 to 125 per cent, but by the third week it has fallen to the usual 70 to 80 per cent.

The erythrocytes run from 6 to 7 millions and the leukocytes are more numerous, viscid and deliquescent than in the adult. The average leukocytosis in the infant is from 18,000 to 20,000 at birth, falling rapidly until after the fourth day, when the count again rises to about 12,000.

The coagulation time is generally lengthened on the third day after birth, and one or two days succeeding, so that circumcision and other operations are best postponed until after the first week.

Endocrine System.—The thyroid and thymus glands are relatively large in the newborn, particularly the latter, which sometimes is sufficiently hypertrophied to cause pressure upon the trachea, with a peculiar crowing respiration and attacks of cyanosis, occasionally resulting in fatal asphyxia. The development of such symptoms should be followed by immediate roentgenologic investigation of the thymus and an x-ray treatment if this is found unduly large. Both glands usually recede to their normal size in the first month after birth.

The child after birth tends, for a time, to retain its attitude of universal flexion—the fetal ellipse—but within a few hours lies relaxed and extended in sleep.

The molded head rapidly resumes its normal oval contour and the subcutaneous edema which has marked the caput succedaneum is absorbed in a day or two.

The stump of the cord undergoes a dry necrosis and is usually separated by the fifth day. Occasionally the cord remains moist and may have to be cut free at the end of the tenth day. After separation the umbilicus is usually well healed but a central area of granulation may persist and require cauterization with lunar caustic to promote epithelization.

Management of the Newborn Child.—Attention to the eyes and the cord have already been described.

A great essential in the proper care of the newborn is the maintenance of bodily heat. The child should be warmly wrapped in blankets as soon as born, and if resuscitation of a partially asphyxiated infant is necessary, the body of the child should always be kept warm during the manipulation.

The Bath.—Tradition demands that the child should be anointed with olive oil or other fatty substances to dissolve and remove the vernix caseosa, which is the sebaceous material that accumulates in the skin folds and on the body of the fetus.

The oiling is followed by a gentle sponge bath with soap and warm water after which the baby is dressed and placed in its crib.

In hospitals, where epidemics of impetigo contagiosa are always feared, the oiling and bath are not done, the baby being well rubbed with an ointment of 5 per cent ammoniated mercury. Subsequently the child is treated with a 2 per cent ointment of ammoniated mercury in lanolin and is then duly oiled daily with one of the sterile oils marketed for the purpose.

IV. OBSTETRICAL PATHOLOGY

It has been stated that though reproduction is theoretically a physiological process without possessing any inherent pathological factors, nevertheless, the tissue changes are so profound and the trauma of birth so considerable, that lesions of greater or less degree may occur at any time during pregnancy, labor or the puerperium.

Obstetrical pathology is divided into the pathology of pregnancy, of labor, of the puerperium and of the newborn child. The first of these groups to be considered is the pathology of pregnancy, which consists of two divisions of abnormal condition:

1. The diseases or lesions *incidental to pregnancy;* that is, those in which pregnancy must necessarily be present, as for example, abortion, extra-uterine pregnancy, etc.

2. The diseases or lesions *accidental to pregnancy;* that is, those in which pregnancy is merely a coincidental occurrence, although having some bearing upon the progress of the disease as, for instance, appendicitis, pneumonia, or pyelitis occurring in the pregnant woman.

The diseases incidental to pregnancy may conveniently be subdivided further into: A. Local conditions. B. General or systemic lesions.

There is one group of diseases incidental to pregnancy which combines both general and local factors and which is of extreme importance to obstetricians in that 16 per cent of all maternal deaths from obstetrical causes are included in it, the mortality from this cause being exceeded only by that from puerperal sepsis.

This important group is known as the toxemias of pregnancy.

CHAPTER XVII

THE TOXEMIAS OF PREGNANCY

THE Toxemias of Pregnancy is the title assigned to a series of pathological conditions, specific in their nature, differing widely as to symptomatology, morbid anatomy and even as to the tissue attacked, but having as a common factor the presence in a woman of a living embryo and its appendages.

More than one half of all pregnant women become toxic to some degree during the course of gestation and about 1 in 10 are definitely affected.

Etiology.—The reason for these intoxications in association with pregnancy is not clear, although an immense amount of experimental work has been done and an impressive array of theories promulgated.

Whether the toxins originate from unreduced albumin of ovular origin, or whether they arise as the result of a sort of endocrine activity of certain rapidly growing fetal cells as the syncytium has not been proved. Some observers hold that bacterial action is causative, others that deficiency in functions of the excretory organs, the kidneys and liver, will furnish the explanation.

Recently there has grown a steadily increasing tendency to regard eclamptic toxemia as due to hyperfunction of the hypophysis, probably as a result of insufficient secretion of the antagonistic ovarian hormone. Pituitrin has a known antidiuretic and pressor action. Experiments have shown that this antidiuretic secretion exists in cases of hypertension and edema, while it cannot be demonstrated with certainty in the blood of healthy, pregnant women. The most exhaustive studies along chemical lines have been performed and have yielded an imposing amount of information, none of which has thrown any light upon the cause of the toxemia.

Indeed the whole question of etiology may well be summed up in the words of Ballantyne, in his closing of a somewhat similar matter. "It is clear that this subject is obscure. So much alone is clear; therefore, in God's name, let us leave it."

It must be understood that any toxic process developing during the course of gestation is truly a toxemia of pregnancy; thus the various skin eruptions, the constipation, the mild headaches, etc., all properly are to be classified under this generic term. There are, however, certain definite symptom groups, which in the frequency of their occurrence, the importunity of their clinical aspects and their tremendous importance as to the life and health of mother and child are usually studied and managed under the title of Toxemias of Pregnancy. These syndromes are:

1. The Toxemia of Early Pregnancy (Hyperemesis Gravidarum).
2. The Toxemia of Late Pregnancy:
   a. Low reserve kidney.
   b. Nephritic toxemia.
   c. Preeclamptic toxemia.
   d. Eclampsia.
   e. Acute yellow atrophy of the liver or hepatic toxemia.
   f. Miscellaneous toxemias.

This classification is admittedly imperfect and arbitrary, but it at least offers a logical approach to the study of the various types of toxic manifestations.

It is the opinion of the writer that the toxemia of early pregnancy, the so-called "pernicious vomiting," is an entirely different process from the toxemias of late pregnancy.

Because a woman suffers from this type of intoxication, it does not necessarily follow that she will develop preeclamptic toxemia, although she is somewhat more likely to do so than the woman who has not so suffered. In a recent study made in the author's clinic at Kensington Hospital for Women, Missett found that the incidence of late toxemia is definitely increased in cases presenting the physiologic nausea and vomiting of the first trimester. Forty-one per cent of multiparae and 51 per cent of primiparae experiencing this form of early toxemia were toxic in the last trimester.

THE TOXEMIA OF EARLY PREGNANCY

Pernicious Vomiting of Pregnancy; Hyperemesis Gravidarum

This form of toxemia was known to the acients, Soranus of Ephesus describing it in 20 A. D. The paper of DuBois (1852) still remains as a classical description of the condition.

Definition.—The toxemia of early pregnancy is an exaggeration of the morning nausea and vomiting which is regarded as almost a characteristic of normal pregnancy, but which is probably always a manifestation of toxemia to a mild degree.

It occurs in about 40 per cent of pregnancies and consists only of nausea and vomiting, with their obvious sequelae of dehydration, starvation, acidosis and exhaustion from loss of rest.

It is generally self-limited, terminating spontaneously at the end of the third month of gestation, although rarely, it may persist in some measure thoughout pregnancy.

The severity of this toxemia is very variable, most patients recovering without permanent systemic damage, although abortion, irreparable liver injury and death may occur.

Frequency.—Nausea and vomiting of lesser or greater gravity appearing a few weeks after conception and persisting until about the end of the third month is so usual an event during pregnancy that it has come to be regarded as an important subjective diagnostic factor in determining the existence of gestation. Indeed some writers speak of this condition as physiological, a decided misnomer.

Cases wherein the vomiting becomes so constant and severe that the patient may be regarded as seriously ill, occur about once in 600 pregnancies in the United States, whereas those terminating fatally are uncommon.

Etiology.—The cause of hyperemesis gravidarum is shrouded in obscurity, many theories having been advanced concerning its pathogenesis, none of which are entirely satisfactory. Older writers divided the cause into *reflex*, the exciting factor being some irritation in the pelvic organs, as a retroverted uterus, erosion and laceration of the cervix, adhesions about the tubes, hyperexcitation of the uterine nerve fibers by their being widely stretched as the organ enlarged; *neurotic*, when the vomiting was due to fear of the outcome of the pregnancy, mental unrest in women illegitimately pregnant or worry of any sort, and *toxic*, when absorption of some toxic agent was responsible. Later, hepatic degeneration was found on autopsy in patients dying of this condition, the lesions being those characteristic of acute yellow atrophy and the most constant finding being a necrosis of the central lobule, the periphery remaining intact. J. W. Williams and others have differentiated between this histological picture and that found in the liver of eclamptics, when the degenerative process begins in the periportal spaces.

For a time a high ammonia coefficient in the urine was regarded as highly significant, a much larger proportion of the total nitrogen being excreted in the form of ammonia than is usual. Normally the ammonia coefficient during pregnancy varies between 4 and 5 per cent, but in toxemic vomiting it may rise to from 20 to 50 per cent.

Glycogen deficiency in the liver of the mother has been strongly suggested as the cause of pernicious vomiting, it being believed that the morning vomiting is due to starvation during the night and a resulting hypoglycemia in the morning. This view has been opposed, the finding of hypoglycemia being uncorroborated by several experimenters.

A view quite generally accepted at present and subscribed to by the writer is that during the early months of gestation, the syncytium is the most active and specialized tissue of the developing ovum. The syncytial cells, with their property of eroding and in a measure digesting the decidua, exert a powerful influence and indeed seem to act in an almost endocrine manner, precipitating some agent into the blood stream which has a specific action upon the nervous centers controlling vomiting.

Corroborative evidence is furnished by the frequency and severity with which hyperemesis appears in association with certain diseases of the chorion, in which the syncytial cells grow in an atypical manner and in which the uterine vascular spaces are penetrated to a considerable extent by these cell masses. Thus Pinard reports a true hyperemesis in 19 instances out of 27 cases of hydatid mole and among 6 cases of this condition studied by the writer toxic vomiting of a grave nature was present in 4.

This view will explain the gradual cessation of vomiting, spontaneously, toward the end of the third month, as the syncytium becomes more and more inert and its secretive activity less. Furthermore, it is in consonance with the fact that vomiting ceases almost universally when the ovum dies as in cases where pregnancy has been therapeutically terminated for the relief of the symptoms.

It is the conviction of the writer that all vomiting in pregnancy is primarily toxic in character usually aggravated by a strong neurotic factor, and that reflex irritations are entirely secondary. While it is true that the reposition of a retroverted uterus or, indeed, simple dilatation of the cervix with the finger have affected cures, it is reasonable to suppose that in these cases the normal resistance of the body forces against the toxemia was just overbalanced by the added reflex irritation and that elimination of this added load restored the balance, the symptoms ceasing forthwith.

Retroversion of the uterus, constipation, laceration of the cervix, are all extremely common conditions but very, very rarely is persistent nausea and vomiting found accompanying any of them *per se*. Only with the occurrence of pregnancy in these women does vomiting appear, continue during the first few months, and then spontaneously cease. Furthermore, since in a large majority of the most marked cases of hyperemesis, no pelvic lesion of any sort is discoverable, it seems illogical to ascribe the vomiting to such cause.

Undoubtedly there is a strong psychic element underlying pernicious vomiting, even though the direct exciting factor be a toxemia, and in many instances, when suggestive therapeutic measures have successfully eliminated the neurotic factor, the normal bodily resistances readily overcome the toxemias, whatever they may be and the symptoms clear up.

Foci of infection remote from the birth canal sometimes are important etiological agents since they tend to overthrow the delicately balanced metabolisms in pregnancy and to reinforce the inroads of the toxic elements.

Cases in which prompt relief from hyperemesis has followed the extraction of abscessed teeth or the removal of infected tonsils illustrate this mechanism, although here again, the possibility of suggestion playing a part cannot be ignored.

In brief then, any degree of vomiting during pregnancy is due, apparently, to the circulation through the tissues of some form of toxin derived primarily from the ovum.

In the majority of instances the normal physiological readjustments of metabolism readily overcome the toxic invasion and the vomiting is spontaneously held in control, ceasing at about the end of the third month.

In a minority of instances the balance is thrown against the normal readjustments and the vomiting becomes pernicious. Reflex sources of irritation and focal infection may add to this imbalance but are in no sense causal. A strong neurotic element is present in greater or less degree in most cases, if not in all.

Prognosis.—Although women who suffer from hyperemesis often become very ill, recovery is the rule, fatal results being very uncommon unless some accident supervene as cardiac dilatation from the effort of almost continual retching or cerebral hemorrhage from the same cause.

When death results from the vomiting itself, there are always found a group of pathological findings whose incidence seems to be due to another set of etiological factors. I refer to the acute yellow atrophy of the liver, which is by no means a constant accompaniment of pernicious vomiting but which seems to be associated with it in a certain percentage of cases.

Pathology.—There are no organic lesions directly associated with hyperemesis so far as is known, since most patients recover and present no sequelae which point to any permanent tissue damage.

In fatal cases, unless the death be, as it were, accidental from cardiac failure, cerebral hemorrhage or from starvation, there are regularly noted profound changes in the liver and occasionally in the kidneys. The hepatic lesions first described by Matthews Duncan in 1879 have been repeatedly confirmed, the work of Ewing, Stone, Williams, Winter and Hofbauer being especially noteworthy. Williams in his terse and accurate summary of the findings says in effect that the liver changes are identical with those observed in acute yellow atrophy. There is a profound necrosis of the central portion of the lobules, while the periphery remains intact. In other cases the necrosis is absent but the entire liver has undergone marked fatty degeneration, so that upon staining fresh specimens with sudan red, practically the entire specimen seems to be filled with fat. The renal lesions are degenerative in character and are practically limited to the convoluted tubules, whose epithelium in many cases is necrotic and whose lumina are filled with débris. As a rule the renal changes occur only in the terminal stage of the disease. The stomach may show small petechiae and areas of hemorrhages caused by the violent vomiting. Inasmuch as hepatic lesions of the character described are almost always fatal, and since, as has been said, so few cases of hyperemesis reach a lethal termination, it seems clear that these so-called "liver cases" belong to a distinct type, that these changes are not characteristic of hyperemesis and that accordingly, this group should be classified as a special variety of toxemia, closely akin to acute yellow atrophy of the liver.

There are a series of chemical changes accompanying severe vomiting of pregnancy, the most prominent being decreased blood chlorides, high ammonia coefficient in the urine, increased nonprotein nitrogen, increased uric, amino and lactic acids and great increase of acetone bodies in the blood stream. All of these changes may be accounted for by starvation and dehydration.

Symptoms.—The toxemia of early pregnancy varies from cases of very slight indisposition wherein the "morning sickness" amounts to nothing more than a distressing nausea during the early hours of the forenoon with perhaps occasional attacks of vomiting, to the very grave cases where the exhaustion and starvation acidosis attains a severity which places the patient in deadly peril of her life, and which indeed may result fatally.

The symptoms are best grouped in periods of stages of the disease as suggested in the old classification by DuBois, in 1852.

First Stage.—The morning sickness becomes rapidly more intense until the patient vomits all food taken, even water being almost immediately rejected. After a few days, attempts at vomiting may be almost continuous even though nothing has been taken by mouth. There is rapid emaciation, marked restlessness, insomnia by reason of the continuous vomiting although the patient may be very sleepy. Anxiety is intense, many of these unfortunate women beseeching the attendant for relief from their intolerable nausea. The urine is concentrated, small in amount, rich in urea, its ammonia coefficient steadily rising until it may reach to 10, 20 or even 40 per cent. There is usually some bile in the urine, and albuminuria may occur although this is by no means a constant factor and is not an essential finding.

The blood pressure is consistently low, 90 minimum systolic being a very ordinary reading.

The pulse is elevated, its rate usually rising from day to day in an irregular but continuous upward curve.

Slight jaundice is common, the tongue is thickly furred, the coating becoming brownish and there may be considerable tenderness in the epigastrium.

The temperature is normal or subnormal, the breath heavy, and the bowels obstinately constipated, the feces hard and dry.

Second Stage.—With the progress of the disease, signs of dehydration appear, the features being pinched and wizened, and the emaciation rapidly becoming intense.

Sordes develop about the mouth, gingivitis with small hemorrhages from the gums is present. The pulse rapidly increases, a rate of 120 to 130 per minute being frequently noted. The heart sounds become weak and distant. Acidosis develops, acetone and diacetic acid are found in the urine, the breath assumes a sweetish odor and a low delirium may supervene.

Third Stage.—In untreated cases this third stage is the terminal one. Delirium becomes more marked and may be maniacal in type.

The vomiting is of a coffee-ground character and may contain free blood from a developing gastric ulcer. The pulse becomes very small and rapid, the urine is intensely concentrated and may be almost suppressed. Jaundice becomes marked and death results from cardiac failure or pure toxemic exhaustion.

Happily the great majority of cases never progress beyond the first stage, a few reach the second and the proportion of women seen in the terminal stage is small indeed.

Management of the Mild, Ambulatory Case of Hyperemesis Gravidarum.—While prophylaxis in the true sense of the term is impossible in the toxemia of pregnancy, prompt attention to the first days of vomiting may so reduce the all-important neurotic element that the more advanced stages of the disease may never appear.

Careful explanation of the phenomenon to the patient and her family and the assurance that the vomiting is but a phase of pregnancy and that it most certainly disappears after the third month, if not before, does a world of good. Physical examination will reveal reflex causes, foci of infection, etc., which must be corrected at the outset. The daily life of the woman should be ordered in detail. She should not have any association with the preparation of food, and if possible should not rise in the morning but take a light breakfast in bed.

There should be short intervals between meals which themselves are but small in amount and eaten with a minimum of fluid accompaniment. The smaller meals may consist of soda or salted crackers, popcorn, Zwieback or dry toast, with a little jam or marmalade, a dry cereal. Some items of food should be eaten at two-hour intervals during the entire day, with a little nibbling from a bedside tray if the woman should be wakeful. Plain candy, peppermints, etc., supply some needed sugar and are often well tolerated as is ice cream.

Fluids should be taken in abundance, not with food but rather in the intervals between meals. Carbonated water and ginger ale are often more acceptable than plain water.

Milk is often refused and its use at this time should not be enforced. The prescribed meals of the day, luncheon and dinner, may consist of the ordinary mixed menu, no article being specially interdicted, but the amount should be small, and the fluids restricted.

Daily rest in the afternoon is essential, with long hours of sleep at night and as much gentle outdoor exercise as the patient may accomplish without undue fatigue.

Medication.—Mild sedatives and alkalis are usually indicated. The effervescent tablets of bromide now on the market are valuable. Three tablets daily, the usual bromide content of each being 15 grains, will suffice.

Insomnia is met by the use of barbiturates in small amount. Pentobarbital sodium in ¾-grain doses or phenobarbital ¾ grain at bedtime is safe and efficacious.

The old soda mint mixture is often highly regarded by patients.

℞ Sod. bicarb. .... 10 gr.
    Spts. ammon. aromat. .... ½ ʒ
    Aquae menth. pip. .... 1 ʒ

The effervescent alkalines sold under many trade names are also elegant and useful preparations.

Constipation should be controlled by the administration of milk of magnesia, ½ to 1 ounce doses, mineral oil or if necessary the vegetable cathartics as fluidextract cascara sagrada, 20 to 30 minims.

Occasionally there is a deficiency of hydrochloric acid and improvement results from the exhibition of the agent possibly in connection with a tonic

℞ Acid. hydrochlor. .... 10 ℳ
    Tr. nucis vomicae .... 10 ℳ
    Tr. gent. comp. .... 1 ʒ

before meals diluted.

As time goes on and the symptoms improve, the meals may be larger, the intervals between them longer and the patient may gradually resume her usual way of life.

The management of the more severe forms of pernicious vomiting is based upon:

1. The management of neurosis by strong suggestive therapy.
2. The elimination of associated pathological foci.
3. The control of restlessness and the securing of sleep.
4. The treatment of the dehydration by supplying fluids to replace those lost by vomiting and to compensate for the lack of fluid intake.
5. The supplying of assimilable food to overcome starvation.
6. The control of acidosis by alkalinization of the tissues.
7. The termination of pregnancy if a fair trial of other measures fail.

To these may be added (8) attempts at specific treatment.

The above measures should be combined in a definitely planned course of treatment during which all of the indications are to be met.

Psychic effect should be obtained by a confident and self-assured approach on the part of the physician who should first complete a painstaking history and physical examination. The patient is then to be quietly informed that she will be promptly relieved upon the institution of treatment, provided all ordered details are exactly carried out.

The woman should be absolutely isolated from her family and friends for a trial period of forty-eight hours at least and obviously the best form of isolation is hospitalization which also carries with it a change of room and scene and instills a conviction of active treatment into the receptive mind of the patient.

If removal to a hospital is impossible the cooperation of the family should be demanded in order that isolation may be carried out. A competent nurse is a necessity, who must not be a relative or intimate friend of the patient and who is instructed on no account to discuss with her charge the symptoms of the latter's illness nor indeed may any professional topic be the subject of conversation.

A careful and complete physical examination will reveal any possible foci of irritation which, if found, should receive immediate attention. The retroverted uterus is to be replaced, the eroded cervix painted with phenol or silver nitrate, infected tonsils treated, preliminary to their removal, and abscessed teeth extracted if this be possible. Should constipation be a factor colonic irrigation will dispose of the fecal sources of toxemia.

Restlessness and insomnia are best combated by the bold use of morphine in combination with hypnotics. When the patient has been prepared for sleep and the necessary manipulations are completed, the exhibition of ¼ grain morphine sulphate hypodermically and 15 to 20 grains chloral hydrate per rectum will usually result in a quiet night's sleep, the patient awakening in the morning greatly refreshed and usually in a fairly optimistic mood.

On the second night the morphine may be omitted, the chloral alone being administered, the same plan being followed on the third night, if necessary, which is not usually the case.

Dehydration, acidosis and starvation are controlled by the intravenous administration of glucose. Some authorities believe the maintenance of sugar balance to be an essential in the treatment and others hold that glucose is almost, if not entirely, a specific in this field and, unquestionably, soluble sugar both as a food and as a weapon against acidosis is of prime importance. The glucose should be administered by the intravenous route and the proper therapeutic dosage must be carefully estimated. A careful report by Titus in this connection summarizes the results of many observations. Dextrose or glucose is best administered in hypertonic solution. Twenty-five per cent concentration being the most satisfactory for general use, although as Titus points out, in the dehydrated patient suffering from pregnancy toxemia, to whom water is a great necessity, more dilute solutions, say 10 per cent, are advisable. The amount of glucose to be used is of great importance, since it has been shown that excessive dosage so overstimulates the pancreas that a hypoglycemia is produced with symptoms similar to a moderately severe insular shock. Underdosage, on the other hand, fails of its therapeutic purpose.

It has been found by Titus and his coworkers that 75 Gm. in 25 per cent solution is the optimum dose for a woman of average size, the amount being increased or decreased in direct ratio to marked variations from this average.

The rate of injection is also important since too rapid administration simply produces a rapid loss of sugar through the kidney. No more than 0.8 Gm. of glucose per kilogram of body weight should be injected per hour, according to the accepted findings of Wilder and Sansum. This means that at least thirty minutes should be allowed for the injection of 25 Gm. of glucose, and a slower rate is even somewhat better.

Dehydration may be so marked as to require further measures of restoring fluid balance and this may be accomplished by the rectal instillation of normal saline, further alkalinized by the addition of 5 per cent sodium bicarbonate if acidosis be marked.

An ordinary douche bag to the tube of which a fair-sized rubber catheter is attached forms an acceptable apparatus, the fluid being allowed to flow at a rate of from 30 to 40 drops per minute, at a temperature of 100° to 104° F. The temperature in the bag may be maintained by attaching one or two lighted electric bulbs to the outside of it and covering the whole with a Turkish towel. In hospital practice, of course, the usual proctoclysis apparatus will be utilized.

Neither food, water or drugs are administered by mouth, though annoying thirst may be allayed by giving small pieces of ice.

In a very large proportion of cases, such treatment carried out with minute attention to detail for from twenty-four to forty-eight hours will result in an entire reversal of the clinical picture. Vomiting ceases, restlessness disappears and the patient lies quiet and expectant, awaiting with confidence the next step in her management.

Feeding may then be resumed, and here again great attention to the psychological element is necessary.

Inasmuch as hyperemesis is in no sense an expression of any gastro-intestinal lesion, but purely a reflex phenomenon, no special foods are required or interdicted.

The first meal consists of a carefully selected lamb chop or beef steak, free from fat and daintily broiled, a baked potato and a small portion of green vegetable, string beans or spinach. The invalid tray is set up with the most delicate china and the crispest napery available decorated, if possible, with a flower or two and presented without previous information that the taking of any food is contemplated. Patients after fasting will regard such a tray at first with some anxiety and then with delight and often will make an excellent repast without any recurrence of vomiting whatsoever.

In a minority of instances the food will be ejected and the nausea return, in which case the treatment should be repeated from the beginning, another twenty-four or forty-eight hours being allowed to elapse before further attempts at feeding.

Induction of Abortion.—If after this time there is no improvement it is probable that severe hepatic lesions are present, and after consultation with a professional colleague, the pregnancy should be terminated.

The rapidity with which women who are apparently in extremis recover their strength and health after termination of pregnancy in these cases is amazing.

The anxious, restless, sometimes delirious woman, with a pulse rate of alarming rapidity, shallow respiration, extreme acidosis and emaciation, will often eat a large meal within a few hours after emergence from the anesthetic and within a few days will have put on an astonishing amount of weight with corresponding improvement in her vitality.

The decision as to the proper moment to induce abortion is most difficult and important, since the patient may not be possessed of sufficient recuperative powers to withstand the necessary traumatism, if the procedure be delayed too long, and on the other hand, many infant lives will be unnecessarily sacrificed if too prompt surgical intervention be practiced. The indications for therapeutic abortion are:

1. Steadily rising pulse rate.
2. Marked evidence of starvation, as evidenced by dehydration.
3. Acidosis
4. Delirium
5. Progressive jaundice.
6. Increased weakness.

There are two difficulties attending upon therapeutic abortion in the treatment of toxemia:

1. That abortion is done too soon, before necessary.
2. That it is done too late when the patient is of such low resistance that she will succumb in spite of therapeutics. To judge the proper time requires experience.

The combination of toxic and neurotic symptoms exhibited by these women is most striking, and treatment to be successful must attack both these widely divergent etiological factors in combination. It is probable that all cases of pernicious vomiting are primarily toxic in their nature, the psychic features being secondary and varying with the mental stability of the individual.

Furthermore, inasmuch as but a small number of these patients die, and as late hepatic disease is unusual among the many who recover, it is fair to assume that the changes in the liver are morphologically slight and temporary.

Those cases which result fatally, and which on autopsy disclose the characteristic lesion of acute yellow atrophy of the liver, belong from the outset to another group in which the symptoms may be similar but the pathology far different.

There are several cautions to be observed and certain well-marked danger signals which present themselves in patients suffering from hyperemesis.

Excessive alkalinization must be avoided lest the serious acidosis be replaced by an even more serious alkalosis, and to this end the dosage of sodium bicarbonate should be kept within very moderate limits; Williams warning against the exhibition of more than 2 or 3 drachms per day.

Jaundice which deepens rapidly usually predicates severe liver damage and is an indication for prompt termination of pregnancy

A steady increase of the pulse rate from hour to hour and day to day suggests a toxic myocarditis and here again termination of pregnancy is the only means by which permanent cardiac disability may be prevented.

Specific Therapy.—From time to time various specific agents have been advocated in the management of pernicious vomiting.

The intramuscular administration of adrenalin was proposed in 1909 by Rebaudi and has had some success.

Extract of corpus luteum in 1-cm. doses given intramuscularly daily for from eight to twelve days was warmly recommended by J. C. Hirst, who reported a large percentage of cures. His results have not been generally corroborated.

Placental extracts, the serum of healthy pregnant women and serum from the cord blood have all been used with variable results.

Of late there is a growing literature concerning the employment of insulin in this condition, though no definite series of cases has yet been published, though attention is directed to the suggestive article of Andre Weill and Laudat.

Pilocarpine hydrochloride as a specific has been successfully employed by Levy-Solal and Le Loup, who base the use of this agent upon its special action on anaphylactic phenomena and who hold that hyperemesis is an expression of a colloidoclastic activity.

These authors are enthusiastic regarding this method of treatment and report several brilliant successes.

Specific therapy may be dismissed from the present with the statement that no one agent has proved itself sovereign in the treatment of hyperemesis, but that such encouraging results in scattered instances have followed the use of various sera or glandular extracts that it seems fair to believe that the control of this form of toxemia is to be found somewhere along such lines of investigation.

Blood transfusion as originally advocated by Garnett has recently been employed by Bissell, who successfully treated two marked cases by the transfusion of 250 cc. of blood. The serum of normally pregnant women has been utilized with success by Fieux and his followers and normal human serum has also been used. The results of these agents are not uniform and their value as specifics still awaits confirmation.

THE TOXEMIAS OF LATE PREGNANCY

Mild Hypertensive Toxemia (Low Reserve Kidney); Preeclampsia (More Advanced Hypertensive Toxemia); Eclampsia; Nephritic Toxemia; Hepatic Toxemia

DEFINITION

The toxemia of late pregnancy may be defined as a symptom complex occurring during the latter half of pregnancy, all of whose manifestations are referable to changes in the renal function, although on autopsy most marked lesions are present in the liver.

It is characterized by hypertension, albuminuria, edema and, untreated, eventuates usually in convulsions, coma and death, unless spontaneous recovery should follow the delivery of the child.

Low Reserve Kidney.—This is a term suggested by Stander and Peckham to include a large group (35–40 per cent) of the milder toxemic cases and which takes in those formerly designated as "kidney of pregnancy," "simple albuminuria," "hydrops gravidarum," etc.

It is a condition characterized by albuminuria in mild degree, rarely more than 2 Gm. per liter, usually less than 1 Gm.; by moderate hypertension from 150 to 160 mm. systolic with 90 diastolic or thereabouts. A few casts are present in the urine and there is moderate edema.

The blood chemistry shows no change and there may be no subjective symptoms whatever although some patients complain of malaise and headache. Excessive weight gain usually accompanies this condition.

Etiology.—There is no known explanation for the low reserve kidney. In normal individuals about one half the glomeruli function, the remainder constituting a reserve for unusual kidney strain. In the condition under discussion, it is believed that this normal reserve has been reduced for some reason, so that while the kidneys may function perfectly under the usual conditions of life, they cannot respond to the added stress of pregnancy.

There is no permanent damage to the kidney in low reserve toxemia, the function returning to normal within a few weeks after delivery and curiously enough, the condition may not appear during subsequent pregnancies.

It is probable that in most instances, however, low reserve kidney, if unrecognized and untreated, will eventuate in preeclampsia and even in eclampsia in its true sense.

Preeclampsia.—This rather confusing term is best applied to those cases of sudden toxemia, developing generally during the last two months of pregnancy, presenting all the evidences of renal insufficiency, often terminating in true eclampsia, sometimes improving rapidly after treatment.

Hypertension is marked, a sudden rise of systolic pressure to 200 mm. or more being common. Albuminuria is a constant finding. Five to 20 Gm. per liter being the rule. Edema of the feet and hands and also of the face may be expected, and retinal hemorrhages, or edema, with choked disk is a serious but common finding.

The patient may be dull and apathetic or restless as if a convulsion were impending and in some instances twitching of the extremities is noted.

The blood chemistry is not altered except for an increase in its uric acid content and some lowering of the CO_2 combining power.

Etiology.—This remains entirely unknown, though recent writers emphasize hyperpituitary function as causative.

Eclampsia (to flush, or shine out) may be defined as a toxic disease of late pregnancy, characterized by intermittent convulsions, generally clonic, sometimes tonic, which are followed by ever deepening coma, and carry a high mortality rate. The convulsive attacks are preceded by marked albuminuria, hypertension, edema, epigastric distress, visual disturbances, headache and constipation. In a word, eclampsia is the final stage of preeclamptic toxemia, which almost always precedes it, for a longer or shorter period.

Eclampsia may occur during late pregnancy, antepartum eclampsia; during labor, intrapartum eclampsia; or after delivery, puerperal eclampsia. As to the relative frequency of the time of onset, it is probable that most cases begin before labor, and that the profound systemic stimulation of the convulsive seizures originate uterine contraction, the patient going into labor. Hence the statistical statement that eclampsia most often occurs during labor, which is in error.

Nephritic Toxemia.—This term is used to designate those cases in which the toxemia of late pregnancy is superimposed upon a preexisting nephritis. Any form of nephropathy may occur among pregnant women, chronic glomerulonephritis or some form of nephrosclerosis being the most common.

It does not follow that because a woman has a chronic nephritis she must necessarily become toxic during pregnancy, but it is true that damaged kidneys withstand the added strain of pregnancy badly, that under this strain the severity of the disease may be greatly aggravated and it is probable that each succeeding pregnancy tends to increase the renal damage. It is also true that with careful management of pregnancy and labor, many nephritic women may enjoy offspring without any appreciable exacerbation of the nephritis.

Preexisting kidney disease is present in from 10 to 20 per cent of all women presenting signs of the toxemia of late pregnancy and its presence should be carefully sought for in the antenatal study of the patient.

Etiology.—Chronic nephritis may be due to some infectious diseases of childhood, may be the result of focal infection in the teeth or tonsils, etc., or it may follow renal injury developing after preeclampsia or eclampsia in a previous pregnancy.

Hepatic Toxemia.—Acute yellow atrophy of the liver or icterus gravis is happily an uncommon complication of pregnancy, only about 100 cases having been recorded.

Etiology.—This remains entirely unknown.

Pathology.—On autopsy there is always atrophy of the liver, with central necrosis of the lobules, which may, indeed, involve the entire lobule. There is also usually an associated acute nephritis. Prognosis is most grave, the disease usually having a fatal termination.

Recapitulation.—The toxemias of late pregnancy, with the exception of the late hepatic type, present the same clinical picture in a general sense.

In some instances the symptoms develop gradually and steadily, in others there is a fulminating onset, some cases never go beyond a mild course, some come on with incredible violence and severity.

A woman thought to be suffering from low reserve kidney with its benign symptomatology may suddenly become preeclamptic and so on.

It may be said then, that from the practical standpoint, these toxemias may be best considered as different manifestations of the same process in different individuals whose reactions vary with their personal resistance to the inroads of toxins. The management is the same in all of them, varying only with the severity of the disease.

FREQUENCY

The toxemia of late pregnancy is said to occur about once in every 500 labors, but if the preconvulsive stage be included, it is probable that at least 2 pregnant women per 100 disclose some evidences of its presence.

Statistics on this point are very variable, as witness the 0.7 per cent incidence in 120,000 labors at the New York Lying-in Hospital reported by McPherson as compared with the 2.5 per cent incidence of Lichtenstein's cases. Hospital reports are, of course, unreliable, since many of the less severe cases are not hospitalized and escape notice.

In Philadelphia, eclampsia is much more common among the foreign born and negro elements of the population than among native Americans, this being possibly accounted for by the less careful attention to diet and the neglect of prenatal care in these women.

The seasonal variation is striking as has been well shown by Harrar, who analyzed the eclampsias admitted to the house during a period of ten years and was able to construct a curve showing the peak of occurrence during the early spring, and a corresponding low point in the late fall.

Climatic influences have been further studied by Oppenheimer, who showed that the absolute air pressures have no effect upon attacks of eclampsia, while temperatures well above the monthly mean do favor it. High temperatures probably necessitate an increased metabolism and, with it, an increase in residue, which overbalance the adaptability of the already weakened excretory system.

The disease seems to be more common in cold climates than in the tropics and has been stated to occur with greater frequency in rural than in urban communities.

Primiparae are more prone to the toxemia of late pregnancy than multiparae, the ratio being almost four to one.

Recurrence.—Eclampsia and preeclamptic toxemia may recur in subsequent pregnancies, although the disease seems to create a relative immunity. Recurrence occurs in about 2 per cent of eclampsias, and Williams believes that a woman who has had eclampsia is less liable to it in future pregnancies than one who has never had it.

MORTALITY AND PROGNOSIS

The death rate in eclampsia remains far too high though considerable reduction has been brought about by the gradual abandonment of the more radical and traumatic methods of treatment and their substitution by some form of conservative therapy.

Statistics naturally vary with the nature of the work done in different institutions. The city hospital, with its constant population of neglected cases among undernourished individuals of poor heredity and worse environment, will show a far higher mortality than the institution where prenatal care is the rule and emergency cases form but a small minority of the admissions.

The average mortality for the mother is still about 20 per cent, when eclampsia develops, but naturally is far lower when the toxemia is recognized and treated in its early stages. The statistics vary from the 5.31 per cent of Strogonoff to the 45–7 per cent of Buttner.

In a well run hospital service the mortality should be under 10 per cent. The disease is very destructive to the infant, 20 to 30 per cent being the usual death rate. The infant deaths are due to prematurity, toxemia, asphyxia from convulsions of the mother and birth injuries resultant upon hasty and traumatic delivery.

Death in eclampsia is the result usually of cardiac failure, respiratory failure during a convulsion, apoplexy, or overwhelming toxemia.

Dilatation of the heart is by far the most common lethal factor, with toxemia second and arrest of respiration responsible for but few fatalities.

The *prognosis* depends chiefly upon the condition and behavior of the heart. Given a strong, firm cardiac muscle with full, regular and not too rapid pulse, the prognosis is good no matter how many the convulsions, or how marked the urinary changes.

Conversely, in cases where the albuminuria is moderate, the blood pressure is not excessive and the convulsions few or, indeed, not present, the prognosis is uniformly grave when the heart muscle is weak, the valve sounds distant and flapping and the pulse rapid, irregular and of small volume. One cannot determine whether convulsions will continue and toxemia become more intense but the condition of the heart muscle is a fairly definite indication of the outcome and prognosis may be based upon this fact alone.

ETIOLOGY

The cause of the toxemias of late pregnancy remains shrouded in obscurity.

An immense literature has accumulated upon the subject but our knowledge as to the true cause has not advanced in the slightest. Some of the more attractive theories as to the etiology are as follows: *absorption* of the end-products of Fetal Metabolism: (Fehling and Dienst followed by other workers.) Not proved.

Toxemia derived from substances formed by an autolysis of the placenta, or by the absorption of enzymes developed in the syncytia.

Bacterial Invasion.—Strogonoff thought that eclampsia was an infectious disease of respiratory tract origin; various bacteria have been isolated from the blood of toxemic patients.

Endocrine Origin.—A pressor and acute diuretic agent presumably of pituitary origin has been found in the blood of toxic women (Anselmino and Hoffman).

Dysfunction of the thyroid, adrenal and parathyroid glands has also been invoked as a cause. Not proved.

None of these diverse views have been shown to be correct and the whole subject of etiology is best dismissed with the simple statement —unknown. For a detailed discussion of this matter the reader is referred to the monograph of H. J. Stander, and the scholarly résumé in the late Prof. J. W. Williams' "Obstetrics."

In considering the etiology of this most baffling lesion, one fact stands out; that the presence of a living fetus and its envelopes, the former approaching maturity, are essential factors since no condition comparable to eclampsia has been observed in other than pregnant women. Inasmuch as the disease is very rare in the early months of gestation there is evidently some source whose output of toxins increases with the maturity of the fetus. Furthermore, since eclampsia is not common among women carrying dead fetus, it follows that the toxic agent is associated with a living, growing embryo.

PATHOLOGY

The pathological findings in the toxemias of late pregnancy only add to the confusion as to the etiology, since though the symptoms and course of the disease would seem to predicate overwhelming vascular and renal lesions, the organ most damaged is the liver. However, kidney changes are found in over 95 per cent of eclamptic patients coming to autopsy (Drutz) although there is still dispute among pathologists as to whether these changes are primary or secondary.

The characteristic autopsy finding is peripheral necrosis of the liver lobule, with thrombosis of the smaller, interlobular periportal vessels, with hemorrhagic and anemic necrosis and occasionally diffuse thrombosis of the portal vessels with degenerative changes in the liver (Fig. 160).

The kidneys are almost always damaged in eclampsia, the common lesion being a glomerulonephrosis (Fahr, Lubarsch), viewed by many pathologists as significant of pregnancy toxemia and differing from the glomerulonephritis of infectious origin. There are degenerative changes in the tubules and a distinct decrease in the lumen of the capillaries caused by thickening of the capillary basement membrane. There may also be a necrosis of the renal cortex (Fig. 161).

The Brain.—Almost any cerebral lesion may be found in patients dying of eclampsia.   Hyperemia or anemia, softening, with or without edema, capillary hemorrhages or thrombosis and in some instances massive hemorrhage occurs.

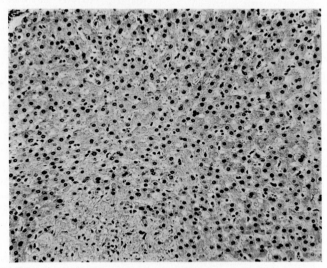

Fig. 160.—The liver in eclampsia showing degeneration of the liver cells with peripheral necrosis of the lobules.

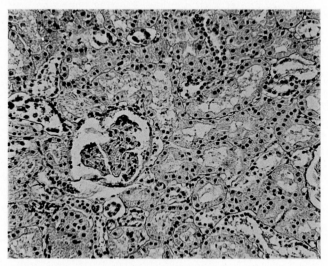

Fig. 161.—The kidney in eclampsia, showing degeneration of the tubular epithelium and marked cloudy swelling.

The Heart.—In about 95 per cent of all cases, the heart is found to be more or less affected. Degenerative changes in the myocardium are common, varying from cloudy swelling to fatty change.   There may be coronary thrombosis or small thrombotic areas scattered through the heart muscle.

The Lungs.—May be normal, though pulmonary edema is common, and masses of syncytial cells have been demonstrated in the capillaries of the lung. This is probably an accidental finding, usual in pregnancy.

DIAGNOSIS AND SYMPTOMATOLOGY

It has been previously stated that the toxemia of late pregnancy is generally a progressive process, usually beginning insidiously and if untreated proceeding with greater or less rapidity to a grave state, wherein the classical symptom of convulsion, marked albuminuria, retinal hemorrhage, etc., develop in all their terrible aspects. The first evidence of an oncoming toxemia may be considered under six heads:

1. Changes in the circulatory system.
2. Changes in the urinary system.
3. Chemical changes.
4. General systemic changes.
5. Eye lesions.
6. Changes in the nervous system.

Changes in the Circulatory System:

a. Hypertension.

b. Edema.

Hypertension during pregnancy is *always* suggestive of beginning toxemia and may never be ignored in obstetrical practice.

The onset of hypertension may occur at any time during gestation, depending upon the degree of preexisting kidney damage. Thus in patients suffering from glomerulonephritis of the infectious type, the blood pressure may be elevated even before conception and may be found above normal at the first examination by the obstetrician. This finding is always suggestive of dangerous kidney disease and should demand a careful study of the renal function (q. v. differential diagnosis). In most cases the hypertension first appears at the sixth or seventh month and may be gradual or sudden in development.

Any persistent elevation of blood pressure of 10 mm. or more in a pregnant woman is sufficient basis for a diagnosis of at least impending toxemia.

The rise may be quite slow and gradual, a woman whose normal pressure is 110/60, one day disclosing an elevation to 120/68. Within two weeks the elevation may reach 130/75–140/80, etc., with a steady increase until an alarming hypertension ensues.

In other cases the rise may come with great speed, an increase of 40 to 50 mm. in systolic pressure occurring in two or three days.

Edema; Swelling.—When such edema is present upon arising in the morning and extends well up the leg, it is significant of toxic change. This is particularly true when the edema affects the upper portion of the body, the hands and face. Puffiness of the latter, with

18

a complaint of marked swelling of the hands is highly suggestive of toxemia. There has been described a "hidden edema" (Willock), in which there may be an accumulation of fluid in the tissues, with a sense of fulness and swelling of the hands, and some smoothing of the lines of the face, but no demonstrable edema.

The amount of swelling and the rapidity with which it occurs, offer a fair index as to the severity of the toxemia, although it is true that patients with the most widespread and marked edema usually suffer from less marked and more infrequent convulsions than do those in whom the swelling is less marked.

Also there are cases of severe toxemia in which little or no edema is present. Excessive gain in weight is a common finding among toxic women. This increase is in part due to lack of dietary control in unsupervised patients, in part to the accumulation of fluid in the tissues.

In a series of cases studied at Kensington Hospital, the average weight gain of nontoxic women during pregnancy was 24 pounds, while in the toxic group 38 to 40 pounds was the rule.

Urinary Changes.—Albuminuria in varying degree is a fairly constant finding in the toxemia of late pregnancy. In general the amount of albumin rises in direct ratio to the elevation of blood pressure, until from a "faint trace" it may reach 40 Gm. per liter at which point the urine boils solid. Slight or moderate albuminuria alone is not necessarily alarming since it may simply be an expression of the low reserve kidney, or as it was formerly known, the kidney of pregnancy. Albuminuria associated with hypertension, however, is always significant of the onset of true toxemia. The urine may contain casts, which are usually small in number but which may be abundant in cases of chronic nephritis and which may be present in very large numbers in the violent, fulminating type of eclamptic attack.

Pus and blood cells may be present, in which case pyelitis should always be suspected and sought for.

The amount of urine voided in toxemia is usually decreased. With the growth of edema there is a corresponding diminution of urinary output, until in severe eclampsia there is practically complete anuria. Excretion of from 2 to 4 ounces in twenty-four hours is not uncommon and sometimes catheterization of the woman having repeated convulsions, will secure but a drachm or two of immensely concentrated urine, solid with albumin and containing many hyaline and granular casts and erythrocytes. With the subsidence of the symptoms and after appropriate treatment, the urine gradually returns to normal both in amount and content.

Changes in the Body Chemistry.—Blood and urine chemistry is subject to great variations in the toxemia of late pregnancy, depending upon the stage and severity of the intoxication and upon the effects of the toxemia upon the organs of different individuals. In the milder phase as the low reserve kidney, there are no appreciable chemical changes except albuminuria. In patients suffering from chronic nephritis upon which a pregnancy toxemia has been super-imposed, there may or may not be disturbances of the nitrogen parti-tion of the urine, with a drop in the urea nitrogen and an increase in ammonia nitrogen, while nitrogen retention in the blood may not ap-pear until the nephritis has attained a grave degree of advancement.

In the acute and quickly developing preeclamptic toxemia, without preexisting nephritis, examination of the blood will reveal a lowered CO_2 combining power and a steadily growing uric acid content. Otherwise the blood chemistry is usually unaltered.

In true eclampsia with or without convulsion, there is increased uric acid, decreased CO_2 combining power and markedly lowered pH of the blood. The blood sugar is variable, some investigators as Titus and his followers finding a persistent hypoglycemia, though it is gen-erally believed that there is usually an increased blood sugar.

The variations in the other constituents of the blood are still under investigation and no generally accepted changes have been described. True, acidosis, due to an uncompensated alkali deficit, is a common finding and is sometimes severe enough in itself to cause death (Stander).

General Symptoms.—The woman with a developing toxemia usually feels dull and listless although in patients who have presented the picture of fatigue and weakness which is associated with persistent hypotension, there may be a great apparent improvement in general health due to the elevation of the blood pressure. The skin usually becomes dull and vague headache begins, there may be "heartburn" and a gaseous indigestion with sometimes a return of the nausea and vomiting of the early months.

Constipation is common, and hemorrhoids often add to the distress of the patient. The gain in weight and edema have been mentioned already.

Eye Changes.—Early in the course of toxemia, the patient may complain of floating spots before the eyes—muscae volantes—later amblyopia and amaurosis may occur, but retinitis and retinal detach-ment are the most important lesions met. These retinal changes simply predicate some disease of the general arterial system with hypertension. The so-called "retinitis" is dependent upon a construc-tion of the lumen of the capillaries, brought about by toxic spastic contraction.

This may be followed by complete stasis, localized edema and hemorrhage, with sometimes diffuse, albuminuric retinitis. Detach-ment of the retina to varying degree also occurs.

These lesions may improve rapidly after the subsidence of the toxemia, or they may persist with permanent impairment of vision, rarely almost complete blindness.

Changes in the Nervous System.—Headache and dizziness are fre-quently precursors of toxic invasion, and as the poisoning proceeds there may be mental and nervous irritability, the onset of convulsions often being preceded by twitchings of the extremities and sometimes nystagmus. Often, too, the patient becomes dull and listless, slow in mental reaction, going into what has been termed "mental hebetude."

THE CLINICAL PICTURE OF THE ADVANCED TOXEMIA—ECLAMPSIA

This phase of the disease is characterized by a marked rise of systolic blood pressure, 200–240 mm. being not infrequently seen. The pulse tension remains fairly constant.

The patient usually is of a dull or fairly icteric color, the tongue is thickly coated, edema is prominent. In this stage vulvar edema is sometimes a significant and troublesome complication, the labia sometimes being distended with fluid to many times their normal size, and being almost translucent.

Headache is severe and constant, and spots before the eyes are a prominent complaint. The urine is loaded with albumin, sometimes boiling solid in the test tube, casts, hyaline and granular may be present, acetone and diacetone in the very grave cases. The amount may be very small, a drachm or two of turbid thick fluid composing the entire output for hours.

There is usually marked indigestion, with more or less epigastric pain and perhaps vomiting, anorexia and constipation are constant factors and the patient complains of feeling weak and ill. Some degree of mental hebetude, a laziness and delay in the mental processes are often noted. This sluggishness is apt to alternate with intense restlessness, insomnia and a fear of impending events. On auscultation the fetal heart sounds may be found retarded in rate, a sign portending grave danger to the fetus.

At this time there may be considerable disturbances of vision and ophthalmoscopic investigation will reveal either a beginning albuminuric retinitis or retinal hemorrhages with areas of detachment in some cases.

Should the patient recover, under these conditions, there will obviously be more or less permanent interference with vision, and the extent of ocular damage as demonstrated by the ophthalmoscope should be an important factor in determining the treatment.

When a woman presents the foregoing clinical picture, the utmost energy and recourse is demanded of the medical attendant, lest the toxins continue to accumulate in the blood, until their concentration eventuates in that dread explosion, the eclamptic convulsion.

This termination may occur at any moment during the course of such toxic state, and indeed, the seizure sometimes occurs with startling suddenness. The patient, who may have been conversing with her attendant a moment before, is seen to stare into space with fixed eyes. Almost immediately there develops a twitching of the eyelids rapidly spreading to the other muscles of the face, the lips drawn back and the mouth set in a rigid and sardonic smile. The true convulsion then begins with a general muscular contraction, the respiratory muscles and the diaphragm being fixed and immobilized. Respiration is arrested and the face becomes cyanotic, the lips purple and swollen, the sclera injected until the entire picture is one of impending death from respiratory arrest. The pulse becomes rapid and may be irregular. This stage while seemingly endless, in reality lasts from but ten to twenty seconds, rarely so long and is at once succeeded by violent tonic and clonic convulsive movements involving the entire body, but more particularly the upper extremities and the head and face. Sometimes the convulsive movements are so rapid and violent that it is with the utmost difficulty that the patient is kept in bed. The champing of the jaws and the irregular and stertorous respiration causes a frothy saliva to issue from the mouth, which may be blood-stained should the tongue or cheeks be bitten.

The active convulsion may last for a minute or more when the movements become less violent and are succeeded by a period of coma, when the respiration is snoring and slow, the air being expelled with loud puffs from the swollen lips. The cyanosis gradually clears and the pulse slows and becomes more regular. In some cases the period of coma is absent, the patient recovering consciousness at once, upon the cessation of the convulsion, but in most instances there is a period of unconsciousness followed by a muttering state which either gradually fades or is succeeded by another and usually more severe and protracted convulsion. The number of such seizures is variable, some patients experience but one, most having from four to six, while more than 100 have been reported during the course of a single attack. One noteworthy case in my experience suffered 66 definite convulsions in a period of thirty-six hours, completely recovering thereafter, with no evidence of permanent kidney damage.

After an interval of time which may vary from a few minutes to a day, during which the patient may be conscious or semiconscious, lying quietly with puffing respiration and slow full pulse in some instances, or becoming extremely restless with muttering delirium in others, the convulsion again appears. Each succeeding attack lasts a little longer with a more protracted period of coma following until the scene is ended by death, or the toxins being eliminated, gradual improvement takes place, convulsions becoming shorter, milder and finally ceasing altogether. The French, who have intensively studied eclampsia, divide the attack into the stage of invasion, that of contracture and that of convulsion. The temperature in eclampsia is extremely variable, as is the case in most renal affections. Possibly remaining normal or slightly subnormal, in some instances, the temperature rises to 106° F. or even as a terminal condition to 108° F. There has been some discussion as to the cause of the fever, but it is now generally assumed to be toxic and due to some disturbance of the heat center. Occasionally a patient experiences an attack of eclampsia without going into labor, subsequently delivering a living

child. This termination is most unusual, the fetus either dying undelivered or the woman going into labor during the attack.

In fatal cases, the convulsions come on with increasing frequency
and severity, coma becomes constant, there is almost complete anuria,
the skin begins to leak, the pulse becomes rapid and thready, the temperature rises and death comes usually with pulmonary edema, and
cardiac failure. The fatal result is sometimes accelerated by the exhaustion of the expulsive efforts of labor.

A favorable outcome is suggested by a decline in the severity of
the convulsion, the reestablishment of urinary secretion, decrease of
edema and of hypertension and the birth of the child, which generally
hastens the recovery.

The cause of eclamptic convulsions has not been definitely proved
but it seems clear that they follow the irritating qualities of the specific toxin, whatever that may be, upon the nerve center, with special
affinity toward the cortex of the anterior brain.

Convulsions are often brought about by external stimuli, noise,
handling of the patient, the irritation of an indigestible meal, etc.

Some observers consider the convulsions as merely due to increased
intracranial pressure from edema of the brain.

THE DIAGNOSIS OF TOXEMIA OF LATE PREGNANCY

Is based upon the three evidences of albuminuria, edema, hypertension developing in a pregnant woman. If all three are present, the
diagnosis is absolute, whereas any one alone is not sufficient to permit
such diagnosis. Of the three, increasing hypertension is by far the
most important, edema and albuminuria following in order.

Differential Diagnosis.—In the earlier stages the one important
differential in the toxemia of late pregnancy is whether or not it is
accompanied by a preexisting nephritis, and this sometimes offers
great difficulty. A history of rheumatic disease in childhood associated with edema or, indeed, the history of any grave infectious disease
is suggestive. It may be that the woman is known to have had an
attack of nephritis, which of course will clear up the diagnosis.

Clinically, the early appearance of hypertension, edema and albuminuria arouses the suspicion that nephritis is present, but in many
cases these evidences are vague and indefinite.

Kidney function tests seem to offer the best approach to a recognition of the true condition, but here again, these tests are by no means
infallible. The phenolsulphonphthalein, the Mosenthal concentration
test and others have been utilized with generally unsatisfactory results.
The one functional test that does seem to have some appreciability is
the urea clearance based upon Ambard's law of urea excretion the test
itself having been well developed by Van Slyke and others.

The diagnosis of nephritic toxemia, unfortunately, is often reached
only after the completion of pregnancy and the puerperium, when it

is found that kidney function is definitely and permanently impaired, a state of affairs only true when the nephritis antedates the pregnancy.

Differential Diagnosis of Eclamptic Convulsion.—Convulsions may arise from causes not associated with pregnancy as epilepsy, major hysteria, strychnine or other poisoning, cerebral syphilis, brain tumor, meningitis, encephalitis, diabetes and uremia.

These differentiations offer but little difficulty, if one realizes the nature of the eclamptic convulsion, which is associated with complete unconsciousness, with intervals of lethargy or coma, with elevation of temperature, albuminuria, edema and hypertension.

Epilepsy may usually be eliminated by the history of prior attacks and the absence of signs of kidney involvement although rarely an initial seizure of grand mal occurs during pregnancy or it may even be inaugurated by an attack of toxemia (DeLee).

Hysteria, in which the patient is conscious during the convulsion, the muscular movements of which are uncoordinated and irregular, together with the absence of other symptoms should clear up the matter.

Diabetic convulsions may be recognized by the hyperglycemia, acetonuria, lowered blood pressure and so on.

Brain tumor, meningitis and encephalitis may cause difficulty, but here again the absence of the concomitant signs of pregnancy toxemia, the eye changes, muscular spasticity, conditions of the spinal fluid as shown by lumbar puncture, should aid.

True uremia cannot be separated from eclampsia, and, indeed, requires no differentiation since the management of the two conditions is identical.

MANAGEMENT OF THE TOXEMIAS OF LATE PREGNANCY

The treatment of the toxemia of late pregnancy is one of the outstanding achievements of modern medicine. While it is true that when the degree of intoxication has been reached which eventuates in eclampsia, the mortality is far too high, still the ravages of the disease have been immeasurably cut within the last generation. Further progress in this direction depends upon a more clear understanding of the pathology and the causative lesions.

The treatment may well be divided into four phases:

1. Prophylaxis.

2. The management of incipient toxemia as evidenced by rise of blood pressure, more or less albuminuria and possibly some malaise.

3. The treatment of the severe toxemias including the eclamptic state.

4. The care of a woman who has recovered from an attack of toxemia.

Prophylaxis.—It is by the prevention of eclampsia and the detection and treatment of toxemia in its earliest manifestations that prenatal care has won its place in obstetric art and indeed the results of such care justify the dictum that a death from eclampsia of a patient who has during her pregnancy been under the care of a physician is almost always absolutely inexcusable. This matter has been fully considered in the chapter upon the management of pregnancy and will be but briefly recapitulated here.

A pregnant woman should be seen by her accoucheur at least once monthly during the first seven months and twice monthly thereafter. If any evidences of ill health develop during this period the patient must be kept under the closest observation since any slight and otherwise transient infection, the common cold, a mild influenza may precipitate an attack of toxemia.

At each visit the patient is questioned as to her general health, with especial reference to headache, indigestion and constipation. Pretibial and facial edema is to be sought for, and a careful urinalysis is to be made. The blood pressure should be carefully taken and recorded.

A persistent rise of 10 mm. or more in the systolic pressure of a pregnant woman is invariably strong presumptive evidence of a beginning toxemia.

Albuminuria, if slight, is a sign of secondary importance, but must always be regarded as additional evidence. Should the albuminuria at any time increase in amount, the trace becoming a cloud, toxemia in some degree may be assumed to have begun.

Pretibial, facial and manual edema, when present serve to corroborate the more definite findings, and when in addition to the foregoing the patient complains of headache, malaise, some inertia and presents a muddy or faintly jaundiced complexion, the diagnosis is assured, particularly if corroborated by chemical change in the blood and urine. The symptoms rarely occur synchronously, a slight rise in blood pressure being usually the first change noticed. This is followed by mild albuminuria, within a week or two, the other signs rapidly developing. Many cases of toxemia, however, are manifested by rise of blood pressure alone, prompt eliminative treatment precluding the development of the associated conditions. Whenever, during pregnancy, the above clinical picture presents itself, immediate treatment should be instituted. The patient is instructed to return to her home, and invalidize herself until further investigation proves that the impending toxemia has been dissipated.

The diet should be very light, skim milk, green vegetables, lettuce with French dressing, spinach, asparagus and kale, and potatoes sparingly. No meat or eggs of any kind are to be taken, no rich soups, no pastry. Butter and other fats are to be sharply restricted. Sweets as ice cream, fruit juices and candy in moderation are allowed, salt is greatly restricted.

Great emphasis should be laid upon the question of diet, both the character and the amount of food to be indulged in, being specified. It is my plan to advise that the patient eat only one half the quantity of any permitted food that she would ordinarily regard as a portion. It is the constant observation in maternity hospitals that patients admitted in eclampsia have grossly overeaten of foods rich in proteins, just previous to the attack. The material obtained via the stomach tube in some of these women being amazing to quantity as well as to character.

The bowels should be kept quite free, preferably by the use of saline cathartics, followed by enemas or colonic irrigation if the latter be procurable. An initial draught of 1 ounce magnesium sulphate, followed by the daily administration of from 1 to 3 drachms of the effervescent sodium phosphate is a valuable procedure. The skin should be utilized as an eliminant, by sweating. This may be accomplished˶ by having the patient wrap herself into a cocoon of blankets with what hot-water bags are available, each afternoon, the position to be maintained for twenty minutes after free sweating starts. She is then to be vigorously toweled and dressed warmly enough to prevent chilling. When a bath cabinet is available, it may be utilized to obtain the necessary sweating.

If after three days of such treatment, the blood pressure has receded, the albuminuria disappeared or become greatly reduced in amount, the patient may cautiously increase her diet, avoiding all meat and potatoes, however, until the termination of her pregnancy.

The sweats may be discontinued and the woman may go out, provided the weather is favorable. The use of mild saline laxatives is to be continued for several weeks after all evidences of toxemia have disappeared. Such plan of treatment if scrupulously carried out will arrest a great majority of all toxic attacks and will return the patient to health. She is however, to be regarded as a potential eclamptic and observed with the closest scrutiny, until the completion of her puerperium ends the danger. There is usually no indication for drug therapy, unless some associated pathology becomes apparent. If restlessness and anxiety be excessive bromides may be utilized in moderate dosage. If the symptoms do not abate, the patient should be hospitalized for further study.

THE TREATMENT OF ECLAMPSIA

At the onset it may be said that in the management of a case of advanced toxemia of pregnancy, all of the resources of the medical attendant are called into requisition. Unremitting care, the almost constant observation of the patient in order to detect and combat new phases of the disease are an absolute essential for success.

The treatment is based upon the following essentials:

1. The elimination of toxins.
2. The control of convulsions.
3. The maintenance of the circulation.
4. The prevention of injury to the patient during periods of unconsciousness.

5. The preservation of the life of the child if possible.

6. The prevention of permanent damage to the kidneys.

There are certain facts of a general nature which govern the treatment and which must ever be kept in mind.

Most patients in eclampsia go into labor spontaneously either shortly after the onset of the attack or some time during its continuance. Induction of labor is therefore superfluous in the majority of instances.

Toxic patients though apparently in a sthenic state bear traumatism very badly, and succumb to shock or to an intense aggravation of their illness when radical measures are instituted. This point was well brought out by Cragin who rightly insisted upon the gentle and nontraumatic management of these cases.

General anesthesia leads often to a final kidney breakdown, due to the superimposition of the irritant anesthetic agent upon an already overstrained mechanism. The use of such anesthesia is therefore usually inadvisable.

Obstetricians are still somewhat divided in their methods of attack in grave toxemia—one group advocating prompt emptying of the uterus, either by induction of labor or by cesarean section, while a second and much larger group hold that medical treatment, permitting the pregnancy to take its natural course, offers a far greater hope of success, except in the presence of special indications. For the reasons before stated, the writer is in accord with the latter plan.

The management of eclampsia may proceed along one or a combination of several of four general plans.

1. Sedative treatment.

2. Eliminative treatment.

3. Surgical treatment.

4. Other methods.

Examination of the fundus oculi should be a routine procedure in order to determine the existence and extent of retinal damage.

Whatever plan of treatment is carried out there are certain general measures which are essential.

1. The patient must be isolated in a quiet, darkened room, *always* under the observation of an attendant.

2. All disturbances, noise, manipulation and examination must be reduced to an absolute minimum.

3. The patient must be sedulously guarded against injury.

Since there are violent uncoordinated movements during convulsion some form of restraint must be utilized, either by means of sheets fastened to the bed or in severe cases the leather restraint straps to control arms and legs.

The tongue and lips are often injured by the spasmodic biting motions of the jaws, which should be separated by means of a padded wooden tongue depressor or other similar appliance managed by the attendant.

4. The bladder should be emptied by catheter, the urine measured and subjected to immediate examination.

Sedative Treatment.—The sedative treatment was originated by Veit and developed and popularized by Stroganoff of Leningrad, who has reported the lowest mortality in a large series of cases ever recorded, 5.31 per cent, but it is more than probable that some of these cases were less severe than those usually included in statistics of eclampsia since no one has been able to equal Stroganoff's results.

Stroganoff's method includes the use of chloroform in the convulsion, together with large doses of chloral hydrate. These drugs are considered as contraindicated in eclampsia in the writer's clinic and the sedative method has accordingly been considerably modified in consequence. The details are as follows:

The general measures described above having been instituted, the patient is given a hypodermic of morphine sulphate, ¼ grain. This drug is repeated in the same dose at intervals of from one to four hours, depending upon the response of the patient, until restlessness and convulsions cease or until the therapeutic limit has been reached as shown by:

a. Respiration dropping to 12 per minute.

b. A pulse rate of 60 or thereabouts.

This medication is continued for an indefinite time, until distinct improvement occurs or until signs of increasing toxemia render more active measures imperative. In addition to the morphine, magnesium sulphate intravenously administered is of great value in reducing the number and severity of the convulsions.

This treatment, warmly advocated by Lazard and others, consists in the intravenous administration of 20 cc. of a 10 per cent solution of magnesium sulphate, the sterile ampules of this solution which are prepared by various pharmaceutical houses being best for the purpose. From 8 to 10 cc. of magnesium sulphate may be given in twenty-four hours but not more. Phenobarbital, or pentobarbital, in doses not to exceed 6 grains may act as a satisfactory adjuvant to the morphine.

The Eliminative Treatment.—This depends in principle upon ridding the patient of toxins, by utilizing all possible sources of elimination. Upon admission, in eclampsia, the same general rules as outlined above are put into effect without any drug therapy, after which the patient receives:

Gastric lavage, repeated until the washings are clear. It is amazing to note the masses of undigested food, so often found in the stomach of eclamptic women. At the completion of the lavage 2 ounces of saturated solution of magnesium sulphate is introduced through the stomach tube and allowed to remain.

Colonic Lavage.—The emptying of the colon should be thorough, the irrigation being carried out by means of a rectal tube or better, a two-way colonic irrigator. From 6 to 10 gallons of hot water are generally required to cleanse the colon completely, and a surprising increase in the urinary output occurs immediately following this procedure.

The Use of Glucose Intravenously.—Fifty Gm. of glucose in 500 cc. Ringer's solution is given as soon as the gastric and colonic lavage is completed. The glucose serves several purposes in that it assists elimination, supplies fluid to the patient unable to swallow, combats acidosis and replaces the sugar deficiency brought about by the accompanying liver damage.

Sweating.—This old-fashioned procedure still seems a desirable addition to eliminative treatment. The patient is wrapped in hot dry blankets and placed in one of the electrically heated cradles, to remain for twenty to thirty minutes until free cataphoresis occurs. She is then carefully rubbed dry with gentle skin friction and covered with a dry warmed blanket. This constitutes the treatment by elimination.

Surgical Treatment.—This implies immediate delivery, either from below by instrumental, bag or manual dilatation of the cervix, followed by forceps extraction or version; or by immediate abdominal cesarean section. The method has been abandoned generally by reason of its high mortality, but cesarean section in individualized cases still has a definite place as will be explained later.

Other Methods.—*Water balance* or *dry treatment* was first urged by Zangemeister, some years ago, who maintained that increased intracranial pressure played an important rôle in the production of eclampsia.

Recently Arnold and Fay have revived the viewpoint and report excellent results from their "Temple" plan of treatment which consists in:

Lumbar puncture with drainage of 40 to 80 cc. at four- to six-hour intervals.

The administration of *hypertonic solution* by vein every four or six hours (50 cc. 50 per cent glucose, alternating at two to three hours with 20 cc. 10 per cent magnesium sulphate solution). Free purgation by magnesium sulphate. The skin is kept warm, but hot packs are avoided. If spinal puncture is not available, venesection, in 20- to 30-ounce amounts is substituted.

No morphine or barbiturate is given except to facilitate the spinal tap.

No fluids are given for from twenty-four to forty-eight hours, then according to output and mental status; with strict regard to water balance.

Veratrum viride in large doses up to 1 cc. of the fluidextract or mixture repeated subcutaneously until there is a satisfactory fall in blood pressure. This treatment is now but rarely used.

Plasmapheresis in which the patient is bled 1 liter into a citrate solution and the blood so obtained is centrifuged, the supernatant plasma pipetted off, the cells washed in normal saline solution, and after repeating the washing and centrifuging several times, the blood cells are taken up in 1 liter of saline solution and reintroduced into the patient intravenously. This method is advocated by Irving and others but has not as yet been accepted.

The Management of Complications of Eclampsia

Maintenance of the Circulation.—It has been stated that cardiac failure is one of the common causes of death in eclampsia. Increasing rapidity of the pulse, which becomes soft and sometimes dichrotic, is a dangerous sign, and the heart should be vigorously stimulated with digitalis, given hypodermically in large enough dose to affect the heart definitely.

Venesection is a measure of the greatest value, when indicated. Given a patient with a dilating right heart, labored cardiac action, cyanosis and beginning pulmonary edema, the effect of the withdrawal of perhaps 1000 cc. of blood is often most gratifying. The cyanosis disappears, the heart resumes its normal tones and the râles disappear.

Treatment of Pulmonary Edema.—This alarming and often terminal condition is heralded by the development of moist râles, soon becoming bubbling, respiration becomes rapid and labored and deepening cyanosis begins.

Atropine sulphate in doses of $\frac{1}{100}$ grain hypodermically, ammonium chloride as suggested by Mussey, venesection, and, if possible, the utilization of continuous endobronchial respiration by means of a device applied by a skilled bronchoscopist are the measures available for the control of this complication.

Acidosis.—May be suspected when coma is early and persistent and its presence may be ascertained by studying the CO_2 combining power of the blood. Should this fall below 30 volumes per cent, acidosis is present, and if it reaches a level of 15 volumes per cent, probably fatal acidosis is present. Sodium carbonate, by bowel or intravenously in 5 per cent solution, glucose and insulin are the weapons with which a threatening acidosis may be combated.

The Clinical Application of the Several Modes of Treating Eclampsia

It is rarely advisable to restrict oneself to any single plan of treatment in dealing with eclampsia.

In the writer's clinic, the usual plan is to combine the sedative and eliminative treatment with recourse to surgical measures under certain conditions.

The routine, if the word may be used in connection with a therapy so intensely individualized, as is that of eclampsia, is as follows:

On admission, or when the truly eclamptic woman is first seen—

1. Morphine sulphate, ¼ grain, hypodermically, repeated as described above.

2. Isolation in a quiet, semidarkened room. P. R. T. recorded. Patient protected from injury.

3. Blood pressure estimated, catheterization and urinalysis, blood chemistry.

4. Gastric lavage.

5. Colonic lavage.

6. Hot dry pack.

7. Glucose, 10 per cent, 500 to 1000 cc. intravenously.

8. Eyeground examination.

9. Nothing by mouth unless the patient is completely conscious and able to swallow.

10. Repeated blood pressure and urine examination to determine the effect of treatment.

From twelve to twenty-four hours of this management will usually show a distinct effect. The convulsions grow less severe and the intervals between them longer. Coma recedes and urine output increases.

Commonly the patient falls into labor and delivers, either spontaneously or by the aid of outlet forceps.

In other cases, however, not only does improvement not occur, but the toxemia grows worse, the convulsions and coma more marked, the blood pressure either maintaining its level or rising. Severe ocular damage which presupposes permanent impairment of vision also demands prompt delivery.

In such event prompt delivery is indicated and here the judgment and skill of the obstetrician is put to the test. If the patient is a multipara, if there is no disproportion and particularly if the cervix is effaced and partially dilated, labor may be induced from below, by simple rupture of the membranes under aseptic conditions, or by bag induction. As soon as the pains are well established and the cervix dilated, delivery may be accomplished by forceps or version and extraction. Nitrous oxide and oxygen is the only permissible anesthetic and if the patient is in coma or even semicoma, even this anesthesia becomes unnecessary.

Cesarean Section in Eclampsia.—Cesarean section in the management of eclampsia has a limited but a very definite place. The operation should always be considered:

a. When there is an obstetrical indication, *i. e.,* disproportion.

b. When the patient is a primipara not in labor, with an uneffaced cervix, and is not definitely improving after say twelve hours of conservative treatment.

c. In a multipara, not in labor in whom the eclampsia is of a fulminating type, rapidly becoming more severe.

Many sets of statistics have been adduced, regarding the so-called "radical treatment" of eclampsia, all of which show that the mortality following operative delivery is far greater than that of the conservative treatment.

These facts are quite true, yet the statistics are valueless in determining the relative results. This is so because in many clinics section is regarded as a procedure of last resort, when the patient has been treated conservatively for some time and has failed to improve, also because cesarean section is often done in eclamptics, in desperation, by operators not competent in abdominal surgery. It is perfectly true that the operation is indicated in only a small proportion of cases, but it is equally true that when indicated it is a life-saving measure of the greatest value.

When cesarean section is determined upon it should be done by the classical method, unless previous vaginal manipulation renders this dangerous, and only local anesthesia should be used. This is of the greatest importance, since any inhalation anesthetic adds to the trauma and introduces more toxic elements to be eliminated. In skilled hands spinal anesthesia is permissable.

The operation should be performed when the patient has still some hope of surviving for as Deaver once said, "The resources of surgery are seldom of avail, when practiced upon the dying."

The Termination of Pregnancy in Nephritic Toxemia, Preeclampsia and Eclampsia

It has been stated that preexisting nephritis complicates the toxemia of pregnancy, always produces increased and permanent kidney damage and Stander and others believe that the life expectancy of nephritics is materially reduced by child-bearing. Hence there is a school of thought that in all women who suffer from demonstrable nephritis, pregnancy should be terminated upon the establishment of the diagnosis, and that the patient should be sterilized to prevent further risk.

The more generally held opinion, however, is that with careful supervision and management, nephritic patients, for the most part, can be carried through one or two pregnancies without much aggravation of this renal pathology, and that the question of termination and possible sterilization should be left to the discretion of the patient and her husband, after a careful explanation of the possibilities involved.

In preeclampsia and eclampsia, the question of termination of pregnancy is resolved by the progress of the disease. If after appropriate treatment there is little or no improvement and the toxemia deepens the interests of the mother usually demand delivery, but if improvement takes place the pregnancy may be permitted to continue until term, or until some fresh indication for interference arises.

Induction of Premature Labor in the Interests of the Child.—The accepted practice has been for obstetricians to endeavor to carry the toxic woman to as near term as possible, in order to avoid excessive prematurity in the infant but it has been shown that in the more severe grades of toxemia, it may be safer for the infant to take its chance of being delivered as a premature fetus than to run the risk of being stillborn, should pregnancy be allowed to continue. Clifford feels that the child of a toxemic mother is generally well developed but undernourished, and that pregnancy may be allowed to continue when the blood pressure is under 180 mm., until the fetus reaches an approximate weight of 5 pounds. When the blood pressure of the mother is well over 180, pregnancy should be terminated, regardless of the size of the fetus, provided it be viable.

The Management of Puerperal Eclampsia

When eclamptic manifestations first appear after delivery, the treatment consists in narcosis by morphine, catharsis by salines, preferably magnesium sulphate, the use of this salt intravenously as before described and the free administration of fluids. Venesection is rarely indicated, but cardiac stimulation is often urgently required.

Convalescence in Eclampsia.—In favorable terminations, the convulsions gradually become less, both in number and violence, the blood pressure falls within forty-eight hours, and the excretion of urine reaches larger amounts. The temperature rapidly drops to normal, and persistent fever should always engender suspicions of pneumonia, sepsis or pyelitis.

Within a few days a light diet of milk, cereals, etc., may be allowed, this being gradually increased to ordinary mixed diets, without alcohol or highly spiced foods. The recovering eclamptic may nurse her child although in some instances the milk seems to possess toxic qualities and breast feeding must be stopped.

The After-care of Eclampsia.—There is always danger of permanent kidney damage after pregnancy toxemia and the patient, being advised of this, should be observed for one year after delivery, monthly visits for the first three months postpartum, then quarterly examination should be insisted upon, the blood pressure, urinalysis and if necessary blood chemistry determining the degree of renal disease, if any exists. In the latter case, the treatment is that of nephritis in general.

Acute Yellow Atrophy of the Liver. Hepatic Toxemia

Fortunately, this type of toxemia is uncommon. When it does develop the mortality is very high, and treatment is of but little avail.

The *diagnosis* may be made by the history of a prodromal stage, characterized by slight jaundice, malaise, vomiting and constipation, with slight mental confusion, great weakness and epigastric pain. This is shortly followed by a deepening icterus, delirium followed by coma and sometimes convulsions, bloody vomitus and stools, great thirst and severe epigastric pain and with death in a few days. Identical symptoms may follow poisoning with chloroform, phosphorus, etc. The temperature is variable, sometimes reaching 104° to 105° F., in other instances remaining persistently subnormal. The pulse is rapid and thready. The urine is diminished and contains variable quantities of practically all the elements denoting renal and hepatic degeneration, albumin, casts of all kinds, acetone and diacetic acid, indican, peptone, rarely sugar, leucine and tyrosine, etc.

The liver steadily diminishes in size, the reduction being clinically demonstrable, and there is marked tenderness over the liver area.

The tongue is typhoid in type, the face slightly cyanosed, the eyes sunken. Death occurs from overwhelming toxemia, usually with cardiac failure.

Treatment.—There is no definite treatment. Pregnancy should be terminated at all costs as soon as the diagnosis seems clear. The fetus requires no consideration since it is practically always lost in the presence of this disease.

Glucose in large amounts is theoretically indicated, but offers little hope of a successful outcome.

OTHER MANIFESTATIONS OF TOXEMIA

Various symptom groups occur in pregnancy which are best explained by the influence of some toxic factor, but the underlying pathology of which remains unknown.

The most noteworthy examples are:

Chorea gravidarum

Psychosis in pregnancy.

Neuritis.

Ptyalism.

Chorea gravidarum is an uncommon but exceedingly serious complication of pregnancy. It may be primary in pregnancy, but generally there is a history of chorea in childhood, hysteria, severe nervous shock or possibly an infection of low grade and long duration. Rheumatic fever and endocarditis precede chorea gravidarum in about one third of the reported cases.

When the disease develops during pregnancy in a woman who has previously been choreic, the symptoms are usually mild and amenable to treatment but when the symptoms first appear during gestation, they may become so severe as to prevent sleep or eating. Indeed the patient may become maniacal and usually aborts, with a favorable termination unless exhaustion or cardiac failure is overwhelming.

Willson has collected 906 cases, most of which occurred in young women, the average age being twenty-two and four-tenths years. He shows that the prognosis varies, in direct ratio with the time of onset, there being no mortality when the disease antedates pregnancy with a steadily increasing death rate as it appears in the first, second or third trimester.

The average mortality is about 15 per cent.

Pathology.—On autopsy endocarditis is found in over three fourths of the cases. There may be meningeal exudates but no definite morphological change has been noted.

Diagnosis.—The incoordinated spasmodic movements and twitchings, occurring at any time but generally increasing with efforts at

19

mental or muscular concentration will establish the diagnosis. Careful anamnesis may disclose a predisposing cause, and may serve to exclude hysteria.

If the disease progresses to an advanced degree, emaciation, bed sores, jaundice, purulent skin lesions and dehydration may occur. Elevation of temperature and incontinence of urine and feces are danger signs. The fetal mortality is 50 per cent or more.

Treatment.—Sedative drugs as bromide in large doses, the barbiturates or chloral hydrate are of benefit. Isolation in a quiet darkened room, with the exclusion of visitors is important. If after a few days of such simple medical management, the patient grows progressively worse, therapeutic abortion should be performed. This is the more strongly indicated since permanent mental disturbances may follow severe attacks of chorea gravidarum.

Psychoses.—Psychoses developing during pregnancy are most frequently of toxic origin. (See Diseases of the Nervous System.)

Neuritis of toxic origin is often encountered in pregnancy. Pain and tingling in the sciatic, ulnar and trifacial nerves is annoying and may be confused with tetany (*q. v.*). The pain may be followed by slight paralysis, tenderness over the nerve trunk and some loss of tactile sensibility.

When the optic or auditory nerves are involved, permanent blindness or deafness may result if the pregnancy is not promptly terminated. One of the author's patients, the wife of a physician, has been rendered totally deaf from an auditory neuritis, which developed late in pregnancy and when symptoms at that time were not seriously regarded.

Polyneuritis.—A very dangerous form of polyneuritis associated with the toxemia of early pregnancy may develop usually during the fourth or fifth months. This condition has been studied by Plass, who has seen 12 patients 9 of whom died promptly. The first symptoms are increasing weakness, especially of the legs, with at first acceleration then weakening and final disappearance of the deep reflexes. Finally voluntary motion may be lost completely. The legs are more frequently affected than the arms.

Plass thinks that involvement of the vagus frequently leads to a persistent tachycardia, sometimes ending in paralysis of one half of the diaphragm. Death may result from bulbar paralysis, the muscles of respiration and deglutition being paralyzed.

The diagnosis may be made from the rapidly increasing weakness and loss of muscle tone, the persistent vomiting, tachycardia, ocular movements as nystagmus, loss of deep reflexes and pain over the deep nerves.

Autopsy reveals cloudy swelling of the viscera, degeneration of the affected nerves, with atrophy of the nerve fibers, and possibly degeneration and vacuolization of the spinal cord.

Should the patient recover from the acute attack, with or without termination of the pregnancy, there may be persistent muscular weakness and atrophy, with pain and tingling in the course of the involved nerves.

Treatment consists in the relief of pain by salicylates, opium and external heat. Later massage and diathermy are of value. Elimination of toxins, by catharsis and low diet is also indicated. Termination of pregnancy should not be too long delayed.

Ptyalism.—One of the most inexplicable and annoying toxic manifestation in pregnancy is the excessive secretion of saliva, which sometimes becomes so marked as to destroy appetite, prevent rest and actually produce dehydration from the amount of fluid expectoration.

Levoff reported a case in which 1500 cc. was secreted daily and in one of my patients 18 ounces was expectorated in one day between arising and bed time. The constant spitting not only prevents social intercourse, but the woman may develop distressing sordes and the unpleasant odor of the saliva may accentuate the already objectionable nausea and vomiting of early pregnancy.

The cause is probably interwoven with that of hyperemesis gravidarum and the detailed mechanism of the process is not known.

Treatment.—Astringents as alum and tincture myrrh as mouth wash may be employed, belladonna and sedatives seem to be beneficial, but the most useful treatment in the author's experience is the free use of glucose intravenously, in 25-Gm. doses daily, and in having the patient munch small quantities of salted food. Saltines, salted peanuts, etc., seem to restore the chloride balance and in some way to decrease the oversecretion of saliva.

In one patient, the loss of fluids and nausea became so marked that therapeutic abortion became necessary, although so radical a measure is rarely indicated, since the ptyalism usually ceases by the end of the fourth month.

CHAPTER XVIII

ABORTION AND PREMATURE LABOR

ABORTION is the termination of pregnancy from any cause, before the child is viable, *i. e.*, the twenty-sixth to the twenty-eighth week. After this period the interruption of pregnancy before term is called premature labor.

The old term "miscarriage" sometimes used to differentiate spontaneous from criminally induced abortion is obsolete and is no longer in scientific use.

Abortion may be spontaneous, surgically induced for therapeutic effects or criminally produced.

Frequency.—It is probable that nearly 40 per cent of parous women have had an abortion, and Hirst states that the average incidence is one abortion to every four pregnancies. Statistics upon the frequency of this accident are very variable, from Taussig's 43.4 per cent of full-time birth to Mocharloff's 10 per cent. None of these figures represent the true state of affairs since so many abortions are unrecorded but general experience shows that 25 per cent of full-time births is probably a fairly accurate estimate.

The frequency of abortion varies in relation to the duration of pregnancy. Most abortions occur during the third month, the second month follows and the number then steadily diminishes as pregnancy progresses. This does not take into account the many unrecognized abortions occurring in the very early weeks of gestation.

Parity.—Abortions are more common in multiparous than in primiparous women, but this may be due to the fact that multiparae have had more opportunity for the accident than primiparae.

ETIOLOGY

The causes of abortion are legion, sometimes clear, sometimes obscure and for convenience of description they may be divided into:

Fetal.

Maternal.

Paternal.

Fetal Causes of Abortion.—*Imperfection of the Ovum.*—Mall states that one third of aborted fetuses submitted to him for examination are teratologic. The deformity may be due to inherent deficiency of the germ plasm, or to disturbances resulting from placental disease, anomalies of the cord or of the membranes.

The mechanism of abortion following fetal death is not understood, but the most generally held opinion is that there is a cessation of the hormonal secretion of the growing embryo and a consequent regression of the corpus luteum of pregnancy, with the loss of its inhibiting action on ovarian stimulation.

Maternal Causes.—Endometritis or deciduitis probably explains many abortions. Following an extensive inflammation of the endometrium, the utricular glands are injured and the decidual formation is defective. There may be hemorrhages into the decidua, which interfere with the penetration of the villi; there may be actual bacterial invasion of the ovum but this is uncommon. Chronic metritis, which is often a corollary of endometritis, may be causative by interference with the blood supply of the uterus.

Displacement of the Uterus.—Retroversion, once accepted as a prime cause for the premature expulsion of the embryo has been largely discredited as an etiological factor, but nevertheless it is probably true that on many occasions, the rapidly increasing passive congestion of the growing uterus tends further to exaggerate the torsion of the uterine veins which accompanies retroversion and so disturbs the blood supply that little hemorrhages appear in the decidua with consequent detachment of the ovum from the uterine wall.

Malformation of the uterus may bring about abortion, especially if the pregnancy is in an undeveloped horn of a double uterus. However, it is true that women with double uteri are extremely fertile and that many of their pregnancies go to term.

Hyperpyrexia from the infectious diseases may readily bring about abortion. It is said that the fetus in utero cannot withstand a maternal temperature above 105° F., although this is not quite accurate.

Occasionally the organisms of infectious disease reach the endometrium through the blood stream and act in the same manner as endometritis. Malaria, pneumonia, typhoid and influenza are the chief offenders, the abortion rate during the epidemic of influenza in the United States in 1918–19 reaching 80 per cent of all pregnancies in certain areas.

Poisons.—The metallic poisons, lead, arsenic, phosphorus and mercury are responsible for many interruptions of pregnancy in women subjected to their action. Workers in match or paint factories are extremely liable. The metallic salts seem to act by producing coagulation necrosis of the placenta, with hemorrhages into the placental area and finally degeneration and separation of the trophoblast (Datnow).

Roentgen Rays and Radium.—Women subjected to prolonged irradiation for any cause are apt to abort and in other instances to bring forth monstrous infants.

Syphilis.—Formerly thought to be possibly the chief factor in the etiology of abortion, recent investigation has shown that syphilis rarely operates early in pregnancy. After the twenty-eighth week, premature labor and the delivery of dead or luetic infants occur in well over 50 per cent of the cases.

Tumors of the Uterus.—Myomata and fibromata may cause abortion by reason of circulatory change, but in my opinion, the number is less than that usually stated, namely about 30 per cent.

Endocrine Disturbances.—Various abnormalities of the endocrine system are probably provocative of the early termination of pregnancy, but our knowledge is as yet insufficient to permit of more than the broadest generalizations, hypopituitarism, hyperthyroidism, ovarian dysfunction and so on may all be responsible.

Dietary Deficiencies.—Insufficient calcium ingestion, and a lack of vitamin E in the diet have been shown as cause for abortion. These are not of especial importance in the United States where the people enjoy a generous and well varied diet. In certain cases of repeated abortions, without apparent cause, the application of a diet rich in vitamins has been shown to result in the birth of full-term, healthy children.

Emotional Disturbances.—Severe nervous shock, such as the sudden tragic death of a husband or child or overmastering terror, may and does bring about abortion especially in women of highly sensitive temperament.

Brucella Abortion.—Upon the discovery that contagious abortion in cows was due to the bacilli of Bang, it was thought that this organism must be responsible for many human miscarriages, but investigation proved that to be untrue, only one group of observers having isolated this organism from an aborted human fetus, although cases of unexplained abortion have been reported among farm women living where contagious abortion in cattle was prevalent.

Focal Infections.—Sometimes but not often, bacteria from a distinct focus as teeth, tonsils, etc., enter the blood stream and produce a deciduitis with local necrosis and interference with the proper nidation of the ovum.

Trauma.—Many abortions are explained by women as being due to injury of greater or less degree. However, when one considers the very grave lesions which may be endured by pregnant women without interruption of gestation it becomes obvious that in the absence of some additional etiological factor such as deciduitis, trauma alone is not a common cause for premature termination of pregnancy. In one of the author's cases, the three months pregnant woman was in an automobile accident in which she suffered a fracture of the skull and seven distinct fractures of the pelvis with laceration of the urinary bladder, and yet she went on to term, being delivered of a healthy, full-sized infant. In certain women, however, even slight trauma, a stumble or a light fall results in abortion, but here again, predisposing factors must be taken into account.

Spasmodic Muscular Action.—The older writers laid great stress upon continuous spasmodic movements as producing abortion. Chorea, uncontrollable vomiting and coughing, epileptic convulsions, etc., may act by the constant succussion of the abdominal muscles or by the extreme exhaustion which develops. This cause of abortion is uncommon, possibly because the provocative conditions are uncommon.

Constitutional Disease.—Systemic diseases, resulting in great debility, may carry in their train such circulatory weakness that adequate nutrition of the embryo is impossible, hence its early death and extrusion. Advanced tuberculosis, profound anemias, and grave cardiorenal disease are sometimes responsible. It is probable that here either oxygen deficiency or possibly some toxic action may be responsible.

Irritable Uterus.—This term has long been used to designate a condition wherein the slightest abnormal effort seems to stimulate the uterus to contract. Coitus, dancing, even ordinary household activities may excite uterine action. In most instances, however, close investigation will disclose some decidual lesion as underlying the hypersensitivity of the uterus.

Induced Abortion.—The greater number of abortions are those either performed by the woman herself or induced at the hands of a criminal abortionist. It is a lamentable fact that surveys show the great majority of such criminal procedures (75 to 80 per cent) to occur not among girls illegitimately pregnant, as would be supposed, but in married women, having one or more children. Economic stress or the mere desire to avoid the responsibility of rearing more offspring is at the root of their disastrous act.

The obstetrician should be on his guard, and if called to a woman whom he does not know and who is suffering from an abortion, he should be prepared to notify the authorities if any untoward symptoms develop, so as to avoid suspicion of complicity should a fatal result bring about an investigation.

Also, local treatment, curettage, etc., must be avoided in these cases unless demanded by urgent hemorrhage.

Paternal Causes.—Defective spermatozoa may be the result of chronic sepsis in the male genital tract, there may be an inherent deficiency of these cells, or acute toxemia as alcoholism or the effects of metallic poisons may so lower the individual vitality of the spermatozoa that the fertilized ovum is itself defective and pathological implantation occurs. Sexually exhausted men, and those who have been much exposed to irradiation also produce defective sperm.

Undiscoverable Causes.—In from 25 to 40 per cent of all spontaneous abortions, no true cause can be isolated. This simply means either that the investigation has not been thorough, or that there is some underlying mechanism to explain these cases, which has not yet been demonstrated.

THE PATHOLOGY AND MECHANISM OF ABORTION

The mechanism and pathology of abortion varies with the stage of pregnancy at which the accident occurs. During the first six weeks, the little ovum lies entirely within the decidua, which is thick and friable and firmly attached to the uterine wall. Hence in abortion in the early weeks, the decidua remains relatively undisturbed, whereas the ovum, detached from its imperfect implantation, escapes sometimes almost intact.

After the sixth week, the placenta has begun to develop, the area of implantation has grown enormously, the chorionic villi have penetrated deep into the decidua basalis and meantime large venous spaces have appeared in the uterine wall and the intervillous spaces in the decidua are very vascular.

Now, if abortion occurs, the ovum is not usually expelled intact, but portions of the sac are extruded, while that part of the placenta which is firmly attached by the anchoring villi will remain in position together with most of the remaining decidua, free bleeding from the open blood spaces and the torn villi being characteristic (Fig. 162).

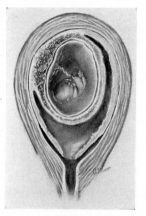

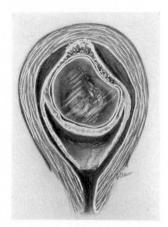

Fig. 162.—Beginning abortion. Blood seeping into the decidual spaces.

Fig. 163.—Inevitable abortion. All layers of decidua being separated by blood.

After the third month, abortion takes on the aspects of labor at term. The fetus is usually expelled first, through a rupture in the membranes and the intact placenta, by this time very large in comparison with the embryo is expelled later by a more or less imperfect mechanism.

The uterine contractions are not vigorous enough to detach and expel the placenta at once, separation is slow and as a result of prolonged squeezing in the contracting uterus, the placenta is often converted into a cylindrical roll, with a stump of umbilical cord dependent from it. This may be extruded from the uterus, but commonly is found wedged in the cervical canal, from which it may easily be withdrawn by ring forceps.

Litzenberg has well classified these three mechanisms of abortion as:

1. The decidual stage, or early abortion, the first six weeks.

2. The attachment stage, or intermediate abortion, the second six weeks.

3. The placental stage, or late abortion after complete placental formation and before the twenty-eighth week.

During the decidual stage and early in the stage of attachment, the entire ovum may be expelled intact, the sac containing a small fetus and being surrounded by the shaggy coat of the chorion frondosum (Fig. 164).

Sometimes the entire decidua is detached and cast off as a triangular cast of the uterine cavity.

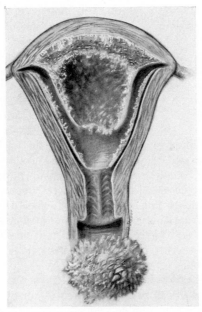

Fig. 164.—Early abortion. The ovum in its shaggy coat has been expelled intact.

In the placental stage, the ovum is but rarely extruded entire, but the fetus escapes first, followed by portions of the decidua and the placenta. The portions remaining in the uterus are invaded by saprophytes and become necrotic and decomposed, the cells losing their morphological characteristics, some liquefaction occurring, with a peculiarly pungent foul odor.

THE SYMPTOMATOLOGY AND DIAGNOSIS OF ABORTION

The cardinal symptoms of abortion are:

Pain.

Hemorrhage.

Dilatation of the cervix.

If to this be added the expulsion of any portion of the ovum, the symptom-complex is complete.

Pain.—The pain in abortion is akin to that of dysmenorrhea or labor pains. Sometimes beginning as a mere heaviness in the pelvis it becomes colicky or severe and cramplike. The pains may assume regular intervals as in full-term labor or they may occur in series with a considerable rest period alternating with a group of severe contractions of short interval and fairly long duration. Occasionally complete separation and extrusion of the ovum may take place with surprisingly little distress but this is uncommon. The pain may take the form of backache and may extend down the thighs as in dysmenorrhea.

Pain may be the initial symptom in impending abortion, but usually it is preceded by hours or days by some type of uterine bleeding.

Bleeding.—Hemorrhage of varying degree is a constant symptom of abortion. It may begin as a little irregular spotting, followed in a day or so by a moderate discharge of blood which simulates a menstrual period. This seemingly irrelevant and inconsequential bleeding may persist for several weeks, before the onset of frank hemorrhage and uterine pain heralds the completion of the process of expulsion of the ovum. Again, the hemorrhage may be sudden and alarming, so much blood escaping in a few hours that the patient becomes exsanguinated and presents a picture of extreme collapse; pallor, thirst, yawning, sweating, shallow rapid respiration, rapid thready pulse with marked restlessness and anxiety depicted upon the face.

Depleting though the hemorrhage may be, it is rare to encounter a fatal termination from this cause alone. Infection supervening in a profoundly anemic and bled-out woman is extremely dangerous, the combination of these two factors being responsible for most of the deaths from abortion.

Dilatation of the Cervix.—There is always some effacement and dilatation of the cervix during the course of an abortion. In early cases, the effacement is negligible and the dilatation may be retarded, thus retaining the products of conception and causing greater uterine effort and consequently more pain in nature's attempt to expel the products of conception. The later the abortion, the greater the tendency for cervical dilatation, since as time goes on the mechanism of expulsion more nearly approaches that of labor at term.

Expulsion of Portions of the Ovum.—When fragments of decidual portions of the embryo or the placenta are expelled from the uterus, the diagnosis of abortion may be made with absolute certainty, although this is not a necessary sign to establish the true condition.

The diagnosis of abortion depends then, upon the presence of the three cardinal symptoms occurring in a woman who is *known to be pregnant*. The signs of pregnancy should be sought for and if there is doubt as to this point, an Aschheim-Zondek or Friedman test may be employed.

TYPES OF ABORTION

For clinical purposes, abortion has been arbitrarily divided into:

Threatened.

Inevitable.

Complete.

Incomplete.

Afebrile.

Infected.

Threatened Abortion.—This term includes those cases wherein the life and attachment of the ovum are threatened but not beyond hope of a normal termination of pregnancy. There may be colicky pain, slight cramps and a little spotting. The cervix is soft but not appreciably dilated, and there may be a heavy mucous discharge, blood-tinged or not.

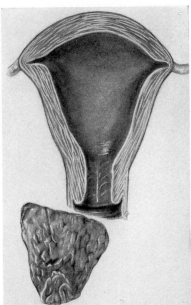

Fig. 165.—Complete abortion. The ovum and decidua have been expelled, the uterus being left clean and empty.

Inevitable Abortion.—When the symptoms of threatened abortion grow steadily worse, the bleeding becomes profuse, the pain severe, recurring at short intervals and closely resembling labor pain at term, and when the cervix is distinctly dilated and partially effaced, the abortion becomes inevitable. Should the membranes rupture and amniotic fluid escape, or should portions of the ovum or decidua be extruded, the question is settled beyond question, but in general the increase in the extent of the cardinal symptoms is sufficient to determine the outcome.

Complete Abortion.—Sometimes the entire ovum is expelled either en masse or in fragments, but in either case the cavity of the uterus is completely emptied within a few hours, leaving only a scattering remnant of bits of decidua adherent to the musculature (Fig. 165). These small tags are either resorbed, or becoming detached they escape in the discharge of blood and mucus that follows abortion. In such cases the symptoms though they may be violent are of short duration, and the patient usually recovers rapidly and without further treatment.

Incomplete Abortion.—This term is used to describe those cases (the majority of all forms of abortion) in which a portion of the

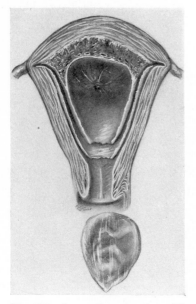

Fig. 166.—Incomplete abortion. The fetus and membranes have been extruded; the placenta remains attached.

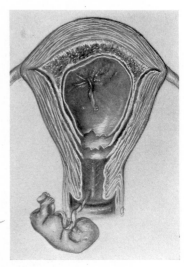

Fig. 167.—Abortion incomplete. The fetus has escaped, the placenta and membranes remain.

products of conception is extruded, the rest remaining within the cavity of the uterus for an indefinite time (Fig. 166). In the earlier weeks of pregnancy, the ovum is apt to be expelled entirely, carrying with it its chorionic covering, the shaggy coat, and in these instances there is but little left in the uterus. However, if the membranes are ruptured and the embryo alone escapes, there may remain sufficient decidua to cause prolonged bleeding, with constant danger of infection (Fig. 167).

Later in pregnancy, that is, after the third month, incomplete abortion is the rule. The fetus is usually delivered, all or a considerable portion of the placenta remaining, together with the decidua vera.

As stated above, the expulsive efforts of the uterus may cause the placenta to be rolled into a tightly compressed cylinder which is slowly forced into the cervical canal from which it is still more slowly expressed by continued uterine contraction, aided by some degree of voluntary pressure exerted by the abdominal muscles. Less commonly, the placenta is expelled, the fetus remaining in the uterus, where it prevents firm contraction thus favoring continuous hemorrhage, until uterine effort finally dislodges it.

Incomplete abortion is the variety usually coming to the attention of the specialist, the patient giving a history of pain, bleeding and the passage of some sort of tissue, which usually has been lost. The diagnosis must be made by the size and consistency of the uterus—if empty it is fairly hard and small, if retention is present, it is large, boggy, often retroverted into the cul-de-sac and bleeding with more or less rapidity. There may be a portion of the placenta attached to the uterine wall and protruding from the cervix.

If the diagnosis remains obscure, digital exploration of the cavity of the uterus under rigid asepsis may be undertaken.

Afebrile Abortion.—Includes most spontaneous ones, in which the temperature is rarely elevated above 99.5° F. unless the patient has had some previous focus of pelvic infection.

Septic Abortion.—Includes most of the criminally induced cases, and those resulting from direct trauma to the uterine contents. The importance of the distinction lies in the management, which differs much in the two conditions.

Cervical Abortion.—When the ovum becomes detached from its implantation in the fundus uteri, and lodges firmly in the canal of the undilated cervix, the phenomenon is termed "cervical abortion." The fundus may be large and boggy, distended with blood, but the cervix remains obdurately contracted, imprisoning the mass of tissue. A trickle of blood usually escapes from around the plug of ovum. Reimplantation of the ovum in the cervix has been reported but is improbable.

THE DIFFERENTIAL DIAGNOSIS OF ABORTION

Abortion must be distinguished from ectopic pregnancy.

Tumors of the uterus—fibroid and carcinoma.

Functional menstrual disturbances.

Hydatidiform mole.

Of these, the distinction between intra-uterine abortion and ectopic pregnancy is of the utmost importance and will be considered under the discussion of that lesion.

From fibroid tumors the diagnosis is made by the age of the patient, the previous history of the presence of a tumor, the palpation of irregular nodules, the absence of the usual signs of early pregnancy and a negative Aschheim-Zondek test.

When pregnancy is superimposed upon a fibroid tumor, the diagnosis may offer great difficulty, and the dual condition may be explained sometimes, only after careful biological tests (Friedman-Aschheim-Zondek).

From cancer of the cervix abortion may be differentiated by the discovery of a typical eroded carcinoma of the cervix, and if the nature of the lesion is in doubt, biopsy will clear the issue. Carcinoma of the body of uterus, with its intermittent bleeding, moderately enlarged uterus and sometimes slightly softened cervix, may offer difficulties in differentiation, but here again, the biological test will determine the presence or absence of pregnancy.

The coexistence of pregnancy and fundal carcinoma is very, very rare, although the writer has seen and reported such a case.

From functional uterine bleeding, abortion may be separated by the absence of the usual phenomena of early pregnancy, the duration of the bleeding and by biological tests. Also in functional bleeding the uterus tends to remain small, and the cervix hard and pale.

Hydatidiform mole may be distinguished from abortion by the size of the uterus, which far exceeds that of the normally pregnant organ at the same period of gestation. In mole the bloody discharge is apt to contain some of the little thin-walled cystic bodies whose discovery makes the diagnosis absolute.

The signs of pregnancy are present in both conditions, but the biologic test offers a striking difference, since in the presence of a mole, the hormone content of the urine is so great as to cause marked reaction in rabbits' ovaries with dilution equal to one tenth of the amount of urine from the normally pregnant woman required to effect a like reaction. The toxemia of early pregnancy—hyperemesis—is usually more severe in mole than in normal pregnancy.

THE PROGNOSIS IN ABORTION

It has been stated above that few patients bleed to death from abortion. It is equally true that the more profound the anemia the lower the resistance to invasion by pyogenic bacteria and that infection following hemorrhage is the great cause of fatal terminations. Actual figures are difficult to state because so many abortions are unreported that the relation of the deaths to the total number is undeterminable.

The mortality of septic abortion admitted to hospitals may reach 10 per cent in certain districts at times when the invading bacteria are peculiarly virulent, but generally the rate remains about 2 to 3 per cent.

In spontaneous abortions, not infected, the prognosis is good, but few of these cases terminating fatally. The prognosis as to health and future child-bearing is much more serious, subinvolution, persistent endometritis and metritis being common sequelae, and occlusion of the fimbriated extremity of the tubes by a plastic exudate renders subsequent sterility a common occurrence.

Obviously where gross instrumental brutality has been practiced, either by the patient herself or the criminal abortionist, the prognosis is grave indeed. Perforation of the uterus with the curet, a metal catheter or other instrument is common, as is multiple laceration of the cervix from attempts at hasty dilation. Peritonitis, bacteremia and widespread cellulitis naturally follow. These infections will be discussed more fully in the chapter dealing with puerperal sepsis.

THE TREATMENT OF ABORTION

Prophylaxis.—Much can be done to prevent abortion. In parous women the lacerated and infected cervix should be repaired, either by cautery or plastic operation, the retroverted uterus should be replaced by a well-fitting pessary, the relaxed, pendulous abdomen supported by a girdle.

Serologic studies and appropriate treatment if indicated will eliminate syphilis as a cause, and careful prenatal instructions as to the evils of excessive coitus, too violent exertion, etc., will be of great aid. It is the moral duty of the physician to advise his patients against the all too prevalent practice of induced abortion, and to explain to them the physical disability which is so prone to follow this form of assault as well as the irreparable damage to society and to personal character from an extension of the practice.

The Treatment of Threatened Abortion.—Upon the first appearance of any disturbance of the uterine contents, during the early months of pregnancy, the essentials of treatment are sedation and rest. Prospective mothers should be warned of the significance of colicky pains, of a dragging heavy feeling in the pelvis and most of all, bleeding, however slight. At the onset of any of these symptoms, the woman should be placed at rest in bed at once, with an ice-cap applied to the lower abdomen. The diet should be light and all laxatives are avoided, the bowels being evacuated by simple soapsuds enemas, when necessary. The nervous tension and anxiety as to loss of the child may be combated by the administration of general sedatives, as sodium or potassium bromide in doses of 30 grains, given four times daily. For the uterine irritability, opium is the drug of choice. Morphine sulphate, ¼ grain, by mouth and repeated when the effects have worn off, that is, at six- to ten-hour intervals, may be used for one or two days. Paregoric in drachm doses every three or four hours is a favorite remedy, which often acts very satisfactorily. Under such management either the pain disappears, the bleeding ceases and the threat of abortion is over, or in spite of what has been done, the reverse is true. The symptoms become more severe, hemorrhage grows profuse and the abortion becomes inevitable.

If the desired result of cessation of symptoms occurs, the woman should be allowed to resume her usual life habits gradually, avoiding all strenuous exercise and the use of drastic laxatives. Mineral oil, or the milk of magnesia supplemented by enemata, if necessary, are sufficient to control constipation. Upon the recurrence of symptoms, the treatment must be repeated until all danger seems past.

Sometimes the pain ceases, but a more or less continuous bleeding persists, for weeks. In such cases, the life or death of the fetus may be ascertained by a biologic test, and if the embryo is dead, there is no longer occasion for delay and the case should be regarded as one of incomplete abortion and so managed. If the biologic tests reveal that the embryo is still living, further expectant treatment is indicated in the hope that the bleeding may cease. After three or four weeks of this it is wiser to consider that the fetus has at least suffered great injury from an error in attachment of the placenta and the uterus should be emptied.

Treatment of Inevitable Abortion.—If, despite treatment, abortion appears inevitable and imminent, the uterus must be aided in expelling its contents as quickly and as completely as possible; hence all sedation is abandoned, to be replaced by the use of oxytocic drugs in order to facilitate uterine contraction. Fluidextract ergot or better, the ergonovine may be given in doses of 1 drachm by mouth three times daily. Pituitary extract in ½-cc. dose hypodermically often causes firm uterine contraction with rapid expulsion of the products of conception. If after a day or two of this treatment, the abortion is not completed, spontaneously, the case becomes one of incomplete abortion.

The Treatment of Incomplete Abortion.—As has been stated, abortion is often attended by severe blood loss and if the hemorrhage from the uterus has ceased, or greatly diminished, the obstetrician may devote his attention to measures designed to restore blood, and to combat shock before proceeding to empty the uterus.

Blood transfusion is of paramount importance, large amounts, 500–600 cc., being given if possible. Lacking donors for blood transfusion, glucose in 10 per cent solution may be utilized intravenously up to 2000 cc. Gum acacia in 5 per cent solution is also valuable to supply the tissue with the necessary fluids.

Morphine for restlessness, digitalis or caffeine to stimulate a failing heart and the administration of an abundance of hot liquid food, broth, milk, tea, coffee, may all be required to relieve the effects of severe hemorrhage.

Meanwhile, if vaginal bleeding continues the vagina should be firmly packed and for this purpose I prefer absorbent cotton to gauze.

The technic is as follows: with the patient in the lithotomy position, or if the packing must be done on a bed, in the Sims position. The vulva is gently scrubbed with green soap and water, the pubic hair shaved or cut. The cervix is exposed with a Sims or weighted speculum, the vagina gently wiped dry and then pledgets of absorbent cotton, which have been soaked in a 4 per cent solution of mercuro-chrome or a 1 per cent solution of lysol, are squeezed dry between the fingers and introduced to the vault of the vagina with dressing forceps. The pledgets when squeezed dry should be about 2 inches in diameter by ⅛ inch thick.

Under the eye, these bits of cotton are fitted into the vault of the vagina, until the fornices are filled, then the cervix is covered in and finally the packing fills the lower vagina to be held in place by a **T** bandage. If the hemorrhage has been severe the foot of the bed may be elevated, and the patient, warmly wrapped up, left to rest.

After twenty-four hours, the packing is removed and in many in-stances the uterine contents will be found either in the vagina, or caught in the cervical canal, whence they may be withdrawn easily, upon being grasped by ring forceps. If this is not the case, the uterus must be evacuated by the following technic:

It is presupposed that the patient is afebrile. After the usual pre-operative preparation of a cleansing enema, shaving of the pubic hair and the assurance that the urinary bladder is empty, the patient is placed in the lithotomy position preferably on an operating table, although any ordinary table equipped with leg holders or a Glover's crutch may be utilized.

Anesthesia is induced with nitrous oxide and oxygen or ether, and the entire pudendal region carefully scrubbed with tincture of green soap, followed by 1 per cent lysol or other skin antiseptic. The opera-tor, being scrubbed, gowned and gloved, sits between the patient's thighs and a weighted speculum is introduced into the vagina. The an-terior lip of the cervix is grasped with a ring forceps or tenaculum and the cervix gently dilated to 3 cm. either with Goodell's or Hegar's grad-uated dilators. Great gentleness must be exercised to avoid laceration of the soft cervical tissue. When the dilatation is completed, the depth of the uterus is ascertained by the gentle introduction of a uterine sound to the fundus. The finger may then be introduced to loosen as much of the ovum from its detachment as possible and to explore the cavity.

The ovum is then grasped with placental forceps, care being taken that the uterine wall is not included in the bite of the instrument. The forceps are withdrawn, emptied, and again introduced until the bulk of the ovum has been extracted. A fairly large, sharp curet is then introduced to the fundus and the entire cavity of the uterus is gently curetted to remove adherent fragments of placenta and decidua.

The uterus is then packed with 2-inch gauze packing, and a light pack fills the vagina. The packing is removed at the end of twenty-four hours and the patient kept in bed for five days, under the usual postoperative régime.

Comment.—Dilatation and evacuation is an operation of consider-able danger. Perforation of the soft uterus is a common accident and may lead to serious consequences, especially if unrecognized. In

20

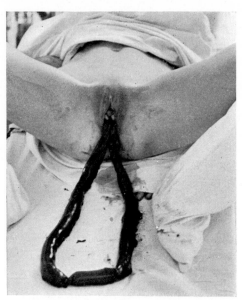

Fig. 168.—Perforation of the uterus in the treatment of incomplete abortion. Four feet 2 inches of ileum, stripped from its mesentery, was dragged through the rent in the uterus, with placental forceps. On admission the patient denied any operative interference. (Kensington Hospital for Women.)

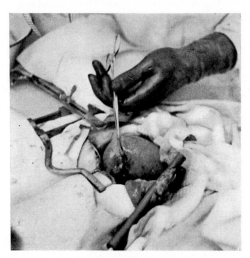

Fig. 169.—The same case, showing the rent in the posterior wall of the uterus and the loops of gut, cut off and held in intestinal forceps. Uncomplicated recovery.

this event the placental forceps may slip through the perforation and omentum or even intestine be drawn out of the vagina. For this reason, this operation should never be performed with the woman drawn across a bed, for the buttocks sink into the mattress, and the vagina points upward causing an angulation between its axis and that of the uterus (Figs. 168 and 169).

Furthermore, the position of the uterus, whether acute or retroverted, must always be known, as in the latter case, the dilator or curet may easily perforate the anterior uterine wall under the attachment of the bladder (Fig. 170).

To avoid this danger, emptying of the uterus with the finger has many advocates. In the experience of the writer, this is an unsatisfactory procedure, since oftentimes the fundus cannot be reached nor the uterus completely emptied by this method.

The sharp curet, intelligently used, is preferable to a dull instrument as the decidua is sometimes quite firmly attached and the blunt curet slides over the adherent fragments. The operation should never

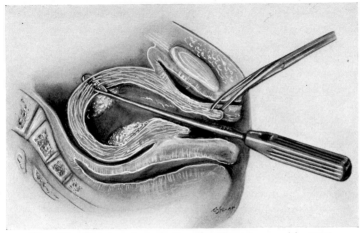

Fig. 170.—Showing danger of perforating uterus with curet.

be done in the presence of acute infection of the uterine contents, as in this event lymph and blood channels are opened, the protective layer of lymphocytes and fibrous exudate is torn away and the further invasion of pyogenic bacteria is facilitated.

Anesthesia is always indicated, although in special circumstances, as where no skilled assistance is available, the procedure may be carried out without anesthesia. This is not advised.

When the fetus is known to have been discharged and the rolled-up placenta presents in the cervical canal, it may be grasped with ring forceps, and gently pulled out, without anesthesia.

Rigid asepsis is a sine qua non for success.

The operation may be followed by sharp hemorrhage, and sterile packing should always be at hand, to be used in most cases.

The Treatment of Complete or Nearly Complete Abortion.— Watchful expectancy, rest in bed, the restoration of blood by hema-tonics or, if necessary, transfusion, with the exhibition of ergot to favor uterine contraction will suffice in most cases. This treatment is also available in incomplete abortion where there is but slight bleeding and it is thought that only a little decidua remains in the uterus.

Septic Abortion.—Many cases of induced abortion and a few spontaneous ones result in infection of the ovum and the decidua. The infection is apt to spread to the uterine musculature, the pelvic cellular tissue, the peritoneum and there often is a true bacteremia.

These cases are extremely grave, the mortality being exceedingly high as shown in the three years' survey of maternal deaths by the Philadelphia County Medical Society and the Obstetrical Society of Philadelphia in which it was found that septic abortion was responsible for over one fifth of all the maternal deaths reviewed. There were in the three years 162 deaths from this cause of which 102 followed illegal induction and many of the others were presumably due to the same cause, although the facts could not be brought out.

The patient suffering from septic abortion is often very ill when first seen in hospital or by the attending physician.

Pallor, a rapid thready pulse, rigors occurring several times each day, a temperature typically septic and ranging from 105° to 97° F., and vaginal bleeding constitute the usual ensemble of symptoms. The sedimentation time is rapid, the leukocytosis may reach 20,000 to 30,000, the Schilling index tends toward the left, and all too often there is a positive blood culture of hemolytic streptococcus, Streptococcus viridans or staphylococci.

If peritonitis be present, the usual signs of pain, tympanites, vomiting and paralytic ileus may be found. If salpingitis or pelvic cellulitis has developed, pain may be intense, but generally these women experience little or no pain and are often unaware of the gravity of their condition.

The further complications most to be feared are pyemia with multiple abscess, acute bacterial endocarditis and septic pneumonia.

Treatment.—Septic abortion must always be reported to the nearest legal authority, the district attorney, the coroner or the local health officer. In most cases a crime involving manslaughter has been committed and in the interest of the community as well as to safeguard the physician himself, prompt reporting is absolutely required.

The medical treatment is that of general sepsis from any cause. Blood transfusion, cardiac stimulants, the intravenous use of glucose in 10 per cent solution to combat dehydration, morphine to insure rest and if possible, the exposure of the patient to fresh air and sunshine, constitutes the treatment. The Fowler position may aid drainage. In the case of positive blood-stream infection, the use of solution of metaphen or mercurochrome in an attempt to sterilize the blood stream may be utilized, as may the so-called "immunotransfusion" (see treatment of puerperal sepsis).

Local Treatment.—It is an obstetrical rule that in septic or potentially infected abortion, the uterus should never be invaded, by finger or instrument, except upon two indications:

First: to remove masses of débris from the cervical canal (not the cavity of the uterus) in order to insure better drainage.

Second: when profuse hemorrhage must be controlled, where the interference must be limited to temporary, twenty-four-hour packing if possible. Only in the most exceptional circumstances is it permissible to attempt intra-uterine manipulation to extract the infected products of conception.

This is true because any intra-uterine manipulation tends to break down the protective wall of fibrin and leukocytes which has been set up, and so facilitates the invasion by bacteria of the deeper tissues and the blood stream.

Habitual Abortion.—Repeated abortion without discoverable cause is known as habitual abortion, and so far has eluded all attempts to demonstrate its etiology. In true examples of this state of affairs, local lesions are absent in both parents, syphilis cannot be shown to be present and in fact there is nothing to explain the recurring accidents. It is probable that some endocrine imbalance is responsible but this has not been proved.

Treatment.—The most painstaking examination of both husband and wife to eliminate syphilis, local pelvic disorders in the latter and lesions of the genital tract in the former, must be carried out.

Basal metabolism estimation may disclose hypo- or hyperthyroidism in either parent, when treatment by thyroid extract or iodine may be instituted.

When the woman does become pregnant, she should remain at rest in bed at the time when the menstrual period would be due. She should refrain from all violent exercise and is to employ a diet rich in all the vitamins, and in calcium. Between pregnancies, an outdoor life, with vigorous exercise and change of scene may be beneficial. As Litzenberg says, "What an attractive field for research."

Missed Abortion.—A term first used by Matthews Duncan to describe cases of retention of the ovum beyond the usual time of expulsion, after its death. Litzenberg has placed an arbitrary but correct limit of two months after the death of the fetus as the borderline between abortion and missed abortion.

Etiology.—The causes for retention of the dead ovum and its later expulsion are not understood but, here again, further elucidation of the physiology of the endocrine mechanism of pregnancy will probably clear up the question one day.

Frequency.—Over **200** cases have been collected, and doubtless many more remain unrecorded.

Pathology.—If death of the embryo occurs in the early weeks, the decidua and the chorion may continue to grow since they receive their nourishment from the maternal blood, but since this growth is atypical there may be many areas of hemorrhage into the tissues, until the whole uterine cavity may be filled with a soft mass of decidua, containing many small round cells and infiltrated with blood. This is called a blood mole, and may give rise to severe, even fatal hemorrhage should the large blood vessels of the uterus undergo advanced degeneration.

In later cases the placenta itself may go on growing even though the fetus be dead and at the final expulsion a little dried-up embryo is found attached to a large, succulent placenta with local areas of necrosis, hemorrhage, and infarction.

Rarely the soft parts of the fetus become resorbed only the skeleton remaining and this becoming calcified, is converted into a lithopedion (*q. v.*) which may remain in the uterine cavity for many years.

Again the amniotic fluid may be discharged or absorbed and the fetus becomes compressed and desiccated in the uterine cavity, where it is termed "fetus compressus," and if this process goes on long enough, the fetus may assume a parchment-like appearance called "fetus papyraceus."

Maceration of the fetus occurs when the bones of the skull collapse, the abdomen distends and the skin is exfoliated in large patches, leaving a dull red subcutaneous surface. In the very early weeks, the embryo may be entirely dissolved and reabsorbed so that no trace of it is ever discovered.

Symptoms and Diagnosis.—At first the symptoms are slight. A little bleeding, and some abdominal pain give rise to the suspicion that threatened abortion is in progress after which all symptoms subside. Some time later, the patient complains of malaise, headache, loss of weight, constipation and possibly a little irregular bleeding or the discharge of some brownish mucus. On examination the uterus is found not to have grown as in normal pregnancy, but it may even have become smaller. It has a peculiar soft yet dense consistency, and there may be a definite afternoon rise of temperature.

A history of early pregnancy, without definite abortion, plus the general invalidity of the patient should give rise to the suspicion of missed abortion.

Treatment.—When the diagnosis is established, the contents of the uterus should be removed instrumentally, the patient being prepared as in the treatment of incomplete abortion, the cervix dilated under an anesthetic, and the uterine contents carefully removed with placental forceps and curet. Because of the danger of hemorrhage from degenerated vessel ends, the empty uterus should be firmly packed with gauze, which is to remain for twenty-four hours after operation.

The material recovered must be submitted to searching microscopic examination to exclude the possibility of chorionepithelioma which sometimes closely simulates missed abortion.

THERAPEUTIC ABORTION

Sometimes it becomes apparent that a pregnant woman will not survive the continuation of her pregnancy and in the interests of her life gestation must be terminated and the fetus accordingly sacrificed.

Religious interdiction makes such procedure impossible in certain families and the physician should be on his guard never to run contrary to the question of faith. If he is morally convinced that termination of pregnancy is essential to the life of the woman, and if he be prevented from acting upon his conviction by religious scruples, of the patient or her family, he should withdraw from further connection with the case.

Therapeutic abortion is a serious matter, involving the deliberate destruction of a living human entity, and it should be entered upon only after the most careful deliberation and never without consultation with a medical colleague. The conditions for which such abortion may justifiably be performed are:

Grave systemic disease, the progress of which is obviously being hastened by pregnancy, as: acute progressive tuberculosis of lungs, kidney, etc. Severe cardiac disease with increasing decompensation. Nephritis, with rising hypertension and evidence of renal destruction. Chorea and other marked neurological lesions occasioning uterine hemorrhage. Hyperemesis gravidarum which progresses to a stage where the life of the patient is endangered. Other conditions might be mentioned but the above will serve as a criterion of the type of condition in which therapeutic abortion is permissible. The physician must always be wary of designing women and their husbands, who desiring to avoid an unwanted child seek to beguile the medical attendant into performing an abortion by inventing disease or grossly exaggerating the severity of a condition which is actually present.

Technic.—Therapeutic abortion being determined upon by a consultation of 2 or 3 physicians, the patient should be hospitalized if at all feasible. This is important by reason of the greater safety and ease with which operative procedures may be carried out, and because it makes the entire conduct of the case open and known and avoids any suspicion of misconduct. The patient being prepared as for any plastic operation, abortion may be induced by one of three methods:

1. The cervix (after surgical cleansing) may be gently dilated, just a little, with the finger or a Hegar dilator, and a strip of gauze packed firmly into the canal. The vagina is also to be packed. In successful cases pain comes on within a few hours and abortion follows. Some operators prefer to introduce a sound into the uterine cavity to rupture the membranes and to break up the ovum a little.

2. Under anesthesia and prepared in the lithotomy position as for any plastic procedure, the cervix may be seized with a tenaculum, dilated with Goodell or Hegar dilators and the ovum removed by placental forceps followed by the curet and firm uterine packing.

This procedure is more surgical, the work is done at one sitting, but it has the disadvantage of sometimes giving rise to dangerous hemorrhage. It should never be undertaken except in the most favorable surroundings and with sterile packing within reach and ready for immediate use.

In the later weeks of pregnancy it may be necessary to supplement the dilatation by incising the anterior face of the cervix after first displacing the bladder from its attachment to the anterior surface of the uterus.

3. Abdominal hysterotomy with removal of the ovum and tubal sterilization. This method is applicable particularly where it is desired to combine sterilization with therapeutic abortion, in cases of grave and uncurable systemic disease.

Many conditions which formerly were regarded as indications for abortion are now treated differently. Contracted pelvis, pelvic tumors, placenta praevia and so on, are to be managed by cesarean section at term, and not by the termination of pregnancy before the viability of the fetus.

PREMATURE LABOR

This term is used to designate labor and delivery before the maturity of the fetus, but after it has become viable, that is between the twenty-sixth and thiry-eighth weeks.

The causes are syphilis in more than one half of the cases, nephritis and other toxemias of pregnancy, hydramnion, incidental acute infection as influenza, pneumonia, etc., and sometimes traumatism, especially if this be associated with rupture of the membranes.

Occasionally severe heart disease with its disturbances of circulation may cause premature labor, as may severe bronchitis with its incessant coughing.

Course of Labor.—The course in premature labor differs from that of delivery at term only in that the uterine contractions may be less efficient, the small baby may present in a transverse or other pathological position and the third stage is apt to be slower, the placenta separating with some difficulty. Postpartum hemorrhage is possibly more common and subinvolution of the uterus may prove a complication.

The management of premature labor is that of labor at term, with especial reference to the possible abnormalities described above.

CHAPTER XIX

DISPLACEMENTS OF THE UTERUS

THE uterine displacements which may produce disturbances during pregnancy are anteflexion and version, retroflexion and version, prolapse, and rarely lateral deviation.

The normal position of the uterus is one of acute anteversion, the fundus tilting forward and the cervix pointing backward toward the sacrum.

ANTEFLEXION AND ANTEVERSION

Pathological anteflexion may be a cause of sterility especially as it is ofttimes associated with an infantile uterus and defective ovaries. When pregnancy does take place the angulation at the cervicofundal juncture usually straightens out and gestation proceeds undisturbed. In late pregnancy the uterus becomes markedly anteverted due to its distention, and at this time it lies against the anterior abdominal wall. Should the latter be relaxed, from poor musculature, the stretching of multiparity or possibly as a result of congenital defect of the abdominal parieties, the muscles become markedly relaxed, the uterus falls still further forward in what is termed "pendulous belly." This condition is quite uncommon in primiparae and in women who have enjoyed pre- and postnatal care, and is generally found in the undernourished multipara of the clinic, whose life has consisted in arduous toil even during pregnancy and too soon after delivery.

Pathologic anteversion during pregnancy may sometimes be caused by deformities of the spine, kyphosis or exaggerated lordosis, in which the uterus is thrust forward against the abdominal wall by the angulation of the spine. It also occurs in cases of marked contraction of the pelvic inlet, the head being unable to descend into the pelvic cavity, the growing uterus being forced anteriorly to find room for further expansion. *Pendulous abdomen* may cause discomfort and a dull heavy pain in the abdomen during the late months of pregnancy and may cause dystocia, because the uterine contractions force the presenting part backward against the promontory of the sacrum, rather than into the pelvic brim. The result of this abnormal mechanism may be rupture of the uterus (rare) or the production of malpresentation as shoulder, complete transverse, etc.

The management of pendulous abdomen is simple and efficacious. A well-fitting binder worn during pregnancy, even at night, will splint and supplement the defective abdominal wall. During labor, the binder should be even more firmly adjusted and if need be, the hand

313

on the uterine fundus may draw it backward and upward during a pain, so as to thrust the birth canal into line and direct the head into the pelvic brim. Some writers advocate the squatting position with the thighs pressed against the abdomen during the first stage of labor, but I have never found this necessary.

Upon the completion of the puerperium, the patient should strengthen the abdominal muscles by systematic exercise to avoid a repetition of the trouble. Sometimes there is marked diastasis of the recti muscles and the uterus slips between them, only covered by peritoneum, thinned-out fascia and skin. This is not an alarming state of affairs and is controlled by the binder as before stated.

Antefixation of the Uterus.—It was formerly the practice to correct retroversion of the uterus by suturing its fundus to the anterior abdominal wall. This results in a firm connection between the two and the anterior uterine wall is unable to expand with the advent of pregnancy.

It consequently becomes much thickened, the cervix is pulled upward and backward until it and the lower portion of the anterior wall of the uterus covers the pelvic inlet. In the meantime the growing embryo stretches and expands the free posterior wall until it becomes markedly thinned out, eventually being converted into a thin-walled sac, the so-called "posterior sacculation of the uterus."

Fortunately the operation of ventrofixation of the uterus has been abandoned in child-bearing women, and this dangerous complication only takes place when accidental adhesion of the fundus uteri to the abdominal wall follows some form of suspension operation or other pelvic procedure.

Course of Pregnancy.—Abortion is common in cases of antefixation. Sometimes the pull of the growing uterus breaks the adhesion to the abdominal wall, with sharp pain and possibly a mild pelvic peritonitis, sometimes premature labor results, and occasionally such patients go to term with uterine inertia as a result of the stretching out of the posterior wall, malpresentation, and even spontaneous rupture of the thin-walled uterus.

The diagnosis is made from the history of a previous suspension operation, the continued pain just above the symphysis and radiating to the flanks, and the palpation of a thick band of uterus filling the anterior vault of the vagina with the cervix pulled upward and backward. Abdominally the thin, tender posterior uterine wall may be felt as a conical mass, the point upward and the base toward the vagina.

Treatment.—When one is certain that anterior fixation exists, it is best managed by laparotomy and freeing of the uterine adhesions during the early months of pregnancy, before sacculation becomes marked.

If labor comes on, vaginal examination will determine the degree of mobility of the cervix. If this can be brought into the axis of the birth canal and the presenting part be made to engage, vaginal de-

livery probably with the aid of forceps may be permitted. If, however, the cervix remains high, and the os lies directly posterior,
cesarean section is the method of choice in securing delivery. This is
particularly so, because of the ever-present danger of rupture of the
thinned-out uterine wall.

In these cases, version should be avoided if possible, or attempted
with the greatest care and gentleness, in order to minimize the danger
of rupture.

RETROVERSION AND RETROFLEXION OF THE PREGNANT UTERUS

Authorities agree that from 15 to 20 per cent of women have some
degree of retroversion, and this condition is probably responsible for
some sterility and a definite proportion of spontaneous abortions. On
the other hand, most women with uncomplicated retroversion conceive
without difficulty and go through pregnancy to a successful delivery.

When conception takes place in a retroverted uterus, the commonest termination is spontaneous correction of the retroversion, As
the uterus expands the fundus slips over the promontory of the sacrum
and the organ lies in the body axis—not forward as normally, but
no longer in retroversion. As pregnancy progresses, the uterus more
nearly assumes its normal anteversion until near term it lies in its
proper position. When the optimum result does not occur, by reason
of dense adhesions binding the fundus down (most adhesions are
stretched, torn or absorbed during pregnancy), pressure from pelvic
tumor, or possibly a deformed promontory with a beaked projection
which holds the fundus down, two terminations are possible—abortion
and incarceration of the uterus below the promontory of the sacrum,
with marked stretching of the anterior wall—anterior sacculation.
DeLee describes a third termination called partial restitution in which
a part of the fundus is retained in the pelvis while the remainder
becomes the container of the ovum and rises into the abdomen.

Abortion in retroversion is probably due to circulatory changes in
the uterus resulting from torsion and partial obstruction of the veins
in the broad ligament, plus the chronic hyperplastic changes of the
endometrium which so often accompany this condition. It is seldom
caused by the pressure of the confined and growing uterus upon the
ovum.

Incarceration of the fundus behind the sacral promontory constitutes a serious and dangerous but uncommon complication, the
chief symptoms being referable to the bladder. Traction upon this
organ and the urethra by the upward growth of the anterior uterine
wall induces great congestion about the trigone at the internal urethral
sphincter. Urination is impossible and the bladder becomes enormously distended, 2 gallons of urine having been withdrawn in one
reported case. As a result of overdistention, there may be some
dribbling of urine from the urethra—the incontinence of retention.
The dysuria causes intense pain and if unrelieved the bladder may

rupture intraperitoneally with resulting peritonitis, its walls may become gangrenous, or there may be rupture into the pelvic cellular tissues with extravasation of urine and resulting necrosis and sloughing, all of these accidents resulting fatally in most instances. Uremia may develop from retention of urine in the kidneys.

If the uterus has grown to a considerable size, its thinned-out anterior wall may rupture in its attempt to expel the ovum. The bowel may be subject to such pressure from the incarcerated uterus that symptoms of partial intestinal obstruction appear, or at least there may be marked tympany and constipation.

Diagnosis.—Incarceration of the uterus presents little difficulty in diagnosis. Dysuria or dribbling of urine in a pregnant woman should excite suspicion and a vaginal examination will disclose the cervix pushed high against the symphysis pubis while the dense compressed fundus fills the cul-de-sac, the promontory of the sacrum being buried in the uterine wall.

Abdominally the distended bladder may be palpated as a fluctuating, tender tumor, sometimes extending to the umbilicus and disappearing after catheter withdrawal of an excess amount of urine.

The differential diagnosis must be made from an accompanying pelvic tumor, as a large ovarian cyst, or fibroid, and from ectopic pregnancy.

Treatment.—Retroversion of the uterus, recognized at the first obstetric examination, may be disregarded if no symptoms are present. If the uterus remains in retroversion after the third month, the woman is carefully watched for bladder symptoms. In most cases reposition of the uterus occurs spontaneously when the ovum has grown large enough so that the fundus is forced over the promontory of the sacrum and into the abdomen.

In the small minority, incarceration occurs and dysuria is at once noted. When the diagnosis of incarceration has been made it is a mistake to temporize, since abortion, severe cystitis with possible pyelonephritis and gangrene of the bladder may result from delay. Immediate laparotomy should be done, care being taken to avoid the bladder which has been displaced upward.

The uterus is then dislodged from its imprisonment and fastened anteriorly by some form of round ligament suspension.

If laparotomy is impossible the uterus may be emptied from below, although reaching the cervix may present some difficulty since it is displaced so far forward and upward. Sometimes the patient may go to term, and during labor podalic version and extraction may terminate the case satisfactorily. Rarely it may be possible to perform a posterior wall hysterotomy, when the fundus projects far down in the cul-de-sac.

No matter what the treatment, attention must be focused upon the bladder, and as soon as this organ cannot empty itself, catheterization must be resorted to. In neglected cases, with a long, distorted

Incarcerated retroversion with pregnancy.	Fibroma uteri with pregnancy.	Ovarian cyst with pregnancy.	Ectopic pregnancy.
Usually a young woman in her first pregnancy.	Older woman, who has been pregnant or who has married late.	No point of differentiation.	No point of differentiation.
Increasing dysuria with some incontinence.	Absent unless tumor is very large when they may appear in slight degree.	Absent or inconsiderable.	Absent.
Complete amenorrhea.	Complete amenorrhea.	Complete amenorrhea.	Irregular menstruation or missed period followed by spotting.
Uterus can be felt as a continuous tumor, smooth and symmetrical.	Tumor may be nodular; may feel uterus as a separate growth.	Tumor smooth and fluctuating, may feel uterus as a separate growth.	Vague mass in cul-de-sac uterus slightly enlarged or not at all.
Vaginal examination discloses cervix pulled upward and against symphysis. Canal at right angles with pelvic floor. Fundus uteri in hollow of sacrum. Not tender on movement.	Cervix may be displaced forward or backward but remains in line of pelvic cavity. Not tender on movement.	Cervix may be displaced forward or backward but remains in line of pelvic cavity. Not tender on movement.	Cervix slightly displaced, tender to movement.
In moving the cervix the enlarged uterus moves with it.	May move uterus while tumor remains fixed.	May move uterus while tumor remains fixed.	No clear cut tumor. Mass does not move with cervix.
Pain comes on gradually, referred to bladder, steadily becoming worse.	Pain from pressure only, not apt to be acute.	Pain from pressure only, not apt to be acute.	Sudden lancinating pain when rupture or tubal abortion occurs.
Leukocytosis comes on slowly, not marked until severe cystitis.	Inconsiderable leukocytosis.	Inconsiderable leukocytosis.	Leukocytosis may be very high.
Urine contains blood cells.	No.	No.	No.

bladder whose walls are congested and infected, catheterization some-times offers great difficulties, but can usually be accomplished by the use of a metal catheter, using great gentleness to avoid making false passage. In extreme cases the bladder should not be emptied at once, for fear of hemorrhage into its overdistended walls, and in all instances of marked distention a permanent catheter should remain in place for several days.

Prolapse of the Pregnant Uterus.—Procidentia may be present in the early months of pregnancy, but the uterus usually retracts upward later, or abortion takes place.

If the uterus does not retract spontaneously, it must be replaced and held in position by gauze packing or soft rubber pessary, until its increased size prevents further descent. Naturally, ulceration of the cervix must be treated by cauterization with strong silver nitrate solution (10 per cent).

Hernia of the Uterus.—The pregnant uterus may occupy the sac of an inguinal or ventral hernia, several cases being reported some years ago. This accident is of no special obstetric significance, since the uterus can be either pushed out of the hernial opening which is then temporarily closed by adhesive plaster strapping, or in the event that this is not possible, pregnancy may go on with the uterus still occupying the hernial sac.

Axial Torsion of the Uterus.—Reis and Chaloupka have gathered 16 cases of axial torsion of the uterus at term. The accident is an exaggeration of the physiological dextrotorsion, and if it develops gradually and the degree of twist is not too great, may produce no symptoms.

When it comes on suddenly, however, and the torsion exceeds 180° there are prompt evidences of shock and intraperitoneal calamity, and such cases usually end fatally.

The condition is probably due to some asymmetry of the uterine musculature.

PELVIC TUMORS COMPLICATING PREGNANCY

Fibromyomata, ovarian tumors and uterine carcinoma may co-exist with pregnancy and their presence gives rise to certain pos-sibilities of pathological change.

Fibroid tumors are very common during the childbearing age, possibly 30 per cent of pregnancies having this association (Fig. 171).

If the tumors are small, their presence causes little disturbance although sterility and abortion may occur, due to the alteration in the uterine circulation produced by the tumors. In large tumors, bleeding during pregnancy and postpartum hemorrhage are common. Pain and pressure symptoms occur, and sometimes necrobiosis of the tumor makes its immediate removal imperative (Fig. 172).

Interference with rhythmic uterine contractions if not absolute ob-struction from the tumor itself, complicates labor (*q. v.*).

Management.—Diagnosis is important, since all too often a large, low-lying fibroid nodule is mistaken for the fetal head and the mistake

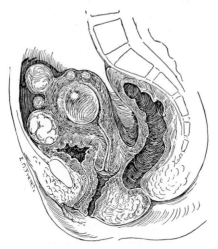

Fig. 171.—The type of fibroid which does not interfere with development of pregnancy. (Polak in Surg., Gynec., and Obstet., vol. 46, 1928.)

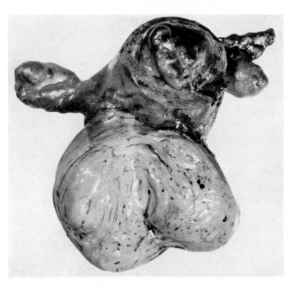

Fig. 172.—Large cervical fibroma complicating pregnancy in a woman of forty-three years. Degeneration of the tumor necessitated hysterectomy at the third month. (Kensington Hospital for Women.)

not recognized until rupture of the uterus has occurred after long and tumultuous uterine contractions have failed to force the presenting part past the tumor.

Usually the only treatment necessary during pregnancy is abundant rest and close attention to vaginal bleeding. Pain and pressure symptoms or evidence of infection in the tissues may necessitate myomectomy during pregnancy, this operation being always preferred to hysterectomy, unless the tumor is sessile and so large that the resulting wound in the uterine muscle might rupture during the subsequent delivery.

During labor cesarean section may become necessary (*q. v.*).

Ovarian Tumor.—Usually ovarian cysts are uncommon in pregnancy, although large ones have been reported. Because of the danger of torsion of the pedicle, or rupture of a large cyst during labor, these growths should be removed upon diagnosis. The pregnant uterus is so tolerant of the excision of ovarian growths that little danger of abortion need be feared. Unless pressure or torsion takes place, ovarian cysts rarely cause symptoms during pregnancy.

Solid tumors of the ovary are rare at best, and usually produce sterility. Campbell reports a very large ovarian carcinoma in a young woman of twenty-eight who was sterile. He removed the ovary and at the end of two years, the patient became pregnant and produced a living child.

Dermoid cysts of the ovary grow rapidly under the stimulus of pregnancy, and are quite liable to torsion of their pedicle. Such tumors should be removed upon discovery.

Carcinoma of the Cervix.—This condition is rare in pregnancy. Unless the lesion is in its incipiency sterility is the rule. The frequency is not known, statistics being extremely variable as the 1 in 2000 cases found by Werther as opposed to the 1 in 15,000 cases reported by Glockner.

When pregnancy does supervene upon a cervical carcinoma, the growth of the latter is much accelerated by the general increase in pelvic vascularity. Hemorrhage may be fatal even during the early months.

The diagnosis may be confirmed by biopsy and when positive, early panhysterectomy should be performed, without regard for the child and the operation followed by thorough irradiation. It has been advised to wait until the child is viable and then perform cesarean section with complete hysterectomy, but this plan of management results in such extensive growth of the carcinoma, that the mother is invariably doomed to early death.

Carcinoma of the fundus uteri coexistent with pregnancy has been reported by the writer, who observed a pregnant multipara with uterine bleeding. Curettage disclosed adenocarcinoma and upon hysterectomy the uterus was found to contain high in the fundus a two-months fetus with sac intact. The area of carcinoma lay below the site of the pregnancy.

Comment.—Pelvic tumors complicate labor rather than pregnancy.

Fibroid tumors are common among pregnant women. They may

have no effect, or their presence may result in abortion, deformities of the fetus, hemorrhage during pregnancy, postpartum hemorrhage, disturbances of uterine contraction during labor and puerperal infection as well as actual obstruction to delivery.

Pain and pressure symptoms during pregnancy may necessitate myomectomy.

Ovarian tumors tend to rapid growth, torsion of the pedicle, and necrosis during pregnancy and should be removed.

Carcinoma of the cervix is rare in pregnancy, but when found should be subjected to radical extirpation plus irradiation at once.

21

CHAPTER XX

EXTRA-UTERINE PREGNANCY

Extra-uterine pregnancy, tubal pregnancy, ectopic pregnancy or eccyesis, is the condition which results when the fertilized ovum is implanted anywhere outside the cavity of the uterus, the most frequent site for such aberrant implantation being the fallopian tube.

Frequency.—Ectopic pregnancy occurs in a ratio of 1 to 300 intra-uterine pregnancies. The incidence being slightly greater in urban than in rural districts. It effects women at any time during the child-bearing age, younger patients being the most frequent sufferers. Race seems to play no part in the development of this lesion.

Sites of Ectopic Pregnancy (Fig. 173).—Faulty implantation of the ovum may occur in the intramural portion of the fallopian tube,

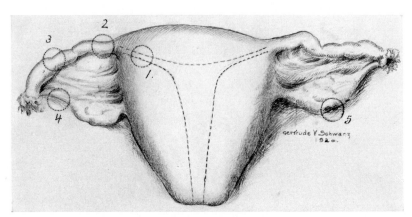

Fig. 173.—The sites of implantation of the ovum in extra-uterine pregnancy. 1, Interstitial; 2, isthmial; 3, ampullar; 4, tubo-ovarian; 5, ovarian. (Author's book on "Extra-Uterine Pregnancy," D. Appleton-Century Co., Publishers.)

the isthmus, the ampulla, or the ovary itself. These are primary locations. Secondarily, the ovum may be implanted anywhere in the abdominal cavity, the posterior leaflet of the broad ligament and the parietal peritoneum being the commonest areas for such secondary implantation. There are a few cases on record of implantation of the ovum on the parietal peritoneum but these are so rare as to be of but slight clinical significance.

Etiology.—Extra-uterine pregnancy depends upon some factor which delays the passage of the fertilized ovum to the uterine cavity, the delay permitting the ovum to grow to such size that it cannot possibly pass the area of contraction. The delay may be due to an obstruction of the tube from without, obstruction of the tube from within, diverticula of the tube and tubal endometriosis.

Obstruction of the tube from within is usually the result of a healing salpingitis in which some of the delicate mucosal processes of the tubal lining have become coalesced and form a sort of network in which the ovum becomes enmeshed. Rarely fibromata of the tubal musculature may impinge upon the lumen and so reduce its size.

Obstruction of the tube from without involves kinking of the tubes as a result of the adhesions following a perisalpingitis, pressure from adjacent uterine fibroids or ovarian cysts. *Congenital anomalies of the tube:* accessory ostia with a blind ending; accessory lumina running parallel with the main lumen and either rejoining it or ending blindly, or diverticula and pockets in the tubal mucosa, may all act to retain the fertilized ovum within the tube, until it undergoes implantation in the false decidua.

A persistence of the fetal type, the tubes being long and possessing many convolutions with wide variations in the size of the lumen, may act in a similar fashion.

Decidual Reactions and Tubal Endometriosis.—It is probable that a false decidua develops in the tubal mucosa occasionally, but studies of tubes removed during pregnancy show only scattered areas of decidual cells which have been thought to be of fetal and not maternal origin.

Endometrial implants may, and do, undergo a true decidual change and offer a suitable bed for implantation of the tubal ovum, but true endometriosis of the tube wall in connection with ectopic pregnancy is very uncommon.

Repeated Ectopic Pregnancy.—There seems to be a tendency for the recurrence of tubal pregnancy in women who have had one tube removed for this condition, the etiology being probably identical in both instances. The incidence of recurrence is somewhere in the neighborhood of 15 per cent.

Twin and triplet ectopic pregnancies have been reported but are uncommon and of no diagnostic or therapeutic importance.

Combined intra-uterine and tubal pregnancy is not too rare, more than 300 such cases being recorded.

PATHOLOGY OF TUBAL PREGNANCY

Changes in the Uterus.—The uterus undergoes the hypertrophic changes, characteristic of pregnancy, and the endometrium becomes converted into a decidua parietalis. Since no ovum is implanted, there are neither capsularis nor basalis formations.

The uterus may attain the size of a two months' pregnancy, the decidua remaining intact, until the ovum perishes, when it is discharged either in fragments with more or less bleeding or sometimes as an intact decidual cast of the uterine cavity.

The cervix is soft and succulent but rarely becomes cyanotic.

Changes in the Tube.—The tubal mucosa reacts somewhat to the stimulus of pregnancy, its mucosa becoming thickened, its cells low and cuboidal and its surface rendered irregular by the presence of finger-like cytoplasmic projections from the nonciliated cells, but there is never a true decidual formation. The walls of the tube are thin, and their musculature offers little depth for the invasion of anchoring villi.

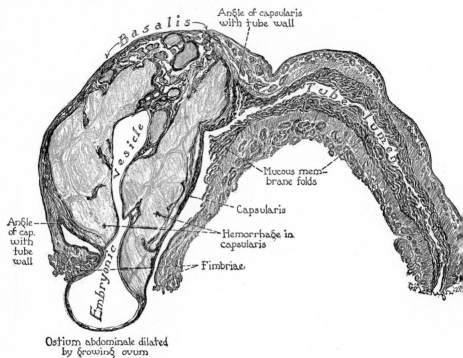

Fig. 174.—Composite drawing made from various longitudinal serial sections brought by the artist to one plane. Showing nidation near fimbriated end of tube. (Ovum bulging through ostium abdominale by growth and not by tubal abortion. Capsularis is not ruptured. No bleeding from tube.) (Litzenberg in "Nelson Loose-Leaf Living Surgery," vol. 7.)

The ovum passes through the several changes characteristic of early uterine pregnancy. The trophoblast develops into the chorion, with its villi which exert their normal erosive action in penetrating the mucosa and opening blood spaces (Fig. 174).

The ovum burrows into the vascular tube walls, a capsule being formed by the chorionic cells, the residue of the partly destroyed and displaced muscular and connective tissues and fibrin. This capsule is termed the "pseudodecidua capsularis."

The chorionic villi, seeking adequate nutrition, erode deeper and deeper into the tube wall, which is soon perforated by them, a tiny rupture of the tube resulting. Hemorrhage from the site of perforation leads to hemorrhage about the ovum and within its cavity, to the death of the embryo and to the formation of an ovoid mass of blood clot, degenerated tube wall tissue and the dead ovum itself.

Even when the tube wall is not perforated hemorrhage into the ovum takes place from the failure of a decidua basalis to receive the open ends of the eroded tubal vessels and to form a blood sinus (Fig. 175).

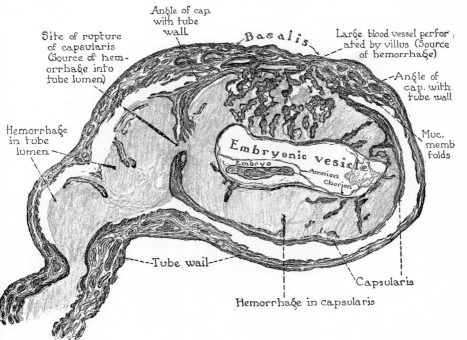

Fig. 175.—Composite drawing of various serial sections brought to one level, showing rupture through capsularis, with blood flowing through the tube. The ovum is still firmly attached to the tube wall, showing that the bleeding is from an internal rupture and not a tubal abortion. (Litzenberg in "Nelson Loose-Leaf Living Surgery," vol. 7.)

In most cases, these factors cause the death of the embryo, with attendant hemorrhage in from six to twelve weeks, but very rarely the tube may be sufficiently elastic and vascular to provide an area for placentation and the unruptured tubal pregnancy may go to term.

THE TERMINATIONS OF TUBAL PREGNANCY

Tubal pregnancy may primarily eventuate in:
   1. Early death of the ovum with complete resorption and a restoration of the tube to its prepregnant condition.

2. Death of the embryo with the formation of tubal mole (Fig. 176).

3. Tubal abortion.

4. Rupture of the pregnant tube, either into the peritoneal cavity or between the folds of the broad ligament.

5. The growth and development of the embryo may proceed to term, when either the fetus dies as a result of nutritional failure, or is delivered by abdominal section.

6. If the pregnancy be interstitial, the fetus may gradually be extruded into the uterine cavity, the placenta remaining

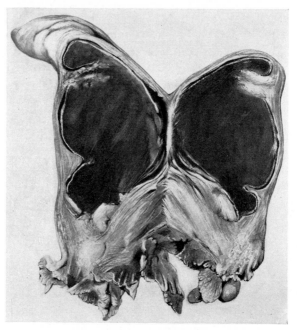

Fig. 176.—A tubal mole. All gross evidence of pregnancy has disappeared, the distended tube being filled with organized clot. On microscopical examination, distinct placental shadows could be seen in the tube wall. (Author's book on "Extra-Uterine Pregnancy," D. Appleton-Century Co., Publishers.)

attached to the cornual wall, and the pregnancy may terminate by spontaneous vaginal delivery, as in normal intrauterine gestation, the placenta being also spontaneously expelled.

These are the primary terminations of tubal pregnancy.

Secondarily, the embryo may be expelled from the tube and the placenta remain behind, the pregnancy going to term, with the fetus free in the abdominal cavity and the placenta implanted in the tube—the so-called "tubo-abdominal" pregnancy. Or, the entire living ovum may be expelled, the placenta reattaching itself to any tissue within the peritoneal cavity and pregnancy then going on to term—secondary abdominal pregnancy. In either of these instances the fetus, unless removed by laparotomy, dies and proceeds to suppuration and necrosis, lithopedion formation, mummification, or adipocere. Practically speaking, unless terminated by surgical intervention, every case of ectopic pregnancy results fatally for the child, except the rare case of secondary uterine gestation following a primary interstitial implantation of the ovum.

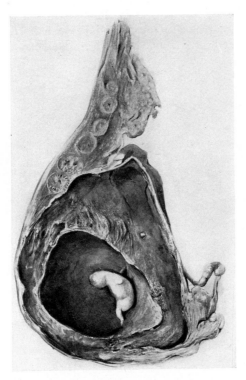

Fig. 177.—A tubal mole, the fetus still intact but undergoing degeneration. Tube greatly distended but not ruptured. A large blood clot separates the fetal envelopes from the tube wall. (Author's book on "Extra-Uterine Pregnancy," D. Appleton-Century Co., Publishers.)

1. **Termination by resorption of the ovum** takes place, in the opinion of the author, much more frequently than is commonly believed. In taking detailed histories of gynecological cases when some operation is contemplated for relief of pelvic symptoms, it is not uncommon to elicit an account of a train of symptoms strongly suggestive of the existence of an ectopic pregnancy at some past period of the woman's life. When, upon subsequent laparotomy, no evidence whatever is found of any lesion of the tubes, or when a small, nodular

area of fibrosis exists in one tube, the fact that resorption of an extra-uterine embryo has at some time taken place is at least suggestive.

Furthermore, the finding of small, absorbing tubal moles upon the examination of certain excised tubes lends additional plausibility to this form of termination of extra-uterine pregnancy. Nothing more definite than the foregoing facts is available, but it seems reasonable in the face of such evidence to consider death and resorption of the ovum as one mode of termination in these cases.

2. **Death of the Embryo with the Formation of Tubal Mole.**—A tubal mole (Fig. 177) results when the fetus dies in the intact tube, with marked hemorrhage about it and between its membranes. At the same time the liquor amnii is absorbed, the blood clot more or less

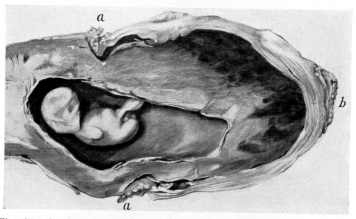

Fig. 178.—Section of a tube showing incomplete tubal abortion. The embryo in its sac which is surrounded by a large clot, is seen partially extruded from the enormously distended fimbriated extremity (a). The uterine end of the tube is shown at (b) (case of Dr. J. M. Baldy). (Author's book on "Extra-Uterine Pregnancy," D. Appleton-Century Co., Publishers.)

organized, and a structure produced which is identical with the moles occurring in uterine pregnancy. Such moles may vary markedly in size, according to the age of the pregnancy and the amount of hemorrhage, and may be retained in the tube for an indefinite period.

3. **Tubal abortion,** one of the two most common terminations of extra-uterine pregnancy, occurs when the ovum becomes detached from its imbedding site in the tube and is expelled from the fimbriated extremity of the tube by tubal muscular contraction, the abortion being complete when the ovum and its envelopes are entirely extruded from the tube and fall into the abdominal cavity, and incomplete when only a portion of the sac protrudes from the free end of the tube, the remainder being still confined within the tube walls (Fig. 178).

Tubal abortion is usually accompanied by severe hemorrhage, and clinically cannot be differentiated from rupture of the tube, although occasional cases are recorded where the hemorrhage was negligible in amount.

4. **Rupture of the Pregnant Tube.**—(a) *Into the Peritoneal Cavity* (Fig. 179).—According to many authorities rupture is the most usual mode of termination of a tubal pregnancy. Such accident happens usually before the twelfth week, most commonly, in the opinion of the writer, before the eighth week following conception. Naturally ruptures occur in almost a direct ratio to the site of implantation of the

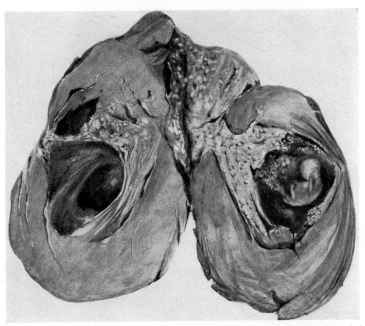

Fig. 179.—A gestation sac with large surrounding blood clot found lying free in the peritoneal cavity, the result of a complete and rapid tubal abortion. There was but little hemorrhage. (Author's book on "Extra-Uterine Pregnancy," D. Appleton-Century Co., Publishers.)

ovum. Ampullar pregnancies are far more prone to end by tubal abortion than by rupture; midtube pregnancies terminate almost equally by these two accidents (Fig. 180), while in isthmial and interstitial pregnancies, the tube usually suffers a rupture of its wall. The tear in the tube is commonly over the site of the developing placenta, and when intraperitoneal, takes place on the free aspect of the tube.

The older writers considered this accident to be due to a simple overdistention of the tube wall beyond the point of its elastic resistance. Close study of the pathology led to a change in thought, and it was held that the rupture was always due to perforation of the tube wall by proliferating syncytial cells (Fig. 181).

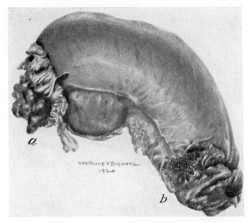

Fig. 180.—Rupture of a pregnant tube occurring subsequently to the development of tubal abortion. At (a) is seen a portion of the clot surrounding the embryo being extruded from the fimbriated extremity of the tube while at (b) is a secondary point of the rupture, which was bleeding freely at operation. (Author's book on "Extra-Uterine Pregnancy," D. Appleton-Century Co., Publishers.)

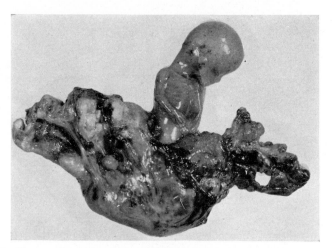

Fig. 181.—Ruptured tubal pregnancy, the ten weeks' fetus half way out of the rent in the tube. (Kensington Hospital for Women.)

My own view is that a combination of these factors brings about the lesion, an area of the tube wall becoming thinned out and weakened by the erosive action of the syncytium, and being the point of least resistance, yielding to the pressure of the growing ovum, or more commonly to the accumulated mass of blood clot gathering in and about the oval sac (Fig. 182).

So far as the writer's personal observation goes, rupture occurs with nearly double the frequency of tubal abortion.

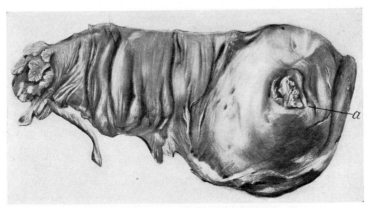

Fig. 182.—Beginning rupture of an isthmial pregnancy, on the inner, posterior aspect of the tube. The rupture is shown at (a) a few fronds of the chorionic villi having been forced through the minute opening. (Author's book on "Extra-Uterine Pregnancy," D. Appleton-Century Co., Publishers.)

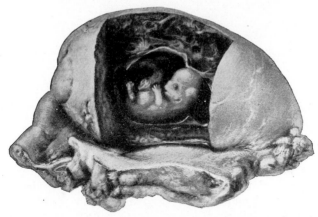

Fig. 183.—The tube has been dissected so as to show the embryo in position. The space between the amnion and the tube wall is filled with a partly organized clot. The embryo appears to be normal. ($\times$ ⁵/₆.) (Mall in "Contrib. to Embryology," 1915.)

(b) *Rupture Between the Folds of the Broad Ligament.*—In exceptional cases the tube may rupture along its inferior aspect, through the mesosalpinx, the hemorrhage thus taking place in the extraperitoneal portion of the tubes, and dissecting between the layers of the broad ligament (Fig. 183).

This type of rupture may eventuate in the death of the embryo and the formation of a broad ligament hematoma, or by the further development of the embryo as a secondary broad ligament pregnancy (exceedingly rare), or if the tension created by the extravasated blood be sufficiently great, there may occur a secondary rupture of the broad ligament, the blood eventually escaping into the peritoneal cavity (Fig. 184).

This variety of rupture is rarely attended by severe hemorrhage, and from the clinical standpoint is to be regarded as by far the most favorable type with regard to the welfare of the patient.

When the growth of the embryo continues after its escape into the broad ligament, the future course depends largely upon the degree of completeness with which the placenta has been separated from its tubal attachment, as pointed out by J. W. Williams, who states that

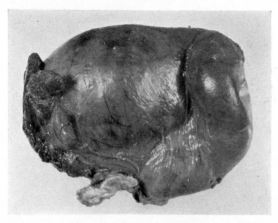

Fig. 184.—An unruptured tubal pregnancy of about eight weeks.

if the placenta remains attached to the tube on the side opposite the point of rupture, it generally becomes displaced upward as pregnancy advances, and comes to lie about the fetus; but when it is situated near the point of rupture, it gradually extends down between the folds of the broad ligament, being implanted partly upon the tube and partly upon the pelvic connective tissue (Fig. 185).

In either event the fetal sac lies entirely outside the peritoneal cavity, and as it increases in size, the peritoneum is gradually dissected up from the pelvic walls. This condition is designated as extraperitoneal or broad-ligament pregnancy.

5. *The Growth and Development of the Fetus to Full Term, While Still Confined Within the Tube.*—This rare and interesting termination of tubal pregnancy is occasionally recorded in the literature, and the writer has had the good fortune to observe a case.

Secondary Terminations of Extra-uterine Pregnancy.—In addition to the foregoing primary terminations of extra-uterine pregnancy, certain secondary end-results may develop.

Tubal rupture or abortion, but far more commonly the former, may be succeeded by:

1. Tubo-abdominal pregnancy.
2. Secondary abdominal pregnancy.
3. Tubo-ovarian pregnancy.
4. Intraligamentous pregnancy.

1. *Tubo-abdominal pregnancy* is that condition which is found when, following a rupture of the tube wall on its free surface, the placenta remains attached to the tube wall either wholly or in part, fetal nutrition in the latter instance being derived from placental

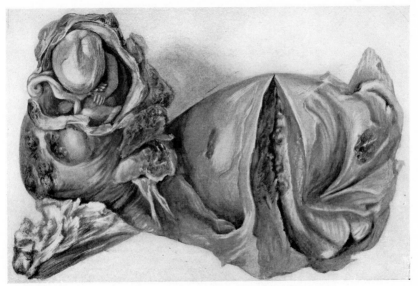

Fig. 185.—Late rupturing tubal pregnancy. (Author's book on "Extra-Uterine Pregnancy," D. Appleton-Century Co., Publishers.)

adhesions to contiguous structures. The fetus meanwhile has been expelled through the aperture in the tube wall and lies free in the abdomen, surrounded by its amniotic envelope, or is in some cases entirely devoid of covering.

Whether fetal life can continue or not, under these circumstances, depends naturally upon the traumatism inflected upon the embryo by the act of tubal rupture, and upon the area of placenta remaining imbedded in the tube and maintaining unimpaired vascular connection with the tubal vessels. It will at once be seen that the possibilities of irreparable injury to the embryo from hemorrhage, as well as the tendency to complete or nearly complete separation of the immature placenta from its abnormal implantation site, are so great that the proportion of tubo-abdominal pregnancy in which development of the fetus continues to term as compared with immediate fetal death following rupture is extremely small. Tubo-abdominal pregnancy is, therefore, a rare condition though by no means unique, as a fairly large number of cases are recorded.

2. *Secondary abdominal pregnancy* is that condition found when, following tubal rupture or abortion (more commonly the latter), the entire ovum is expelled into the general peritoneal cavity and the embryo continuing to live, the syncytia attach themselves to whatever tissue they may and reimbedding takes place in an entirely secondary location (Fig. 186).

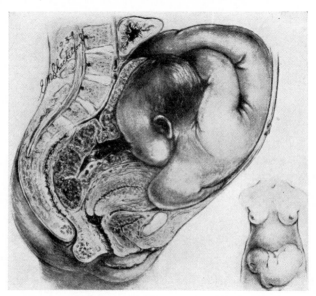

Fig. 186.—Relative position of fetus, placenta and uterus. The upper portion of the placenta had no maternal attachment. (Eisaman and Ziegler, Jour. Amer. Med. Assoc., June 15, 1935.)

3. *Tubo-ovarian pregnancy* occurs when the fetal sac is composed partly of tubal and partly of ovarian tissue. It may originate in a tubo-ovarian cyst, or more commonly in a tube, the fimbriated extremity of which was previously adherent to the ovary.

Pathologically these cases are not distinct varieties, but begin as tubal or possibly rarely as ovarian pregnancies, their subsequent course being due to the accidental attachment of the tubes to the ovary.

4. *Intraligamentary pregnancy* results when the tube ruptures between the folds of the broad ligament and, the placenta remaining fast to its tubal attachment, the fetus develops within the broad ligament. As growth proceeds the parietal peritoneum is dissected away

from the tissues and the entire gestation sac continues to be extra-peritoneal. The term "subperitoneopelvic pregnancy" has been used to describe this variety, and it was considered a common occurrence by the older writers. With more careful study of the anatomy, however, intraligamentary pregnancy has been found to be quite rare.

THE END-RESULTS OF EXTRA-UTERINE PREGNANCY

Untreated or long-standing ectopic gestation may eventuate in:
1. Resorption of the products of gestation.
2. Tubal mole.
3. Hematocele, which may be:
    (a) Diffuse.
    (b) Solitary.
    (c) May become infected.
4. When fetal development continues the fetus may become:
    (a) Lithopedion.
    (b) Mummified.
    (c) Adipocere.
    (d) Skeletonized.
    (e) May suppurate.

1 and 2. *Resorption and tubal mole* have been discussed in the section devoted to terminations and will not be further considered here.

3. *Hematocele.*—The older works on gynecology devote much space to a consideration of this subject, hematocele being considered as a distinct clinical entity.

The formation of an hematocele is one of the favorable terminations of ectopic pregnancy, in that the development of organized clot predicates the passage of sufficient time for active bleeding to have ceased, and the danger of death from hemorrhage to have passed. Hematocele is the result, necessarily, of slow hemorrhage, and it follows therefore that this termination occurs far more frequently where the initial lesion is tubal abortion, with its trickling of blood from the fimbriated extremity of the tube, rather than frank rupture of the tube wall, with is accompanying free bleeding.

The presence of blood in the peritoneal cavity sets up an irritative plastic, aseptic peritonitis, which invites adhesion formation, and in time the entire clot, occupying more or less of the whole pelvic cavity, becomes walled off by intestinal adhesions, the coils being firmly glued together and serving to form a sort of capsule for the clot. It has been held that the development of this so-called "diffuse hematocele" must have been preceded by adhesions between the pelvic organs, but the writer inclines to the view that the adhesions slowly form as a reaction of peritoneal surfaces to the irritation of free blood.

Infected Hematocele.—Hematoceles, from their very nature, are excellent culture media for pyogenic bacteria, and infection of these collections is a frequent and dangerous sequel. The colon bacillus is naturally a common offender. The result of infection by this or other pyogenic organisms is to convert the hematocele into an abscess, which may point into the general peritoneal cavity, with subsequent peritonitis, may rupture into the rectum (a very fortunate termination for the patient), or into the bladder, or happily may sometimes drain into the vagina. Infected hematoceles are among the most serious and dangerous sequelae of ectopic pregnancy.

Cornual or interstitial pregnancy occurs when the fertilized ovum becomes embedded in the thickness of the uterine muscle, at the cornua. It is quite uncommon and does not differ from other varieties of tubal pregnancy, except in so far that the hemorrhage after rup-

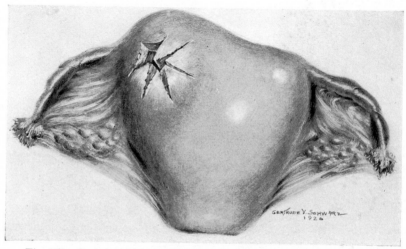

Fig. 187.—An interstitial pregnancy which had ruptured, literally blowing the anterior uterine wall into fragments. Very profuse hemorrhage into the peritoneal cavity. (Author's book on "Extra-Uterine Pregnancy," D. Appleton-Century Co., Publishers.)

ture is much more violent by reason of the increased vascularity of the uterine wall. Rarely interstitial pregnancy may, by extension of the placenta along the lines of least resistance, become intra-uterine (Fig. 187).

THE PATHOLOGY OF ADVANCED ECTOPIC PREGNANCY

It has been previously stated that far advanced tubal pregnancy without rupture of the tube is a rare occurrence. Under these circumstances, the pathology is that of a marked distention of the tube wall, the thinning out of the muscular layer, and the wide distribution of connective tissue in and between the muscle bundles. The tube becomes involved in a reactive inflammation and is usually found more or less densely adherent to surrounding structures. Otherwise, there is no noteworthy change.

The common forms of advanced ectopic gestation (and these, too, are most infrequent) are either the secondary abdominal types, which follow rupture of the tube with the expulsion of the embryo into the peritoneal cavity, or the quite rare type which develops when the entire ovum is extruded from the tube and becomes secondarily implanted upon tissues possibly remote from the original site. Most cases of abdominal pregnancy seem to follow either rupture into the broad ligament, development continuing between the folds of this structure, or the rupture taking place on the posterior aspect of the tube, the placenta remaining partially attached to its original site within the tube lumen and partially becoming secondarily attached to the posterior surface of the broad ligament. In cases reported in the literature, the fetal sac is frequently described as ending in a pedicle, composed of the tube and the broad ligament on the affected side.

An analysis of the literature leads to the conclusion that while the fetus in these cases is usually enclosed in a sac which may be composed either of the fetal membranes or of a fibrinous exudate, evidently of secondary formation, there may be no evidence of any embryonic covering whatever, with normal growth and development of the fetus.

Placental attachment in these cases is usually in the tube or along the border of the broad ligament, though occasionally the entire ovum may have been extruded from the tube and the ovum have become secondarily implanted at a point remote from its original site.

Extraperitoneal abdominal pregnancy results when the ovum continues to develop after a rupture of the tube between the folds of the broad ligament. As the embryo grows, the leaflets of the broad ligament are dissected widely away from the pelvic walls, and the sac develops under the peritoneum and becomes what Hart has termed a "subperitoneal pelvic pregnancy," until the pelvic brim having been passed by the steadily growing fetus, the gestation becomes subperitoneo-abdominal.

When abdominal pregnancy goes on to term, an attempt at labor usually occurs, the contractions of the uterus being more or less marked for several hours and then subsiding. After the subsidence of labor pains, fatty degeneration of the placenta takes place, resulting in the death of the fetus, which may then undergo various changes in its composition.

In this connection, it is interesting to note that abdominal pregnancy, terminated by operative interference, has in some instances resulted in the delivery of a living child. The majority of the children in these cases lived but a few hours after delivery and many of them were deformed. A few, however, survived.

The Fate of the Embryo in Ectopic Pregnancy.—In the great

22

majority of cases of extra-uterine gestation the embryo is destroyed during the early weeks of development. A careful study of the matter is that of Mall, which will be freely quoted here: "In normal implantations in the tube most of the ova are destroyed in the early stages by the hemorrhage which is produced for their nourishment. If the dam built up by the trophoblast is sufficient to check the flood in part, enough villi will remain to nourish the ovum. When the tube ruptures into the broad ligament the space for the chorion becomes sufficiently large for new villi to grow and attach themselves."

It is noteworthy that among the specimens studied by Mall far more tubes ruptured, when they contained normal embryos, than among those in which the embryo was pathological; showing that a live, normal, tubal embryo is probably far more dangerous to the mother than a pathological one. Pathological ova without embryos are very frequently encountered in examining series of specimens of tubal gestation.

Terminations of Abdominal Pregnancy.—The usual end-result of abdominal pregnancy is the death of the fetus, and its subsequent surgical removal.

In some instances, as has been seen, living babies are delivered from the abdominal cavity by laparotomy. If the condition remains unnoticed as is sometimes the case, the fetus may be retained for months or years, finally developing into a calcified mass, presenting the outline of the fetus and termed lithopedion, or the soft parts may be absorbed, a mummified skeleton remaining, or the entire body may be converted into a soapy mass called adipocere.

SYMPTOMATOLOGY AND DIAGNOSIS

Tubal pregnancy, in which there has been no hemorrhage into the ovum, gives rise to no symptoms other than the subjective signs of early pregnancy. These may be a missed menstrual period, some nausea or at least gastric discomfort, increased frequency of urination and pain and tingling in the breasts. There is no localized pain and no uterine bleeding.

This state of affairs may last for two or three weeks to three months, and very, very rarely to term, if the tube should not rupture and the fetus survive (some 4 cases of this type are in the literature).

In the great majority of instances the process of implantation and beginning placentation lead to hemorrhagic lesions in the ovum, or in the tubal lumen about the pseudodecidua. As soon as such an accident occurs, usually from three to twelve weeks after fertilization, symptoms begin, pain and irregular vaginal bleeding being the chief evidence of the existence of ectopic gestation. When the tube wall has ruptured as a result of the intratubal accumulation of blood and the erosive action of the syncytium or when tubal abortion has begun, following rupture of the pseudocapsular decidua, the symptoms become more marked and characteristic.

Pain.—Before rupture or tubal abortion but after hemorrhage into the pelvis, the pain may be slight, a mere heaviness in one or the other iliac fossae. The pain may extend down the thigh, and should a very little blood escape into the peritoneal cavity, there is a generalized abdominal ache. The symptoms at this time are not particularly severe, and may not impel the patient to seek the advice of a physician.

Symptoms When Rupture or Abortion Occurs.—On the occurrence of either of these terminations of tubal pregnancy, the pain becomes very definite and may assume one of two varieties:

(a) A sudden, lancinating violent pain, which may cause syncope and shock, and which is followed by an increasing generalized abdominal pain as the escaping blood irritates the peritoneum. In cases of tubal abortion, the first violent attack may be followed by remittent cramplike pain, as the peristaltic action of the tube seeks to dislodge the ovum and its surrounding blood clot. After such accident has occurred the patient is found in collapse, of greater or less degree, the skin pale and leaking, the face anxious, the nostrils twitching. Respirations are shallow and rapid, the temperature is subnormal, the pulse rapid, running and small. The abdomen is scaphoid and tender in its lower aspect and the blood pressure is low. There may be nausea and vomiting. There is usually some bleeding from the vagina, but this may be a mere spotting and may have preceded the attack by several days. Very rarely is the bleeding profuse. On vaginal examination, the cervix is tender to motion, a spindle-shaped mass may or may not be palpated in one or the other vaginal fornices and there may or may not be a doughy, bulging mass in the cul-de-sac, depending upon whether or not there has been time enough for the free blood in the abdominal cavity to have gravitated into the pelvis.

Examination of the blood during the first hours following rupture is negative, there being no immediate change in the blood picture. Later evidences of primary anemia present themselves and the leukocytes rise, sometimes reaching 30,000. The sedimentation time is generally shortened. If untreated, the patient may die from blood loss and shock, or the bleeding may cease temporarily, and recovery from the state of shock may ensue. This is the classical picture of ruptured ectopic pregnancy and is sometimes called the asthenic form. It is seen in slightly less than one half of all cases.

The *sthenic variety* of symptom-complex follows tubal rupture or abortion, when the rupture is small and the hemorrhage slow, is characterized by the occurrence of pain which is sudden in onset, not lancinating and violent but a steadily increasing dull and throbbing ache, which does not subside and which frequently gives rise to the mistaken diagnosis of inflammatory disease of some type. When blood accumulates in the cul-de-sac there is severe pain on defecation and when the cervix is moved during examination. The clinical picture is often that of an acute salpingitis or appendicitis, the temperature moderately elevated, the pulse full, its rate about 100 per minute.

The abdomen is rigid and tender, and may be slightly distended. There is no external evidence of hemorrhage other than the slight or moderate uterine bleeding.

The vaginal examination is as before, and study of the blood usually reveals a slight primary anemia with a moderate to high leukocytosis. In this type of case slow recovery, if untreated, is the rule, the hemorrhage ceasing with the death of the ovum, and the free blood being slowly resorbed. Sometimes painful adhesions, or infection of an hematocele constitute sequelae which invite operative interference and clear the diagnosis.

In other cases hemorrhage may recur and the patient go into secondary shock and collapse.

The diagnosis of ectopic pregnancy depends upon (a) the past medical history of the patient; (b) the menstrual phenomena; (c) nature of the attack; (d) the evidence that pregnancy exists; (e) findings upon physical examination.

(a) The past medical history is of great importance because tubal pregnancy so frequently occurs in a damaged tube.

Hence, history of attacks of pelvic inflammation, either puerperal, postabortal or other, together with a record of a period of sterility after the last previous pregnancy point to tubal inflammatory disease. Previous pelvic operations, with their sequelae of peritubal adhesions, are suggested factors. Recurrent ectopic pregnancy is not rare, so that a history of a preceding tubal gestation is in some degree corroborative.

(b) Menstruation is generally disturbed in tubal pregnancy. A missed period, a delayed period, one which apparently begins normally but after a day or so the flow ceases, only to return after the passage of a few more days, all point to the possibility of ectopic gestation.

(c) The nature of the attack has already been described. It is important to note that the overwhelming majority of cases of this lesion are characterized by vaginal bleeding. This may be a little spotting for days or even weeks before the attack of severe symptoms, or the bleeding may accompany the rupture of the tube.

The bleeding is hardly ever profuse, and I have never seen a massive vaginal hemorrhage in this condition.

(d) The fact that pregnancy exists may be adduced by the presence of the subjective symptoms of pregnancy—nausea, breast changes, etc., plus a positive Aschheim-Zondek or Friedman test.

(e) The findings upon physical examination have been discussed.

The ruptured tube with its surrounding blood clot forms an ovoid or spindle-shaped mass in the adnexal region, which is tender on palpation.

Blood in the cul-de-sac causes a bulging of the posterior vaginal wall and gives the sensation of a semifluctuating, doughy mass to the examining finger.

Movement of the cervix gives rise to great pain.

In examining patients who are suspected of suffering from tubal pregnancy, great care and gentleness must be exercised since it is easily possible to rupture a distended, blood-filled tube by rough manipulation as is evidenced by many case reports. If the diagnosis is in doubt, a long needle may be passed into the cul-de-sac through the posterior vaginal wall, and any fluid contents aspirated with a syringe. The presence of fresh or old blood will confirm the diagnosis of intraperitoneal hemorrhage.

Special Symptoms of Ectopic Pregnancy.—Pain in the shoulder; severe and fairly constant shoulder pain on the same side of the ruptured tube occurs in a definite proportion of cases and when present is suggestive, although in my experience it is neither a constant or definite sign.

Peri-umbilical Ecchymosis (Cullen's Sign).—A definite area of subcutaneous ecchymosis has been described as evidence of intra-abdominal bleeding. I have seen this only twice, once in a case of acute purulent salpingitis, and once in a case of postoperative acute yellow atrophy of the liver with fatal hepatic bleeding. In neither of these patients was ectopic pregnancy present.

Dilatation of the pupil on the affected side has been described, but this sign has never been noted, in my experience, possibly because it is not often enough sought.

Note.—The diagnosis of tubal pregnancy while the ovum is still living and there has been no hemorrhage into its capsule is rarely made, for two reasons.

First, the patient, experiencing no symptoms, does not consult a physician, and second, because even if vaginal palpation should be done, in the course of a routine physical examination, the pregnant tube, having approximately the same density as the intestinal mass and being free and movable, will escape detection. This is not true when hemorrhage into the ovum has taken place, even before rupture.

DIFFERENTIAL DIAGNOSIS

The important differentiations of ectopic pregnancy are from intra-uterine abortion, and from pelvic inflammatory disease, including appendicitis.

Intra-uterine Abortion	Ectopic Pregnancy
1. Subjective signs of pregnancy prominent.	1. Subjective signs of pregnancy vague.
2. Not necessarily so.	2. History of previous pelvic inflammation, operation, etc.
3. Onset gradual, symptoms steadily growing worse.	3. Onset sudden and strong maybe with collapse and shock.
4. Pain, cramplike and intermittent like labor or menstrual pain, may radiate down thighs.	4. Pain sudden, lancinating or may be a generalized abdominal distress.

INTRA-UTERINE ABORTION	ECTOPIC PREGNANCY
5. Bleeding free, may be exsanguinating.	5. Bleeding confined to spotting or a moderate vaginal hemorrhage.
6. Parts of embryo may be discharged.	6. Fragments of decidua; no embryonic tissues discharged.
7. No mass or bulging cul-de-sac.	7. Spindle-shaped mass in iliac fossa. Doughy bulge in cul-de-sac.
8. Blood picture normal or showing primary anemia.	8. Blood picture shows primary anemia with sharp leukocytosis.
9. Sedimentation time unchanged.	9. Sedimentation time decreased.
10. Visible bleeding corresponding to systemic reaction to hemorrhage.	10. Systemic evidence of hemorrhage exceeds visible blood loss.

Ectopic pregnancy of the sthenic type may be differentiated from acute intraperitoneal inflammatory disease by the following points of variance:

ECTOPIC PREGNANCY	INFLAMMATORY DISEASE
1. Evidences of pregnancy (subjective).	1. No such evidence.
2. Biological pregnancy test positive.	2. Negative.
3. Vaginal bleeding in some degree.	3. No vaginal bleeding.
4. Usually some abnormality in menstrual cycle.	4. No such abnormality.
5. Onset sudden and strong. No initial vomiting.	5. Onset, a rapidly increasing abdominal pain, vomiting common.
6. Leukocytosis very variable.	6. Leukocytosis usually 10,000 to 15,-000.
7. Puncture of vaginal vault discloses presence of blood.	7. No blood in vault.
8. Uterus enlarged.	8. Uterus of nonpregnant size.

Ovarian cyst with twisted pedicle, incarcerated retroverted uterus in pregnancy, hydrosalpinx and even sometimes ruptured gastric or duodenal ulcer may be mistaken for ectopic pregnancy or the reverse, but the history and the result of a biological test will usually determine the diagnosis.

TREATMENT

There is no expectant treatment for a pregnant tube, which must be removed by surgical intervention as soon as discovered. Shock and collapse are not contraindications to immediate operation because experience has shown that very few patients die as a result of surgery, while many perish while the medical attendant is awaiting a recovery from shock, which unhappily does not take place. This does not imply the pen-knife type of operation but contemplates proper conditions for aseptic surgery performed by one skilled in such work. Where the patient has survived the first rupture, and has emerged from shock, it may be permissible to defer operation, and indeed some of these patients recover completely with no surgical interference at all. Nevertheless this laissez faire policy is dangerous, as a fatal secondary hemorrhage may develop at any time, so that immediate operation generally offers the best hope of cure.

Inasmuch as the diagnosis of rupture of the tube as opposed to tubal abortion is at best tentative, the two conditions are grouped as one from the standpoint of management.

Operative Procedure.—Local anesthesia in the hands of those accustomed to its use, or some variety of inhalation anesthesia is employed. Through a median incision, the uterus is grasped and elevated and the tubal lesion brought into view. The tube is removed by the standard technic, the ovary left behind, unless the patient is in extremis, when both tube and ovary should be removed, because of the greater rapidity with which such procedure may be performed.

Blood clots in the abdomen which obscure the view are scooped out, but a meticulous toilet of the peritoneal cavity is not performed because it wastes time, and also the remaining blood is usually reabsorbed with advantage to the patient.

Management of the Opposite Tube.—Both tubes should be inspected, and both may contain ectopic ova, in which case they should be removed. If the remaining tube shows evidence of inflammatory change it may be removed if hopelessly damaged and the patient is in good condition. Otherwise it should be permitted to remain since while 12 per cent of ectopics recur, 47 per cent of women who have had one extra-uterine pregnancy subsequently conceive and give birth to normal, intra-uterine children.

Drainage is not employed. I do not practice or advise the collection of abdominal blood and its subsequent reintroduction by transfusion, by reason of the loss of time, the traumatism engendered in recovering the blood and clots and the possibility of infection. The keynote of success with these very ill patients is gentleness and speed in performing the operation.

In those cases where shock and anemia are not factors, more leisurely and detailed operative procedure may be employed.

Preoperative Treatment.—In the interval between the rupture of a pregnant tube and the time of operation, treatment is of the utmost importance. Stimulation by drugs and the intravenous administration of fluids must be avoided, since by this means the low blood pressure will be elevated and the tendency to further hemorrhage increased. Rest and quiet should be secured by the free use of morphine, the foot of the bed is raised if the patient be in collapse, and external heat is freely applied.

When everything is in readiness for operation, and the patient draped preparatory to the initial incision, vigorous stimulation should be started, caffeine, digitalis, etc., to maintain the circulation and blood transfusion, or failing this, the intravenous administration of glucose in 10 per cent solution is begun. By the time that an effect is secured the operation will have been completed and the bleeding point secured.

The postoperative management is that of any pelvic laparotomy plus frequent blood transfusions if anemia be severe.

Treatment of Hematocele and Late Ectopic Pregnancy.—Such cases are rarely emergencies, and their treatment is based upon the peculiar condition involved. Old hematoceles are usually best attacked by the abdominal route, with any necessary attention to adnexal lesions.

Should the hematocele be infected, simple posterior colpotomy with drainage is probably the best method of treatment.

The Management of Advanced Ectopic Pregnancy.—By advanced extra-uterine pregnancy is meant those cases not seen until after the fifth month, the fetus being alive or having perished, as may be. Here the management of the placenta becomes the factor of first importance, together with the fact that a possible infant life is to be considered, as well as that of the mother.

The placenta may occupy any position within the abdominal cavity, although it is most commonly found firmly attached to the posterior fold of the broad ligament and the floor and lateral walls of the pelvis, the villi dipping deep into the pelvic vessels. In other instances, however, the placenta may be found attached to the omentum, the intestines or indeed to any of the intraperitoneal viscera. In such case where the fetus is alive and the placental circulation active, the removal of this organ may be attended by absolutely uncontrollable hemorrhage.

No definite technic for the performance of an operation for advanced ectopic pregnancy can be formulated, since each case is a law unto itself, but certain general directions will be found valuable.

The incision is preferably to be made along the outer border of the rectus muscle overlying the gestation sac, since so many of these placentas are found under and between the folds of the broad ligament that the removal of the fetus and placenta may be accomplished without entering the peritoneal cavity, a matter greatly to be desired, especially if the placenta cannot be removed at the time of operation.

Having reached the sac, it should be incised, the child extracted and the cord ligated as in cesarean section. The sac should then be examined in great detail, in order to ascertain whether it be feasible to attempt ligation of its blood supply and excision, or whether the attachment to great vessels or to vascular viscera is so intimate that attempt at enucleation will result in disaster.

In the former alternative, careful ligation of the vessels supplying the placenta should be performed, before attempts at its removal are instituted. The ligations accomplished, the placenta may be manually pulled off its attachment, bleeding being controlled by ligature and pressure by gauze wrung out in hot saline solution, and the wound closed without drainage.

Should the location of the placenta be such that control of its blood supply seems impracticable, there are two methods for its management. First, the time-honored plan of marsupialization, stitching the edges of the gestation sac to the abdominal wound and lightly packing the cavity with gauze. The gauze packing is changed at forty-eight-hour intervals and the separation of the placenta aided by gentle traction. In the course of a few weeks the tissue has sloughed out and there remains a sinus of varying size, which usually closes spontaneously, although a second operation for the repair of the abdominal wall may be required.

The second and preferable method of treatment is to leave the placenta *in situ,* ligating and cutting the cord at its point of insertion in the placenta, closing the abdomen without drainage, and permitting the placental tissue to be resorbed. Theoretically this procedure would seem open to the objection that detachment of the placenta from its abdominal implantation might occur shortly after the operation, with resulting hemorrhage, but practically this accident does not take place. In a number of reported cases recovery has been rapid and uneventful, nor has there been any later evidence of the persistence of placental tissue in the peritoneal cavity.

In a consideration of the treatment of advanced ectopic pregnancy from the standpoint of the child, two questions present themselves; first, whether the fetus is apt to have suffered some arrest of development which renders its postnatal life doubtful or impossible; second, whether or not the maternal risk is greatly increased by permitting the pregnancy to continue until term or thereabouts.

1. The best time to operate is during the sixth or the seventh month.

2. The added risk in waiting for a well-developed child is slight up to the thirty-ninth week.

3. The danger of a catastrophe is sufficiently great in the last two weeks to warrant interference before this period is reached.

In the interests of the child it is found that the best time to operate is the thirty-eighth week, more infants having survived at this period than at any other. This may be explained by the fact that, as interference is practiced before term, the child, as well as the mother, is spared the danger of spurious labor, and further, that the fetus is subjected to greatly increased pressure during the last two weeks of pregnancy, by reason of the diminution in the amount of the liquor amnii at this time.

Since the risk in waiting for the thirty-eighth week is slight for the mother, and since this is the time of election for the child, it follows that the thirty-eighth week of pregnancy is the best period for surgical intervention from the standpoint of both mother and child.

That these abdominal children are worth saving is beyond a doubt, Cragin finding two normal living infants in his four cases, while Horsley's statistics, previously quoted, amply confirm this.

The Treatment of Advanced Ectopic Pregnancy When the Fetus is Known to Be Dead.—Should the fetus have been dead for a considerable time, immediate removal of the placenta is usually possible, its vascularity having markedly decreased and a partial separation of the villi from their site of implantation having taken place. If the fetus is known to have been dead for a short time, it is advisable to defer operation until some obliteration of the maternal blood spaces about the villi has occurred, since the enucleation of the placenta is greatly facilitated thereby. During the month or six weeks of waiting for the separation to take place, the patient should be under constant observation in a hospital, in order that immediate operation may be performed in the event of any infection of the gestation sac supervening as evinced by an elevation of temperature and pulse rate and an increasing leukocytosis.

Ovarian Pregnancy.—This is a rare variety, less than 100 cases being recorded. In it the ovum becomes fertilized before escaping from the follicle, within whose walls it develops.

The sac is formed of the theca and lutein layer of the follicle, and the embryo may be completely covered by ovarian tissue, or may grow out into the peritoneal cavity. In order to prove the existence of ovarian pregnancy, it must be shown that both tubes are free from any evidence of tubal gestation, and that the embryo is covered with ovarian tissue.

These cases go on to further development before rupture than do the tubal forms, and several are on record in which the fetus was viable.

The diagnosis and treatment are identical with that of tubal pregnancy, from which the ovarian form cannot be differentiated, until the condition is observed at laparotomy.

Prognosis.—In 1872 Parry stated that the mortality from ruptured extra-uterine pregnancy was 85 per cent.

Today in well-organized clinics the mortality falls well below 4 per cent, an improvement due to generally improved diagnosis, and to the formulation of definite and correct methods of treatment.

CHAPTER XXI

DISEASES OF THE EMBRYO AND APPENDAGES

DISEASES OF THE FETAL MEMBRANES

Polyhydramnios, hydramnion or **hydramnios** is the condition in which an excessive quantity of liquor amnii collects within the membranes. Minor degrees of hydramnion are fairly common but occasionally huge accumulations of fluid occur, Kustner having observed 15 liters and Schneider 30 liters, at the fifth and six month, respectively.

The factors influencing the quantitative and qualitative production of liquor amnii are almost unknown—there may be either an excessive production or an excessive retention of fluid. Careful examination of the amniotic epithelium has disclosed no variation from the normal in the histology of the cells in cases of hydramnion. Lessened absorption is a most important factor, the greater part of such absorption taking place in the alimentary tract of the fetus after the liquor has been swallowed. In many cases of hydramnion there has existed an absence of such absorption due to atresias of the upper alimentary tract.

Etiology.—The etiology of hydramnion may be briefly considered under several groupings. The first great causative factor is deformity of the fetus. According to Hinselmann fetal deformities can be grouped into: (1) those having no influence upon the amount of amniotic fluid, as hydrocephalus; (2) those producing an excess of fluid, due either to increased transudation of fluid or deficient swallowing and absorption, as anencephalus, atresia of esophagus, etc., and (3) those associated with oligohydramnios or scanty fluid.

The second etiologic cause is multiple pregnancy, especially uniovular twins, in one of which ova hydramnion is quite frequent.

Third in etiologic significance is the occurrence of moderate degrees of hydramnion in excessively large children and placentae. In one of the writer's cases a child weighing 10 pounds 4 ounces was associated with 3000 cc. of fluid.

Maternal toxemia is another prolific source of hydramnion, especially where there is an associated edema.

Syphilis has been regarded as causative but there seems little evidence to support this contention. In most case series the percentage of syphilis is no greater than in other groups of pregnant women.

Clinical Course.—Hydramnion may be divided clinically into the rare acute variety, the more common chronic form and a third phase in which an existing chronic hydramnion suddenly presents an acute exacerbation. Acute hydramnion arising early in pregnancy may give rise to a rapid accumulation of enormous size, which occasions more or less severe pressure symptoms. Dyspnea so severe as to absolutely preclude the patient's lying down, cyanosis, edema of the lower extremities with pain in the abdomen and back may be present. The skin is tensely stretched, many striae appearing with punctate hemorrhages in the skin from excessive tension. The entire abdomen is hard and tense, fetal parts are not palpable nor are heart tones audible. There may be fever and exhaustion and a fatal outcome may ensue if the maternal heart is the seat of an organic lesion.

Diagnosis.—The diagnosis of acute hydramnion is usually simple if pregnancy is known to exist, but the condition must be differentiated from ovarian cysts, especially in connection with intra-uterine pregnancy, from ascites and from hydatidiform mole. In ovarian cyst, the enlargement is not generally so sudden, there is no history of pregnancy, the small uterus can easily be outlined as playing no part in the enlargement, and the cervix is hard and closed. In ovarian cyst complicating pregnancy, the differentiation is much more difficult, but the demonstration of two tumors, separated from each other, should determine the state of affairs. Frequently, however, this diagnosis is missed and the condition is not made clear until after delivery. In mole pregnancy the rapid increase in size of the uterus is almost always accompanied by more or less severe vaginal hemorrhages or the extrusion of the characteristic hydatidiform cysts in the vaginal discharge, which should serve to clear up the diagnosis.

The chronic form of hydramnion offers little difficulty in diagnosis. The greatly distended uterus, the soft and patulous cervix, through which the fetal presenting part may be palpated, easy elicitation of ballottement, and the presence of fetal movements, although the heart tones are faint and distant, all serve to make the situation clear, although when the distention of the uterus becomes very great, so that the fetus can no longer be palpated, diagnosis is sometimes very difficult and hydramnion may easily be mistaken for very large ovarian cystoma.

Employment of the x-ray will always definitely settle the question. Excessive abdominal enlargement due to ascites may be differentiated by the characteristic movable dulness on percussion, and by the fact that on vaginal examination the uterus is found to be of the correct size in relation to the duration of the pregnancy.

Careful examination is sometimes necessary to determine whether the uterine distention is due to multiple pregnancy or hydramnion alone. The two conditions are frequently associated.

Treatment.—The treatment of acute hydramnion is active and should consist in rupturing the membranes under strict asepsis and allowing the fluid to escape gradually to avoid undue loss of intra-abdominal pressure. The patient is then left to a spontaneous abortion which almost always occurs, other active treatment being determined by special indications which may arise.

It has been clearly shown that hydramnion most commonly occurs in the presence of a deformed fetus and consequently every effort should be made to determine the nature of such deformity if present. Here the x-ray is of prime importance and repeated roentgenological examination should be undertaken, if necessary, to secure a clear understanding of the fetal contours.

General treatment consists of rest in bed to avoid undue cardiac strain and careful search for possible toxic factors such as nephritis. Should the pressure symptoms become extreme, the excess fluid should be drained away by a trocar introduced through the cervical canal. The withdrawal should be slowly done to prevent too great fluctuation in the intra-abdominal pressure. Rigid asepsis must be practiced. The evacuation is probably best accomplished with the patient in the knee-chest position to avoid prolapse of the cord and the too sudden descent of the head into the lower uterine segment. This procedure is usually followed by the onset of labor in a few hours, in which event preparation must be made to combat possible postpartum hemorrhage which is all-too-common a sequel.

The presence of a monster as proved by the x-ray is an indication for immediate evacuation of the fluid and induction of labor at any period of pregnancy.

Oligohydramnion.—This term implies a deficiency or absence of amniotic fluid and is far less common than the excess previously described. The liquor amnii may be represented by a few drachms of thick, viscid, greenish or brownish fluid, often having an offensive and somewhat characteristic odor.

The *etiology* is shrouded in mystery, but it is suggested that urinary tract deformities in the fetus are present in a large number of the cases. Thus Neumann found such deformities to occur in 9 cases among a total of 49.

Oligohydramnion occurring early in pregnancy is attended by serious consequences to the fetus, by reason of adhesions forming between it and the amnion with which it lies in contact. Cranioschisis, gastroschisis, spina bifida, and amputation of extremities, curvatures, clubfoot and skin defects have all been reported. When the diminution in fluid takes place late in pregnancy, the effect upon the fetus is less marked but still severe. Under such circumstances, the fetus clearly shows the effect of long-continued pressure, and minor deformities are usual. Especially characteristic is the dry, leathery skin which may be a result of the oligohydramnion, but which Ahlfeld believed to be causative.

The *diagnosis* is difficult unless the uterus, smaller than normal, may be easily palpated through a thin, relaxed, abdominal wall as irregular in outline and coapted closely to the fetal body.

Taussig well sums up the *clinical characteristics* of oligohydramnion as follows:

1. Proportionately small size of pregnant uterus.
2. Greater frequency among primiparas.
3. Tendency to breech presentation, in which position the fetus adapts itself more closely to the shape of the partly filled uterus.
4. Prolonged pregnancy (from twenty to thirty days overdue).
5. Long, slow labor with frequent necessity for manual or instrumental interference.
6. High fetal mortality during and after labor.

Amniotic Adhesions.—In oligohydramnion and even sometimes when the liquor amnii is present in normal amounts, adhesions may form between the amnion and the fetus. As has been stated, when such adhesions occur early in pregnancy, great deformity results from failure of the embryo to develop in the areas in contact with the amnion (Fig. 188).

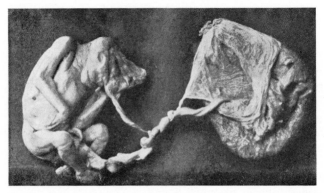

Fig. 188.—Deformed infant the result of amniotic adhesions in oligohydramnios. (Seitz.)

Many instances of failure of development of the abdominal parietes, with eventration of the viscera, are due to this cause. Amputations of extremities from compression by a band of amnion have been reported, though the correctness of this view has been disputed, and the writer is inclined to agree with Ballantyne who believes that the so-called "amniotic amputations" are really due to some form of trophic disturbances analogous to Raynaud's disease in later life.

Amnionitis.—Inflammation of the amnion. During pregnancy inflammatory processes occasionally invade the amnion. They are usually associated with a deciduitis and result from preexisting gonorrhea or possibly from some invasion of the uterine cavity in an attempt to procure abortion.

Intrapartum inflammation is far more common and Siddall has shown in a study of 1000 consecutive placentae from the seventh month to term, that 48 or 4.8 per cent showed a definite inflammatory reaction in the amnion and chorion. In 7 of these placentae, bacteria were demonstrated, although in no case was there clinical or histologic evidence of gonorrhea or syphilis. It is obvious that premature rupture of the membranes permits access of bacteria to the uterine cavity with ample time for well-established inflammatory reaction before the placenta and membranes are extruded. Such inflammation will account for many instances of intrapartum fevers and serves to emphasize the necessity for scrupulous asepsis in vaginal manipulations after the membranes have ruptured. It reveals as well the inherent danger of cesarean section under these conditions.

Cysts of the Amnion.—Years ago Ahlfeld called attention to the occurrence of small cysts, lined by normal epithelium, which form in the amnion. Williams thinks they generally result from the fusion of amniotic folds with retention of fluid.

DISEASES OF THE PLACENTA

Infarct Formation.—Practically all placentae if subjected to careful scrutiny will show few or many whitish, hard, nodular areas occupying the fetal or maternal surface, or both surfaces, and varying in size from the most minute to several centimeters in diameter. These nodules are the so-called "infarcts," or, as they have been variously termed, "hepatization," "scirrhus," "placentitis," "apoplexy," "cirrhosis," and "phthisis."

Several varieties have been described and their mode of origin has given rise to a huge literature, out of all proportion to their clinical significance. J. W. Williams described six kinds of infarcts, and the number has been raised or lowered by other observers.

The more significant varieties of infarcts are the so-called "red infarcts," "white infarcts" and "placenta marginata."

Red infarcts are sharply demarcated oval, or pyramidal-shaped areas, situated on the maternal surface of the placenta, or deep in its structure. They are the result of localized tissue necrosis, probably from thrombosis of the vascular supply in the immediate area.

On microscopic examination they are found to be composed of lamellae of fibrin and coagulated blood, together with degenerated villi. In general they appear like fresh, intravascular thrombi, and vary in size from 1 to 4 cm. in diameter.

White infarcts are round, oval or roughly quadrilateral bodies, usually found on the margin of the placenta, sometimes near the maternal surface, rarely on the fetal surface. They represent an advanced stage of tissue necrosis and may be massive, involving sometimes one fourth of the entire placenta.

Microscopically, white infarcts are composed of closely packed villi with a thin layer of fibrin between and in the older forms, the blood cells have largely disappeared from the intervillous spaces, while the stroma has lost all evidence of cellular structure.

Placenta Marginata.—Sometimes a white ring, varying in width from 2 to 20 mm. and 1 to 4 mm. thick, is found encircling the edge of the placenta just at the site of the subchorial decidua and this formation is called placenta marginata. The condition may be of clinical significance in producing placental retention or adhesion of the membranes, with some of the fragments remaining in the uterine cavity, to cause late hemorrhage or infection.

The frequency of infarct formation is noteworthy, since in Siddall and Hartman's series of 700 placentae there were 67.7 per cent presenting infarcts of some kind, measuring at least 5 mm. in diameter, and it is probable that many more showed these defects of microscopical dimensions.

Thoms, who studied 58 placentae by injection, section and roentgen photographs, says that marginal white infarct formation is so common that it may be considered a normal phenomenon of the mature placenta.

Clinical Significance of Placental Infarcts.—The older writers laid great stress upon the interference with fetal oxygenation which might be produced by extensive infarct formation and cases are recorded wherein the death of child *in utero* was presumably caused by such diminution in oxygenative surface.

In Thoms' series, however, 17 per cent were found infarcted to a degree which actually interfered with the placental circulation. In one case 24 per cent of the placental circulation was thus arrested by the process, yet there was no evidence of material toxemia or ill effect upon the baby. Furthermore, infarct formation seems to bear no relation to the growth and weight of the child as shown by several series of statistics.

The writer has long felt that the tremendous factor of safety provided for by nature in all of her processes must and does apply to the placenta, and that all possible contingencies are so provided for short of complete catastrophic breakdown, as, for example, abruptio placentae.

The Relationship of Infarction and the Toxemias of Pregnancy.— Here lies a fruitful ground for argument among obstetricians. Most textbooks emphasize the relationship. For example DeLee says that infarcts cannot be diagnosed clinically but their existence can be expected in cases of nephritis, heart disease, syphilis, endometritis and when they were present in previous pregnancies.

The writer is of the opinion that no distinct connection can be traced between toxemia and infarct formation and has for years called the attention of interns and students to the absence of marked infarction in placentae from severe cases of eclampsia, while on the other hand, patients with perfectly uneventful pregnancies and with normal, full-size babies, often present such striking areas of infarction as to make the placenta an object of pathologic interest.

Cysts of the Placenta.—Small cystic areas scattered throughout its structure are very common in the placenta. These cysts are usually very small, only a few millimeters in diameter, although they may reach a diameter of 6 cm.

They are generally found in the thickest, central portion of the placenta, somewhat nearer the fetal than the maternal side of the organ. The cysts are rarely spherical, but commonly are irregular in outline, often presenting elongated diverticula; the cyst wall is a whitish fibrin band, a millimeter or less in thickness. The cavity is filled with a clear, creamy, or sanguineous gelatinous material, which may vary in viscosity from a firm jelly to a thin mucoid fluid.

Cysts are usually found in the decidual islands, which are normal constituents of the placenta, being portions of the decidual septa. They may occupy the center of an infarct, are filled with gummy fluid and according to J. W. Williams were mistaken by the older writers for abscesses.

Clinically these structures appear to possess no significance. Paddock and Greer studied 231 cases without any conclusive evidence as to any relationship between these cysts and maternal or fetal mortality and Williams sums up the matter by saying, "Cystic formations, whether occurring upon the fetal surface or in the depths of the placenta, are of interest purely from the pathologic point of view and exert little or no influence upon the course of pregnancy or labor."

Tumors of the Placenta.—All writers upon placental tumors begin by quoting the work of John Clarke who in 1798 reported a case of solid tumor, the size of a man's fist, which made up a large part of the placenta. Since this publication only 131 cases of placental tumor have appeared in the literature. These rare tumors take their origin from the epithelium, connective tissue, and blood vessels of the placental chorion. Their etiology is unknown, although many hypotheses have been advanced concerning them. They consist of masses of chorionic villi with immense hypertrophy and hyperplasia of the terminal vessels and hence belong to the group of chorio-angiofibromata. They are usually single, though four and six separate growths have been described in one placenta. They range in size from a few millimeters in diameter to a weight of nearly 800 Gm. They may appear on the maternal surface of the placenta, but the majority are found as firm elevations just beneath the amniotic surface of the placenta.

These tumors usually possess a pseudocapsule made up of compressed and degenerated villi. They are sharply circumscribed and are readily enucleated. In most cases the only direct connection with the placental tissue is by blood vessels entering the tumor through a small pedicle. The growths are usually single and almost spherical in shape although they may consist of a group of small, compressed lobules easily separable one from the other.

23

Clinical Aspects of Placental Tumors.—These growths seem to have little or no effect upon the prognosis or course of pregnancy in the mother. Among the 131 cases collected by Siddall, the obstetrical history was about as usual except for the impressive number of cases of hydramnion in the group. During the third stage of labor there may be some increase of risk from hemorrhage since in the same group of 131 cases postpartum hemorrhage and operative removal of the placenta or tumor were each reported six times and in four other cases manual removal of the placenta was necessitated by excessive bleeding.

Malignant Tumors of the Placenta.—Such growths are very rare and so far as known are never primary but originate as metastases from a remote primary tumor focus.

Inflammation of the Placenta.—Acute inflammation of the placenta is occasionally noted but is never primary, being due to an extension from the decidua, resulting from an exacerbation of a preexisting chronic gonorrhea or from an acute infection due to the entrance of pyogenic bacteria into the oval sac. Such inflammatory change almost always accompanies general uterine sepsis or is a result of prolonged labor, or frequently, of premature rupture of the membranes.

Very rarely abscesses are found in the placenta, following prepartum infection.

Tuberculosis of the Placenta.—Placental tuberculosis offers great difficulty in demonstration, for neither microscopical nor histologic changes need be present even though the tubercle bacilli may be numerous.

According to Norris tuberculosis apparently exerts no influence upon the size of the organ, nearly all of the described specimens being of average size and weight. When massive lesions do occur they are usually found as yellowish, soft, caseous areas, at the base of the placenta, near the insertion of the cord. The maternal and fetal surfaces are often rougher than usual, and occasionally small tubercles may be present. The cord is generally normal.

Hemorrhages of the Placenta.—Owing to the extreme vascularity of the decidua, hemorrhages are common in it. These bleedings are generally in the serotina and lead to various degrees of placental separations.

Occasionally hemorrhages take place in the decidual septa between the cotyledons and also in infarcts both red and white. DeLee gives the causes of placental hemorrhage as acute and chronic congestion, increased blood pressure, stagnation of the venous blood current, disease of the villi, or of the decidual blood vessels, the blood changes incident to nephritis, toxemia, hemorrhagic diathesis and syphilis, physical or mental shock and local injury. The writer is inclined to place syphilis first on the list.

Clinically, placental hemorrhages are of great importance. If they develop early in pregnancy, abortion is the rule, while if the hemorrhage be not sufficiently massive to cause this result, arrest of fetal development may take place with resultant monster formation.

Later in pregnancy massive serotinal hemorrhages are the first phase of abruptio placentae, and should the bleeding be between the cotyledons or in the subchorial decidua, serious results to the child may be anticipated, as from hypo-oxygenation and insufficient nutrition.

Edema of the Placenta.—Huge edema sometimes occurs in the placenta, and is in most instances associated with hydrops universalis fetus. The writer collected 38 cases of this condition among which the placenta was described in 36, 30 of these revealing massive edema. In Opitz' case the placenta weighed 2280 Gm. The condition is usually present in women who have shown the existence of some form of gestational toxemia, or in whom the presence of such toxic factor is suspected but cannot be confirmed. Syphilis is rarely causative. On examination such placentae usually show great edema with some degeneration of the syncytial cells. The villi are vacuolated, there is separation of the connective tissue by fluid and the syncytial cells are swollen, their nuclei pale and in many instances shrunken.

Clinically, if the edema occurs early in pregnancy, abortion promptly follows. Should the gestation continue, the child usually suffers from general edema, and formidable dystocia may result from this cause.

Calcification of the Placenta.—Small calcareous deposits or flat plaques are frequently found on the maternal surface of the placenta. They are composed of calcium carbonate, calcium phosphate, and magnesium phosphate, and are usually seen in the upper layers of the decidua serotina, especially around the anchoring villi, and are due to the calcareous degeneration of the villi, being in a sense analogous to infarcts. They are probably a phase of senescence of the placenta and have no clinical significance, there being no apparent relationship between the degree of calcification and any maternal disease. DeLee thinks that they render the placenta stiff, which facilitates its separation and expulsion, and that no portion of a calcareous placenta is ever retained.

Placenta Accreta.—Placenta accreta is a condition resulting from an entire or almost entire absence of the decidua basalis, which exposes the muscle of the uterine wall to the erosive action of the trophoblast and to penetration by the villi. This intimate union of placenta and muscle wall entirely invalidates the normal mechanism of placental separation and makes it impossible to locate any line of cleavage for such separation. The frequency of this condition has been made the subject of a number of estimates. Polak places it at approximately 1 in 6000 deliveries, B. C. Hirst, 1 in 40,000. Suffice it to say, then, that placenta accreta is a rare but definite pathologic entity (Fig. 189).

Etiology.—Since placenta accreta is dependent upon an absence of the decidua basalis, one must search for a reason for this absence in order to determine the genesis of the condition. Such atrophy may be produced by previous deep and vigorous curettage, an atrophic endometritis, or thinning of the endometrium overlying submucous myomata. Placentation occurring high in the uterine cornua where the mucosa is thinnest has also been advocated as a cause.

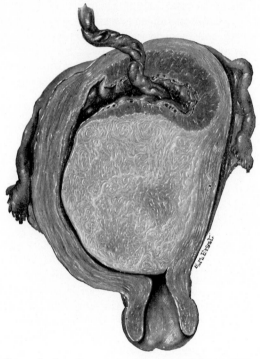

Fig. 189.—Case of placenta accreta. Implanted in uterine cornu, and on atrophic endometrium, over large myoma. (Polak and Phelan in Surg., Gynec., and Obstet., February, 1924.)

In placenta accreta, where there is no basal decidua present and the villi directly penetrate the uterine wall and make with it one continuous structure in which no line of cleavage can be demonstrated, the placenta cannot separate and hence remains as an integral portion of the uterine wall. Furthermore, in the absence of decidua, the chorionic villi erode themselves into the muscle fibers, with a resulting degeneration and thinning of the uterine wall, even to the point of rupture. Indeed, in a case reported by Tennant, the placental villi not only penetrated the serosa of the uterus, but actually invaded the abdominal cavity. On examining a uterus, the seat of placenta accreta, the musculature over the placenta is seen to be relaxed and thin, even perforated in some cases by chorionic villi. There is no line of demarcation between placenta and uterus and attempts at separation result only in the tearing of fragments of placenta out of the uterine wall.

Microscopically, the decidua basalis is entirely absent, the villi directly entering the uterine muscle and generally there may be demonstrated groups of syncytial cells in and between the muscle fibers, while other masses of these cells split the uterine wall into ragged fragments.

Clinically, placenta accreta must be distinguished from: (1) retained separated placenta, and (b) simple adhesions of the placenta. Retention of the separated placenta is characterized by uterine bleeding, descent of the cord and the typical globular contour of the uterine fundus. In simple adhesion and in placenta accreta, there is no uterine bleeding, since the retroplacental blood spaces remain plugged by the placental villi. There is no descent of the cord, and, according to Polak (*q. v.*) the fundus assumes a characteristic shape, being broader from side to side and intermittently relaxed, but assuming the firm contraction and ball-like shape present when the placenta has separated.

Simple adhesion cannot be differentiated from placenta accreta except by attempts at manual removal. If the former condition be present a distinct line of cleavage will readily be found and complete separation may be attained by the exploring fingers, whereas, if the adhesion be due to an accreta no cleavage is discovered and attempts at manual removal result only in piecemeal extraction of ragged portions of the placenta with intractable hemorrhage.

The diagnosis of adherent placenta, whether simple or due to an accreta, may be inferred when the placenta has been retained in the uterus for more than two hours following the delivery of the child, without uterine bleeding, descent of the cord or the rise of the globular fundus uteri (Fig. 190).

Differentiation of simple adhesion from accreta can only be made after manual intra-uterine exploration as described above.

Prognosis.—The mortality of placenta accreta is difficult to estimate because of the imperfection of records and the rarity of the condition. Polak reported 4 cases of his own, 3 dying from hemorrhage or sepsis after attempts at manual removal, while the fourth patient recovered after hysterectomy. The cause of death is either hemorrhage or sepsis or both. If manual removal is attempted and portions of placenta torn off, the bleeding is usually so severe as to necessitate abandonment of the attempts at removal, and uterine packing, which often fails to control the hemorrhage. In addition, owing to the great thinning of the uterine wall, perforation may result, with intra-abdominal bleeding as a sequel.

Sepsis, of course, is always to be dreaded and is usually associated with hemorrhage in effecting the literal termination of these cases.

Treatment.—From the foregoing description a definite management of unexpelled placenta may be formulated. Whenever the placenta remains unexpelled for two hours, in the absence of uterine bleeding and descent of the cord, the delay should be viewed with

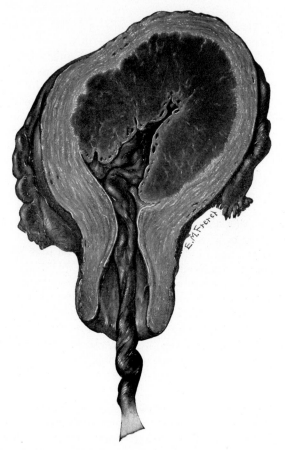

Fig. 190.—Case of adherent placenta. Cornual implantation. (Polak and Phelan in Surg., Gynec., and Obstet., February, 1924.)

suspicion and no attempt at Credé expulsion should be made. Aseptic manual exploration of the uterine cavity under anesthesia should be made in these cases and a line of cleavage sought.

Should such cleavage be demonstrated, simple adhesion is the causative factor and the placenta may readily be peeled from its uterine attachment and extracted, the uterus being then firmly packed with gauze. Should it be impossible to detect a line of cleavage, attempts at manual removal should at once be abandoned and the patient immediately subjected to abdominal supravaginal hysterectomy, since by this procedure only can the excessive mortality from sepsis and hemorrhage be avoided.

Abnormalities of the Placenta.—The normal placenta is a flattened disk, varying from 15 to 20 cm. in diameter and from 2 to 3 cm. in thickness. In the later months of pregnancy the placenta may vary considerably in size and exhibits also many abnormalities in its form. Occasionally the organ is divided into several parts which may be entirely distinct or more or less closely united. This phenomenon may be an atavistic form since the placenta of many of the higher apes is always double though but a single fetus is present. Rarely the placenta may be roughly rectangular in shape with an aperture near the center, this variety being termed placenta fenestrata. Some-

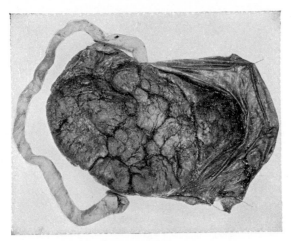

Fig. 191.—Placenta succenturiata. (Author's case, Kensington Hospital for Women, Philadelphia.)

times it is composed of several lobes, placenta bipartita when there are two divisions, and tripartita when there are three. Rarely there are a number of small lobes, their vessels uniting to furnish the adequate blood supply for the fetus, as many as seven small lobes having been described. Sometimes the cord, usually inserted near the center, is attached to the very margin of the placenta, the so-called "battledore placenta." These variations in form have no clinical significance.

Placenta Succenturiata (Fig. 191).—In this anomaly one or more accessory lobules are developed in the membranes at a greater or less distance from the margin of the main placenta. Usually these accessory lobules are connected to the placenta by their blood vessels but occasionally they are entirely separate and if, as is usually the case, the accessory lobule is expelled with the main organ it has no clinical significance, but should it not be so expelled, rather serious complications may occur. First there may be immediate postpartum hemorrhage from rupture of the vessels between the accessory lobule and the main placenta. Second, the accessory lobe may remain in the uterus and give rise to marked delayed hemorrhage. Third, by its retention the accessory lobe may occasion sepsis. The diagnosis of placenta succenturiata may always be made if the extruded placenta be closely examined. If evidences of a torn surface or, particularly, if torn blood vessels are found at the margin of the membrane, this anomaly must be considered and manual exploration of the uterus must be performed in order to remove it.

Placenta circumvallata (Fig. 192) is a condition in which there is a more or less complete circular ring upon the fetal surface of the

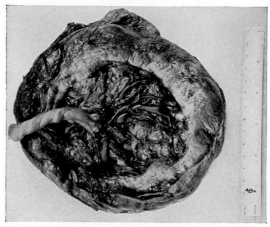

Fig. 192.—Placenta circumvallata. (Author's case, Kensington Hospital for Women, Philadelphia.)

placenta at varying distances from its margin. The ring, about 1 cm. in width, is slightly elevated upon the general surface of the placenta, and usually presents a white or yellowish appearance. It divides the fetal surface of the placenta into two distinct regions, the central portion bounded by the internal margin of the ring, and a peripheral zone outside the ring. The central area is that of a normal placenta containing the attachment of the cord and the large fetal vessels, which latter are always absent from the peripheral portion of the placenta, their terminal branches turning directly downward into the substance of the organ before reaching the edge of the ring.

The mode of origin of placenta circumvallata has given rise to a large literature, there being many theories regarding it. The whole matter has been very well reviewed by Williams, who surveyed the literature and came to the conclusion that the essence of the abnormality lies in the restricted area of the chorionic plate, the folding of the membrane and the presence of a layer of decidue upon the extrachorionic portion of the fetal surface of the placenta. This strik-

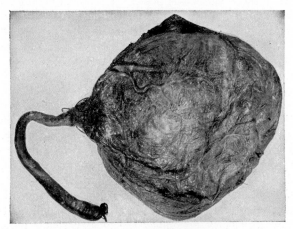

Fig. 193.—Battledore placenta.

ing anatomical anomaly has no clinical significance except in its occasional association with widespread placental infarction (Fig. 193).

DISEASES OF THE UMBILICAL CORD

Variation in Length of the Cord.—The average length of the umbilical cord is given by Naegele as from 34 to 48 cm. while Lariot gives from 50 to 60 cm. as the normal length. Von Winckel says that the cord is approximately as long as the fetus or about 50 cm. in a mature child.

Very marked variations in length may occur, a cord of 198 cm. having been recorded, while rarely it may be so short that the abdomen of the fetus is in contact with the placenta, but under such circumstances a congenital umbilical hernia is always present.

Too long cords have no clinical significance other than their tendency to prolapse or to coil about portions of the infant.

Short umbilical cord may give rise to severe dystocia and constitutes a very definite peril to the infant intrapartum. From the clinical standpoint short cords are divided into the absolutely short, 32 cm. or less in length, and the relatively short, 35 cm. in length. To these must be added the shortened cord, which, originally of normal or even greater length, has been shortened by looping or coiling about parts of the fetal body.

Variations in Insertions of the Cord.—The umbilical cord is usually inserted eccentrically upon the fetal surface of the placenta, nearer the center than the periphery, while a truly central implantation is less common. Occasionally the insertion is at the margin of the placenta, the so-called "battledore placenta" (*q. v.*). Williams gives a series of 2000 placentae examined as to cord insertion, finding 73 per cent eccentric, 20 per cent central and 7 per cent marginal and adds that these variations possess no clinical significance.

Velamentous Insertion.—Occasionally the vessels of the umbilical cord separate at varying distances from the placenta and reach their placental termini by taking their course between the amnion and chorion, or are enveloped in a fold of the former tissue. This condition, termed "insertio velamentosa," has been estimated by various observers as occurring in from 0.4 to 0.9 per cent of all cases. Williams found it in 1.25 per cent of the series described above. The condition is much more frequently observed in multiple than in single cases, Miranoff giving the occurrence as 5 per cent in twins.

The genesis of this anomaly has given rise to much speculation. The theory of Franque is now generally accepted, that is, that the abdominal pedicle ordinarily extends to the fetus from the most vascular portion of the chorion, usually that in contact with the decidua basalis, and hence the cord becomes inserted into the placenta. Sometimes, however, in early pregnancy the most vascular portion of the ovum may be in the decidua capsularis, in which case the abdominal pedicle takes its origin from this tissue. As pregnancy advances, however, the decidua basalis eventually becomes the most vascular area and while the abdominal pedicle retains its original position, the vessels extend from its maternal end to the placental margin.

Velamentous insertion of the cord is of some clinical importance, several cases of fetal death from rupture of such cords being recorded. Kosmak reports a typical case in which free vaginal bleeding occurred at term, with loss of fetal movements and heart tones. On cesarean section (performed in the belief that abruptio placentae was present), there was found a velamentous insertion of the cord with rupture of its vessels and consequent fetal death. The diagnosis of this condition is naturally very difficult but its presence may be suspected when moderate bleeding occurs during the first stage of labor, with no evidence of placenta praevia or abruptio placentae. Absolute diagnosis is possible only when the pulsating cord vessels (vasa praevia) are palpable within the cervix, over the bulging membranes. Should the anomaly be suspected, prompt delivery by the most available method is the only treatment.

Torsion of the Cord.—The cord may become more or less twisted as a result of fetal movements. The condition is found frequently in aborted fetuses but is uncommon in the mature infant.

The twisting is sometimes marked, 380 turns being noted in a case of Schauta's, such extreme torsion being obviously incompatible with fetal life. When a twisted cord is found in the presence of a dead fetus, it is generally impossible to determine whether the torsion caused fetal death or whether the twisting occurred during the active movements of the fetal death agony, or, indeed, whether the twisting occurred after the death of the child.

A certain degree of torsion is physiologic, the veins being twisted about the deeper lying arteries, usually from right to left; and in thin cords, with little of Wharton's jelly present, this torsion may readily become so marked as to interfere with the fetal blood supply and, indeed, to cause death from asphyxia. Cases are recorded wherein the torsion was so marked as to almost divide the cord, a thin pedicle alone uniting the ends.

Diagnosis is impossible except that a suspicion of late torsion may be aroused, should the fetal heart rate change in character rather suddenly during the latter weeks of pregnancy. The only suggested treatment is prompt delivery if any form of cord obstruction is suspected.

Knots of the Cord.—True knots of the umbilical cord are said by some writers to occur quite frequently, but Browne regards them as uncommon. He quotes von Winckel as stating that they are present in 0.4 to 0.5 per cent of all births. These knots have been held to be developmental anomalies, but modern opinion holds that they are due to the movements of the fetus, causing it to pass through a loop, and most frequently occur early in labor. Very long cords and some degree of hydramnion are contributing factors in knot production. When knots occur late in pregnancy or during labor, they are of no clinical importance, rarely becoming tight enough to interfere with the circulation, but should they develop during the early months, they may gradually be drawn so tight as to produce fetal asphyxia and death. Browne collected 26 cases of this accident.

False Knots of the Cord.—Occasionally piling up of the jelly of Wharton into irregular masses along the course of the cord gives rise to little nodules which are called false knots. Since the vessels of the cord are longer than the cord itself, they may become folded upon themselves, also giving rise to nodulations which are designated as false knots. These conditions have no clinical significance.

Solid Tumors of the Cord.—This excessively rare condition has only been reported eight times in the literature and according to Browne no case has been published since 1891.

Of these eight tumors three proved to be telangiectatic myxosarcoma, two were teratomatous in origin, one a myxangioma, and in two histologic investigations were not carried out.

Varices of the Cord.—This rare tumor of the cord has been described five times in the literature, according to the exhaustive article of Adair. These vascular tumors, though rare, are of clinical importance because of the grave danger to the fetus, whose life is dependent upon the integrity of the tumor wall, which may or may not rupture as pregnancy proceeds.

The varices differ in size, the smallest one reported being the size of a hazel nut while the largest was some 12 cm. in diameter, and among the five reported cases three types of varix may be differentiated, three being of the thin-walled type with a relatively large cavity, one a small tumor with thickened walls and one a simple dilatation of the umbilical vein as it entered the umbilicus. Four of the five infants were stillborn.

Edema of the Cord.—Edema is rarely present with a living infant in good condition, but is common in certain fetal diseases, notably general edema, as reported by the writer, and it is also often found with dead and macerated fetuses. Sometimes an undue increase in the amount of the jelly of Wharton present in the cord produces an erroneous impression of edema. The condition seems to be of no clinical significance, except as a part of a general fetal dropsy.

Inflammation of the Cord.—Inflammatory lesions of the cord, exclusive of those of syphilitic origin, are rarely met with as long as the child is alive but are reasonably common after its birth. In most instances, the cord becomes inflamed after premature rupture of the membranes, in the presence of intrapartum fever, and in leukocytic infiltration of the placental chorion and amnion. Siddall made a study of 1000 cords from consecutive deliveries and found inflammatory reactions in 6 per cent. Both ends of the cord were usually affected but the intensity of the changes were greater at the placental end and in the umbilical vein. The lesions were usually leukocytic and small round cells infiltrated the vessel walls and the adjacent connective tissue. Siddall believes that inflammation of the cord occurs most frequently in the absence of syphilis and is, therefore, of little value in the diagnosis of this disease.

The immediate prognosis for the child is not affected by the presence of such inflammation.

DISEASES OF THE DECIDUA

The decidua may be affected by a variety of inflammatory lesions, all of them prototypes of more or less similar changes occurring in the nonpregnant endometrium, most of them being simply continuations of an inflammatory process present before conception occurs. Occasionally such inflammation may originate during pregnancy, especially where criminal abortion has been unsuccessfully attempted.

True endometritis is usually associated with sterility. Although minor disturbances of the endometrium may not interfere with conception, abortion, placenta praevia and other abnormalities are frequent sequelae of conception occurring under these conditions.

Diffuse Thickening of the Decidua.—Under this term Williams describes a generalized hyperplasia of the decidua, in which, as pregnancy advances, this structure becomes much thicker than normal and is exceedingly vascular. Areas of hemorrhage are present, there is always more or less degeneration and microscopically there is considerably round-cell infiltration. Sometimes the hypertrophy occurs in isolated patches, giving rise to irregular polypoid projection of the decidua and hence called by Virchow "tuberous or polypoid endometritis deciduae." Certain writers consider this a common lesion and Williams quotes Nyulasy as reporting 100 cases in his own practice. Williams himself, however, had never seen a case, nor has the writer.

Glandular Hyperplasia of the Decidua (*Endometritis Deciduae Glandulare*).—This condition occurs when the uterine glands are hypertrophied and increased in number, the ducts usually remaining patulous. It results in a more or less profuse yellowish discharge (the endometritis deciduae catarrhalis of Schroeder), the amounts varying up to 500 cc. as reported by Ahlfeld. The continued secretion prevents the union of the vera and the capsularis, which remain separated during the entire pregnancy. The discharge has been termed hydrorrhea gravidarum.

Atrophic Endometritis Deciduae.—Certain writers have described a condition in which large portions of the decidua vera and capsularis undergo atrophic change, similar to that which normally occurs outside the placental site after the third month. Very little is known of this condition or its clinical effects.

Acute Endometritis Deciduae.—The decidua may suffer infection by the gonococcus, or by the pyogenic bacteria which gain access to the uterine cavity in attempts at criminal abortion, sometimes by coitus with a patulous cervix. It may also follow the acute infectious diseases, such as scarlet fever, typhoid, measles, etc. Occasionally a purulent exudate is formed which almost inevitably terminates in abortion.

Hydrorrhea Gravidarum.—Under this term has been mentioned the discharge which follows glandular deciduitis.

Decided differences of opinion exist as to the origin of the fluid. Stoeckel and others believe it to be due to premature rupture of the membranes, which then retract over the child's body and lie in folds upon the surface of the placenta, the baby occupying the uterine cavity not covered by membranes, the so-called "extramembranous pregnancy." Under these circumstances the amnion continues to secrete and there results an intermittent flow of fluid.

Cases have been recorded wherein sufficient quantities of fluid escaped to permit collection and analysis, and the amniotic origin has been demonstrated on microscopical examination by the presence of lanugo hairs.

The clinical aspects of deciduitis are important, inasmuch as an infected or defective decidua leads to imperfect nidation of the embryo with a definite tendency toward abortion, and, since abortion leads to further endometritis, a vicious circle is established. Monster formation, arrest of development, placenta praevia and finally mole formation may all follow this inflammatory process.

Treatment.—There is no treatment for deciduitis during pregnancy, but after delivery or abortion thorough curettage should be performed in order to excise every portion of the infected endometrium.

HYDATIDIFORM MOLE

Hydatidiform mole, also known as cystic degeneration of the chorion, vesicular mole, or myxoma chorii, is a lesion of the chorion in which the terminal extremities of the chorionic villi are converted into transparent cysts of varying size and having clear viscid contents. These cysts are usually very numerous and their size varies from a few millimeters in diameter to 2 or 3 cm.

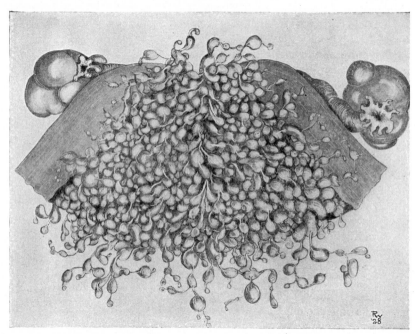

Fig. 194.—Uterus containing an hydatid mole, showing the vesicles. (Dept. Obstet., University of Pennsylvania. Schumann in "Nelson's Loose-Leaf Surgery.")

Each small cyst terminates in a delicate pedicle which represents the proximal portion of the villus, and these pedicles in turn spring from the villous stems, from which the cysts hang in clusters, closely simulating a bunch of small grapes of various sizes. Although the entire chorion may be invaded, usually only a portion of the tissue is involved in this cystic degeneration. In some instances a small cluster of vesicles constitutes the entire growth while in others the mole may attain the size of five or six months' pregnancy, the mass weighing several pounds (Fig. 194).

Etiology.—The true cause of the development of hydatidiform mole is not known. Since moles are entirely a disease of fetal structure, and inasmuch as endometritis is at best a very questionable pathologic entity, the author is not in accord with the theory that the latter is an important etiologic factor in mole formation. The decidua is not involved and it is difficult to associate mole development with any lesion of maternal tissues, except insofar as trophic or nutritive errors may be causative.

The true etiology seems to lie in some specific fault in development of the chorionic villi, rather paralleling the development of general edema of the fetus and similar degenerative and proliferative phenomena whose modes of origin remain entirely unsolved.

Frequency.—A true estimate of the frequency of these cases is impossible, because so many occur outside hospitals and are either un-

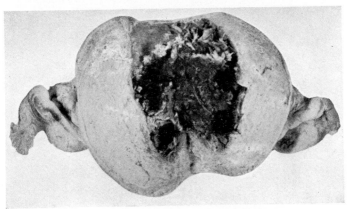

Fig. 195.—Uterus after expulsion of hydatidiform mole. Note areas of deep invasion of uterine muscles. (Schumann, E. A.: Amer. Jour. Obstet. and Gynec., 4: 386, 1922. C. V. Mosby Co., Publishers.)

diagnosed or are not reported. A century ago Madame Boivin believed that moles occurred once in 20,000 pregnancies. Brodhead and Kasselbohm found 6 moles in 12,030 cases of labor and abortion. Gordon, of Bellevue, found moles in one out of every 214 cases of labor or abortion. At the Frauenklinik at Lund the proportion was 3 per 1000, according to Essen-Möller. In short, the statistics vary in such wide degree that no definite conclusions are possible.

Meyer makes the statement that "mole formation is a rare disease at or near term, but it probably is the commonest of all diseases of the ovum during the earlier months of gestation. The typical large hydatidiform mole is an end-result which it has taken long months to develop. No one seems to have followed its evolution, although hydatidiform degeneration whether total or partial is, of course, gradual in its advent" (Fig. 195).

Morphology and Pathology.—The microscopical appearance of hydatidiform mole varies from the development of a few tiny vesicles in an aborted ovum or a partial degeneration of the chorion in the decidua of a full-term pregnancy, to the characteristic masses which are clinically asociated with the lesion. A well-developed mole consists of a number of transparent cysts, varying in size from a few millimeters to 2 or 3 cm. in diameter (Fig. 196). Its weight may be from 300 to 600 Gm. Each cyst is attached to a delicate pedicle which represents the stalk of the villus, and the pedicles are attached to each other and not uncommonly to a dense area of decidua

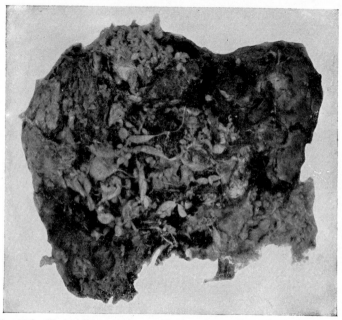

Fig. 196.—Hydatidiform mole expelled spontaneously from uterus shown in Fig. 195. (Schumann, E. A.: Amer. Jour. Obstet. and Gynec., 4: 386, 1922. C. V. Mosby Co., Publishers.)

which occupies the center of the mass. Scattered between the vesicles in an expelled mole are masses of cellular débris, fibrin, and blood clot (Fig. 197).

Histology.—Each individual cyst is a swollen and edematous chorionic villus. The ectoderm covering the villus is represented by more or less proliferated Langhans' cells, exuberant and irregular buds of syncytium, and a delicate stem. The stroma may contain calcareous or hyaline areas. The stroma of some cysts has a tendency to become necrotic and takes the stains poorly.

Moles may show marked variation as to the relative proliferation of Langhans' cells and syncytium, and different vesicles in the

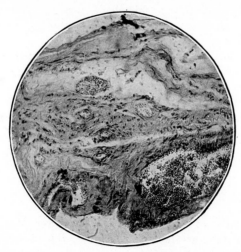

Fig. 197.—Section from wall of uterus shown in Fig. 195, showing implantation of nests of syncytial cells deep in the muscle, together with several small intramural hemorrhages. (Schumann, E. A.: Amer. Jour. Obstet. and Gynec., 4: 386, 1922. C. V. Mosby Co., Publishers.)

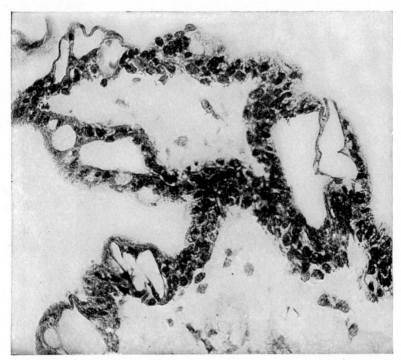

Fig. 198.—Hydatidiform mole, showing a distended villus with syncytium. (Lab. Gynec. Path., University of Pennsylvania. Schumann in "Nelson's Looseleaf Surgery.")

24

same specimen may present histologic textures varying widely one from another. One may find perfectly healthy and normal villi scattered throughout a mole (Fig. 198).

All moles must be regarded as rapidly growing tumors, of embryonic origin and of potential malignancy. There is no cellular arrangement in moles which might give information as to their probable benign or malignant nature, and Hirschmann stated definitely that there are no morphological criteria of value in establishing a prognosis.

Diagnosis.—Bleeding during the early months of pregnancy usually impels the patient to seek medical advice. Even then the characteristics of the disease are so vague that an immediate diagnosis is difficult. The most definite evidences of the presence of a mole are as follows:

1. Enlargement of the uterus to a size greater than that of a normal pregnancy of corresponding duration, the uterus having a soft and elastic feel.

2. Intermittent hemorrhage without known cause, which may vary from a slight spotting to profuse hemorrhage.

3. The extrusion of one or more typical vesicles from the uterus which, of course, is positive evidence.

4. The palpation of the mole through the cervix uteri. Negatively there is absence of a fetal body and fetal heart sounds, and the patient feels rather ill. Multiparae are more often affected than primiparae, although Moltor reports a case occurring in a girl nine years of age. Ordinarily, however, moles develop in women during the middle of the child-bearing period.

Systemic disease, as syphilis and cardiac lesions, have no significance, but there seems to be some association with nephritis. The relation of lutein cysts of the ovaries will be discussed later, and such cysts, when present, may be utilized as corroborative factors in the diagnosis of mole.

The diagnosis of hydatidiform mole and chorionepithelioma has been greatly facilitated by the development of the various hormone tests, notably that of Aschheim and Zondek.

There is an extraordinarily high concentration of the anterior hypophysial hormone present in the urine and blood of women with hydatidiform moles, and a minute quantity of the urine will give a positive hormone test. Often one tenth or even one twelfth of the usual amount of urine injected into the test animal will provoke a positive reaction.

Furthermore, the excess of hormone in the urine disappears in two weeks, after the termination of intrauterine pregnancy, whereas it persists much longer after the expulsion of a mole.

Prognosis.—The embryo is almost universally destroyed early during mole formation, and in many instances is undiscoverable in the extruded moles. Occasionally when only a portion of the chorion is involved, a dead, well-formed fetus is discovered in the mole (Fig. 199).

The mortality from hydatid mole alone depends upon the ravages of hemorrhage occurring before, during or after the expulsion of the mass, upon sepsis developing in the uterus after a mole, and upon peritonitis resulting either from spontaneous rupture of the uterus or perforation by the invasion of syncytial masses.

If cases of secondary chorionepithelioma are disregarded, a primary mortality rate of between 10 and 15 per cent is fairly accurate.

Clinical Course.—The view held previously that moles occur near the end of the reproductive cycle, or near the menopause, is erroneous. An analysis of reported cases shows that moles occur most com-

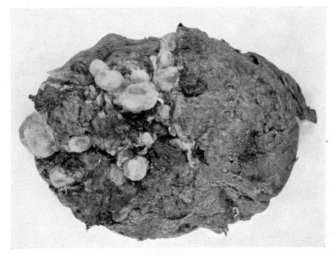

Fig. 199.—Hydatidiform mole surrounding a sac which contained a fetus. (Courtesy of Dr. Paul A. Gempel.)

monly in the middle of the child-bearing period, the average age being about thirty years. All statistics agree that multiparous women are more susceptible than primiparous women, the proportion being about 3 to 1. American reports disclose a marked preponderance of white over negro patients.

Size of Moles.—Those which come to the attention of the gynecologist will average probably about 500 Gm. in weight, although they may vary in size within wide limits, from the minute degeneration in very young villi to numerous clusters of vesicles weighing 1200 Gm. or more.

Relation of Lutein Cysts of the Ovary.—A majority of patients having hydatidiform mole present bilateral cysts of the ovary sometime attaining the size of a fetal head. At least a portion of the walls of these cysts are formed of flattened lutein cells, and the contained fluid is prone to be turbid or blood stained (Fig. 200).

Lutein cysts develop as a result of the excessive amount of anterior pituitary sex hormone present in moles, and they tend to regress promptly upon the removal of the mole.

No other treatment is necessary in most instances, though occasionally the cysts may remain and even continue to grow, under which condition it may be necessary to excise them.

Symptomatology.—The presence of hydatidiform mole presents no definite syndrome. There are the early signs of pregnancy, such as amenorrhea, uterine enlargement and breast changes, and there is an increased tendency toward toxemia among these patients. Sud-

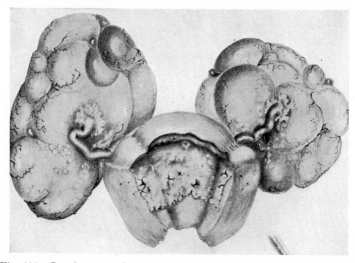

Fig. 200.—Lutein cysts of ovary associated with hydatidiform mole. (Dept. Obstet., University of Pennsylvania. Schumann in "Nelson's Loose-leaf Surgery.")

denly the uterus may begin to enlarge rapidly, and there may be associated acute abdominal pain and repeated sharp hemorrhages, coming on without warning. If pregnancy has advanced to the fifth month or beyond, the patient may notice the absence of fetal movements, and this may direct her mind to the possibility of some abnormality in the pregnancy.

Treatment.—The mass must be immediately and completely removed as soon as the diagnosis is made. The inherent danger of hemorrhage and sepsis as a result of the invasion of the uterine musculature, and the high ratio of chorionepithelioma after mole pregnancy, combine to make this form of management urgent and absolutely necessary.

The profuse hemorrhage suffered in most of these cases renders the patients poor surgical risks. The possibility of sepsis developing in the uterine cavity, in which there are many areas of more or less necrotic decidua, further adds to the risk.

The ordinarily accepted plan of treatment is to evacuate the uterus from below, the patient being lightly anesthetized. Under the most painstaking and rigid asepsis the cervix is dilated sufficiently to admit two fingers, which are used to gently peel the growth from its uterine attachment; extreme gentleness in operating is imperative, since the uterine wall is so thin in many of these cases that perforation with the curet or even the finger is a constant danger.

The use of the curet and the placental forceps is to be avoided whenever possible, first because of the danger of perforation by this means and second because of the danger of distant metastases, as to the lungs, being produced by instrumental removal.

After evacuating the uterus of its mole, a careful exploration is made to detect the possible presence of a beginning chorionepithelioma. If such a malignancy is encountered immediate abdominal hysterectomy is to be performed. The evidence of a beginning chorionepithelioma is based on the discovery of a soft, friable hemorrhagic area into which the finger sinks, and from which small necrotic masses may be shelled out.

In cases where previous hemorrhage has greatly reduced the resistance of the patient, preliminary blood transfusion is a measure of the greatest value and should be regularly practiced. During the operation the blood loss may be alarming and packing of the uterus with gauze is advocated to prevent further bleeding. Whenever possible, the interior of the uterus should be carefully explored with the finger after the removal of a mole to insure against the retention of a portion of the material.

In women who are exsanguinated, and consequently poor risks for the hemorrhagic operation of vaginal removal of the mole, abdominal hysterotomy under local anesthesia is a valuable procedure. Morphine sulphate, $\frac{1}{4}$ grain, scopolamine $\frac{1}{100}$ grain, hypodermically, one hour before operation, and then local infiltration with 0.5 per cent novocain solution, or if local anesthesia is not well borne, a light inhalation anesthesia. The uterus may be opened on its anterior aspect with but little blood loss, the mole removed under the eye, and the uterine wall carefully inspected for areas of marked thinning, intramural hemorrhage, or widespread and deep invasion of the uterine muscle by the proliferative process. If the uterine muscle is in relatively good condition, the cavity may be swabbed with iodine and firmly packed with gauze, the end of the pack being thrust through the cervical opening and the wound in the uterus carefully closed by layer suture, after which the abdominal incision is closed.

Supravaginal hysterectomy is the procedure of choice when the uterus has undergone massive invasion with syncytial elements, or where many hemorrhagic areas are present.

This method of treatment is especially indicated in women near the climacteric, and in cases where the bleeding is profuse and the cervix rigid.

The dangers of recurrence should be brought to the attention of the patient and she should be under careful observation for two years. If irregular bleeding should occur during this time, a diagnostic curettage should be performed. Immediate hysterectomy is performed if the scrapings reveal any histologic findings suggestive of chorionepithelioma. Observation of the patient is necessary regardless of hemorrhage, since vaginal or vulvar metastases may occur without any uterine involvement whatever. If these metastatic nodules occur they should be excised but experience has shown that the uterus is rarely affected in these cases and consequently hysterectomy need not be done.

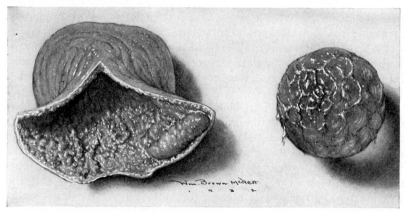

Fig. 201.—Early Breus's mole. The specimen shows expulsion of the entire mole, the unruptured ovum containing no remnant of fetus. (Author's case.)

Radium alone or with deep x-ray therapy is indicated in all cases of hydatid mole arousing any suspicion of malignancy. The embryonal cells which make up the bulk of both moles and chorionepitheliomata are of the type which succumb readily to radiotherapy and this adjuvant to treatment must never be neglected.

Breus's Mole; Mole Tuberosa.—In 1892 Carl Breus described a series of 5 cases of retained ova, expelled at a late stage of pregnancy, and with certain definite characteristics which distinguished them from ordinary retained ova. Breus called them "moles tuberosae," but they are commonly described under the name of their first observer.

The characteristics of these moles are the small size of the ovum as compared to the duration of pregnancy, the small size of the fetus (9.5–17 mm.) in proportion to the large size of the egg, and the peculiar protuberances which mark the limits of the placenta and which are hemispherical or pedunculated, often distended with blood and covered with fetal membranes (Fig. 201).

Clinically, Breus's moles occur in cases of missed abortion, in which an early pregnancy terminates with a greater or less amount of pain and hemorrhage. Presently these symptoms subside and recovery is good, although no products of conception have been expelled. Such moles are ovoid or bean-shaped masses, measuring usually about 8 by 4 cm. or thereabouts, and shown on section to consist of a small dead fetus, surrounded by an organized blood clot, and in one portion of the mass a series of rounded purplish-blue or dark-red prominences ranging in size from a pea to a large cherry. These prominences may or may not be pedunculated and appear to be dilated intervillous cavities, the ovum and chorion being usually clearly distinguishable. The cause of this formation is as yet unknown.

CHORIONEPITHELIOMA

Chorionepithelioma may be defined as a highly malignant tumor which develops after the formation of fetal cells, and may, therefore, follow full-term labor, abortion or hydatidiform mole, and in some cases may develop coincidentally with mole pregnancy.

Frequency.—It is difficult to estimate the frequency of chorionepithelioma. There are several hundred cases in the literature and many are unrecorded. In Philadelphia, admission to hospitals revealed 18 cases of known chorionepithelioma among about 140,000 deliveries.

Etiology.—The etiology of chorionepithelioma remains obscure, although in most instances cells of fetal origin must be present before the growth can develop. There are isolated cases, as mentioned by Vineberg, where fetal tissues are not demonstrable, as in very young females, or, indeed, in males.

In almost all cases, pregnancy in some form has antedated chorionepithelioma. The disease is essentially one of fertile women, and the frequency of its occurrence naturally bears a direct ratio to the degree of fertility.

As to the character of the pregnancy next previous to the chorionepithelioma, more than one half the cases of chorionepithelioma follow mole pregnancy, and one third abortion, with the remainder scattered.

Pathology.—On a basis of their clinical and anatomical distinctions, Ewing has divided chorioma into three divisions:

1. Chorio-adenoma destruens. Destructive placental mole.
2. Choriocarcinoma.
3. Syncytioma and syncytial endometritis.

1. *Chorio-adenoma Destruens.*—This tumor, more commonly referred to as "malignant mole," has the following characteristic gross appearance: the uterus is usually considerably enlarged, with thick walls, and the mole presents either in a cavity in the musculature or in small areas scattered throughout. Perforation has occurred in 7 cases, with 6 deaths.

When the mole remains *in situ* the bulky tumor mass is found adherent over the implantation site. Evidences of hemorrhage or suppuration are frequently present. After expulsion of the mole, coarse shreds of necrotic tissue or large lobulated masses resembling blood clot adhere to a portion of the wall and are continuous with the distended sinuses.

Sometimes the diagnosis of malignant mole can be made from inspection of the expelled material. The occurrence of great variation in the size of the vesicles, with many small, opaque nodules in material which comes away in fragments with difficulty and in rather reduced amounts, is a suggestive sign. (Abstract from Ewing.)

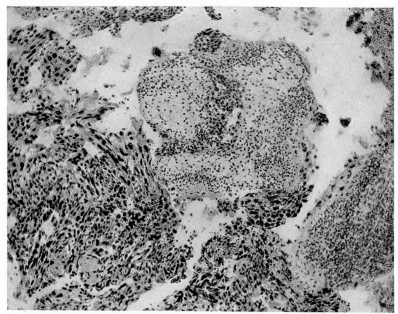

Fig. 202.—Typical chorionepithelioma, showing masses of syncytia and Langhans' cells. (Lab. Gynec. Path., University of Pennsylvania. Schumann in "Nelson's Loose-leaf Surgery.")

Histology.—Malignant moles are essentially overgrowths of Langhans' cells, the syncytia, and the connective tissue, which latter is but slightly vascular and while often edematous, is not generally subject to mucinous change. The Langhans' cells are greatly multiplied and occur in masses or plates about the bases of the villi. The syncytium appears as definite, well-defined buds of strongly acidophile cytoplasm with abundant compact hyperchromatic nuclei.

Metastases.—Metastases are, uncommon and when they do occur the two sites are the pelvic tissue and the lungs. In the vagina they form small bluish nodules, firm in consistency and densely adherent to the surrounding structure.

2. *Chorionepithelioma, Choriocarcinoma.*—This is the most malig-

nant of all tumors. Histologically, the cellular structure is markedly disorderly. The original description by Marchand cannot be improved upon. He divided chorionepithelioma into a typical and an atypical form.

Typical Form.—The typical form is that of a reproduction of the normal trophoblast in early pregnancy, with syncytial masses, interwoven with plates or layers of Langhans' cells, together with areas of necrosis and hemorrhage. Erosion of maternal blood vessels takes place, masses of cells may be demonstrated in the tumors of veins, and as Frank points out, nowhere is there any indication of a newly formed connective tissue or vessel such as is seen in other neoplasms.

Atypical Form.—The atypical form is characterized by a less regular arrangement by the absence of syncytium, by the comparative

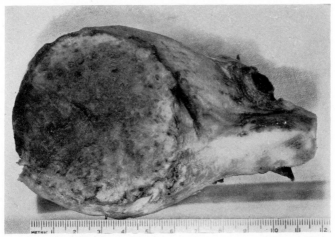

Fig. 203.—Chorionepithelioma, showing a large solid tumor in the fundus uteri. (Courtesy of Dr. Paul A. Gempel.)

scarcity of Langhans' cells, and by the presence of and invasion of the muscularis of the uterus by large mononuclear and polynuclear cells called "wandering syncytial cells." The uterus in these cases is considerably enlarged, and its walls are laden with cell masses, areas of necrosis, and necrotic débris (syncytioma of Ewing) (Fig. 202).

Metastases are almost universal and of very rapid occurrence, as the cell masses are directly transplanted by the blood stream. These metastases are most frequent in the lung, and then in the vagina, liver, and vulva, in order. Poten and Vassmer (quoted by Lynch) excised two vaginal tumors five days before the primary growth was detected in the uterus (Fig. 203).

3. *Syncytioma.*—Some authors have described purely syncytial tumors, but Marchand believes it likely that at least in some portion of these growths, Langhans' cells can be discovered.

Metastases.—Rapid and widespread metastasis is one of the most prominent characteristics of chorionepithelioma. Occasionally metastatic nodules appear in the vagina before the diagnosis of an intrauterine growth has been completed (Fig. 204).

Ovarian Change in Chorioma.—The coexistence of lutein cysts of the ovary, varying from small multiple cystomata to large tumors, is a regularly observed phenomenon, paralleling exactly the development of these cysts in association with hydatidiform mole, which has been discussed in detail.

Diagnosis.—The diagnosis of chorionepithelioma is frequently very difficult, the physical findings being vague and indeterminate until the growth has progressed to such stage as to be beyond any hope of removal. Certain factors, however, tend to suggest the presence of

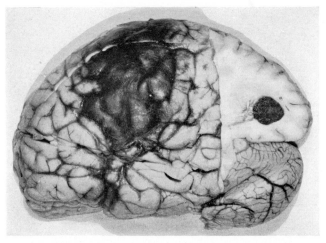

Fig. 204.—Cerebral metastasis in the case illustrated above. (Courtesy of Dr. Paul A. Gempel.)

this destructive neoplasm. Hemorrhage, slight or severe, at any time following the expulsion of an hydatidiform mole, is always most suspicious and should lead to active surgical interference. Persistent hemorrhage following abortion is not suspicious per se, unless fairly definite histologic findings obtained from a diagnostic curettage are present. Bluish or purplish nodules on the vagina or at the vulvar orifice, which tend to ulcerate and bleed easily, are almost certain to be chorionepitheliomata, either primary or metastatic in origin. Sometimes attention is first attracted by pulmonary metastases, with hemoptysis, chest pains, and rapid cachexia. In general, however, it may be said that the diagnosis depends almost entirely upon the occurrence of persistent uterine bleeding in women who have been pregnant in some manner.

Inasmuch as chorionepithelioma so commonly follows hydatidiform mole, the thorough and complete evacuation of the uterus of any hydatid mole tissue must be carried out. Vaginal hysterotomy as proposed and carried out by Vineberg, or abdominal hysterotomy as advocated by the writer, will in a large measure obviate the development of chorionepithelioma, since all hydatid tissue can be detected by sight. Also, this plan of operation will disclose the existence of a chorionepithelioma should its formation occur synchronously with the mole.

The detection of an elevated, fairly hard nodule in the uterine wall, with an excavation in its center, is almost pathognomonic. Should such tumor be suspected shortly after a full-term pregnancy and labor, the uterine cavity may usually be explored through the persistently patulous cervix. When the cavity will not admit the

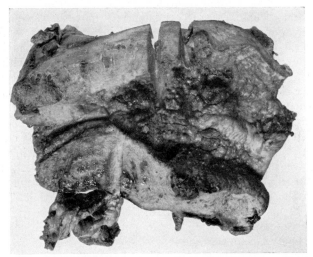

Fig. 205.—Chorionepithelioma. A tumor which persistently presented negative Aschheim-Zondek reaction.

finger, it must be dilated or incised until thorough palpation becomes possible. In cases where chorionepithelioma follows abortion, the diagnosis is most difficult, since bleeding, irregular in duration and amount, is so characteristic of both lesions. Diagnostic curettage must be resorted to under such circumstances, and even this procedure, though the material obtained be studied by a competent pathologist, may prove most misleading.

The persistence of a positive hormone test from the urine of women who have suffered from hydatidiform moles or abortion is a valuable aid to diagnosis, and may be said to be almost pathognomonic. The reverse is not true absolutely, however, since in a case under my observation, the hormone test was negative during the development of a chorionepithelioma until within a few weeks of death from metastases, when it became positive (Fig. 205).

Histologic Diagnosis.—The histologic appearance of chorionepithelioma is clear and definite, where a portion of the uterine musculature is available. Where, however, the material for diagnosis consists solely of curettings, great difficulty frequently arises in reaching a conclusion. Trophoblastic tissue without villi, discovered in the uterus shortly after pregnancy, is the usual criterion for a diagnosis of chorioma. When villi are present, the diagnosis is immediately in doubt since there is no definite knowledge as to the amount and character of epithelial overgrowth which will justify a diagnosis of malignancy.

Differential Diagnosis.—The most important differentiation to be made is the separation of chorionepithelioma from infected incomplete abortion. The symptoms, clinical course, and history are identical with those of chorionic tumor. In infected abortions, the necrotic decidua and secundines are permanently removed by the curettage, although this operation may increase the incidence of systemic infection. In chorioma, the tumor masses rapidly reform, and in a few weeks after curettage the uterine cavity is again filled with friable, bleeding and necrotic tissues. Degenerating fibroids, sarcoma, and sometimes fundal carcinoma may simulate chorionepithelioma, but the absence of recent pregnancy and the histologic picture will usually clarify the diagnosis.

Persistence of the anterior pituitary hormone tests, as outlined in the discussion of hydatidiform mole, is most important in the prognosis of chorionepithelioma. Should the anterior pituitary hormone remain absent from the patient's urine following operation or radiation for chorionepithelioma, it may be assumed that the active chorionic elements have disappeared. The hormone test (*q. v.*) is also of great value in determining the presence of chorionepithelioma after abortion or hydatidiform mole.

Prognosis.—Death within one year of the onset of this most malignant tumor known to pathologists is the rule. The metastases are usually widely disseminated. On the other hand, there are several reported recoveries after simple curettage.

There are several recorded cases, notably among them that of Hirschmann and Christofoletti, in which an attempted hysterectomy was abandoned because of the extent of the tumor, which involved the vagina and bladder and which had infiltrated through the pelvis. This latter patient improved rapidly, although the operation was incomplete. One month later there was no sign of the uterine tumor and seven years later the woman was in perfect health.

Neither the pulmonary nor vaginal metastases imply a high mortality although patients who develop cough and hemoptysis rapidly succumb.

There seems to be a great divergence in the malignancy potential in chorionepitheliomata. If we accept Ewing's classification, it follows that while his group of chorio-adenoma or syncytioma are of low malignancy value, those coming under the classification of chorio-carcinoma are almost invariably fatal. In order to arrive at a true estimate, all excised tissue material must be systematically studied by an experienced pathologist who is competent to differentiate the several varieties of the tissues.

At any rate, the mortality is distressingly high and chorionepithe-lioma must continue to be regarded as one of the most malignant and fatal of known tumors.

Treatment.—Prophylaxis consists in the complete evacuation of every hydatidiform mole, not by curettage and packing, but by hysterotomy, preferably by the abdominal route, with removal of the mole under the eye, and immediate hysterectomy if evidences of chorioma present themselves.

The curative treatment consists in prompt and widespread pan-hysterectomy, with the removal of all pelvic veins and glands which are susceptible of excision, as soon as the diagnosis has been made. If a curettage be necessary to determine the diagnosis, a rapid study of the curettings should be instituted so that hysterectomy may be performed with as little loss of time as possible.

Radium has been suggested and utilized in some of the recent cases, but there are, as yet, insufficient data upon which to base a conclusion. Inasmuch as the tumor is of fetal origin, and hence presumably ex-tremely susceptible to radiation, it would seem that this method of attack offers great possibility of success.

Vaginal metastases should always be excised, but no method of treatment of visceral metastases has as yet been offered. Deep x-ray therapy may give some relief.

CHAPTER XXII

PLACENTA PRAEVIA

PLACENTA praevia exists when all or a portion of the placenta is embedded in the lower uterine segment in the zone of dilatation below the fetus, either partially or completely covering the internal os of the cervix. The condition must be separated from low implantation of the placenta which exists when its lower border is less than 10 cm. above the internal os, while the bulk of the organ is above the isthmus uteri.

Historical.—Placenta praevia was first recognized by Paul Portal in 1679, who graphically described the sensation to the examining hand of a placenta completely covering the internal os. In 1775 Rigby differentiated between placenta praevia and premature separation of the normally implanted placenta, giving to the former condition the name "unavoidable hemorrhage." Since this time the lesion has been well known as a clinical entity.

Etiology.—*Predisposing Causes.*—Placenta praevia occurs much more frequently in multiparae than in primiparae, and in most cases careful anamnesis will disclose a history of abortion, of infection following labor, subinvolution possibly of gonorrhea, irregular menstruation or leukorrhea. In other words there has existed some abnormality of the endometrium.

The increased frequency in multiparae (10:1) may be partially due to the fact that among pregnant women, multiparae outnumber primiparae by more than 3 to 1.

The direct causes of placenta praevia are:

    a. Gravity.

    b. Reflexal placenta.

    c. Overgrowth of the placenta.

    a. *Gravity.*—In normal cases the placenta is most commonly found attached to the posterior uterine wall, next frequently to the anterior wall, then the lateral walls and only rarely is true fundal implantation found. It would seem, then, that the fertilized ovum drops from the uterine orifice of the fallopian tube and falls into a convenient niche of the decidua where it remains until embedding begins. If now, owing possibly to some decidual anomaly following an old endometritis, there is no well marked folding on the upper aspect of the uterus, the ovum may drop low in the cavity, even possibly to the internal os, before it finds a lodgment for its nidation.

It is also possible, that in exceptional cases vigorous peristalsis of the muscle at the uterine ostia of the tube may propel the ovum into the uterine cavity with considerable force, so that it is literally tumbled down to the lower uterine segment.

In such case, the way in which the placenta grows over the cervical opening must be explained. The internal os is a tiny opening and it is quite conceivable that the growing ovum, splitting the decidua, may push the reflexa across the small opening and that this reflexa may become adherent to the decidua vera or the opposite uterine wall, then completely covering the cervical opening.

b. *Reflexal Placenta.*—This mode of development of placenta praevia originated in the classical contribution of Hofmeier and Kaltenbach in 1884.

They held that in a low implantation of the placenta it is possible that the villi frondosa of the chorion, which are in contact with the decidua reflexa, do not atrophy as is generally the case, but for some reason, possibly increased vascularization or extra thickness of the reflexa, they continue to grow. Placental cotyledons are then formed all around the ovum instead of being restricted to the decidua basalis.

As the ovum grows, this placenta-bearing reflexa is gradually forced into contact with the vera on the opposite side of the uterus to which it adheres, forming in effect an extension of the decidua basalis. The villi on the upper aspect of the reflexa now atrophy, leaving a large, broad placenta covering the lower uterine segment, and occluding the internal os.

c. It has been held (Strassman) that since low implantation of the placenta is due to defective decidual formation, it follows that the blood supply of such placenta is poor, and that, seeking vascular space for embedding, the villi of the placenta spread out, the end-result being a thin placenta, larger in diameter than the normal. This view is borne out by the fact that many placentae praeviae are thin, broad structures having very extensive maternal surface. It is held that this increase of area tends to cause a portion, at least, of the placenta to occupy the lower uterine segment and even to encroach upon the region of the internal os.

Frequency.—Statistics as to the frequency of placenta praevia vary widely. In the writer's experience, it occurs about once in 700 pregnancies.

Varieties.—The varieties of placenta praevia simply refer to the extent to which the internal os is involved.

Thus these have been described:

1. Marginal placenta praevia.
2. Partial or lateral placenta praevia.
3. Complete or central placenta praevia.
4. Low implantation of the placenta.

The term *marginal placenta praevia* means that the placenta is implanted on the lower uterine segment, its lower edge just approximating the edge of the internal os (Fig. 206).

Partial placenta praevia is present when the placenta covers a portion of the os, but there is a space remaining which is free from placental attachment (Fig. 207).

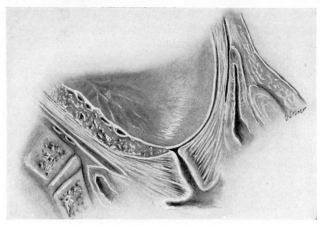

Fig. 206.—Placenta praevia marginalis.

Complete or central placenta praevia implies the complete occlusion of the os by placental tissue. It is not required that the center of the placenta lie over the os, a very rare occurrence (Fig. 208).

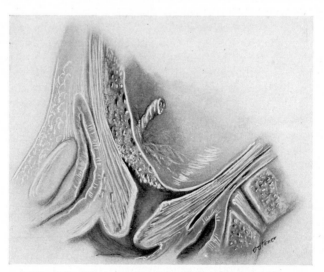

Fig. 207.—Placenta praevia partialis with separation.

Low implantation of the placenta simply means that the organ is situated on the wall of the isthmus uteri or on the lower segment, but not in contact with the os (Fig. 209).

It must be remembered that all of these placental locations are relative as to the stage in labor when they are described. Dilatation

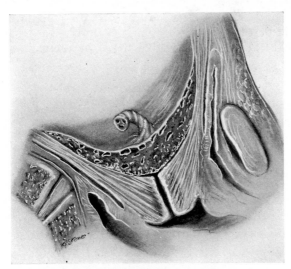

Fig. 208.—Placenta praevia centralis.

and effacement of the cervix, and disappearance of its canal may convert a marginal placenta praevia into a partial and so on.

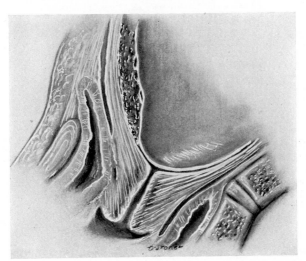

Fig. 209.—Insertion of the placenta in the lower uterine segment.

Pathology.—The reason for the importance of placenta praevia as an obstetric complication is, that with beginning dilatation of the cervix and uterine contraction the placenta is detached from its site, in

25

greater or less degree, either pushed off by the descending head, or the cervix being pulled away from the placenta by the contraction of the upper segment, and, inasmuch as the child is still undelivered and the uterus cannot contract sufficiently to obliterate its blood space, free hemorrhage occurs, becomes more profuse as more and more placenta is detached, and persisting until the uterus is empty and

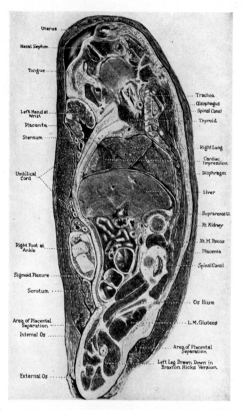

Fig. 210.—Placenta praevia after version of Braxton Hicks. Right half of uterus. Placental attachment extends high on wall of uterus, while left leg drawn down through cervix effectively tampons against further hemorrhage. Area of placental separation is comparatively slight for such profuse hemorrhage. (Titus and Andrews, Amer. Jour. of Obstet. and Gynec., vol. 7, 1924. C. V. Mosby Co., Publishers.)

strong contraction may occlude the blood vessels. Even then the danger of hemorrhage is not over because the lower uterine segment never contracts strongly and bleeding may continue, even though labor is over, and the upper uterine segment remains firmly contracted (Fig. 210).

Symptoms and Diagnosis.—There is but one cardinal symptom of placenta praevia: painless bleeding during the second half of preg-

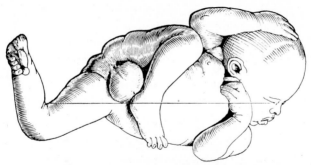

Fig. 211.—Sketch showing posture of fetus in utero after version. Line indicates direction of section through fetus, view being at right angles to that in Fig. 210. (Titus and Andrews, Amer. Jour. of Obstet. and Gynec., vol. 7, 1924. C. V. Mosby Co., Publishers.)

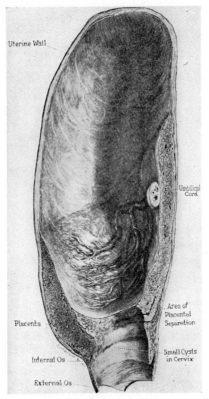

Fig. 212.—Placenta praevia after version of Braxton Hicks. Left half of uterus. Portion of sectioned fetus lifted out to show cavity of uterus with placenta attached over entire lower segment. Area of compression of placenta is seen over internal os, where thigh of fetus had been delivered to check hemorrhage from placental separation. (Titus and Andrews, Amer. Jour. of Obstet. and Gynec., vol. 7, 1924. C. V. Mosby Co., Publishers.)

nancy. It is perfectly true that placenta praevia may exist in the early months, but when this is so, the bleeding is usually followed by abortion, and the praevia is not recognized as the exciting cause. It is probably true also, that these cases of complete abortion, wherein bleeding continues after the uterus is known to be empty, are probably examples of early placenta praevia (Figs. 211 and 212).

However, for clinical purposes, painless hemorrhage during the latter half of pregnancy suffices to describe the cardinal symptom of the condition.

The hemorrhage may occur absolutely without known existing cause. In a desperate case under the care of the writer, a woman lay quietly asleep in her bed and did not awaken until air hunger and extreme rapidity of her pulse with "pounding heart" disturbed her and led to the discovery of an exsanguinating hemorrhage.

The bleeding may occur during ordinary physical activity or it may follow excessive exertion, a fall, or a blow upon the abdomen. Coitus is not infrequently a causative agent.

Happily the first hemorrhage in placenta praevia is usually slight, sometimes a mere spotting, more commonly a frank but negligible blood loss. The initial hemorrhage is followed by others, occurring at irregular intervals but steadily becoming more severe, until there is bleeding on any bodily activity whatsoever or even though the patient be quiescent there may be sudden, painless, massive hemorrhage.

Sometimes the first hemorrhage may become fatal before medical aid may be enlisted and the amount of blood loss in some of these patients is amazing.

On account of the importance of this single symptom of painless hemorrhage, every pregnant woman should be adjured by her physician to report *immediately* any bleeding seen during pregnancy, no matter how slight. It is important to remember that continuous slight bleeding for a long time may not seem dangerous, but the blood loss may be very great and the patient may be so lowered in resistance that she cannot withstand the added trauma and hemorrhage of labor.

Physical Signs Other than Hemorrhage.—The placental bruit, in placenta praevia, may sometimes be heard over the symphysis pubis, while absent over the fundus uteri. On vaginal examination there may be increased pulsation of vessels in the vaginal fornices and more particularly the placenta may be palpated as a soft, doughy mass occupying the lower uterine segment and being interposed between the uterine wall and the presenting part.

Diagnosis.—Painless uterine hemorrhage in the later months of pregnancy, will almost alone establish the diagnosis of some variety of placenta praevia, and if to this there be added the sensation of an indefinite soft mass between the examining finger and the fetus, the diagnosis is practically certain.

An important addition to the diagnostic armamentarium has been proposed recently by Ude and Urner. This consists in a roentgenological examination, to disclose the low lying placenta, displacing the head from its position in the lower uterine segment.

The technic consists in instilling about 40 cc. of sodium iodide solution (12.5 per cent) into the previously emptied bladder and, after withdrawal of the catheter, making an anteroposterior x-ray film.

If the placenta is normally situated the outline of the fetal head will be found close to the bladder margin as outlined by the opaque medium, and lying some 6 to 8 mm. above it. If placenta praevia be present, the concave mass of the placenta will be found to form a distinct gap between the head and the bladder margin.

This procedure is still under observation but seems to offer great hope of making an accurate diagnosis in suspected cases, without contamination of the birth canal, or any danger of exciting hemorrhage by vaginal manipulation.

Differential Diagnosis.—Placenta praevia must be differentiated from premature separation of the normally implanted placenta, hemorrhagic lesions of the cervix as polyp, erosion, carcinoma; ectopic pregnancy, rupture of the uterus.

DeLee speaks of the confusing sensation imparted to the vaginal finger by the presence of a monster with anencephalus and exposed brain, thickened membranes, etc., but these conditions are not associated with painless bleeding which after all is a sine qua non for a positive diagnosis.

In examining a woman with placenta praevia, it is well to attempt to ascertain whether the praevia be central, partial or marginal, by gently sweeping the finger about the cervical opening. This procedure is dangerous because some detachment of the placenta may be inaugurated by the questing finger and severe hemorrhage follow at once.

Intensive examination should be done only in a hospital where facilities are at hand for any necessary operative procedure which may be necessary immediately.

Effect of Placenta Praevia on Pregnancy and Labor.—Abortion is said to be rare, but it would seem that a number of abortions are probably due to low implantation of the placenta with imperfect attachment of the ovum.

Premature labor is common, following early rupture of the membranes due to adhesions about the lower uterine segment.

Since the placenta blocks the lower uterine segment, malpresentations are frequent, the presenting part being shunted away from the cervix by the mass of the placenta. Inertia uteri is a fairly common complication. Postpartum hemorrhage is very often seen, because the lower uterine segment is composed of tissue poor in contractile power and hence the sinuses remain open after delivery.

Late postpartum hemorrhage also occurs because the placenta is so often imperfect in structure that portions remain adherent to the uterine wall, to be detached later with bleeding.

Puerperal infection is to be feared for two reasons: the resistance of the patient has been lowered by a gradually increasing anemia from hemorrhage, and also placenta praevia usually implies some form of operative intervention during labor, with the increased danger of infection from this source. Furthermore the placental site lies in the cervix, very close to the vagina and its bacterial flora.

The child is apt to be premature, to die of asphyxia secondary to maternal hemorrhage, or to be poorly developed as a result of imperfect imbedding of the placenta praevia and consequent poor blood supply to the infant.

Prognosis.—Placenta praevia is a grave complication of pregnancy, the maternal mortality ranging from 5 to 18 per cent according to different sets of statistics, while the fetal death rate may reach the distressing height of 50 to 60 per cent.

In a survey of maternal deaths in Philadelphia during the years 1931–33, there were 25 attributable to placenta praevia or 3.6 per cent of the total number of deaths occurring in the three-year pediod. In Kensington Hospital for Women there were no deaths from this source in the last 5000 cases studied.

Death usually follows massive hemorrhage and shock, although sepsis accounts for a considerable proportion of the fatalities. Rupture of the uterus may occur but is quite uncommon—as is air embolism.

Treatment.—*General Statements.*—1. Placenta praevia is a lesion requiring expert surgical management and should never be treated in a home or by an inexperienced medical attendant. Conditions in the United States are such today that in most communities, the facilities of a proper hospital and of a trained obstetrician are available, and there is no more excuse for attempting delivery in recognized placenta praevia in the home of the patient than there is for the treatment of ruptured ectopic pregnancy or acute appendicitis without resort to all available facilities for correct and timely management.

2. There is no expectant treatment for placenta praevia. Immediate termination of the pregnancy as soon as the diagnosis has been determined will result in the lowest possible maternal mortality.

While the above statement is wholly true, it must obviously be modified in practice.

Given a woman six and one-half months pregnant, ardently desirous of a child, who has experienced one or two small hemorrhages and in whom placenta praevia has been recognized, one hesitates to advise immediate termination; especially since there is no manner of foretelling whether more and dangerous hemorrhage will develop before the viability of the child is established or not. Expectancy is therefore almost the rule although the situation should always be explained to the prospective parents in detail, the risk outlined, and the responsibility for delay placed upon them and not upon the obstetrician.

3. Taken by and large, all cases considered, cesarean section in

placenta praevia offers the best hope for the lives of mother and child.

It is presumed that the section will be performed under good surgical conditions by a trained obstetric specialist.

It will be seen in the discussion of treatment in detail that by no means all cases of placenta praevia should be managed by section, but it is a fair statement that one regrets not having resorted to abdominal delivery in these cases, more often than the reverse.

The Management of Placenta Praevia in Its Various Phases.—Patients suffering from placenta praevia may be divided into a series of groups, according to various factors which must control the therapeutic approach.

1. Duration of pregnancy, whether before or after viability of the child, *i. e.*, before the twenty-eighth week or after it.

2. Parity, primipara or multipara.

3. Uterine contraction, whether patient is in labor or not.

4. Condition of the cervix, effaced or partially dilated, or long and canalized.

5. Type of praevia, complete, partial or marginal.

6. Amount of blood loss, trifling hemorrhage or exsanguinated.

7. Associated and additional complications. Contracted pelvis, toxemia of late pregnancy, advanced systemic disease of pulmonary tuberculosis, cardiopathy, etc.

Whatever the type of case and whatever treatment is contemplated, there is one general rule which may not be ignored, that is, all placenta praevia patients should have a properly matched and typed blood donor in constant readiness, for the probably essential transfusion, and all patients who have lost much blood as evidenced either by clinical signs of anemia or a suggestive blood count, should have a preliminary transfusion of 500 cc. of blood before active treatment is begun.

Methods of Treatment of Placenta Praevia When Bleeding Has Begun.

1. Leaving the case to nature and spontaneous delivery.

2. Vaginal tamponade.

3. Simple rupture of the membranes, with or without small doses of pituitrin to maintain uterine contraction.

4. The use of the dilating bag (metreurynter), either intra- or extra-ovular application.

5. Braxton Hicks version.

6. Delivery by forceps.

7. Cesarean section.

1. *Leaving the Case to Nature.*—In either primiparous or multiparous women, in whom labor is progressing satisfactorily and in whom there is slight bleeding, a dribble during the interval between contractions and a little gush with each pain, vaginal examination will disclose the cervical canal open, the presenting part descending and perhaps just a thinned-out edge of placenta palpable at one or the

other lateral aspect of the cervix, perhaps no placenta whatever palpable.

Under such conditions, labor may be allowed to proceed and terminate spontaneously, blood donors being in attendance, and the obstetrician prepared to combat postpartum hemorrhage with sterile uterine packing, which is in readiness, together with packing forceps, bivalve speculum, tenaculum, etc., should the bleeding become alarming.

2. *Vaginal tamponade* has but small place in placenta praevia. Its use should be restricted to cases with considerable hemorrhage, when a fairly long trip to the hospital is imminent, or when some time must elapse before the necessary apparatus, assistants, etc., may be gathered, to undertake active measures. Under such circumstances, the pubic hair having been shaved, and the parts carefully scrubbed as for delivery, the vagina may be very firmly packed with 2-inch gauze packing, of approved sterility. Tamponade is in no way a treatment of placenta praevia, the packing simply serving to compress the lower uterine segment and its attached placenta between the gauze and the presenting part, until more active measures can be instituted.

3. *Simple Rupture of the Membranes.*—This maneuver, long a standard method of treatment in the Dublin Rotunda and well known to Mauriceau, has much to commend it in certain cases. When the cervical canal is partially or completely obliterated, and when placental tissue may be felt on one side of the os or the other, while bulging membranes are palpable in the remainder of the orifice, rupture of the sac by the amniotome or other sharp instrument, results in almost immediate descent of the presenting part, so as to make pressure against the low-lying placenta while, at the same time, uterine contractions are established, the patient commonly falling into active labor within a few hours. Pituitrin in doses of 2 to 3 minims every thirty minutes aids in stimulating the uterine muscles and in maintaining a sufficient degree of tone to insure constant pressure of the head against the placenta. This method, like all those designed to minimize bleeding by any sort of compression of the placental area, exerts a distinctly deleterious effect upon the infant, who suffers from asphyxia in direct ratio to the amount of pressure brought to bear upon its placental source of oxidation. Despite this the rupture of the membrane is a most rational procedure in those cases wherein it is indicated.

4. *The Use of the Dilating Bag.*—Braun's colpeurynter or Voorhees' bag may be employed either extra- or intra-ovularly. If the bag be inserted external to the ovum, there is danger that the placenta may be further detached by the pressure upon its lower pole and hemorrhage increased. Furthermore, if the bag must remain in position for some hours, lying as it does directly upon the uterine wall, and against the open blood spaces, there is considerable danger of infection. If the colpeurynter be placed within the ovum it lies

against the fetal surface of the placenta and the membranes which tissues are expelled during labor, thus lessening the possibility of infection (Fig. 213).

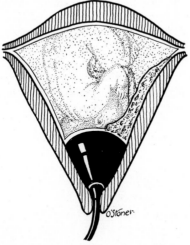

Fig. 213.—Dilating bag in marginal placenta praevia. Extra-ovular use of the bag.

The bag should be utilized in cases of partial and lateral placenta praevia when mother and child are in good condition and when there is room for its insertion alongside the placental edge. In certain in-

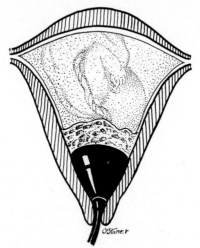

Fig. 214.—The extra-ovular use of the dilating bag in central placenta praevia.

stances of complete or central placenta praevia, the bag may also be used, the collapsed instrument being thrust through the placenta while held in dressing forceps. The cervix must be dilated to 2 or 3 cm. and usually the membranes must be ruptured in order to place the bag properly. When in position, resting upon the fetal surface of the placenta, the bag is distended with 1 per cent lysol solution or other mild antiseptic by means of a piston syringe. The distention is performed slowly and when complete the attached tube is clamped and gentle traction is made upon it from time to time to further dilatation of the cervix. When the bag is expelled, or when it may be pulled out of the cervix by moderate pressure, it is removed and the delivery completed by forceps if the head presents, a foot is pulled down in breech presentation or podalic version and extraction is performed. Great care must be taken that the cervix is dilated or disastrous hemorrhage may result (Fig. 214).

5. *Braxton Hicks Version.*—This procedure which bears the name of the distinguished British obstetrician who popularized it in 1864

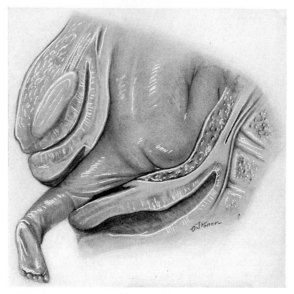

Fig. 215.—Braxton Hicks version in placenta praevia.

(although it had been employed by Wright ten years previously) is of great value in the hands of a trained man, when hemorrhage is severe and necessity for prompt hemostasis is urgent, especially if the infant is dead or in trouble or is quite premature. In order to perform it the cervix must admit at least two fingers (three is better) and a considerable infant mortality is to be feared.

The patient is anesthetized, and the finger introduced either alongside the placenta or through it, if central. A foot of the child is grasped and version performed, the turning being assisted by the external hand. As soon as the knee reaches the vulva, traction ceases and the buttocks of the child compress the placenta and prevent further bleeding (Fig. 215).

The anesthesia is stopped and the case left to nature, plus transfusion and any necessary stimulation. It is very rarely possible to complete delivery by extraction after this type of version, since the mortality from hemorrhage is so great.

Should bleeding recommence, gentle traction is made upon the exposed leg in order to increase the pressure against the placenta. Braxton Hicks version is inadvisable at or near term, or when the infant is in good condition. Cesarean section offers a far better prognosis under these circumstances.

6. *Delivery by Forceps.*—In cases where the hemorrhage is slight, and comes on late in the first or early in the second stage, betokening a marginal or low implantation of the placenta, forceps delivery is justifiable as soon as the cervix is fully dilated and the biparietal diameter of the skull has passed through it.

By this means delivery is hastened and the blood loss minimized. The technic is that of the usual forceps delivery.

7. *Cesarean Section.*—At first condemned by most thoughtful obstetric authorities, abdominal hysterotomy has steadily gained advocates until now it is widely used in the management of placenta praevia throughout the world. In a well conducted clinic the maternal mortality from cesarean section in placenta praevia should not exceed 4 per cent and when the cases are properly selected and operated upon under the best conditions, the mortality should be less than 2 per cent. For the infant, the prognosis is immeasurably better in section than by any other form of treatment and should remain under 6 per cent.

The indications for abdominal hysterotomy in placenta praevia are as follows, it being understood that a trained operator and good conditions are available:

  a. A viable infant in good condition.
  b. A cervix undilated and still canalized.
  c. The placenta covers a considerable portion of the internal os.
  d. The patient is clean, and not infected by previous vaginal manipulation.

The exception to these indications are that even in the presence of a dead fetus section is advisable when the hemorrhage is furious, the placenta central and the cervix undilated and uneffaced.

Also section is permissible even after vaginal manipulation, when it appears that attempts at vaginal delivery will probably result in disastrous bleeding. Under such circumstances the prognosis is grave, whatever the treatment, and one should risk possible infection rather than invite almost certainly fatal hemorrhage.

The preoperative preparation consists in having blood donors always in readiness and in a preliminary transfusion if there has been considerable blood loss. In addition, the ordinary surgical preparation for laparotomy is carried out.

Local anesthesia is of paramount value here and is indicated whenever its use is possible.

Type of Operation.—The classical section is best in treating placenta praevia as the low cervical operation invades the field of placental attachment and so predisposes to excessive bleeding. Also the

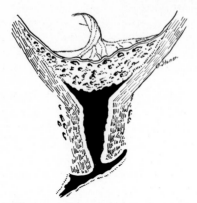

Fig. 216.—The varieties of placenta praevia with respect to treatment. Central type with undilated cervix. Cesarean section is indicated.

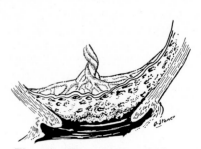

Fig. 217.—The varieties of placenta praevia with respect to treatment. Central type with dilatation and effacement of cervix. Cesarean section is indicated.

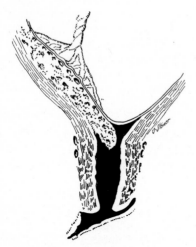

Fig. 218.—The varieties of placenta praevia with respect to treatment. Partial type, with an area of membranes palpable. Rupture of membranes or possibly cesarean section.

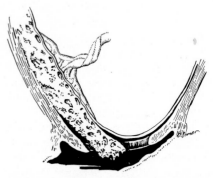

Fig. 219.—The varieties of placenta praevia with respect to treatment. Partial type with membranes exposed and cervix dilated and effaced. Rupture of membranes indicated.

latter operation is more time-consuming and therefore disadvantageous. In potentially infected cases the low, two-flap section should be chosen. (For technic of hysterotomy see Chapter XLIV.)

Postoperative Care.—Because the placental site is in the noncontractile lower uterine segment, all cases of placenta praevia should have the uterus firmly packed from fundus to external os, whatever the manner of delivery. After laparotomy the gauze packing is introduced through the uterine wound, and may be impregnated with a mild antiseptic as 2 per cent mercurochrome, or 1 per cent metaphen, etc. If the delivery has been by the vaginal route, the packing should be carried out from below. Many cases of placenta praevia are lost as a result of late postpartum hemorrhage, the additional blood loss being just sufficient to overcome the vital forces of the already depleted woman. The packing may be removed in twenty-four hours.

If the hemorrhage has been great, repeated blood transfusion plus hematinics, liver extract, and so on during the puerperium will combat anemia.

Summary of Treatment (Figs. 216, 217, 218, 219):

TREATMENT OF PLACENTA PRAEVIA

PRIMIPARAE

Time of pregnancy.	Condition of cervix.	Type placenta praevia.	Treatment.
Before viability of child, 6 to 6½ months.	Long and uneffaced.	Central or partial.	May treat expectantly if hemorrhage not too severe, and with full understanding that such treatment carries increased risk for the mother, rest in bed, no coitus, prevent constipation.
Between seventh and ninth, child living.	Long and uneffaced.	Central or partial.	Elective cesarean section.
At term or nearly so.	Effaced, not dilated beginning labor.	Central.	Elective cesarean section.
At term or nearly so.	Effaced, not dilated beginning labor.	Partial.	May rupture membranes and wait. Section better.
At term.	Effaced and partly dilated, severe hemorrhage.	Central or partial.	Transfusion and section best. May do transfusion or insert bag, or in emergency Braxton Hicks version.

MULTIPARAE

6 to 6½ months.	Undilated and uneffaced.	Central or partial.	May treat expectantly as outlined above.
Between seventh and ninth months.	Undilated and uneffaced.	Central or partial.	Cesarean section.
At or near term.	Undilated and uneffaced.	Central or partial.	Cesarean section.
At or near term.	Dilated and effaced in labor.	Central.	May introduce bag or Braxton Hicks version bringing foot through placenta. Section much preferable.
At or near term.	Dilated and effaced in labor.	Partial.	Rupture membrane. Introduce bag if time. May early require Braxton Hicks version.

CHAPTER XXIII

PREMATURE SEPARATION OF THE NORMALLY SITUATED PLACENTA; ABRUPTIO PLACENTAE; ABLATIO PLACENTAE; ACCIDENTAL HEMORRHAGE

Definition.—Premature separation of the normally implanted placenta implies that partial or complete detachment of the organ from the uterine wall has occurred prior to the third stage of labor, *i. e.*, during pregnancy, at the onset of labor or during its progress.

The term "accidental hemorrhage" was originated by Rigby in 1775, who used it to differentiate premature separation from the "unavoidable" hemorrhage of placenta praevia.

The terms abruptio placentae and ablatio placentae while now accepted in the literature do not present a true definition of the condition since they may also apply to premature separation of a placenta praevia, for example. Abruptio will be used here however as synonymous with premature separation of the normally implanted placenta by reason of its brevity.

Frequency.—Abruptio placentae is said to occur once in 500 pregnancies. This conclusion must be modified by dividing the cases into those of mild or severe hemorrhage. Separation of the lower pole of the placenta, particularly if the placental site is abnormally low, occurs in a fair proportion of labors, possibly 1 in 200. The symptoms are slight bleeding before the onset of labor, and a constant scant dribble of blood during the entire process. On delivery the lower aspect of the placenta is found to be covered with fragments of well-formed clots. On the contrary, the severe cases, in which detachment is complete and the uterus is distended with blood are uncommon and occur in a ratio of less than 1 to 800 pregnancies.

Multiparae are slightly more prone to this accident than primiparae (after correction by reason of the preponderance of multiparous labors) and age seems to play no part.

Etiology.—Here one must limit the discussion to theoretical grounds since the definite cause of this accident has not been discovered.

There are three probable origins.

    1. Trauma (obviously).

    2. Diseases of the decidua or the placenta itself.

    3. Toxemia or toxins of specific character acting upon the utero-placental circulation.

1. *Trauma.*—While violent injury and compression of the abdomen may cause detachment of the placenta, trauma is very rarely opera-

tive *per se*, the pregnant uterus being surprisingly resistant to even major concussions. However, when placental disease or toxemia is present even the slightest injury may prove the final force necessary to cause detachment. A light blow, a fall, coitus, abdominal straining from lifting, sometimes even sudden turning in bed, may induce actual separation of the placenta although the stage has been set for the accident some time before.

2. *Diseases of the Decidua and Placenta.*—Alteration in the size and arrangement of the placental vessels and corresponding variation in the uterine blood space may produce local engorgement and congestion and predispose to retroplacental hemorrhage.

Following this there is an effusion of blood in and between the uterine muscle bundles, which may be very extensive and which tend

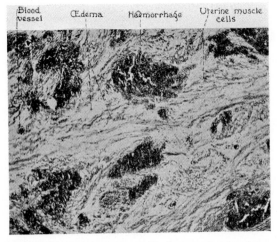

Fig. 220.—This section of uterine wall shows extensive hemorrhage, edema and dissociation of uterine musculature. × 35. (Davis and McGee in Surg., Gynec., and Obstet., vol. 53, 1931.)

to prevent uterine contraction even after the organ is empty (Fig. 220).

3. *Toxemia.*—It has been held that abruptio placentae is commonly associated with the lesions of eclampsia, but this is not so in the experience of the writer, toxic symptoms being absent in 60 per cent of his cases (Fig. 221).

It may be that there is a form of toxemia which affects the placental circulation, but which gives rise to no other sign; thus Hofbauer believes that excess of histamine in the tissues is responsible, an observation which has not been corroborated.

In my own experience this accident seems to have happened most often to women who in most instances were undergoing an apparently normal pregnancy, and in whom the hemorrhage appeared, without demonstrable cause, comparable to spontaneous abortion in seemingly healthy women. Indeed, the phrase "abortion at term" describes this condition very well.

Pathology.—Abruptio placentae is always accompanied by hemorrhage, occasionally slight but usually severe (Fig. 222).

The blood may take on one or more of four directions: (a) the central portion of the placenta may separate, leaving the margin still attached, with the formation of a huge hematoma under the placenta, forcing this structure into the sac of the ovum and bulging outward the uterine wall over the placental site. (b) The upper portion of the placenta may separate and open the amniotic cavity, which then becomes distended with blood mixed with liquor amnii. (c) The upper edge of the placenta may separate and the blood extravasate between

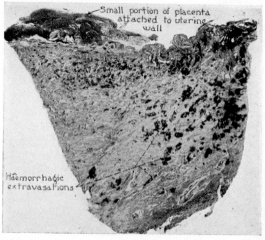

Fig. 221.—Section of uterine wall from a case of uteroplacental apoplexy, showing extravasation of blood into the uterine musculature. × 5. (Davis and McGee in Surg., Gynec., and Obstet., vol. 53, 1931.)

membranes and uterine wall, until the ovum is detached from the decidua all the way round (Fig. 223). (d) Particularly if the lower pole of the placenta separate first, the blood may dissect a passage downward between membrane and uterine wall and escape from the cervix (Fig. 224).

The first three mechanisms give rise to concealed, the fourth to frank hemorrhage. Sometimes the presenting part or the membranes close the cervical canal preventing the exit of blood. The seriousness of the lesion depends much upon which portion of the placenta first becomes separated; if the lower border, the blood may escape by gravity, the loss being moderate, and there being no mechanism present to compel further placental separation. If, on the other hand, the center or the upper pole of the placenta first becomes detached

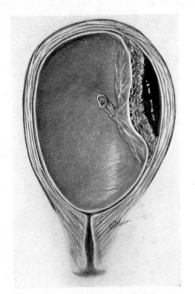

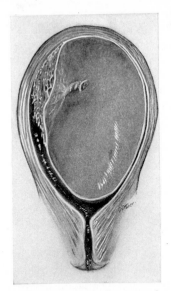

Fig. 222.—Abruptio placentae. Central separation, the margins still attached; concealed hemorrhage.

Fig. 223.—Abruptio placentae; lower pole separated; frank hemorrhage, the blood extravasating between membranes and uterine wall.

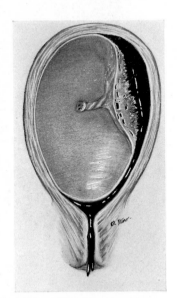

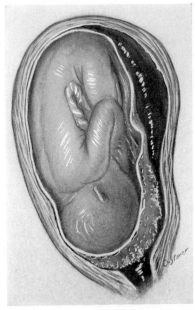

Fig. 224.—Abruptio placentae; complete separation with visible hemorrhage.

Fig. 225.—Abruptio placentae; complete separation of a placenta praevia.

26

the pressure of the accumulating blood will steadily force more and wider separation until the entire placenta is detached and lies free in the uterine cavity, together with the fetus and its sac (Fig. 225).

In these severe cases, uteroplacental apoplexy is common. The blood under pressure seeps between the muscle bundles, separating them with hematomata of various sizes. Sometimes the entire thickness of the uterine wall is filled with extravasated blood until subserosal hematomata make their appearance.

Under such circumstances the uterus presents a mottled, plum-colored appearance, is soft and doughy, fails to contract even after delivery, and must often be removed by supravaginal hysterectomy, by reason of the danger of necrosis, hemorrhage and infection of the blood-riddled muscular walls.

The Placenta.—Upon examination after delivery the placenta may present many areas of infarction, but as these are also frequently noted in the absence of abruptio, they cannot be regarded as significant. Little areas of fibrinized blood clot, lying on the maternal surface of the placenta, make the obstetrician suspicious of the partial separation with small hemorrhages, earlier in pregnancy. Sometimes the placenta is thinned out and fragile giving the impression of some inherent defect in structure which might predispose toward premature separation.

Prognosis.—Premature separation of the placenta in its more severe phase is probably the most dangerous complication of pregnancy. In complete separation 50 per cent maternal and 90 plus per cent fetal mortality may be expected.

Conversely, there are many mild cases, involving separation of the lower pole of the placenta only, which are either wholly unrecognized clinically, or in which the symptoms are so trifling that they cause no alarm.

Between these extremes there are many cases in which the blood loss is dangerous, the symptoms acute, but in which prompt and thoughtful treatment serves to avoid a fatal issue.

However, it is understood that abruptio placentae is a very grave accident in which both mother and babe stand in deadly peril of their lives.

Symptoms and Diagnosis.—During pregnancy there may be repeated, inconsequential bleedings, occurring after unusual physical strain, coitus, fatigue, etc., but ceasing after a few hours. After delivery the placenta of a patient who has experienced these little hemorrhages will disclose a few areas of old detachment, on its lower border, with bits of organized clot clinging to the villi.

In the serious cases, the onset is usually sudden and characterized by a tearing pain in the lower abdomen, which subsides after an hour or two to a steadily growing ache.

Within an hour or two labor usually comes on, and may be violent and tumultuous in character, in which case prompt delivery before too great exsanguination has occurred, tends to a termination favorable for the mother, but extremely grave for the child.

Sometimes, in mild cases, the blood under the decidua inaugurates labor, and a fairly normal delivery follows, noteworthy only by reason of the excessive amount of clotted blood in the uterine cavity which appears after the birth of the child. It is also notable that the placenta is delivered with the baby, thus proving its premature separation.

In another and the most dangerous group of cases, labor pains are weak, irregular and ineffective. The abdominal pain continues, the uterus definitely increases in size and becomes of a curious wooden consistency, the so-called "ligneous" density.

Shortly the evidences of massive internal hemorrhage appear in their order, pallor, a leaking skin, rapid shallow respiration, subnormal temperature, a pulse at first rapid and bounding, later very rapid and thready, syncope, restlessness, thirst and hunger, and loss of vision, all these followed by convulsions or coma, vomiting, delirium and death if the case remain untreated.

At first there may be no vaginal bleeding whatsoever, the hemorrhage being confined to the interior of the uterus, but as the tension increases, first blood serum then frank blood appears at the vagina. Secondarily, the vaginal hemorrhage may be quite considerable.

The uterus becomes extremely tender to palpation, the woman complaining bitterly even at the pressure of a stethoscope. This, together with the characteristic feeling of a solid, noncompressible mass in the abdomen, constitutes almost a complete clinical picture.

Fetal movements and heart sounds fade rapidly until both are absent in a short time as the infant succumbs to asphyxia. At the onset of the separation, fetal movements may be violent and excessive as the anemia begins to affect the infant's blood supply.

Very small separation may be apparent at first, during labor. Bleeding during the first stage of labor, more in amount than would be expected from a dilating cervix, coming on in little gushes with the uterine contractions, and becoming marked as the second stage approaches, suggests a separation of the lower placental pole.

When the presenting part has passed through the cervix, the bleeding may become still more pronounced, when delivery by forceps should be performed in order to permit the expulsion of the placenta and the contraction of the uterus before uteroplacental apoplexy sets in.

Diagnostic Characteristics and Summary.—During pregnancy— slight uterine bleedings after exertion, etc.

Shortly before term or at term—acute separation.

Mild Cases.—Sudden pain in uterus, rapid onset of labor with tumultuous pain and excessive vaginal bleeding. If delivery is prompt child may live, and symptoms cease with the expulsion of the placenta and the contraction of the uterus.

Still Milder Cases.—Slight excess of vaginal bleeding during labor, possibly some difficulty in resuscitating child.

Delivery by forceps usually effective.

Severe Cases.—Sudden tearing pain in lower abdomen followed by severe ache, and very marked tenderness of the uterus to palpation. Rapid changes in tone and form of uterus. Density ligneous, hard and unyielding. Fundus broad, anterior curvature flattened. Signs of fetal life rapidly disappear. May be violent labor pain, may be weak, irregular and ineffective contractions. Serum, then blood appears at vagina, but never in sufficient quantity to account for the physical evidences of blood loss. All the signs of internal hemorrhage rapidly progressing to the point of fatality.

Treatment.—One rule governs the management of all cases of abruptio placentae; *i. e.*, delivery must be effected as soon as possible and with a minimum of further blood loss. This naturally divides the treatment into those of mild cases, during labor, severe cases before labor and during labor.

The very mild cases already referred to need but little treatment during pregnancy, after the hemorrhages have begun to manifest themselves. Rest and avoidance of untoward exertion, with the induction of labor, should the bleeding become at all alarming, will usually suffice.

If the small separation is first noticed during labor, early resort to forceps delivery will tend to minimize the loss of blood. It is in the severe cases that one's obstetrical skill and knowledge are put to the test. When the separation occurs at the onset of labor or before, when the cervix is as yet uneffaced and undilated, abdominal hysterotomy is the procedure of choice regardless of the condition of the child. Whether the infant be living or dead, the uterine blood spaces will continue to pour their contents into the uterine cavity, which cannot contract because of the presence of the fetus.

Immediate cesarean section then is the one procedure of choice. It is frequently necessary to remove the uterus at the hysterotomy, by reason of the infiltration of blood between the muscle bundles.

Whenever the uterus is soft and boggy and especially if there are little hematomata under the serosa, hysterectomy should be performed, since the uterus so impregnated with blood fails to contract and is most vulnerable to infection and necrosis. Obviously the laparotomy should be prefaced by blood transfusion and further supplies of blood should be in readiness in the person of matched and typed donors. When the conditions are such that cesarean section cannot be attempted, recourse must be had to some substitute procedure. If the cervix be undilated, a metreurynter may be employed, until sufficient room is obtained to perform version and extraction (the Braxton Hicks version is dangerous since the empty fundus of the uterus may fill with blood). Craniotomy and extraction or forceps delivery may be utilized.

The outlook for the mother is extremely bad when cases of complete placental separation in the presence of an undilated cervix must be treated in any manner other than immediate laparotomy.

When the cervix is partially dilated 2 to 3 cm. and is to some extent effaced, dilatation may be completed with the bag, or by manual dilatation and the uterus immediately emptied by forceps extraction, version and extraction or craniotomy.

The greater the degree of dilatation and effacement, the greater the hope of success.

It is a fortunate thing that placental separation frequently inaugurates immediate labor and sufficient cervical obliteration obtains for rapid vaginal delivery, since otherwise many more women would perish from this accident.

Violent dilatation of the cervix—accouchement forcé—is to be deplored as too shocking and traumatic, although if there be any place at all for this procedure in obstetric practice, it lies in the management of abruptio placentae, where there are no facilities for section and where the cervix is insufficiently dilated.

After delivery, the uterus should be emptied of its blood clots, and firmly packed from fundus to os, to insure against the postpartum hemorrhage which may follow uterine relaxation. More blood transfusions and stimulation may be required to sustain the patient and the accoucheur must be on his guard against puerperal sepsis developing in the blood-engorged uterus.

CHAPTER XXIV

THE LOCAL DISEASES ACCIDENTAL TO PREGNANCY

THE LOCAL INFLAMMATIONS

Gonorrhea.—Gonorrhea and pregnancy may be coexistent under three conditions:

1. The gonorrheal infection may antedate the occurrence of impregnation.
2. The gonorrhea may have been acquired at the same coitus which resulted in conception.
3. The gonorrhea may have been acquired after conception has occurred.

In cases belonging to the first group, and including by far the greater number, the infection has passed its acute stage and is chronic, the organisms being limited to the deep tissues of the cervix, bartholinian glands, and possibly the endometrium and the fallopian tubes. The latter two groups of cases comprise the acute and subacute forms of the disease.

When may a gonorrheic woman undertake pregnancy? This question is a very common one, when a married woman has been treated for the disease or when a former patient, having married, is desirous of becoming a mother.

As a general rule, the writer is content with three negative smears at one-month intervals, taken as follows:

A cervical or urethral smear in the intermenstrual period, one on the day following cessation of the menstrual flow and one five days later. These three smears being negative, the same process is repeated after one month, and if again negative, the patient is regarded as safe to undertake reproduction.

The influence of pregnancy upon a preexisting gonorrhea is usually quite marked. The congestion and succulence of the tissues which are a part of the gravid state furnish abundant stimulus for the rapid multiplication of gonococci, whether the organisms are of recent introduction or have been present for a long time.

In this manner, an old, latent gonorrhea, the existence of which is ofttimes entirely unsuspected by the patient, may flare up and give rise to active symptoms.

Pregnancy seems to predispose to a widespread upward extension of the disease, since endometritis and deciduitis are not infrequent, and the invasion of the tubes occurs quite often, as may be shown by the instances of acute salpingitis during pregnancy, the tubes often being found completely occluded at their fimbriated extremities.

406

The influence of gonorrhea upon pregnancy is not usually so marked. Abortion may and does occur as a result of endometritis or deciduitis. But it is by no means the rule. The gonococcus is a fairly negligible factor among abortifacients, its great rôle in this connection being that of a causal factor in sterility. If there be an associated endometritis present, malformation of the fetus may occur as a result of faulty implantation of the ovum.

Puerperal sepsis is an all too common complication of neisserian infection, although fortunately gonorrheal sepsis is more generally productive of morbidity than mortality, its usual manifestations being a prolonged and stormy puerperium.

Pure gonorrheal sepsis is uncommon, but if the infection becomes mixed, the streptococcus, staphylococcus or colon bacillus being superimposed upon the original gonorrhea, serious lesions of the pelvic tissues almost invariably follow.

Symptoms and Diagnosis.—The symptoms of gonorrhea during pregnancy are those of the disease in general, although made more severe by the congestion present.

The diagnosis is usually easy. In the great majority of cases, when the disease is recognized as having been preexistent to the pregnancy, a history will be volunteered in the interests of the child. In all cases, the advent of pregnancy is attended by a leukorrhea more or less profuse. The discharge varies from white to greenish-brown in color, it may or may not be offensive and, on microscopic examination, it presents the characteristic gonococci in varying numbers. If the infection be acute and severe, there will be a marked congestion of the vagina with burning pain, and even occasionally some exfoliation of the vaginal mucous membrane, with serous discharge or slight bleeding.

Sometimes the urethral infection is rekindled by the congestion about the pelvic tissues with purulent discharge from the meatus and frequent micturition. If the internal genitalia have been involved there may develop a mild pelvic peritonitis of low-grade type. In most of the cases, however, the chief symptom is the profuse and intractable leukorrhea.

Condylomata, if present, undergo very marked and active growth and become extremely vascular. Indeed, these growths spread with such speed and become so numerous and large as often greatly to alarm the patient. Excision, which sometimes becomes necessary, is made difficult by the vascularity, hemorrhage becoming very severe in some instances. Ligation of the base of pedunculated condylomata, and removal of sessile growths by fulguration under local anesthesia, will usually be sufficient safeguard against this combination.

Various remote complications, as arthritis, endocarditis and sometimes general peritonitis, are noted during pregnancy with rather more frequency than among nonpregnant women.

Treatment.—During pregnancy the local treatment should follow the general line of gonorrhea therapy, with the exception that large douches or vaginal tampons should not be employed.

If the disease be acute and present itself as a violent inflammation of the vaginal mucosa and the cervix uteri, frequent applications of a fairly strong silver solution are indicated. A good practice is to thoroughly coat the vagina with a solution of silver nitrate, 20 grains to the ounce, at two-day intervals, a cleansing douche to be used by the patient on the alternate days. The douche should be mildly antiseptic, small in amount (not to exceed 1 quart) and given with practically no pressure of the stream, 0.5 per cent formalin making an excellent solution for this purpose.

Abscesses developing in Bartholin's glands must be evacuated under local anesthesia and the cavities thoroughly disinfected with a strong silver nitrate solution or pure iodine. Such a plan of treatment will usually control the more violent type of infection.

Where the gonorrhea presents itself in the usual chronic form, manifested only by a profuse leukorrhea with a moderate thickening and congestion of the vaginal mucosa, treatment by means of the instillation of a drachm of brewer's yeast, or the dry yeast spores marketed under several trade names, offers the greatest hope of relief.

The applications should be made every other day, the yeast held in place by a small pledget of absorbent cotton, placed just within the vulva, not in contact with the cervix. Cleansing douches, as outlined above, should be used on the alternate days. Gentleness of manipulation and avoidance of pressure on the cervix or fundus uteri are essential to success.

Should a pelvic peritonitis supervene, absolute rest in bed and the application of heat, together with the ordinary general therapeusis of infection, is the plan of treatment to be followed.

The use of antigonorrheal vaccine or serum has been advocated and good results reported, but I personally feel some hesitation in administering sera during pregnancy, fearing a pronounced reaction with injury to the embryo.

Vulvitis.—Acute inflammation of the vulval tissues is seen sometimes in obese and slovenly women, rarely in those who have regard to general body cleanliness.

In the former group, the accumulation of vaginal mucus, smegma, etc., produce an acute dermatitis of the eczema type. The tissues become reddened, dry and swollen, a pseudomembrane may form or occasionally rather deep, punched-out ulceration may be present, and mycotic infections may occur with their vegetative membranes.

Acute vulvitis may be so severe as to give rise to marked discomfort, with fever and a sharp rise in leukocytes.

Management.—Gentle cleansing, with a weak soap suds, or better still a warm sitz bath, painting the surface with 1 per cent gentian violet solution and the generous application of a mildly antiseptic ointment for a few days will usually ameliorate the symptoms; 2 per cent phenol in petrolatum is a favorite ointment. If deep ulceration or warty outgrowths are present these may be treated by the application of the electric cautery. When the acute inflammation has subsided, the vulval surfaces tend to become moist, and now a dusting powder of equal parts zinc stearate and boric acid is quite efficacious. Instruction in personal hygiene is probably the most important phase of the cure.

Vaginitis.—The above description might nearly apply to vaginitis of filth origin, but the vagina is more commonly attacked by the Trichomonas vaginalis.

This organism, a frequent offender, gives rise to a frothy, yellowish, profuse discharge with considerable irritation of the vaginal and cervical mucosa, most apparent upon the posterior wall. The diagnosis can readily be made by examination of the fresh material in a hanging-drop preparation, under low power and unstained, when the characteristic ameboid bodies with their flagellate movements will be discerned. The treatment of Trichomonas vaginitis is to carefully dry the vagina and cervix with cotton pledgets, then to paint the entire surface with 1 per cent boric acid, 1 per cent chinosol, dilute Lugol's solution, etc. The vagina is then tamponed with 10 per cent boroglyceride solution and the treatment repeated in two days. Coating the vagina and cervix with a powder of silver picrate is often of value.

Endocervicitis and Cervicitis.—Cervical pathology is uncommon in primiparae, excepting always gonorrheal lesions. The ordinary cervical erosion and eversion with polypoid formations are the prerogative of multiparae and are the result of cervical injuries during previous labors.

Owing to the increased vascularity, cervical erosion may give rise to slight but persistent bleeding, which is easily stopped by the application of 10 per cent silver nitrate solution to the cervical mucosa at intervals of one week for several weeks. Annoying leukorrhea may accompany the cervical lesion and is often intractable. Instillation into the vagina of a powder composed of equal parts fuller's earth and soda bicarbonate is useful, as is a mildly alkaline douche.

Endometrial polyps may protrude from the cervix and sometimes these growths bleed freely from erosion of their delicate epithelial wall. Polyps may be snared off during pregnancy without difficulty but they should always be subjected to histological study to eliminate the possibility of malignancy.

Granuloma Inguinale.—This chronic ulcerative inflammation (Fig. 226) seems to be increasing in frequency especially among the negro population. The lesion usually begins as a small noninflammatory papule on the vulva, which papule later ruptures and exudes a purulent fluid, after which the process spreads by a slow proliferation. The typical advanced lesion is that of exuberant granulomatous tissue, soft in consistency and red in color. There is marked tissue destruction in the center of the area, while the edges are raised and overlap

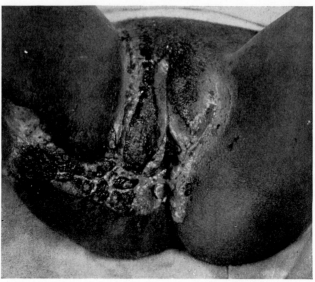

Fig. 226.—Granuloma inguinale. An extensive lesion involving the buttock. (Livermore and Schumann, "Gonorrhea and Kindred Affections," D. Appleton-Century Co., Publishers.)

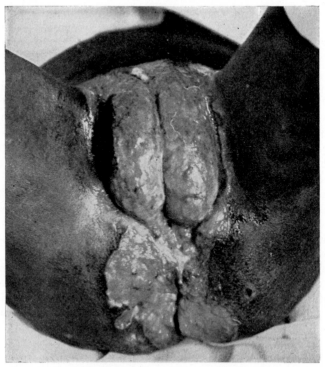

Fig. 227.—Granuloma inguinale. Note the edema and hypertrophy of the labia majora. (Livermore and Schumann, "Gonorrhea and Kindred Affections," D. Appleton-Century Co., Publishers.)

the healthy skin. The disease spreads slowly but widely, with areas of cicatrization where healing has occurred, interspersed with large ulcers of indolent growth.

During pregnancy there is marked exacerbation of the inflammatory process, the ulcer growing rapidly until the whole pudendal region may be involved. Delivery in such instances should be by cesarean section, but as these women are anemic they are apt to prove poor operative risks. The diagnosis is confirmed by the demonstration of the Leishman-Donovan bodies in the secretion (Fig. 227).

Treatment.—Tartar emetic is a specific in granuloma, while excision of the growth and local treatment are of no benefit whatever, topical application to promote cleanliness, absorb discharges and destroy offensive odors being the only occasion for such management.

Tartar emetic is used intravenously in doses of $\frac{1}{10}$ grain dissolved in 1 drachm of salt solution and exhibited once weekly in ambulant cases and every other day in hospital patients. The cure is exceedingly slow and recurrences are common.

CHAPTER XXV

MALFORMATION OF THE UTERUS AND VAGINA

Of all abnormalities of the female genitalia, these are the ones of greatest clinical moment, since serious disturbances in menstrual function, in pregnancy, and in labor so often result from their presence. The genesis of incomplete fusion of Müller's ducts has given rise to much ingenious speculation, but it is probably true that the whole process is one of arrest of development and that inasmuch as the theory of evolution has made it clear that man is the highest animal type yet known, and that our species has gradually been evolved during a long course of development, it naturally follows that when such development occurs in an atavistic form, or a reversion to a lower type, there will be found analogous conditions among certain lower forms of animal life.

Failure of fusion of the müllerian ducts in women always assumes one of a definite number of forms and as the writer has pointed out, every one of these forms has its direct analogue in the normal anatomical formation of the uterus and vagina in one or more of the lower orders of mammalian life; further, the lower the species in the mammalian scale the less the tendency to fusion of the two sides of the genital tract.

If the embryology of the genitalia be reviewed, it will be found that the ovary, ovarian ligament, and round ligament are derived from the genital ridge, and need be no longer considered from the standpoint of these studies, which deal especially with the lower portion of the genital tract. At the time when the wolffian body has almost reached its greatest development, a second longitudinal duct makes its appearance in close proximity to the wolffian, and is known as the müllerian duct. The two fuse together to form a single tube in the lower part of their course, but remain distinct above, each duct retaining its original opening into the peritoneal cavity. The fold of peritoneum surrounding the wolffian body becomes transformed, in the degeneration of that structure, into the broad ligament, the transverse portion of which, in the adult, is due to the fusion of the lower portions of the müllerian ducts.

In the female the müllerian ducts persist and become converted into the uterus and vagina below, and into the fallopian tubes in the upper part of their course. From the margin of the openings by which the ducts communicate with the peritoneal cavity, projections develop at an early period and give rise to the fimbriae. It has been seen that the lower portions of the müllerian ducts fuse together and form a single canal, and it is from this that the uterus and vagina are differentiated, the histological distinction of the two portions commencing to manifest itself at about the third month.

Failure of the development of the various parts just described to be completed in the normal manner leads to various abnormalities in connection with the reproductive organs, which, in so far as they concern the uterus and vagina, will be considered in detail. There have been described five chief varieties of developmental errors of the uterus. Many classifications of these abnormalities have been devised, but a modification of Kaufmann's system is simple and conforms to the clinical varieties of the lesion. This classification is as follows (Fig. 228):

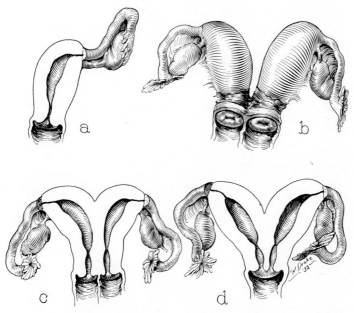

Fig. 228.—*a*, Uterus unicornis; *b*, uterus didelphys; *c*, uterus bicornis duplex with double vagina; *d*, uterus bicornis septus. (Masson and Rieniets.)

(1) *Uterus didelphys* or double uterus. Here there are two distinct organs each one having its fallopian tube and ovary in connection with it, and each possessing a cervix and vagina. This form is very rare.

(2) *Uterus Duplex Bicornis.*—Here the uteri are joined externally but are distinct as to their cavities; the two cervices are joined, and the vagina may be double or possess a septum in its upper portion.

(3) *Uterus Bicornis Unicollis.*—This occurs when the fusion is complete to a point above the cervix, the uterus being widely bicornuate with one cervix and one vagina (Fig. 229).

(4) *Uterus Septus.*—Here the only external evidence of the de-

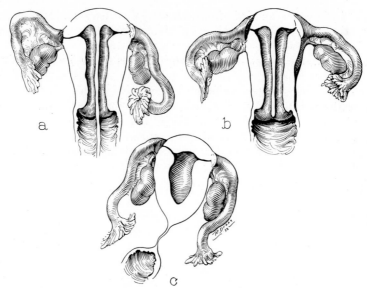

Fig. 229.—*a*, Uterus septus duplex with vaginal septum; *b*, uterus septus duplex; *c*, partial symmetrical congenital atresia; absence of cervix. (Masson and Rieniets.)

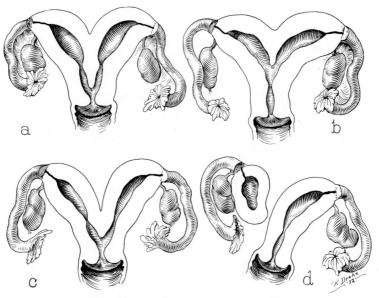

Fig. 230.—*a*, Uterus bicornis unicollis; *b*, uterus arcuatus subseptus; *c*, uterus bicornis unicollis; *d*, bicornate uterus, with one or the other horn rudimentary, and partially hollow. (Masson and Rieniets.)

formity is a depression in the fundus, although a septum may extend either the entire length or through a portion of the cavum uteri.

(5) *Uterus arcuatus* or *cordiformis,* with a heart-shaped fundus, the cleft in the upper portion being the only remainder of the septum.

It must be remembered that these malformations are rarely symmetrical, one horn being usually much further advanced in development than the other, the more primitive one sometimes being merely rudimentary and without evidence of cavity (Fig. 230).

These deformities of the uterus are of great clinical moment because of their effect upon the sex life of the bearer, and a rich and voluminous literature has accumulated, based mainly upon clinical experience with the conditions. All may be discussed under the common head of Uterus Didelphys (double uterus).

UTERUS DIDELPHYS

Clinical Aspects.—The first mention of this condition in the living adult was Fränkel's report, in 1873, of the cases of Ollivier and Bounet as the only two recorded cases. Then Pfannenstiel, in 1894, published 12 instances and Giles, in 1895, 21 cases of the condition. Since that time interest has steadily grown until reports are now a regular part of contemporary obstetric literature.

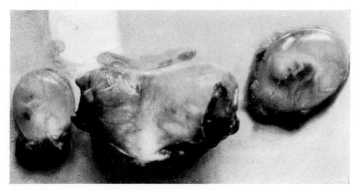

Fig. 231.—Uterus bicornis unicollis with a pregnancy in each horn. (Kensington Hospital for Women.)

Findley has well said that the doubling of the uterus has little clinical significance other than in the event of pregnancy. The malformation is compatible with a normal sexual life save in exceptional instances, and one is impressed by the number of cases wherein the anomaly was not recognized even when pregnancy and labor did occur.

In uterus didelphys the fundi are completely separated, generally unsymmetrical, one being larger than the other. One uterus may lie in front of the other, although they are generally in the same transverse plane. When one uterus is pregnant, the empty one, as a rule, lies behind it. The uterine bodies may be separated by a more or less triangular fold of peritoneum, the rectovesical fold.

The vagina is usually either partially septate or completely doubled, this doubling extending to the vulva, urethra, and bladder in some instances, together with a wide separation of the pubic bones.

Frequency.—Uterus didelphys is an infrequent condition, Stolper reporting 10 cases in 74,000 married women, while Neugebauer found 3 in 19,000 examinations.

Fertility.—Pregnancy and childbirth in cases of uterus didelphys are rather usual, and indeed it would seem that the fertility of women so affected is increased rather than diminished. If one excludes from the reported cases the unmarried women and those in whom conception was inhibited by reason of vaginal deformities, it is clear that fertility is very greatly increased in the presence of double uterus (Fig. 231).

Clinical Course of Pregnancy.—Full-term spontaneous deliveries are common and often the condition is not recognized until after two or more babies. Abortions are more frequent than in normal uteri. Abortion under these circumstances is probably due first to faulty implantation of the ovum in the deformed uterus and second to a secondary torsion or malposition of the gravid horn, leading to active or passive congestion with subsequent uterine contraction and expulsion of the fetus.

Premature labor is another frequent termination of pregnancy in uterus didelphys. This accident is due in general to the same causes that underlie abortion, plus the fact that the nongravid horn sometimes makes considerable pressure in the pelvis, thus tending to uterine irritability.

Superfetation.—Women having double uteri present frequent examples of what may properly be regarded as superfetation. The two uteri have the power to function independently of each other, as is proved by the regular occurrence of menstruation from the nonpregnant side while pregnancy goes on undisturbed in the gravid horn. Dubierre reports a case of twin pregnancy with fourteen weeks' interval between deliveries.

Moench, in a discussion of superfetation in double uterus, reports a case in which a woman gave birth to a living seven-month-old child and three days later again having labor pains, passed a three months' fetus, fresh in its membranes.

Superfetation in single uterus is very rare because the formation of the corpus luteum of pregnancy inhibits the development of other ovarian follicles until the force of its hormone subsides, usually about the fifth month. By this time the uterus is so filled with the fetus, its membranes, and placenta, that the embedding of another ovum is impossible. In double uterus this factor does not prevail, as there is an empty horn perfectly apt for nidation.

Delivery at Term.—Many women having double uteri are capable of spontaneous delivery and the obstetrical attendant should not be unduly concerned regarding the possible accidents of labor, nor should operative interference be practiced until the appearance of some complication discloses an indication.

When dystocia occurs, it is due chiefly to the enlargement and incarceration of the nongravid side behind the pregnant uterus, uterine inertia due to a defective musculature, obstruction by a vaginal septum, rupture of the uterus, postpartum hemorrhage, and toxemia. Breech presentations are frequent, Polak estimating their occurrence at 40 per cent. Malpresentation with faulty rotation is, as is to be expected, of common occurrence.

Obstruction by the nonpregnant uterine horn is fairly common since this structure enlarges parallel to but, of course, in much less degree than the pregnant side. The nongravid horn may encroach directly upon the birth canal and shut it off from the descending presenting part, or it may serve to displace the axis of the pregnant uterus from that of the pelvic canal, and so lead to severe dystocia.

Uterine inertia is rather to be expected, since the muscular structure of these unfused and malformed uteri is usually weak, thin and lacking in contractile power. Inertia, however, unless complicated by obstruction, produces a delay in delivery which is easily controlled by simple forceps extraction. In other cases, morphia, with its attendant rest of wearied muscle fibers, will cause a secondary vigorous contraction with spontaneous delivery.

Obstruction by double or septate vagina requires no detailed discussion. Incision of septa or cesarean section, when the vagina is so deformed as absolutely to preclude the expulsion of the child, will at once overcome the difficulty.

Rupture of the gravid uterus contributes an obstetrical calamity when it occurs, which is usually in those cases in which the pregnant horn is more or less rudimentary (uterus bicornis unilateralis rudimentarius). Here there is a small appendage of uterine tissue connected by a band of fibromuscular tissue, 1 or 2 cm. in width and 7 or 8 cm. long, to the lower or middle portion of an otherwise well developed uterus. In some of these cases a small canal connects the true uterine cavity with that of the rudimentary horn, while in others the only opening to the smaller horn is via its fallopian tube.

Postpartum hemorrhage is a fairly frequent complication by reason of the defective uterine musculature. Its management is difficult because, when packing is indicated, the nongravid horn may obstruct the lower uterine segment of the bleeding side and render the introduction of gauze a matter of some concern. However, the usual treatment of pituitrin subcutaneously and uterine packing, if necessary, generally suffices.

Complications During the Third Stage of Labor and the Puerperium.—Manual removal of the placenta is frequently necessary. Lochial block, owing to obstruction of the parturient horn by the

27

nonpregnant one sliding down posteriorly, is also fairly common. Subinvolution and postpartum retroversion also occur. All of these complications are to be managed in the usual way and require no special discussion here.

In conclusion, it may be stated that from the clinical standpoint, double uterus is chiefly of importance during the course of pregnancy and labor, that delivery by the vaginal route is the rule, malpresentations, breech positions and inertia uteri being common. Abortions are frequent and the complications of the third stage and the puerperium are somewhat more commonly noted than among women with normal uteri.

Diagnosis.—Recognition of double uterus is difficult, and often the condition remains unsuspected during the entire child-bearing period of the patient's life, only to be discovered accidentally in the course of some operative procedure undertaken for a different purpose. Menstrual disturbances, notably dysmenorrhea, and semimonthly menstruation, are suggestive but nonconclusive. Discovery of a vaginal septum, no matter how undeveloped, should at once excite suspicion of uterine malformation. Hematocolpos or hematometra is often found associated with such malformations and suggests the possibility of their presence. Schwarz believes that women with double uteri usually have unusually broad pelves, an observation which has been amply confirmed by many writers.

CHAPTER XXVI

MULTIPLE PREGNANCY

In the human female, the development of a single ovum and the birth of one fetus at each pregnancy is the normal course of events, and multiple births must be regarded as a reversion to lower mammalian forms and therefore in a measure pathological.

Statistics as to the frequency of multiple births among the women of civilized lands have been long established and do not seem to vary much, with further case reports. From two to six fetuses may be born, septuplets having never been reported authentically, although there is a tablet in the town of Hamelin-on-Weser, Germany, which commemorates the birth of septuplets there.

Twins usually occur about once in 80 pregnancies, triplets about once in 6400, quadruplets about 1 in 520,000, while some 32 cases

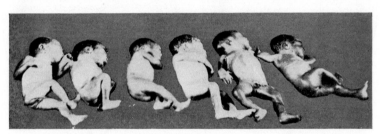

Fig. 232.—Sextuplets: from an old photograph taken in Accra, Africa, by a medical missionary.

of quintuplets are known. D. Hellin's formula of incidence: twins 1 in 80 births, triplets 1 in 80^2, quadruplets 1 in 80^3, quintuplets 1 in 80^4 is a simple and fairly accurate method of expressing the relative frequency.

The famous Dionne quintuplets have greatly stimulated interest in multiple births in America, and much searching of records has followed their advent.

There has recently come to light the birth certificate of a family of sextuplets named Bushnell who were born in Chicago September 15, 1866. This birth certificate, if genuine, states that three boys and three girls were born alive. Of the six, three were living in January, 1935, a fourth died a few years ago and the two others considerably before, but all lived beyond infancy.

Some years ago Dr. Chas. F. Nassau presented the author with a photograph of sextuplets born in Accra, Gold Coast, Africa, the picture taken by his father who was a missionary. The infants were born alive but how long they survived is not known (Fig. 232).

Multiple pregnancy may consist of more than one fetus in the uterus, one in the uterus and one tubal or indeed there may be tubal twinning with or without coincident intra-uterine gestation. The tendency to twinning is a reversion to a more primitive mammalian type, and is distinctly hereditary, the impulse being transmitted through the mother usually, although it seems that the male may have some influence. When both parents possess the hereditary tendency, frequent multiple pregnancies may result and such offspring carry a definite and strong tendency to continue the phenomenon (Fig. 233).

Etiology.—When developed from a single ovum twins are called homologous, identical or uniovular. When two or more ova develop

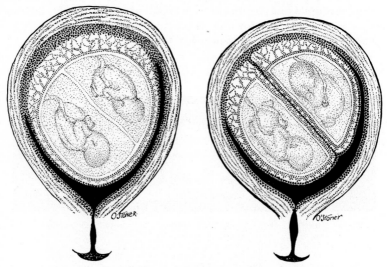

Fig. 233.—Uniovular twins.   Fig. 234.—Binovular twins.

and are fertilized simultaneously, the twins are called fraternal or binovular. Binovular twins occur about four times as frequently as the uniovular variety and may be of the same or opposite sexes, and do not necessarily resemble one another more closely than do other children of the same parents, and are akin to litter mates in the lower animals. Uniovular twins are always of the same sex, and identical in appearance, hereditary characteristics, and even in pathological tendencies. The origin of single ovum twins has been proved by experimental evidence. In certain fishes, the embryonic plate may be separated and two embryos made to develop by a reduction in oxygenation, by heating and so on. Stockard holds that any arrest of development of the fertilized ovum at the onset of gastrulation, the critical moment for twinning, is the underlying cause.

Uniovular twins have a single placenta with free anastomosis of the fetal circulation and, accordingly, should there be some defect in the vascular apparatus of the placenta one twin may develop at the expense of the other, leading to monster formation or to atrophy of one fetus (fetus papyraceus).

They possess one chorion, but usually there are separate amniotic sacs, although the edges in contact may fuse and disappear, leaving a single sac. Each infant has its own umbilical cord, although sometimes a single cord emerges from the placenta, bifurcating at a short distance from its point of origin (Fig. 233).

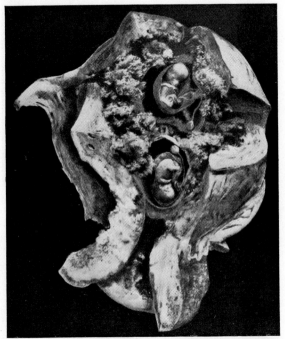

Fig. 235.—Twin pregnancy at three months, showing the relatively large placental area. (Spee.)

Binovular twins have separate placentae although these are frequently fused and give the impression of one long oval organ. The point of fusion can be found, however, and the placentae separated without danger to the cotyledons of either. There are two amnions and two chorions, but here again, sometimes the chorions fuse and create the illusion of monochorionic or identical twins (Fig. 234).

Multiple pregnancies are often repeated as in a patient of the author who had twins four times in succession, then a single birth and finally triplets (Fig. 235).

The individual infants in multiple pregnancy are smaller those of single gestation, but their combined weight is considerably greater.

Sometimes twins are born of different size and degree of development giving rise to the possibility of superfetation or superfecundation (Fig. 236).

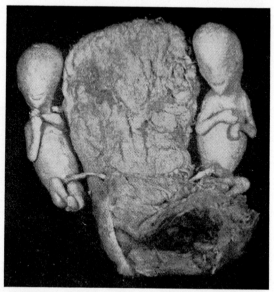

Fig. 236.—Shows deformed twin fetuses with a common sac. (Adair in Amer. Jour. of Obstet. and Gynec., vol. 20, 1930. C. V. Mosby Co., Publishers.)

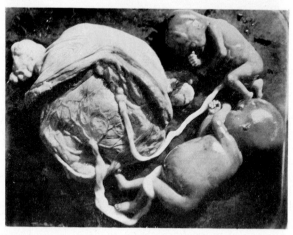

Fig. 237.—Twin pregnancy, one fetus much retarded in growth by interference with its placental blood supply. (Frankford Hospital.)

Superfetation and Superfecundation.—Discussion of multiple pregnancy leads naturally to a consideration of the vexed question of superfetation in these cases (Fig. 237). The generally accepted definition of superfecundation is that condition in which two or more ova belonging to or originating at the same ovulation period are fertilized from sperm from coitus practiced at different times by the same or another male. The ova may originate from one or both ovaries, but in the latter case the ovulation must be practically simultaneous.

Superfetation is the fertilization of two more ova that belong to or originate at different ovular periods by sperm from coitus at the same or different times by the same or another male. This assumes a pregnancy superimposed upon another by the fertilization of an ovum of a later date.

The essential difference between the two terms lies in the fact that in the former instance the ova are separately fertilized but themselves are of the same maturity, that is, they are products of the same ovulation period, while in the latter, the ova are of different ages, products of two ovulation periods. The possibility of the occurrence of these phenomena is still in doubt, the Germans usually denying its existence while the French and American observers credit it.

Diagnosis.—Multiple pregnancy offers so many characteristic features that its diagnosis would seem to be almost routine, but it is remarkable how many times it is not suspected by the medical attendant, until the failure of the uterus to contract after birth of the first child leads to a suspicion of the presence of another.

The diagnosis may be reached by summing up certain factors of suggestion, with others of certainty.

The features of pregnancy suggestive of twinning are:

History of a familial tendency to multiple births.

Excessive toxemia of early pregnancy.

Increased rate of growth of the uterus and its attainment of a size larger than usual in single pregnancies at a corresponding period of gestation.

Change in the shape of the fundus—a globular, very broad fundus as compared to the usual ovoid form is suggestive.

Evidences upon which a definite diagnosis of multiple pregnancy may be reached are:

The demonstration of two or more skulls and spinal columns by radiography (after the twentieth week of gestation) (Figs. 238, 239).

The auscultation of two distinct sets of heart tones, having different areas of maximum intensity and varying in rate by 8 or more beats per minute, when counted by separate observers, both tones being different in rate from that of the maternal pulse.

The definite palpation of two fetal skulls and of more than four extremities.

Differential Diagnosis.—Early in pregnancy, twins must be differentiated from hydatidiform mole. In both conditions, toxemia is excessive and the uterus grows with untoward rapidity. In mole persistent hemorrhage and the extrusion of follicles will clear up the

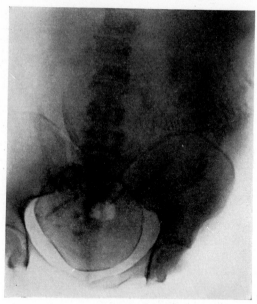

Fig. 238.—Twin pregnancy. One head in the inlet. One high in the uterus. (Kensington Hospital for Women.)

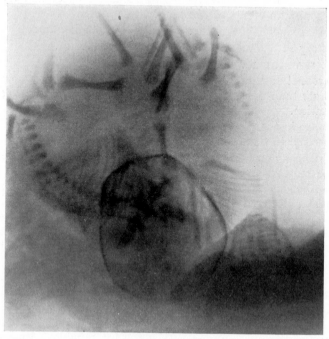

Fig. 239.—Twin pregnancy. Both heads at the pelvic brim. (Kensington Hospital for Women.)

diagnosis, while in twins the radiographic discovery of two skeletons is final evidence.

Double monsters sometimes confuse the issue greatly, but as they are really twins, there is no real error. Careful study of the x-ray picture after the seventh month will frequently disclose evidence of faulty development as acrania, etc., and will establish the presence of some variety of monstrous infant.

Fibroid tumor, ovarian cysts, etc., sometimes are confusing, but usually painstaking abdominal and vaginal examination will localize the complicating tumor and determine the true state of affairs.

Clinical Course of Pregnancy.—Twin pregnancies are apt to prove stormy ones. Discomfort from the oversized uterus, and from the excessive fetal movements vex the woman during the later months,

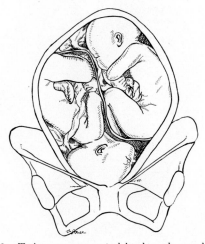

Fig. 240.—Twins, one presented by breech, one by brow.

while marked hyperemesis and a greater tendency to preeclamptic varicosities and edema, toxemia, disturb the earlier period.

Labor in twin pregnancy is marked by uterine inertia, in many instances, although premature labor is rather the rule. While the first stage may be greatly prolonged, spontaneous delivery of the first twin may be anticipated by reason of its small size. The second, however, often requires operative aid to complete delivery, the uterine contractions becoming feeble and infrequent.

The interval between the birth of the first and second twin may be a few minutes, often a half hour, or if the delivery be not assisted, hours or days may intervene.

Twins disturb the normal mechanism of adaptation so that errors in presentation are common.

The frequency of the various combinations of presentation as made up from a composite of several groups of statistics is:

Both cephalic .... 44 per cent
Head and breech .... 30 per cent
Both breech .... 11 per cent
Head and transverse .... 8 per cent
Breech and transverse .... 6 per cent
Both transverse .... 1 per cent

The Management of Twin Labor.—If the first twin presents by vertex or breech, spontaneous delivery should be awaited, and upon birth, the cord must be doubly ligated and cut (Fig. 241).

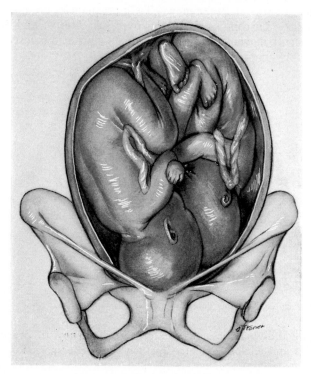

Fig. 241.—Mechanism of labor in twin pregnancy. Engagement of the head of the first twin.

Vaginal examination will then disclose the presentation of the second twin, which frequently lies in a separate sac, the membranes intact. The membranes are artificially ruptured and if the presentation be correct and the uterine contractions vigorous, spontaneous delivery of the second twin may be awaited (Fig. 242).

If there is no progress within fifteen minutes, the obstetrician should change his gloves, the patient be rescrubbed and draped and the remaining infant delivered by version or forceps as indicated by the presentation.

It is unwise to wait indefinitely for the birth of the second child by reason of the possibility of fetal asphyxia from some aberrant circulation, one cord having been ligated, or because the cervix may contract, making a second dilation necessary before the birth of the second child, which may be impossible for the fatigued and inert uterine muscle.

Complications of Labor in Multiple Pregnancy.—Toxemia. Postpartum hemorrhage as a result of overdistention and inertia of the uterus.

Infection from long labor and operative interference.

Dystocia from locking of twins (rare).

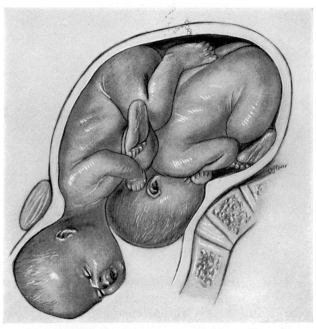

Fig. 242.—Mechanism of labor in twins, both vertex presentations. Delivery of the first twin.

The complications from the standpoint of the babies are:

Toxemia.

Asphyxia from anomalies of placental circulation.

Prematurity.

Injury from operative delivery or interlocking.

Toxemia is managed along the usual lines (q. v.).

Postpartum hemorrhage is avoided by the prompt administration of extract of pituitary gland 0.5 cc. and of a hypodermic preparation of ergot 1 cc. subcutaneously as soon as the last child is born. Packing should always be in readiness and should be used upon the first indication of postpartum hemorrhage.

Locked twins are quite rare. In case of one head and one breech presenting, the chins may become hooked. One child presenting by the breech may sit astride its fellow who lies transversely below it. In cephalic presentation, one head may become impacted against the thorax of the other child and so on (Fig. 243).

If interlocking occurs, the use of surgical anesthesia and the Trendelenburg position will usually enable the operator to ascertain the cause of the dystocia, and by pushing the upper child higher into the uterus, while the interfering parts are separated by gentle taxis usually results in successful delivery.

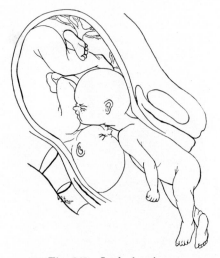

Fig. 243.—Locked twins.

It may be necessary, in rare instances, to perform embryotomy on one of the infants to permit the delivery of both. If the twins are unusually large, and there is true disproportion between them and the maternal pelvis, cesarean section may be obligatory.

Prognosis.—The mortality rate of the mother in multiple pregnancy is slightly increased because of the possibilities of severe toxemia, postpartum hemorrhage and infection.

The fetal mortality is more than double that of single pregnancies for the reasons before stated.

The mortality rate increases enormously with additional number of infants, being very great in triplets and quadruplets.

CHAPTER XXVII

MATERNAL ILLNESSES ACCIDENTAL TO PREGNANCY

ANY illness affecting the pregnant woman is prone to exert a more deleterious effect upon her than were she not pregnant. The added strain of carrying the mass of a fetus and its envelopes in utero, the physiological strain of providing for its nutrition and for the excretion of its waste products imposes a task upon the maternal organism which greatly diminishes its ability to overcome infection or to compensate for degenerative processes. Any disease may occur as a complication of pregnancy, some being acquired after conception and other more chronic conditions may antedate pregnancy by years.

The more common and important diseases in connection with pregnancy will here be briefly discussed. For further details as to the complicating agents the reader is referred to works on internal medicine.

THE ACUTE INFECTIOUS DISEASES

Influenza.—Until 1918 influenza was regarded as a serious complication of pregnancy by reason of its overwhelming toxemia and its tendency to hemorrhagic lesions but the mortality rate was low and abortion was not a frequent sequel to an attack.

In the epidemics of 1918 and 1919, however, the whole picture changed and influenza became the most fatal complication of pregnancy which had yet been known. The mortality among pregnant women was about 28 per cent and in those in which pneumonia supervened the mortality rate reached the appalling figure of 56 per cent.

Abortion occurred in from 30 to 80 per cent according to whether pneumonia developed or not. Since this pandemic the virulence of the influenza epidemics has again abated so that at this time the disease is usually limited to respiratory irritation, malaise, angina, moderate fever and considerable toxemia, all of which symptoms clear up within a few days.

The treatment of influenza in pregnancy is purely medical, but it should be remembered that the patient is profoundly toxic and that anesthesia and trauma will not be well borne, consequently labor, should it come on, must be managed in as conservative fashion as possible, with an avoidance of any operative interference unless that is absolutely necessary.

In the event of an epidemic of the disease, pregnant women should be isolated in their homes, or be sent away from the affected territory as a prophylactic measure because of the increased sensitivity to influenza which is brought about by pregnancy.

Lobar Pneumonia.—When pneumonia is in association with pregnancy, each condition exerts a deleterious action upon the other. The embarrassment of respiration due to the pneumococcic process is aggravated by the diminished excursion of the diaphragm on account of the uterine mass.

On the other hand the disturbed circulation, the high temperature and the toxemia always so evident in pneumonia, tend toward fetal death and toward the induction of premature labor.

It would seem that the termination of pregnancy would favorably influence the course of pneumonia, but such is not the case, the mortality in a series of terminated cases being about four times that of a similar group in which the gestation continued uninterrupted. It is true that the terminated cases may have suffered from a more virulent attack, of the disease, but here again, the rule holds the toxic, ill women do not tolerate trauma well, and the surgical termination of pregnancy necessarily involves considerable tissue injury.

Treatment.—Pneumonia with or without pregnancy is a medical matter, and a competent internist ought always to be called in consultation upon such a case. The recently developed sera have done something to improve the mortality in certain types of pneumonia if used early enough, and the coexistence of pregnancy, is no contraindication to their use. Oxygen should be used early to assist the limited respiratory area.

The Common Cold.—This ubiquitous infection is capable of exerting much harm during pregnancy, since as a result of it, a latent toxemia may spring into undesirable activity, a pyelitis may develop, or less seriously, the patient may be much vexed by a tendency to dribble small amounts of urine under the strain of coughing or sneezing.

Indeed, if the cold be associated with a pharyngitis or bronchitis, the paroxysms of coughing and sneezing may cause premature rupture of the membranes with ensuing labor.

As in all the acute infections, prophylaxis is the dominant note in the treatment. Pregnant women should keep away from crowds when colds are prevalent and if attacked, they should remain in bed for twenty-four to forty-eight hours, following any of the standard plans for treatment.

Inhalation anesthetics are contraindicated during colds because of the preliminary congestion produced and the consequent increased probability of pneumonia setting in. The medical treatment varies widely and may be said to be generally unsatisfactory, though we have had some success in the control of this annoying condition by the early use of morphine in fairly large doses. One-fourth grain of morphine sulphate, being exhibited hypodermically and repeated at intervals of four hours for three or sometimes four doses, sometimes completely inhibits the spread or continuance of the symptoms.

Morphine in pregnancy has no deleterious effect upon the fetus unless labor comes on while the patient is narcotized, when resuscitation may prove difficult.

Acute or subacute bacterial endocarditis may occur in the course of pregnancy and is usually fatal, either as a result of blood stream infection, toxemia, or as the development of pulmonary or central embolism so characteristic of the condition.

Pregnancy is usually ended by the death of the mother, although there are recorded cases wherein living children were born during the course of the disease. Some of these babies were normal and healthy, others showed foci of bacterial growth in heart, brain, lungs or cord, as a result of placental transmission of the pathogenic bacteria.

Typhoid Fever.—With the advent of municipal water filtration, and the development of vaccination, typhoid fever has become an unusual complication of pregnancy, rather than the commonly noted one of forty years ago.

It is probable that the clinical course of typhoid is not much altered by pregnancy, although the onset of labor exerts a decidedly untoward influence upon the prognosis.

On the contrary, typhoid fever is very destructive to the fetus, and greatly increases the probabilities of abortion, premature labor, or the delivery of a stillborn child. The infant suffers by direct placental transmission of the bacteria of typhoid to the fetal blood stream, from the hyperpyrexia and from the toxemia of the mother, which is induced by the disease. The management of typhoid in pregnancy is that of its treatment in those nonpregnant. Prophylactic vaccination should not be done during pregnancy except when contact has been proved, or during an epidemic.

Hydrotherapy is of great value in limiting the excessive fever which is in itself so dangerous to the child. After delivery the infant should be removed from the mother to avoid infection via the milk or possibly the hands.

Diphtheria is common in pregnancy. With prompt antitoxin treatment the course is usually that of the disease in the nonpregnant woman. It is important that transmission of the bacilli to the pelvic organs be prevented, since dangerous genital infection may occur. If cardiac complications set in, pregnancy may have to be terminated with a minimum of trauma.

Malaria.—In malarial districts, or where there is a known latent infection, prophylactic doses of quinine are indicated early in pregnancy, and again near term and immediately after labor. Since quinine exerts a powerful oxytocic action, it must be exhibited in small and frequent dosage, rather than the massive amounts which may produce abortion by the high blood concentration of the drug (3 to 5 grains, three times daily).

Ordinarily malaria is not a serious complication but the more virulent strains of the plasmodium may be responsible for abortion and premature labor, with fetal death from toxemia and insolation.

Placental transmission has not been definitely proved.

Pertussis.—Whooping cough, though not often found in the pregnant woman, is a serious complication in that the paroxysmal coughing causes abdominal distress and may lead to abortion. The insomnia caused by the coughing also tends to exhaustion of the woman, which in one case in the care of the author, became so marked as to necessitate the termination of pregnancy.

Encephalitis Lethargica.—In the unusual instance when the disease comes in pregnant women, the chief difficulty lies in the diagnosis. The lethargic state must be differentiated from beginning coma of toxemia.

Most patients are delivered at term without evidence of painful sensations during labor, while occasionally cesarean section may be necessary.

Induction of premature labor sometimes exerts a favorable effect upon the course of the disease. The mortality rate compares with that of the nonpregnant adult.

Erysipelas, cholera, undulant fever, anthrax, indeed any of the infectious diseases may occur in association with pregnancy but there seems to be no special effect of the interrelationship except probably a greater tendency to abortion.

THE EXANTHEMATA

Smallpox.—The great French obstetrician, François Mauriceau, was born pitted with smallpox, his mother having had the disease some six weeks before his birth, and many additional and less conspicuous cases are on record to prove the placental transmission of the virus of variola.

Pregnancy seems to cause an increased susceptibility to smallpox which is apt to take on the severe hemorrhagic form and carry a high mortality rate. Interruption of pregnancy is common, and the child is apt to show signs of having contracted the disease, or it may escape altogether.

It seems true that vaccination of the mother does not confer immunity on the infant or if it does the effect is transient.

Smallpox is uncommon in the United States and is usually ignored in prenatal care. However in the event of any hint of the disease being reported in the neighborhood, the expectant mother should be vaccinated at any stage of pregnancy, the only real contraindication being severe nephritis. Regardless of the vaccination immunity of the mother, the newborn infant should be vaccinated unless it be in poor condition. The percentage of successful takes in the newborn is very high (80 to 90 per cent).

The treatment of the disease is not altered by the coincidence of pregnancy.

Scarlet Fever.—Scarlatina is so rarely found among pregnant women that this state is believed to confer immunity from the disease.

Occasionally infection does occur and is marked by the usual angina, glandular swellings in the submaxillary region, fever and the regular erythematous eruption, with definite desquamation.   Whether true intra-uterine infection of the child occurs or not is still a moot point, though several apparently irrefutable cases have been reported. Interruption of pregnancy, with a high fetal death rate from prematurity, toxemia, and hyperpyrexia is the rule when the pregnant woman does acquire scarlet fever.

In the puerperium, it becomes difficult to determine whether a erythematous eruption with attendant constitutional signs is true scarlet fever or is a manifestation of a streptococcic puerperal infection.   The differentiation may be aided by the knowledge of whether the pelvic structure or the throat was first affected.   There is generally a two-day interval between the initial rise of temperature and the appearance of the suggestive rash.

If during this interval, the uterus is tender and subinvoluted, and the lochia scant, while the throat is clear, the infection is probably of pelvic origin, whereas if the throat is first affected, true scarlatina is probably present.

In either event, after another day or two both throat and pelvis react to the infection.   It is held that an attack of scarlet fever even in childhood protects the woman in some measure against puerperal sepsis, but this is still subjudice.

Measles.—Uncommon during pregnancy, measles usually brings about prompt abortion as a result of the high temperature, the fetal mortality being over 50 per cent.

Instances of placental transmission have been observed, the infant being born with the characteristic skin eruption.   The dangerous sequelae of pneumonia and puerperal infection increase the gravity of measles, complicating pregnancy.   If a living child be born it carries immunity from the disease during the first years of life.

Varicella.—Chickenpox is rare in pregnancy and generally runs its usual mild course.   Occasionally abortion occurs, and sometimes babies present the skin pustules, denoting placental transmission.

THE CHRONIC INFECTIONS

Tuberculosis.—The reaction of existing pulmonary tuberculosis to the advent of pregnancy has for a long time been the subject of great medical controversy.   Du Bois said, years ago, "If a woman threatened with phthisis marries, she may bear the first accouchement well; a second with difficulty, a third never."   This sage remark is still correct in the main, although the modern sanatorium treatment has lessened the harshness of the conclusion and some women can bear three or more children under especially favorable conditions.

Just why pregnancy should effect tuberculosis unfavorably is not quite clear but probably the increased respiratory rate due to compression of the lungs by the increase in the intra-abdominal mass,

28

the extra strain and stress upon the system brought about by pregnancy and the exertion of labor, all combine to stimulate the activity of the tuberculous foci. When to these factors is added the strain of caring for the newborn baby, and the inability of the young mother to maintain the necessary rest periods, the solution is not far to seek. Women suffering from active pulmonary tuberculosis often show a distinct improvement in their condition, during the course of pregnancy, nor are the symptoms aggravated by labor and the early puerperium, but after six months the disease frequently becomes increasingly progressive and advances with great rapidity.

Tuberculosis has but little effect upon pregnancy, abortion and premature labor being uncommon except in the most active cases.

A number of cases of tuberculosis of the placenta are on record although placental transmission is uncommon, most children of tuberculous mothers being born free of the disease, but the definite number of babies infected in utero must be taken in consideration when planning the management of a case.

The fear that pregnancy will markedly aggravate pulmonary tuberculosis seems ill-founded in the light of careful statistical studies of large series. Forsner found that 86 per cent of first-stage cases, 75 per cent of second-stage cases and even 38 per cent of third-stage cases were either improved or stationary during one year's observation subsequent to confinement.

Barnes and Barnes state that 79 per cent of the incipient cases, 65 per cent of the moderately advanced cases and 28 per cent of the far-advanced cases improved during pregnancy.

Various other students of large case series have reported practically parallel findings. Of the children born to tuberculous women about 80 per cent are alive and well at birth.

The crux of the matter lies in the ability of the patient to maintain the sanatorium type of treatment during and for the first year after pregnancy. If she is economically able and willing to do this, there seems to be no adequate reason to deny her the right to motherhood. If unable or unwilling to subject herself to the rigorous discipline of tuberculosis therapeusis, the woman should not become pregnant, since the ordinary cares of motherhood and the exactions of a housewife's life will probably aggravate the condition. Termination of pregnancy is not indicated except in the very active cases whose progress is enhanced by gestation, and in such patients abortion should be done early, under local anesthesia and with great care to keep blood loss at a minimum level. In far-advanced cases, at or near term, the woman may not withstand the exertion of labor, and here cesarean section under local anesthesia offers the best hope of a living child and exposes the mother to the least danger.

If, in spite of intelligent treatment, the patient declines in health after delivery, subsequent pregnancies should not be attempted, tubal sterilization under local anesthesia being performed if necessary.

Sterilization by irradiation is to be avoided, since the psychic and physical disturbances of a premature menopause impair the success of treatment of the tuberculosis.

Tuberculous women should not nurse their children both by reason of the attendant physical drain of lactation and because the baby may develop tuberculosis from the close handling which nursing implies. About half the babies allowed to remain with and be nursed by tuberculous mothers acquire the disease.

Syphilis.—The discovery of the Wassermann reaction and the application of arsenic salts in the treatment have robbed "the great destroyer" of much of its terror. Before the advent of these measures, syphilis caused more stillbirths than all other causes combined and while it still ranks high on the list, the proportion has been immensely decreased.

The frequency of syphilis among pregnant women varies considerably with the locale and the nature of the group studied. In the clinic type of negro woman the incidence is somewhat around 15 per cent or higher, whereas the average clinic frequency in America is about 6 per cent.

In the Kensington Hospital for Women, located in an industrial district in Philadelphia, and whose clientele is almost all white women, syphilis occurs in 1.1 per cent of all clinic cases.

There are no clinical evidences of syphilis during pregnancy in over 80 per cent of women known to be infected. In the remaining one fifth, there are local lesions all of which effloresce under gestational stimulation. Chancres both of cervix and vagina grow rapidly, may become phagedenic and heal slowly. Secondaries enjoy a luxuriant growth. The skin lesions tend to become confluent, and if broken down the ulcers grow larger and deeper than in the nonpregnant state. Condylomata develop to large size, and the inguinal adenitis becomes very marked.

Generally, however, the pregnant syphilitic is only recognized by the positive serologic reaction. The disease does not seem to affect pregnancy in relation to other complications which may occur, although, occasionally, toxemia may be aggravated or even made manifest by vigorous treatment with arsphenamine.

The great significance of syphilis in pregnancy resolves about the fate of the child. In untreated cases the premature delivery of dead and macerated fetuses may reach 60 per cent, and McCord found lues as the cause of death in 57 per cent of fetal autopsies. The prognosis for the child depends upon the duration of the maternal infection; those women who have had the disease for years giving birth to the greatest number of living children who present slight evidences of lues, whereas in recent infection, especially during the secondary stage when the spirochetae are circulating freely in the blood stream, the child is extremely prone to fall a victim. When the syphilis is acquired after the twentieth week of pregnancy the infant may possibly escape entirely, although this is rare.

The Mechanism of Intra-uterine Infection.—It is now generally held that direct paternal transmission does not occur, but that the disease is acquired by the mother and from her reaches the fetus by way of the placental circulation, and it follows that every woman, the mother of a syphilitic child, is herself syphilitic, and the converse is also probably true, although there are cases in which an apparently healthy child has been born of a syphilitic mother. Most of these children later present stigmata of the disease, but a few never do, and seem to confirm the old law of Profeta.

The spirochetae have been demonstrated in the decidua, the placenta, the umbilical cord and the fetal tissues, but not before the sixteenth week of pregnancy. There may be intrapartum infection of the child from active early lesions in the genital passages.

Syphilis has frequently been referred to as an hereditary disease but, strictly speaking, it is a congenital infection, capable of transmission from one generation to another.

It has been thought that fetal malformations result from old infections or are parasyphilitic manifestations; but this is an error since postmortem examination of monsters and other malformed infants fails to reveal the existence of a syphilitic infection with any greater frequency than in those not so malformed.

Maternal syphilis is not often responsible for early abortion as was formerly thought, except when the infection took place shortly before conception, when the embryo usually dies early and is aborted. The general course is late abortion—after the sixteenth week, and if the patient remain untreated, subsequent pregnancies proceed for longer and longer periods before delivery takes place, until full-term macerated fetuses are born, followed eventually by the delivery of a full-term living child, which usually does, but may not, present the typical lesion of congenital lues. The diagnosis of syphilis is made upon the elicitation of a positive Wassermann or Kahn reaction, which procedure should be carried out on all pregnant women. In private practice this is sometimes difficult, but loss of infant life and the unchecked progress of lues in the mother too often results from failure to exclude the possibility of its presence.

Effect of Syphilis upon Labor.—In most instances the course of labor is not altered by the existence of syphilis. Malpresentations are found as a result of the mobility of the premature and macerated fetus. Occasionally uterine inertia, failure of a fibrous cervix (the so-called "wooden cervix") to dilate and subinvolution are noted.

Syphilis plays little or no rôle in the causation of puerperal sepsis or maternal morbidity.

Treatment.—The resources of antiluetic therapeusis must be utilized to the full in the management of syphilis complicating pregnancy and the life and well-being of the infant is the chief consideration.

Naturally the mother will benefit by treatment, but in her case cure may be deferred until the child is born. Modern arsphenamine treatment has accomplished the happy result of increasing the number of nonsyphilitic children of infected mothers from about 30 per cent to nearly 100 per cent. In one series of cases, every child was free from lues as a result of adequate treatment of the mother during pregnancy.

Three general principles are essential:

1. Every syphilitic gravida must be treated as soon as a positive diagnosis is at hand. Previous treatment or latency of the disease does not alter the rule.

2. The earlier in pregnancy treatment is begun, the better the prognosis for the child.

3. The patient must be closely observed during treatment, in order to prevent possible renal damage. Arsenicals may not be administered in the presence of preeclamptic or eclamptic toxemia.

The medical treatment consists of one, two or three series of injections of arsphenamine, from 6 to 10 injections being given during each series. The initial dose is usually 0.3 Gm. slowly increasing to 0.6 Gm. The arsenic is supplemented by the injection of one of the heavy metals, mercury or bismuth, suspended in oil a few days after each exhibition of arsphenamine and the treatment should be continued to term, regardless of whether the Wassermann reaction has been affected or not.

Hemorrhagic Encephalitis.—One of the dangers of antisyphilitic treatment during pregnancy is the sudden development of acute hemorrhagic encephalitis which is generally fatal. Four such cases were found during the survey of the Philadelphia County Medical Society on maternal deaths in that city, and Plass has recently reported three more.

The symptoms generally appear from a few hours to several days after the injection of an average dose of neoarsphenamine. There is usually early evidence of involvement of the central nervous system, with vomiting, and headache, or dizziness, followed by tonic and clonic convulsions, coma and death. There may be prodromes noted, after previous treatments, as headache, nausea and slight elevation of temperature. In women far advanced in pregnancy the symptom-complex is not unlike that of a fulminating eclampsia, for which the condition may well be mistaken.

The pathological picture, on autopsy, is that of an acute arteritis of the cerebral vessels, with minute punctate hemorrhages, sometimes with edema of the brain.

There is no available treatment, the cases being almost always fatal. It is probable that pregnant women are more susceptible to arsenical toxemia than are other individuals, the susceptibility being more marked according to Plass during the first course of therapy, in latent syphilis, and during the last trimester of pregnancy.

Prophylaxis demands a careful selection of the drugs and the dosages utilized in the treatment of syphilis in pregnant women.

Syphilis Neonatorum.—The effect of syphilis upon the fetus varies considerably, from early fetal death leading to abortion, premature stillborn and macerated fetuses, living children with active manifestations of the disease to full-term babies born without clinical evidence of lues.

In those fetuses born alive, the skin lesions, especially those around the orifices, and on the palms and soles, are most characteristic. Snuffles may be present, and one may demonstrate a large liver or spleen.

Where the product of conception is stillborn or subsequently dies, careful examination, both gross and microscopical and by the *x*-ray, will reveal information of diagnostic and other value. The roentgen examination of the long bones of the older fetuses often shows characteristic pictures of osteochondritis syphilitica. The spirochete seems to disappear rapidly from dead tissues unless incubated. It is the one absolute evidence of the presence of this infection, though there are pathologic changes in the older fetuses and their annexa, which are almost pathognomonic.

The tissue changes which are found occur not only in the fetus itself, but also in the placenta and umbilical cord. Grossly, there is no single constant change which can be regarded as pathognomonic. It has been thought that the ratio between placental and fetal weight is about 1 to 4 in syphilitic, as compared with 1 to 6 in nonsyphilitic fetuses. Attention should be called to the fact that while there is a definite correlation between placental and fetal weight, the ratio is not constant and the placenta is relatively heavier for premature than for mature fetuses. The placenta is sometimes of a pale, pinkish, somewhat mottled appearance, with red and yellowish-white patches. It often has a rather greasy appearance, and, at times, seems softer and more friable (Fig. 244).

The cord shows no characteristic gross changes, though, microscopically, one finds evidence of endarteritis and thrombosis, together with the presence of the Treponema pallidum. Similar changes occur in the vessels of the placenta, and the spirochetes are found both in the maternal and fetal portions of the placenta. Fränkel's disease of the placenta is apparent when the villi are teased in salt solution; they are found to be club-shaped and to have lost their arborescent appearance. Williams found that characteristic placental changes checked with the clinical findings in from 80 to 90 per cent of the cases. These consist of the clubbed villi described by Fränkel together with endarteritis, often with obliteration and proliferation of stroma cells, the latter indicated by the presence of numerous round and plasma cells together with fibroblasts.

Cutaneous changes are frequently observed and are somewhat modified, but are not unlike those seen in acquired syphilis. The primary lesion is rarely seen but may occur in cases where the infection takes

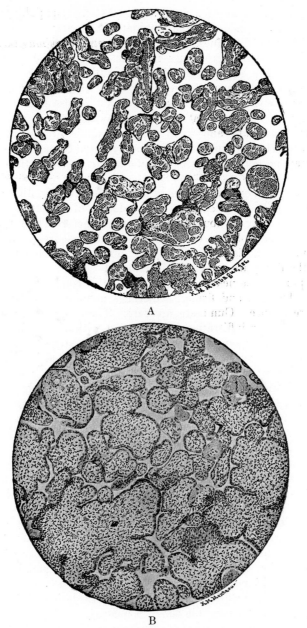

Fig. 244.—Normal (A) and syphilitic (B) full-term placenta. (Williams, "Obstetrics," D. Appleton-Century Co., Publishers.)

place as the fetus passes through the birth canal. Maceration is common in stillborn fetuses and this process affects the skin, as well as other structures. Various observers have found syphilis present in from

25 to 80 per cent of their macerates. Macular, papular, vesicular, bulbous, pustular, nodular, and gummatous cutaneous lesions may all be found in congenital lues. The mucous membranes may be similarly affected. The skin accessories may be involved and more or less alopecia, onychia, and paronychia may result (Figs. 245, 246).

The liver and pancreas frequently show changes due to syphilis. The liver is usually heavier than normal and is also firmer and shows some alteration in color, at times to brownish-red or greenish hue. The color may vary and small opaque granules, representing small miliary tubercle-like gummata, may be scattered through its substance. There may be perihepatitis or gummata, but, usually, the surface is smooth.

Microscopical examination may show some retarded differentiation, with embryonic liver columns and islands of hematopoietic cells. Treponemata may be found in edematous spaces. There are foci of lymphocytic and plasma cell infiltration and less frequently there is pericellular cirrhosis. There may be miliary or isolated gummata, though the latter are especially uncommon.

The pancreas is nearly always involved in congenital syphilis. It is larger, heavier, and firmer, sometimes nodular, and cuts with increased resistance. Gummata are rare. There is more or less characteristic cellular infiltration between and within the lobes and lobules, which causes separation of the glandular structures.

The respiratory tract is very commonly affected, and rhinitis is frequently seen; this may proceed to ulceration and necrosis. The larynx and trachea may be involved. The lungs are frequently involved, and show increased size and weight, with a mottled grayish-white and reddish appearance. They cut with increased resistance. Gummata rarely occur. Pneumonia alba consists mainly of interstitial fibrosis, with desquamation of alveolar epithelium.

The heart may be large, small or dilated. Involvement of the endocardium may occur and the myocardium may show fatty and other forms of degeneration. Miliary and larger gummata have been noted.

Degenerative changes occur in the walls of the vessels, associated with endarteritis and periarteritis.

Gummata of the kidney have been described. Areas of lymphocytic infiltration occur in and beneath the capsule and between the tubules of the kidney.

The more characteristic changes are a retardation of development with a persistent "neurogenic zone," a persistence of new formation of perivascular myeloid cells of a nongranulated type. The principal changes, consisting of perivascular cellular infiltration, occur mainly in the cortex of the kidney.

The central nervous system, including the dural membranes, may show vascular changes, cellular infiltration, and rarely gummata. The spleen shows a quite constant increase in weight. There is a hyper-

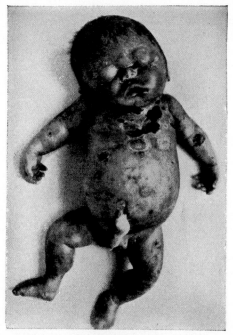

Fig. 245.—Stillborn child with generalized hydrops and papulopustular syphilid. (Reuss in Halban-Seitz, Biol. u. Pathol. d. Weibes, vol. 8.)

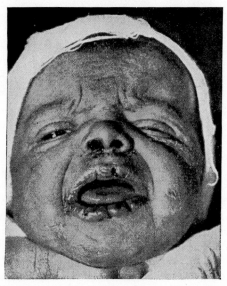

Fig. 246.—Fissures at mouth of congenitally syphilitic baby; also crusts at nose from luetic coryza. (From Riecke, Lehrb. d. Haut- u. Geschlechtskr., 8th ed., Jena, 1931.)

plasia, fibroid changes occur, and gummata have been described. Amyloid degeneration has been found.

The thymus shows some changes which have been known as Du-Bois' abscesses. They are often found in syphilitic fetuses and are supposed to be derived from Hassall's corpuscles.

The suprarenals also show vascular and infiltrative changes and are one of the organs in which the spirochetes can be most easily demonstrated.

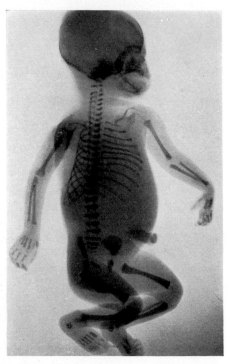

Fig. 247.—Syphilis neonatorum. Note the blurred and velvety appearance of the epiphyses of the long bones, especially the femora.

The skeletal system is most important from a clinical and a pathologic point of view. The cartilaginous bones are commonly affected before birth.

Wegner (1870) seems to be the first to have described the most typical changes of osteochondritis syphilitica. This is the most constant osseous change, as well as the most characteristic, in fetal syphilis. It is due to retarded osseous development with irregular cartilaginous and bony proliferation associated with cellular infiltration. It can be demonstrated grossly as a yellowish, irregular, saw-toothed line at the osteochondral junction of the long bones. It can frequently be shown by the x-ray, in both the living and dead fetus, and it is of considerable diagnostic value (Fig. 247).

There is usually more or less anemia, with a persistence of normoblasts and some leukocytosis, affecting especially the myelocytes and the eosinophils. It has been noted by Adair, and others, that some types of hemorrhagic disease of the newborn are syphilitic.

The special sense organs are sometimes affected, with resultant deafness. Iritis, cyclitis, keratitis, one or all, may occur to produce impaired or lost vision, if the fetus survives.

DISEASES OF THE CARDIOVASCULAR SYSTEM

Heart Disease in Pregnancy.—There is always increased cardiac effort during pregnancy. The weight of the growing uterus, the increased blood volume, the displacement of the heart to a more nearly transverse lie and the embarrassment of respiration due to lung compression by the higher position of the diaphragm, all combine to compel a greater cardiac effort in order to maintain the circulation. Healthy hearts bear this strain without difficulty on account of the enormous factor of safety arranged by nature. Even where considerable heart damage impairs the function of that organ, the majority of women withstand pregnancy and labor without cardiac failure.

Several series of pregnant women with heart disease have been carefully studied and the type of cardiac disability found is similar to that in other groups of young persons, not pregnant.

Rheumatic heart disease furnishes over 90 per cent of all cases, congenital lesions account for about 2 per cent while the rest is made up of various uncommon heart diseases. Of the rheumatic heart disease cases, mitral stenosis is present in the vast majority, mitral stenosis and aortic regurgitation following in frequency.

Cardiac patients make up about 1 to 2 per cent of maternity hospital clientele.

The Effect of Heart Disease upon Pregnancy.—Cardiac damage does not affect fertility, so that many cardiac patients become pregnant—abortion and premature labor are not common unless in terminal cases with congestive heart failure. The incidence of toxemia is not increased nor do these women show any peculiar tendency to give birth to monstrous and deformed infants.

The Effect of the Pregnancy upon the Heart Disease.—Much unnecessary alarm has been felt in the past concerning the prognosis of childbearing in women with heart disease. This is largely due to the fact that the less serious cases were not diagnosed and classified so that statistics were made up from severe cases only.

Nevertheless in the 717 deaths studied in the Philadelphia County Medical Society's survey, there were 16 (2.2 per cent) in which heart disease was a primary factor and 69 (9 plus per cent) in which it was a factor.

In maternities where close study is given patients and where heart lesions are carefully evaluated, the death rate should be well under 6 per cent more nearly approaching 3 per cent.

The vascular complications of pregnancy are much aggravated by coincident heart disease, edema, varicosities, hemorrhoids, etc., being much more frequent.

However, many cardiac patients, indeed a great majority, withstand pregnancy and labor well and are in no worse case after the completion of the puerperium than they were before conception took place.

The Management of Heart Disease in Pregnancy.—The first essential is a correct diagnosis. Hence careful estimation of the capacity and condition of the heart should form a part of the prenatal examination of every patient. In private practice, if the physician is not expert in cardiology, a competent heart specialist should be consulted with regard to the cardiac condition and its prognosis, in view of the established pregnancy.

In maternity hospitals, a cardiac clinic or at least the availability of a consultant cardiologist is an absolute essential.

The diagnosis having been confirmed, the next step is to evaluate the patient as an obstetric risk.

Bad risks are those women who have (a) at the time of examination, congestive heart failure, (b) those who give a history of attacks of decompensation, (c) those who have or have had auricular fibrillation, (d) those who have an accompanying complication as profound anemia, great obesity, nephritis, etc., (e) women with definite heart lesions, who are over thirty-five years of age, (f) those who have had recent manifestations of acute rheumatic fever.

Borderline Risks.—(a) Those women who have definite heart lesions, who have successfully emerged from one pregnancy and who have apparently been uninjured in the process.

(b) Those in whom attacks of congestive heart failure occurred years before but who have since improved.

(c) Women whose heart symptoms improve rapidly under rest and possible digitalization.

Good Risks.—Women with heart lesions who are and have been comparatively symptom-free.

The Management of Bad Risks.—If discovered before pregnancy has occurred such women should be advised not to become pregnant, the dangers of childbearing being clearly described to them and to their husbands. Unfortunately every obstetrician can recall instances where after having been fully enlightened as to the danger, a woman insists upon her right to maternity whether or not the effort costs her her life.

If pregnancy is already present, the bad cardiac should be advised to have the pregnancy terminated, by the vaginal route if before the third month, by abdominal hysterotomy with or without tubal sterilization if after the third month.

When for religious or personal reasons an advanced cardiac patient insists upon going through with pregnancy or when the woman first presents herself after the child is viable, she should be kept under the closest supervision, in bed, preferably in hospital for several weeks before labor, and be delivered by cesarean section under local anesthesia, after digitalization, if indicated.

If decompensation has occurred, the treatment consists of prompt digitalization by the administration of tincture of digitalis in doses of 30 minims at four-hour intervals until slowing of the pulse, diuresis, and regularity of rhythm indicate that the therapeutic effect has been obtained, when the dosage may be appropriately reduced.

Morphine in full doses, $\frac{1}{4}$ grain hypodermically, sometimes gives great relief and if pulmonary edema, cyanosis and marked dyspnea be present phlebotomy with the withdrawal of 500 cc. of blood is highly beneficial.

It is important that operation be deferred until recovery from an attack of congestive heart failure is fairly complete, since patients undergoing operation for delivery while decompensated have but small chance for recovery.

After delivery these women must be kept in bed until all cardiac symptoms have greatly improved and then be kept under close supervision for a long time.

The Management of the Better Risk.—These women, apprised of their condition, are instructed to report immediately any danger signs as hemoptysis, yawning, dyspnea, auricular fibrillation, tachycardia, etc. They should be seen at least once weekly during pregnancy and at the slightest sign of heart failure, especially râles at the base of the lungs, must be confined to bed at once.

If no obstetrical complications are noted, they may be allowed to go into labor spontaneously and delivered according to indication.

Cardiac patients do not have shorter or easier labors than other women and delivery should be expedited in the second stage, if any symptoms of heart embarrassment develop.

Local vaginal and cervical infiltration with novocain 0.5 per cent solution is valuable in these cases, and if complete anesthesia is required, ether is probably as safe as any inhalation anesthetic. Under such management, the mortality of pregnant women suffering from heart disease will be reduced to a minimum.

Arterial Hypertension.—Usually an elevated blood pressure presages toxemia of some type, but occasionally one comes upon cases of essential hypertension in young women, which is not markedly affected by pregnancy. One of the author's cases presented herself pregnant for the first time with a systolic pressure of 160 mm. of mercury which pressure prevailed during this and three succeeding pregnancies, utterly unaccompanied by symptoms. The woman, now in middle life, is perfectly well and still carries her high pressure. Now under observation is a young woman of twenty-four, a primigravida with a pressure of 150 mm. and a record of a similar elevation, recorded at each of her four annual physical examinations while a college student. Here again there are no symptoms.

It is probable that these patients eventually develop cardiorenal disease, but there is no treatment suggested during pregnancy.

Hypotension.—The normal range of systolic pressure in pregnancy is from about 110 to 130 mm. Certain women persistently present a pressure of 100 mm. systolic or less. These patients are usually easily fatigued, somewhat depressed and very possibly have long slow labors from ineffective uterine contractions in the first stage.

Other than this the low pressure has no apparent significance and treatment is limited to the administration of tonics as tincture of nux vomica, etc.

Varicosities.—Varicose veins of the lower extremities are quite common in pregnancy, and masses of varices in the labia are often seen.

The underlying cause of these lesions is somewhat difficult to explain, especially since women note marked variations in their extent during different pregnancies.

It is probable that increased intra-abdominal pressure plays some part, the increase in the total quantity of the blood in pregnancy and the embarrassment of circulation which is often found in connection with them being also responsible.

Varicose veins in the lower leg are easily controlled, by elevation of the limb at intervals and the wearing either of a well applied elastic bandage, or one of the elastic stockings in common use.

When the varicosities are on the thighs, however, they sometimes cause considerable annoyance and pain and are difficult to treat. The old type of men's long, machine-knit underdrawers, cut off at the knee, offer excellent support, and are more convenient than bandages because of the difficulty in adjusting the latter to this region.

Varicosities of the vulva usually require no treatment during pregnancy, but in labor they may rupture, with profuse and, in one case of the writer's, alarming hemorrhage. The torn veins in the labia, with blood clot lying in the loose alveolar tissue, offers a fertile field for infection and should be carefully cleansed with antiseptic solution. If the hemorrhage is slight it may be controlled by simple pressure, but if severe, ligation of the individual bleeding veins must be performed.

Varicosities rarely break down during pregnancy, but sometimes as the result of a blow, rupture occurs with subsequent ulceration. The ulcers are treated by cross strapping with adhesive plaster in the usual manner.

Vaginal varicosities are rare, but sometimes appear, usually on the lateral aspects of the vagina, and may become so large that cesarean section is indicated as the method of delivery, in order to obviate possible dangerous hemorrhage and infection from rupture of the enlarged veins.

Varicosities tend to disappear shortly after delivery and may or may not recur in succeeding pregnancies.

Phlebitis.—Phlebitis is uncommon during pregnancy, but may occur in the veins of the leg as a result of local injury. There is no tendency to an extension of the process but the danger of secondary embolism requires that the affected part be kept at rest. Moist heat with a snugly fitting compress and bandage is the only active treatment required.

Hemorrhoids.—Pregnancy frequently induces the development of hemorrhoids which may be exceedingly annoying, and tend to become much worse during and after labor. Rectal surgery is contraindicated at this time, but if a clot forms in an external hemorrhoid, incision and turning out of the clot may be necessary. If swelling and pain are severe, protruding internal hemorrhoids should be pushed back behind the sphincter with a well lubricated gloved finger, and a pad saturated with tincture hamamelis applied with an ice-cap over it.

When the acute symptoms have subsided an astringent ointment containing powdered opium, tannic acid and ichthyol often gives great relief.

℞ Pulv. opii	1 gr.
Acid. tannic.	10 gr.
Ichthyolis	1 ℥
Petrolat.	q.s. ad 1 ℥

Regulation of habits of defecation is of course indicated.

Edema.—Mild edema of the lower extremities may be expected during the late months of pregnancy as a result of increased intra-abdominal pressure.

If the edema involves the face and hands, water retention is probably present and the cause is usually a beginning toxemia of some type (*q. v.*).

DISEASES OF THE BLOOD

The Anemias.—A moderate grade of anemia is so common in the later months of pregnancy that it has been termed physiologic. This does not seem a reasonable conclusion, and the anemia (hemoglobin of 70 per cent or somewhat less; erythrocytes 3,000,000 to 3,500,00) is more probably due to the change in life habits and diet of the pregnant woman and should be regarded as a pathological manifestation. The blood picture usually returns to normal within a few months after delivery and the condition is rarely a serious one. From the standpoint of the hematologist, much space might be given to this subject, but for the obstetrician, the simple classification of Mussey is completely satisfactory. Practically all pregnancy anemias belong to one of two types of secondary anemia.

Type I, the most common, is apparently due to a deficiency in the activity of the bone marrow. There is a moderate reduction of erythrocytes with a parallel decrease in hemoglobin. The erythrocytes may show polychromatophilia and slight hypochromasia.

Type II.—Here there is a proportionally great reduction in the hemoglobin, resulting in a marked hypochromasia. It has been shown that Type I begins during early pregnancy and though the bone marrow become more active in the later months, the blood picture does not improve, probably as a result of the presence of some hemolytic, toxic agent. Recovery is usually prompt, after delivery. Type II anemia is generally present prior to pregnancy and persists indefinitely after delivery.

The treatment of both types consists in the administration of iron in some form. Blaud's mass, 10 to 15 grains per day, ferric ammonium citrate or ferric citrate 20 to 30 grains three times daily, or ferrous sulphate 12 grains daily usually brings the blood count to a satisfactory condition. Extracts of liver, stomach and bone marrow are not of special value. A well balanced diet and abundant fresh air and sunshine are essential.

True pernicious anemia is a very rare complication of pregnancy, probably always antedates conception but is aggravated by the additional strain.

The management is that of the disease in the nonpregnant state.

Leukemia is also rare, only a few cases being recorded. It is probable that pregnancy exerts a deleterious effect upon the disease. More than half the mothers die and the infant mortality is equally high.

Cases have been reported in which roentgen ray treatment improved the mother and resulted in the birth of living children, but irradiation is so dangerous to the child in utero that early termination of pregnancy is probably wise.

Purpura Hemorrhagica.—Another rare coincidental disease in pregnancy with over 50 per cent maternal mortality, increasing to nearly 100 per cent if the pregnancy goes to term. A small proportion of the children of purpuric mothers develop the disease.

Hodgkin's disease is rare, but the disease may be treated by the *x*-ray and living children result. Termination of pregnancy is not indicated if irradiation therapy is available, though again, the dangers to the child must be remembered.

Polycythemia, aplastic anemia and splenic anemia have been recorded in association with pregnancy but are very rare.

DISEASES OF THE RESPIRATORY SYSTEM

The infectious respiratory diseases have been considered already.

Asthma.—Preexisting asthma is often greatly improved during pregnancy, whereas some patients who have never been troubled by this annoying condition develop it only while pregnant, securing relief promptly after delivery. In these cases a toxic or allergic agent is probably causative. Sometimes chloride retention is responsible, when a salt-free diet brings prompt relief.

The usual treatment by adrenalin or ephedrine is generally successful in abating the attacks, but in one case in the author's clinic, the dyspnea was so constant and exhaustion, from insomnia, so profound that therapeutic abortion was found necessary. In a subsequent pregnancy this patient had practically no return of the asthma.

Immunization against allergic substances may be undertaken during gestation, but possible protein shock must be carefully avoided.

Acute and Chronic Bronchitis.—In the winter months severe bronchitis may be a source of great distress to the pregnant woman. The constant coughing compels involuntary urination, and by the sudden spasmodic increase of pressure against the lower uterine segment, may cause premature rupture of the membranes with labor following. Late in pregnancy severe dyspnea accompanies spasms of coughing. The treatment is absolute rest in bed for a few days, until the acute phase has passed, with the usual remedies to allay cough and the topical exhibition of counterirritants.

Tonsillitis.—Runs its usual course during pregnancy, but should be noted as producing a possible focus which may cause autogenous infection during the puerperium.

Tonsillectomy may never be performed on the pregnant woman, although the drainage of a peritonsillar abscess may be imperative.

DISEASES OF THE ALIMENTARY SYSTEM

Gingivitis.—Inflammation of the gums with bleeding occurs in more than one third of clinic patients and in a somewhat smaller number of women living under conditions of better dental hygiene. The affection usually comes on early in pregnancy and persists, even under treatment until term.

This so-called "pregnancy gingivitis" may assume one or a combination of four forms:

(a) Simple bleeding from the gums under toothbrush trauma.

(b) The free margin of the gums, especially anteriorly, becomes of an irregular, raspberry appearance.

(c) The hypertrophic form in which the swollen and bright red gum papillae grow down and from a sort of sheath over a considerable portion of each tooth.

(d) A single growth, resembling an epulis, reaching several centimeters in diameter.

All these forms are likely to recur with succeeding pregnancies, and the cause is unknown except that there seems to be some connection with the profound endocrine development in pregnancy. Gingivitis is sometimes very annoying, giving rise to bleeding and pain upon brushing the teeth or masticating food.

Treatment.—Careful dental hygiene, gentle cleansing with clean toothbrushes and the free use of an astringent mouth wash as tincture myrrh or a solution of sodium perborate. Attention to carious teeth is important since many of these patients present neglected mouths.

Dental Caries.—It has long been held that dental caries is greatly increased during pregnancy and the old adage "for every child, a tooth" has received the sanction of laymen and obstetrician alike. There is, however, but little authentic evidence upon which to base such a conclusion.

An investigation recently carried out by Mull and Bill is so important and convincing in this connection that it is freely quoted here. These writers studied over 300 prenatal patients at regular intervals during pregnancy, confirming many of the findings obtained upon oral examination, by *x*-ray. Their conclusive findings are as follows:

There is no appreciable change in the teeth of women during pregnancy, or the first few weeks of lactation other than that which would probably occur in a similar group of nonpregnant women during the same period of time. Only 15 per cent of the cases studied showed change.

The levels of the calcium and inorganic phosphorus of the serum of the pregnant woman bear no direct relation to the condition of her teeth.

The vomiting experienced during pregnancy does not seem to have any effect on the incidence of dental caries.

Bacillus acidophilus was not found to be consistently present in the mouths of pregnant women, nor was it always maintained throughout the term of pregnancy in those mouths in which it has been found earlier.

There was no increase in the titrable acidity of the saliva of women during pregnancy.

A general laxity in the oral hygiene was observed, especially following delivery. This condition would probably not be true in other social groups, and may or may not have any bearing on the condition of the teeth.

There is no rise in the average number of missing and carious teeth with the number of pregnancies experienced. There is a distinct increase, however, with age. Examination of the teeth of unmarried women showed them to be no better than those of women who had borne one or more children.

It is evident that there is no connection between pregnancy and tooth decay.

Digestive Disorders.—"Heart burn" and gaseous indigestion are very common nervous complaints, often persisting during the entire course of pregnancy, and very rebellious to treatment. Often they are associated with some measure of toxemia, often not so. The treatment is to some extent dietary, the patient being advised to experiment with various types of food—carbohydrates, proteins, and fruits, sugars, etc., in an effort to ascertain which, if any, produce the disturbance.

Mild antacids as heavy magnesia, soda bicarbonate, or some of the elegant proprietary combinations are valuable, as is the aromatic spirits of ammonia in teaspoonful doses, well diluted. If a nervous element exists, the bromides sometimes give relief. Abundant rest and dry meals, with free water drinking between meals sometimes aid.

Appendicitis.—It is stated that 2 per cent of cases of appendicitis in women occur during pregnancy, but in my experience the number is much smaller. It does seem that gestation has a tendency to activate a previously diseased appendix into acute inflammation.

In the last four months of pregnancy the cecum with the appendix has been pushed upward, until it may be found on a line above the brim of the pelvis. The cecum is also rotated outward to some extent.

The onset of an attack of acute appendicitis during pregnancy is similar to one occurring under other conditions, but as many women suffer from more or less distress in the right lower quadrant while pregnant, the initial symptoms may excite no alarm.

The diagnosis of appendicitis in pregnancy is sometimes confusing because of the leukocytosis of pregnancy and because of the gastric disturbance so common at this time.

Sudden pain, at first over the appendix, somewhat higher than usual, then extending to the umbilical region and finally becoming general, with rigidity of the right rectus and vomiting, together with a mild fever, 100° to 101° F., should permit the diagnosis to be made. If there is a history of previous attacks, the probability is increased that acute appendicitis is the cause of the symptoms.

Differentiation from acute pyelitis must be made always (*q. v.*). When the appendix has ruptured, general diffuse peritonitis is usually the result because the abnormal position of the cecum, coupled with the intermittent contractions of the uterus, renders walling off and the formation of a closed appendiceal abscess improbable.

The management of appendicitis in pregnancy is very definite. *Immediate operation as soon as even a reasonable certainty exists is the only safe rule,* and the incision should be ample. The removal of the unruptured appendix does little harm to the patient and only occasionally results in abortion. The ovaries should never be handled during the laparotomy since even lightly touching the corpus luteum seems to favor the onset of labor.

After operation the patient should be given generous amounts of morphine to quiet the irritated uterus. When the appendix has already ruptured, the problem is far different. Peritonitis in pregnant women is often fatal, and leads to premature labor, with extension of the infection to the pelvic organs.

Hysterotomy should never be attempted in the course of such condition, but the widely open and drained abdominal wound should be strongly protected with gauze pads and an adhesive corset, and the uterus left to empty itself or not as the case may be. A woman known to have had definite attacks of appendicitis should be advised to have the appendix removed before entering upon pregnancy.

Intestinal Obstruction.—Sometimes occurs from any of the usual causes during pregnancy. It is a very dangerous complication and the avoidance of mortality consists in prompt recognition of the lesion and equally prompt operation.

Cholelithiasis and Cholecystitis.—Gallstones are present in many older pregnant women, possibly because of the hypercholesteremia which is present then.

Symptoms may occur at any time but are more often noted during the later months, and treatment may generally be limited to medical measures until the completion of the puerperium.

If imperative symptoms develop—progressive jaundice, empyema of the gallbladder—surgical interference must be practiced and the pregnancy allowed to take care of itself.

Gastric Ulcer.—Happily the combination of peptic ulcer with pregnancy is uncommon but when it does exist the association is very grave indeed. The hyperemesis so characteristic of the early months causes great gastric congestion and consequent aggravation of the ulcer. Alarming hematemesis is the rule with death following all too often. Medical treatment is of little avail by reason of the vomiting and surgery is impossible because of the constant excessive peristalsis.

Prompt termination of pregnancy with subsequent treatment of the gastric condition is the only solution.

When a gastric ulcer ruptures during pregnancy the usual signs and symptoms are present, peritonitis develops rapidly and the absolutely necessary surgical intervention is rendered difficult by reason of the inability to secure proper exposure in the presence of the enlarged uterus which curves the abdominal viscera upward.

Constipation.—The old definition of woman as a constipated biped with a backache is nearly true in pregnancy, constipation being so frequent a complaint.

Treatment.—Regular habit of defecation is the first essential, and this with a diet consisting largely of vegetables and fruits plus copious water drinking, mineral oil or a combination of agar and oil is valuable.

If these measures do not suffice, the continuous use of laxatives may be necessary. Milk of magnesia ½ to 1 ounce at bedtime, the effervescent sodium phosphate in drachm doses on arising, small amounts of fluidextract of cascara sagrada are the laxatives in general use. Drastics must be avoided.

Enemata of soap suds, or a small (3- to 4-ounce) mineral oil injection which is allowed to remain in the rectum over night often give great relief.

DISEASES OF THE URINARY ORGANS

Nephritis has already been considered in its relation to the toxemia of late pregnancy but it must be remembered that nephritis may be active and severe, yet not produce characteristic toxic symptoms even though the advent of pregnancy may affect the preexisting kidney lesion unfavorably.

Acute nephritis may develop at any time as a result of exposure to cold and wet, as a sequel to one of the acute infections or possibly as the result of poisoning by a drug used as an abortifacient. The symptoms and management are those of the disease in general.

Chronic Nephritis.—Either the parenchymatous or the interstitial variety may be present, the former evidenced by widespread general edema, albuminuric retinitis, etc. This type of nephritis may and frequently does produce eclamptic symptoms, but may not. Labor exerts a bad influence upon the disease, and such patients should not undergo pregnancy.

Chronic interstitial nephritis is that form characterized by great hypertension and by a polyuria of low specific gravity. This condition is apt to produce abortion, premature labor, and stillborn or toxic babies. It may, but does not necessarily cause eclamptic symptoms. Abruptio placentae is often seen among these women.

Prognosis.—The mortality of both mother and child are high in nephritis, DeLee giving the figures as 30 and 70 per cent, respectively.

Management.—A woman known to suffer from chronic nephritis should only marry with an understanding that child-bearing is not to be attempted.

If the disease is discovered early in pregnancy, prompt termination offers the best prognosis to the mother, but there are women who insist upon their right to maternity even at their own expense. Under such circumstances the patient must be guarded against exposure to cold, a salt-free diet is directed, and the bowels are kept active. After the seventh month, if the nephritis is being unfavorably affected by pregnancy, labor should be induced, by medical induction plus rupture of the membranes, or if the occasion warrants, cesarean section under local anesthesia gives excellent results. It is better to have a premature baby not yet profoundly saturated with toxins, than a puny full-term child which has been in imminent danger of intra-uterine death for weeks before birth finally occurred (see Chapter XVII).

Pyelitis.—Purulent inflammation of the kidney pelvis is very common among pregnant women and my own experience leads me to believe that its frequency is rather increasing. The disease may occur at any period of gestation but is most frequently noted at the beginning of the sixth month and also near term. It may develop during the puerperium but this is less often noted.

Etiology.—The onset of pyelitis is preceded by a period of urinary stasis. This is brought about by a combination of two factors. There is invariably marked dilatation and kinking of both ureters during pregnancy, the right one being more markedly altered. There is also a dilatation of the pelvis and calyces of the kidneys. Furthermore, there are always hypertrophy of the muscular coat of the ureter, edema, increased vascularity and hypertrophy of the ureteral sheath of Waldeyer; all of which are thought to be of hormonal origin (see Chapter VII).

The second factor in producing stasis is the pressure exerted upon the already softened ureter by the rapidly growing uterus. The right ureter is more affected because of its more exposed course, because of the dextrotorsion of the uterus, and because the left ureter is cushioned by the sigmoid. The pressure is caused by the uterus itself, not the fetal head. Urinary stasis is probably followed by infection of hematogenous origin, from distant foci, and because the constipation so characteristic of pregnant women increases the tendency to passage of the Bacillus coli communis, from the bowel into the blood stream.

Ascending infection from residual urine in the bladder is also a possible cause.

Pathology.—The lesion is that of a pyelo-ureteritis, the parenchyma of the kidney escaping injury in the majority of cases although a true pyelonephritis may develop. The offending bacteria are the colon bacillus most often, though the staphylococcus, streptococcus and indeed any pus-producing organism may be responsible.

Symptoms and Course.—Pyelitis in pregnancy may be acute or subacute. In either case there may be a short period of urinary irritability preceding the onset. One or both kidneys may be affected, either synchronously or the disease attacks the second kidney some time after its occurrence in the first. The right side is much more frequently the seat of the lesion. The attack is ushered in by sudden malaise, dull pain in one or both lumbar fossae, a sudden sharp elevation of temperature usually accompanied by a chill. There may be vomiting, and vesical tenesmus. These is a leukocytosis ranging from 10,000 to 30,000, and while the urine may remain unchanged for a few hours, it soon contains many clumps of bacteria, pus cells, erythrocytes, albumin and much epithelium and cellular débris.

On inspection the urine is cloudy with a heavy sediment.

Sometimes the ureter becomes obstructed, from swelling or urinary débris, with anuria on the affected side. Distention of the kidney, sometimes palpable, together with severe pain, indicates this happening. The temperature becomes septic in type with wide daily fluctuation and the chills may be repeated every day or two.

These acute symptoms may persist for from two to six or eight weeks and are usually rapidly alleviated after delivery, although pyuria may persist for a considerable time.

Continuance of fever, pain and leukocytosis after the birth of the child bespeaks serious damage to the kidney itself and should be investigated carefully.

Subacute Pyelitis.—This is merely a milder form of the same condition and is characterized by bladder irritability, with possibly a slight nightly elevation of temperature, together with pus and bacteria in the urine. The subacute form may continue for a longer period than the acute, and has a tendency to persist longer after delivery.

Diagnosis.—The characteristic onset, the uniformity of the initial chill, lumbar tenderness and the discovery of pus and bacteria in the urine should render the diagnosis simple.

Differential Diagnosis.—There is great possibility of confusing right-sided pyelitis of the acute type with appendicitis and the differentiation between the two conditions is most important.

PYELITIS IN PREGNANCY	APPENDICITIS IN PREGNANCY
Onset generally after the fifth month.	Onset at any time.
Attack often preceded by several days of vesical irritability.	Not so.
Onset sudden, with high temperature (103° to 105° F.), high leukocytosis and chill.	Onset preceded by several hours indefinite abdominal pain, temperature rarely high (101° F.), leukocytosis moderate, chill uncommon.
Pain in lumbar region, radiating down course of ureter.	Pain in umbilical region becoming localized in right iliac fossa.
Rectus rigidity slight if any.	Rectus rigidity pronounced.
Vomiting inconsequential.	Vomiting and nausea a prominent symptom.
Urine contains bacteria, pus, blood and albumin.	Urine may contain a trace of albumin.
May palpate thickened right ureter.	Not so.

Treatment.—Prophylaxis is limited to eliminating the constipation so prevalent among pregnant women, and to encouraging the drinking of abundant quantities of water.

Treatment of Acute Pyelitis.—Absolute rest in bed, an ice-cap to the head and warm covering during the chill are essential. Opiates may be necessary to control pain. A bland liquid diet for the first few days with an excess of water.

Moderate purgation by saline laxatives reduces the bacteria-laden intestinal contents. Colonic lavage is useful.

Elevation of the foot of the bed lifts the kidney in its pouch and straightens the ureter to some extent, so permitting free egress of urine, and in cases of right-sided pyelitis, placing the woman on her left side tends to correct the dextrotorsion of the uterus and thus favors drainage.

Periodical reversal of the reaction of the urine is a valuable aid. Alkalinity is secured by administering sodium bicarbonate 30 grains every four hours, or sodium citrate may be used. After four days, the urine is rendered acid by the administration of sodium acid phosphate, or ammonium chloride in 10-grain doses, four times daily, the process being repeated several times. Hexamethylenamine, by liberating formalin in the urine is a much used drug, although its value is problematical.

In persistent cases small doses of neoarsphenamine (0.1, 0.2 Gm.), intravenously once weekly for two or three weeks, has proved of value in my clinics.

When the colon bacillus is the causative organism, the administration of an autogenous vaccine made from the urine has proved of distinct benefit, especially in refractory cases of long duration.

Ureteral catheterization, with or without flushing of the kidney pelvis with solution of silver nitrate 0.5 per cent, cupric sulphate 1 per cent, etc., is a measure of great importance when the disease is severe. Some authorities feel that the catheter may remain in place for several days, but in my experience this results in ureteral damage, and one hour is about the limit of safety for the indwelling catheter.

Very rarely it becomes necessary to incise and drain the kidney pelvis, through a lumbar incision to secure adequate drainage (pyelotomy).

If the disease continues severe, and drainage to the kidney parenchyma is feared, the pregnancy may be terminated but this is very seldom necessary.

Prognosis.—Most patients recover from pyelitis in a few weeks, and of the remainder the great majority are promptly cured by the advent of labor.

Occasionally the condition is unusually persistent and tends to recur after any infection as influenza, the common cold, etc., such recurrences sometimes coming on periodically for several years. One should suspect pyelonephritis under these conditions and investigate accordingly.

Abortion occurs sometimes as a result of pyrexia and infection but is an uncommon complication, which usually results in rapid relief of symptoms.

DISEASES OF THE DUCTLESS GLANDS

The Thyroid.—The thyroid gland has long been associated with the sexual functions, the connection being even the subject of Roman Law. Recent observations seem to deny any such connection. Marine in particular asserting that there is no cellular hyperplasia unless the iodine supply or the available thyroid hormone be inadequate. Nevertheless clinical evidence supports the older view, although the thyroid enlargement may be merely a temporary congestion.

There is a normal rise in the metabolic rate in the later months of pregnancy (plus 20, plus 25) which is thought to be due to the added heat production of the fetus.

Colloid Goiter.—In goiter regions colloid goiter is common because of the iodine deficiency. The enlargement may have been present before conception, or may first appear in the early months. In the latter case iodine administered in small doses, either direct or as iodized salt, will prevent further growth. Recrudescence to some extent takes place after delivery, but some swelling usually remains and the goiter may resume growth later.

Cretinism and congenital goiter in the infants is common in goiter regions, and the routine administration of iodine to the mother during pregnancy is essential in these areas to prevent this sequel. On the Atlantic coast colloid goiter is uncommon and the precaution is unnecessary.

Surgical intervention is rarely indicated during pregnancy,

Adenomatous Goiter.—The same general principles apply here as to colloid goiter, although thyrotoxicosis is more common in this variety.

Hypothyroidism.—A deficiency in the basal metabolic rate of 25 or more is not an uncommon cause of sterility, and should always be considered in the investigation of these cases. Administration of thyroid extract in small doses (¾ grain daily) is often surprisingly successful in promoting conception in these women. Hypothyroidism in the mother is always a potential cause for cretinism or congenital goiter in the infant, and thyroid therapy must always be maintained during pregnancy.

Hyperthyroidism and Toxic Goiter.—Sterility is the rule in advanced states of hyperthyroidism, but in quite a few instances the disease may have been incipient until stimulated by the general change of pregnancy. In my experience the symptoms of thyrotoxicosis are much aggravated by pregnancy, with special exacerbation occurring during labor. In view of the probable heart damage if the thyroid lesion is not corrected, either prompt surgical intervention or x-ray therapy is indicated in all cases wherein the basal metabolic rate and the symptoms show definite increase during the first few months of pregnancy.

It is true that patients sometimes recover completely after the puerperium but these cases are in the minority and one cannot predetermine which will progress to a dangerous degree and which will recede.

Thyroid surgery today is so safe and the results so uniformly good, that it is the procedure of choice in these patients. Roentgenological treatment is steadily improving and in the hands of an expert the results in hyperthyroidism are excellent. In the Kensington Hospital for Women, x-ray treatment has been the choice of the staff for the past two years, with uniform satisfaction.

In the milder cases and as a preoperative measure, the use of iodine as Lugol's solution 10 to 20 minims daily is indicated.

In the advanced cases, with serious cardiac damage, cesarean section under local anesthesia is sometimes, but uncommonly, required. Termination of pregnancy may be necessary, but rarely so.

It is commonly held that pregnancy should be interdicted for two years after partial thyroidectomy, but the writer has observed two patients who conceived within less than a year after the operation and who both went through an uneventful gestation and delivery.

Diabetes.—Since the introduction of insulin, sterility is no longer the rule in diabetic women, and prenatal clinics note an increasing number of patients who have been or are under treatment for the condition.

During the early weeks of pregnancy there may be some difficulty in stabilizing the carbohydrate metabolism, but in the later months the sugar tolerance is often greatly increased, a phenomenon held to be due to a supplementary insulin supply from the pancreas of the fetus.

The two complications of pregnancy noted in diabetics have been hydramnios and a tendency to oversized babies. Abortion rarely occurs, and termination of pregnancy is not often required.

Close attention to the blood sugar and the usual dietary and insulin treatment should be carried out punctiliously in these women, when pregnancy and labor will generally pursue a normal course.

Diseases of the parathyroids and adrenals are rare in pregnancy, and little authoritative information concerning these glands in pregnancy is available. One case of adrenal shock, with almost total disappearance of systolic blood pressure, occurred after a normal labor at Kensington Hospital. The symptoms were promptly relieved by the administration of adrenalin (no cortin being at hand) and within two hours the patient had completely recovered, the blood pressure rising to normal.

Tetany.—Parathyroid insufficiency manifests itself in a syndrome called "tetany," in which tonic spasms of the muscles of the arms and legs occur, sometimes accompanied by great pain and occasionally by unconsciousness.

Irregular paresthesia, pain and numbness in the hands, together with trophic disturbances, cataract, falling of the hair and nails, sometimes occur. Chvostek's sign may be present.

Tetany is generally aggravated during pregnancy by reason of the calcium deficiency which is usually present. Labor is not altered, although there seems to be a tendency toward fetal death in utero toward the approach of maternity.

The treatment consists in the free use of calcium, the lactate or gluconate being administered in doses of 60 to 80 grains daily.

THE DEFICIENCY DISEASES

Pellagra.—A disease of the southern states; is due to a lack of vitamin B in the diet. Pregnancy and lactation encourage the development of the disease which is marked by diarrhea and persistent stomatitis, together with symmetrical erythema of exposed portions of the skin. Delirium sometimes is present. The treatment consists in the free administration of brewer's yeast.

Scurvy and beriberi are uncommon in pregnancy, although the former is often seen in infants.

Scurvy may follow drastic dietary restriction, but the relief is prompt following the usual citrus-fruit antiscorbutic management.

Osteomalacia is a disease very rare in America but well known in southeastern Europe and China. It has many close relationships with rickets (blood chemistry and nervous symptoms), but is now thought to be due to a deficiency in vitamin D.

Osteomalacia is an adult disease, the youngest patient on record being eleven years old.

It has been thought that some ovarian dysfunction is causal and certainly complete arrest of the disease is secured by castration.

The pathology consists of an osteomyelitis and osteitis involving the whole thickness of the bone, with an absorption of the calcium salts and then replacement by an osteoid substance.

The bones become very flexible and exceedingly vascular. The skeleton becomes almost unbelievably deformed, the limbs bent and distorted, the pelvis irregularly contracted, the spine curved. The disease usually appears during pregnancy, with bone pains, increasing weakness and the early skeletal deformities.

Treatment.—Calcium, cod liver oil and viosterol, foods rich in vitamin D, and sunshine, are the important measures. Cesarean section may be necessary to secure delivery, with castration, if the disease appears progressive.

DISEASES OF THE NERVOUS SYSTEM

The Gestational Psychoses.—This term is in some sense a misnomer, since careful study has shown that pregnancy per se is not a cause of mental change. The associated toxemias are often responsible, and also important is hereditary predisposition toward insanity and neurosis, with exhaustion and nerve strain playing a part

Pregnant women do not infrequently suffer from some form of psychosis, it being stated that from 3 to 4 per cent of all female first admissions to psychopathic hospitals are connected with the pregnant state. R. R. Wilson presents an excellent classification of these conditions:

I. Gestational psychoses:
    a. Pregnancy psychoses.
    b. Toxic states with mental disorders.
    c. Functional disorders.

II. Postpartum psychoses:
    a. Toxic states with mental disorders.
    b. Functional disorders.

GROUP I.—(a) Pregnancy psychoses occur more often in first pregnancies and usually consist of mild and transient emotional states of confusion, melancholia and insomnia, manifesting strong tendencies to spontaneous recovery before gestation is completed.

True dementia praecox may develop during pregnancy or may be precipitated into activity by it. Manic depressive insanity may occur rarely. (b) Toxic states with mental disorders usually occur late in pregnancy and are usually seen in association with eclampsia, pre-eclampsia and some other varieties of toxemia.

The etiology remains in doubt, though hyperpituitarism seems a possible factor. Manic depressive forms, mild or severe confusional insanity and, sometimes, a particularly rebellious melancholia characterize these toxic psychoses.

Group II.—Postpartum psychoses exhibit predominantly the factors of poor heredity and less significantly the elements of toxemia and exhaustive states. Exciting factors are more frequently such accidents as death of the child, improperly conducted labor, severe mastitis, and even domestic situations. More multiparae fall into this group than primiparae.

(a) Toxic states with mental aberrations postpartum often reveal the source of the toxemia only after prolonged study. Most cases run a self-limited course and make complete recoveries, but exhibit tendencies toward recurrence under similar or equal stress when again encountered.

(b) Functional disorders occurring postpartum represent a pathetic group. This includes the paranoic, the schizophrenic, the manic depressive, and the epileptic. Pregnancy as an entity has no peculiar influence in these cases other than it offers a situation of unusual stress. On the other hand, parturition in the insane seems to be remarkably free of puerperal sepsis, difficult labor or accidents of delivery. There seems to be a prevalent impression, however, that episodes initiated by pregnancy have a worse prognosis than if precipitated by other general causes. The number of cases in this group should be relatively small. It is difficult to state that insane women have a reduced fertility, but it is well known that an appreciable number have amenorrheic tendencies—both factors seemingly would contribute to a relatively decreased fertility.

Treatment.—Pregnancy psychoses, other and indeed, including the toxic group, belong in the domain of the psychiatrist and should be turned over to him for management. If a toxemia is causative and present, its treatment by the obstetrician is that of the particular toxemia in general, with special care that the irresponsible patient does not harm herself or anyone else.

If the mentally deranged person is in a maternity hospital, great care must be taken to prevent attempts at suicide, or even homicide. It is far better to have such women transferred to a hospital competent to manage psychiatric cases.

Diseases and Injuries of the Peripheral Nerves.—Mild neuralgias are common in pregnancy, toothache, pain in the sciatic region and trifacial neuralgia being often sources of complaint. Various nerves may be injured from the pressure of the fetal presenting part in spontaneous labor, but more commonly as a result of operative deliveries. Paralyses of the femoral, the sciatic and the peroneal nerves are reported, with much pain and paresthesia and sometimes motor disturbances, foot drop, etc.

The diagnosis of nerve injury is made by the location of the pain and the motor lesions in the muscles supplied by the injured nerve trunk.

The treatment consists in rest, proper splinting, stimulation, massage, etc.

Hemiplegia.—Hemiplegia is rare in pregnancy, only some 30 cases being reported in the literature. The usual causes are the activation of the associated hypertension, embolism, hemorrhage and so on. There is no especial prophylaxis and no definite treatment other than that of hemiplegia in general.

Myelitis occurs, but the influence of pregnancy is doubtful, though it is true that recurring attacks in successive pregnancies have been reported.

The writer observed a case in which myelitis preceded the pregnancy which continued undisturbed, the patient going into labor, and being delivered spontaneously, absolutely without pain.

Epilepsy.—Epilepsy is not caused by pregnancy but is always preexistent. The severity and frequency of the attacks may be greatly improved by the advent of gestation, but in some instances are rendered more severe.

The important feature of this coincidence is the differential diagnosis, between an epileptic and eclamptic convulsion which is sometimes obscured by the fact that an epileptic woman develops eclampsia.

The history of preceding attacks and the urinary and blood pressure findings should clear up the diagnosis.

DISEASES OF THE EYE

Asthenia of the ocular muscles, and an enfeebled accommodation are often complained of by pregnant women and may require the temporary wearing of eyeglasses to correct the defects until full tone is restored after the puerperium which is usually the case.

Optic neuritis may be one of the manifestations of polyneuritis and lead to permanent blindness should the patient recover.

The really common and severe lesions of the eye are those induced by preeclampsia, eclampsia or nephritis.

Here retinal hemorrhages and detachment, albuminuric retinitis, simple edema, sclerosis of the retinal arteries, exudate formation and true optic atrophy all may be found in varying degrees. Naturally these processes generally develop during the last three months of pregnancy when the toxemia becomes well developed. The earlier eye lesions appear, the more severe the toxemia, and under these circumstances interruption of pregnancy must receive serious consideration, first because the toxemia is of so advanced a grade that the child will probably succumb before maturity and second because total blindness may render the mother a complete dependent, incapable of exercising her maternal duties.

Blurring of vision is usually the first sign of optic disease, but frontal headache and persistent spots before the eyes should warn the obstetrician to have the eyegrounds examined and to be on his guard to detect the early evidence of impending toxemia.

Severe hemorrhage may lead to blindness and ultimately end in optic atrophy. The usual prompt blood transfusion will tend to obviate this termination.

DISEASES OF THE EAR

Otosclerosis is sometimes accentuated by pregnancy and in two instances under my observation the disease began during a first pregnancy, underwent some improvement after the puerperium, to be much intensified by a second gestation with very marked and permanent deafness resulting. The presence of well-marked otosclerosis should actuate the patient to give serious consideration to the risk of deafness following further child-bearing.

DISEASES OF THE SKIN

Certain skin changes, as the areas of pigmentation on abdomen, face and mammary areola, are so universal that they are regarded as being physiologic as are the scars of the abdominal surface which mark the striae of pregnancy.

True inflammatory lesions do occur however, but not many are characteristic of pregnancy, or much altered in their manifestations by its presence.

Dermatitis herpetiformis (herpes of pregnancy) is a vesicular, bullous or pustular eruption, the lesions arranged in groups, which sometimes appear early in pregnancy grow worse after delivery, then promptly disappear, only to recur after each succeeding conception.

Nothing is known as to the nature of this disease, the treatment being purely empiric and directed at the symptoms of itching and burning.

Impetigo herpetiformis is an inflammatory disease of the skin characterized by the appearance of miliary pustules arranged annularly or in clusters, attended by constitutional disturbances, high fever and severe rigors, occurring usually in pregnant or puerperal women and generally being fatal.

The lesions are small, superficial pustules which come out in successive crops and are arranged in groups which heal in the center and spread by peripheral extension.

Together with the fever, dry tongue, albuminuria and delirium are to be expected, and the outcome is usually fatal.

The disease is thought to be of toxic or septic origin.

Treatment is based upon general supportive measures, and locally antiphlogistic lotions.

Pruritus.—Generalized pruritus may complicate pregnancy and render its course almost intolerable by reason of the intense and continued itching. It is said to be of neurotic origin, usually disappears after delivery and is amenable only to general sedative drugs and to the use of analgesic ointments or lotions externally. The administration of theelin hypodermically has seemed to improve some of my patients.

When pruritus is limited to the vulva an exciting bacterial cause as possibly the gonococcus or the Trichonomas vaginalis must be eliminated, and diabetic pruritus is also to be given consideration.

V. THE PATHOLOGY OF LABOR

LABOR has been defined as the resultant of two sets of forces; those of expulsion and those of resistance. The overpowering of the latter by the former results in spontaneous delivery, while if the reverse is true, complete obstruction to delivery takes place. Errors and anomalies in these forces, together with accidental complications, involving the mother or child or both, constitute the pathology of labor, which may be studied under three general headings:

1. Anomalies of the forces of expulsion.
2. Anomalies of the forces of resistance.
   (a) Pathological presentations.
   (b) Disproportion between fetus and pelvis of fetal origin.
   (c) Deformity of the pelvis causing disproportion of maternal origin.
   (d) Excessive resistance of the soft parts.
3. Other complications of labor—of both maternal and fetal origin.

CHAPTER XXVIII

ANOMALIES OF THE FORCES OF EXPULSION

THESE forces consist of the contractions of the uterus and secondarily the voluntary contraction of the abdominal muscles.

The uterine contractions may be faulty in (a) too feeble contractions, (b) too vigorous contractions.

Uterine inertia is a term used to denote inefficient contractions of the uterus, the error usually lying both in the quality of the individual contractions and the length of the interval between them. Primary inertia uteri may develop during any of the stages of labor, though it is most common during the first stage, largely because operative delivery is the rule when the cervix is fully dilated.

The causes of the inertia are many. Exhausting systemic diseases such as profound anemia or advanced tuberculosis may be responsible.

Overdistention of the uterus from hydramnios or multiple pregnancy, the muscular atony of rapidly repeated pregnancies, adiposity, relaxation of the abdominal walls with pendulous belly, faulty development of the uterus, all contribute their quota of cases.

The presence of tumors of the uterus, which interfere with the smooth rhythm of muscle contractions, and firm adhesions from previous laparotomies are local causes; elderly primiparae sometimes present this defective muscular action.

Goodall has described an inertia syndrome in which not only the uterus is atonic, but the colon and sigmoid become distended, the urinary bladder is paretic and even the stomach is sometimes involved. The syndrome according to Goodall consists of an abnormal rhythm and tone affecting the hollow viscera of the abdomen, chiefly uterus, bowel and bladder, causing a malfunction of all of these organs.

The cause lies probably in a disturbance of the autonomic system of the splanchnic area and, as the autonomic system is under the influence of the endocrine glands, these latter are the responsible agents. This conclusion is strengthened by the fact that many women suffering from inertia uteri conform to a so-called "endocrine type," being short, adipose and hirsute with many masculine characteristics.

Clinical Course.—Inertia uteri is prone to be preceded by several days of false labor; pains which may be quite severe for an hour or two and then disappear, only to return irregularly. When labor does finally begin the contractions possess the same qualities of irregularity and insufficiency. They are cramplike and annoying to the patient who feels that she is making no progress and is growing fatigued. If the membranes rupture prematurely, the pains may grow much stronger and become regular with the decrease in the size of the uterine contents, and labor go on to completion; or they may continue to be ineffective, in which case the uterus molds itself to the body of the fetus, which is in danger of asphyxia from pressure upon the cord. Thus hours may pass without any progress. Even with intact membranes, infection of the uterus is possible during long labor and when they have been ruptured, the probability of infection is much enhanced.

It follows then that repeated examination and vaginal manipulation must be avoided in inertia uteri.

The cervix dilates slowly, and after long hours of irregular pains may be found as an edematous ring, not well effaced and dilated only to 2 or 3 cm. The patient soon becomes exhausted, and vomiting, acidosis and dehydration evince a dangerous condition, which becomes rapidly worse as the temperature and pulse rate rise.

These eventualities occur more rapidly among weakened and ill women than in those of rugged constitution and great powers of vital resistance.

The fetus is in constant danger, not only from asphyxia, but from infection, and particularly from birth injuries inflicted during the course of a traumatic operative delivery.

Sometimes, in spite of inertia, the cervix becomes effaced and dilated and the head descends to about the level of the ischial spines. The pains continue to be weak and further descent and rotation ceases. At this stage the cord is under pressure, as is the fetal skull, crowded into the cavity of the pelvis, and unless operative delivery is performed fetal death is likely.

Finally, after delivery, the inertia may continue and the uterus fail to contract sufficiently to separate and expel the placenta, with grave danger of postpartum hemorrhage.

Diagnosis.—Diagnosis is based upon the fact that the uterus does not contract strongly and remains soft under the palpating hand, that the pains are irregular in length and intervals, that the woman while suffering is not in severe pain, and that at no time during the labor have these been strong, long, and regular.

Treatment.—The principles of management of inertia uteri are:

1. Maintaining the resistance and morale of the patient and securing rest for her.
2. The stimulation of the uterus.
3. Operative delivery when indicated.
4. The avoidance of infection.

1. Sleep, food, fluids, and relief from pain are desiderata to be obtained. When the woman begins to complain of fatigue, morphine sulphate (¼ grain) hypodermically is safe, if delivery is to be delayed for more than four hours. If less time is to elapse, ⅙ grain is safer for the fetus.

Abundant fluid nourishment, milk, broth, orange albumin, should be administered and if signs of acidosis are present with vomiting and dehydration, 50 Gm. of glucose in 10 per cent solution is given intravenously. After a refreshing sleep in a quiet, darkened room, the woman may awake to an active labor, with normal uterine contractions.

2. If, after the rest, the inertia persists, more active measures must be instituted. Before stimulation of the uterus has begun, a careful obstetric examination must be done. The pelvic measurements are rechecked, a vaginal examination made with the most rigid attention to asepsis will disclose any obstruction to delivery, either from pelvic deformity, disproportion or malpresentation. Auscultation determines the condition of the fetus by an estimation of its cardiac rate and rhythm.

If the birth canal is clear for the passage of a fetus which lies in a normal presentation and position, the uterus may be stimulated, even though the cervix is not fully dilated and effaced. The only drug of value here is pituitrin, the extract of the posterior lobe of the hypophysis cerebri.

Pituitrin may be given subcutaneously in doses of 2 minims every twenty minutes, until nine injections have been administered; the injections being stopped at once upon the occurrence of strong, regular pains. A better plan is the intranasal use of this substance. A small tampon of cotton with a thread bound about it to facilitate removal, is saturated with 0.5 cc. of pituitrin and placed in the nostril, well back to contact the middle turbinate. By this plan not only is the pressor and oxytocic action of the pituitrin increased, but upon any danger sign appearing, the tampon may be withdrawn, the nose flushed with saline and all action of the drug stopped immediately. In my hands pituitrin has been the agent of choice as well as of necessity, since quinine seems practically inert, and ergot may never be used by reason of its prolonged and powerful action.

Under this plan, pains tend to come on within ten to twenty minutes and become strong and regular. If not, the whole process can be repeated in twelve hours, since the effect of pituitrin is fugacious and noncumulative. The question of artificial rupture of the membranes, if these be intact, now arises. The capabilities of the uterus are always open to doubt, and if there has occurred a furtherance of cervical effacement and dilatation under the stimulus of the pituitrin, rupture of the membranes often causes the contractions to continue with unabated force, and allows of spontaneous, or outlet forceps delivery. Per contra, if the pituitrin has not acted well, if the cervix remains undilated, rupture of the membranes will only prepare the way for hour-glass contraction of the uterus, not to mention infection The problem now becomes one of securing cervical dilatation, and leads to

3. Operative Measures.—Rarely the cervix may be dilated manu-

ally, with the patient under surgical anesthesia, but this procedure is productive of so much trauma and infection and is so difficult of performance that it has been largely discarded.

The employment of the metreurynter or hydrostatic bag has general sanction under those circumstances. A large bag of the Barnes or Voorhees type is placed in the lower uterine segment under strict asepsis, filled with an antiseptic solution and a weight of about 1 pound attached to the tube. The cervix is irritated and uterine contraction stimulated. If after a few hours, the bag may be withdrawn from the cervix easily, or is spontaneously expelled, delivery may be completed by forceps or version.

The bag may also be used if the membranes have been ruptured for some time, without cervical dilatation, but here infection is even more to be feared.

In obstinate cases it may be necessary to replace an expelled bag with a larger one in order to secure sufficient dilatation. Occasionally the stripping with the finger, of membranes adherent to the lower uterine segment, will induce stronger pains and facilitate delivery.

Cesarean section is only rarely indicated.

4. *The Avoidance of Infection.*—The probabilities of uterine infection increase in almost direct ratio to the time elapsing after the rupture of the membranes, so that the obstetrician must be increasingly careful if premature rupture has taken place.

All vaginal examinations must be conducted with absolute fidelity to aseptic principles. The patient should lie with the shoulders elevated to favor postural drainage and, in long labors, it is good practice to instill an antiseptic solution into the vagina with a syringe every four hours. Metaphen 1:1000, mercurochrome 3 per cent or lysol 1:200 are commonly used preparations, but the writer prefers 5 per cent argyrol solution. Operative delivery must be considered as a major surgical operation.

Retained placenta and third stage inertia are not uncommon, and packing must always be at hand in these cases to combat faulty contraction after the expulsion of the fetus with the resulting postpartum hemorrhage.

Possibly manual removal of the placenta will be required, and here again the most rigid asepsis is demanded.

Summary of Treatment.—Haste is not obligatory in the treatment of inertia uteri. A long labor is not necessarily a pathological one, and in most instances these women eventually have strong uterine contractions and labor proceeds uneventfully.

During the period of insufficient pain, the morale of the patient must be maintained, abundant food and fluids are given, and periods of sedation and analgesia by appropriate medication, alternated with exercise, walking about the room, etc. The uterus may be stimulated by several doses of pituitrin (never more than 2 minims at a dose if given subcutaneously), and the contractions when established may be maintained by rupture of the membranes. Neither of these measures is permissible until the obstetrician is assured that no obstacle to delivery exists.

Operative delivery is delayed until the cervix has become fully dilated and effaced. Disregard of this principle usually spells disaster and the only condition under which it may be violated is sudden impending disaster to the mother or child.

The maintenance of asepsis must always be a first consideration and postpartum hemorrhage a complication to be borne in mind.

Secondary Inertia. Uterine Exhaustion.—When confronted with a patient in whom uterine contractions are feeble and irregular, the obstetrician must carefully differentiate between primary uterine inertia and exhaustion of the muscle. Whereas in the first instance stimulation of the uterus is indicated, in the second it is strongly contraindicated, since to whip up a muscle already fatigued by attempting to overcome insuperable obstruction is to invite rupture of the uterus.

The diagnosis is simple. A history of the labor will disclose a period of very powerful, long contractions, which continue until the uterine muscle becomes fatigued, loses first its contractile power and finally its tone, relaxing as a soft sac, through which the fetus may easily be felt.

Furthermore, vaginal examination of such a patient will almost always disclose some abnormality of presentation, pelvic deformity, or rigidity of the cervix which will account for the obstruction.

Treatment.—Rest for woman and uterus is the most important consideration. Morphine sulphate (¼ grain hypodermically), glucose intravenously and food and fluids by mouth are given. After the patient has had some rest, another examination will determine the method of delivery, whether forceps or abdominal hysterotomy offers the best hope for a successful outcome. Pituitrin or other oxytocic may never be used in managing uterine exhaustion.

The Use of Pituitrin in Obstetrics.—At first received with great acclaim, pituitrin has proved itself to be an agent of great potential danger, and has fallen into ill repute in many clinics, so much so that its use is often forbidden until the child has been born.

In large doses (0.5 to 1 cc.) pituitrin exerts a most powerful effect upon the uterine muscle. In from five to ten minutes after its subcutaneous administration, the contractions become vigorous, the uterus assuming boardlike rigidity at the height of a pain. The duration of the contractions is much increased, and the interval between them so shortened that they may be almost continuous. The effect begins to lessen in from twenty to thirty minutes and has practically disappeared after forty-five minutes.

If, occasionally, there is little or no effect, it is probable that the preparation used is inert.

Obviously so potent a drug must be used intelligently and certain contraindications at once present themselves.

1. Pituitrin should never be used when there is any mechanical obstruction to labor, as contracted pelvis, malpresentation, disproportion, scars from previous hysterotomy, tumors obstructing delivery, etc.

2. It should never be used to whip up an exhausted uterus, *i. e.*, in secondary inertia.

3. It should never be used in a primipara with a floating head.

4. Doses of more than 3 minims hypodermically are always fraught with danger.

Indications for the Use of Pituitrin.—1. To induce labor, in connection with castor oil, quinine and possibly the rupture of the membrane (*q. v.*) when it is exhibited in 2-minim doses given subcutaneously every twenty minutes until pain begins or 9 doses have been given. The intranasal administration is better.

2. To stimulate a case of primary uterine inertia, *when there is no mechanical obstacle to delivery.* The incompletely dilated cervix is not considered an obstacle in this method of using the drug. The dosage should be as above.

3. To terminate a labor when the head is crowning, and secondary abdominal contractions are not being utilized by a sensitive and uncooperative patient. Dosage as above.

4. After the child is delivered, to promote uterine contraction and placental separation. Here 0.5 cc. may be given with safety. Incarceration of the placenta by a cervix contracted by pituitrin has been reported but must be quite rare.

5. To control postpartum hemorrhage.

Dosage and Mode of Administration.—While the child is in the uterus, the maximum dose of pituitrin for subcutaneous injection should not exceed 3 minims, and 2 minims is better practice.

The injections should not be spaced closer than twenty-minute intervals.

Insufficiency of the Abdominal Muscles.—Primary insufficiency occurs in very fat women with poor musculature, in multiparae with diastasis of the recti and pendulous abdomen, in the presence of large herniae especially ventral herniae, or when the abdomen is much distended with fluid as in ascitic women.

Often nervous, hyperesthetic patients refuse to bear down and so cause voluntary insufficiency.

Secondary insufficiency results when a delicate woman has made unwise and violent efforts at expulsion during the first stage of labor, and the abdominal muscles become utterly exhausted, refusing to contract further even though the patient makes an earnest attempt to utilize their force. In women who have had an analgesic or anesthetic, the contractions are much weakened, although sometimes the action is quite strong and constant.

Abdominal wall insufficiency affects only the second stage of labor, which may be greatly prolonged, the head impinging upon the vulva for hours, without the completion of expulsion.

Management.—Analgesia will encourage the woman to bear down, who previously has failed by reason of her reluctance voluntarily to add to her agony.

The assistance of the nurse or obstetrician, by grasping the hands of the patient and exhorting her to pull powerfully, while she strains with closed lips, during the whole duration of the pain, is of much value as is the old-fashioned knotted sheet affixed to the footboard of the bed as a tractor. When the abdomen is relaxed and pendulous a firm binder applied from the costal margin to the pelvic brim affords a support to the muscles and aids contraction.

The exaggerated lithotomy position, the anterior surface of the thighs resting against the abdomen, also is of value. If in spite of these measures, delivery is delayed, by the insufficiency of the secondary forces, forceps extraction is indicated when the scalp is distending the pillars of the vulva.

Excess of the Powers of Expulsion.—*Clonic Spasm of the Uterus.*—Rarely labor is characterized by a succession of sharp short pains, ceasing for a few minutes and then recurring in similar grouped pains. This is said to be due to irritation of the cervix, as from attempts at forceps delivery before dilatation is complete. The pain is severe, and no progress results. The treatment consists in securing uterine rest by morphine (¼ grain) or better, adrenalin in hypodermic doses of 1 cc. of a 1:1000 solution.

Tetanus Uteri.—Also an uncommon complication due to faulty innervation of the uterus plus the action of an irritant, as manual dilatation of the cervix, the use of bags, premature rupture of the membranes, overdosage of pituitrin, etc.

The condition must be differentiated from obstructed labor. In the latter case, the uterus is firm, but has periods of relaxation and the pains are regular and strong. In addition, examination will reveal the source of the obstruction.

In tetanus uteri the organ is in a stage of constant contraction. Labor comes to a standstill although there is no real obstruction. The uterus is hard and boardlike, and the fetal parts cannot be felt through the abdominal wall. The patients suffer violent pain, sometimes becoming highly excited and even delirious.

On vaginal examination the cervix is hot and dry, and the uterus clasps the child so closely that the hand cannot be placed into the cavity. DeLee believes that spontaneous rupture does not occur in tetanus uteri, but that attempts at delivery may easily cause this accident. The child dies early as a rule and signs of maceration may be present.

Treatment.—Sedative treatment by morphine (¼ grain) and

adrenalin 1:1000 to 3 cc. is indicated but is seldom effective. Immediate delivery is the rule, great gentleness being necessary to avoid rupture of the uterus. Deep surgical anesthesia is an essential, ether or spinal anesthesia producing the most complete relaxation. If the cervix is not sufficiently dilated to permit intra-uterine manipulation the radial incisions of Duhrssen may be required. Delivery is accomplished by craniotomy or other form of embryotomy, it being rarely possible to secure sufficient relaxation for version or forceps delivery.

Sometimes abdominal delivery offers the only hope of success.

Contraction of Bandl's Ring.—Rarely one finds dystocia due to a tonic contraction of Bandl's ring. This isolated ring of muscle, lying between the upper and lower uterine segments, may undergo violent contraction while the parts above and below it remain flaccid. Sometimes the head of the child has passed the cervix before the contraction occurs and the shoulders are imprisoned behind the ring, rendering further progress impossible. Here adrenalin is of great value, but if relaxation does not occur under its influence, deep surgical anesthesia is required, to permit of delivery. Only rarely is cesarean section indicated.

Molding of the Uterus to the Fetus.—Sometimes after premature rupture of the membranes, and in neurasthenic primiparae, the uterus may adapt itself closely to the body of the child, with almost constant ineffective pain, but not the violent contractions of tetanus uteri. Labor comes to a standstill, and the woman rapidly becomes exhausted. Sedatives as above, and operative delivery with cervical incision if necessary is the treatment, which should be prompt if the child is to be saved.

Stricture of the Cervix.—Spasmodic stricture of the cervix either before or after the passage of the head has been described, but is very rare. Apparent spasm is more apt to be, in reality, imperfect dilatation in a cervix, the seat of much scar tissue. Anesthesia, with the possible use of the hydrostatic bag or cervical incision, may be necessary to complete the dilatation.

Precipitate Labor.—This accident is usually due to too strong contractions of the uterus, but sometimes may be the result of intense abdominal contractions after the head has passed through the cervix and is on the perineum. The force of the uterine contractions may be very great, cases being recorded when delivery was complete in a few minutes after the first pain, the cervix being forcibly dilated from within and the child expelled through an unprepared vulvar outlet.

The danger to the child from sudden compression of the head and intracranial hemorrhage is very great, while the mother usually suffers deep laceration of the cervix and extensive damage of the pelvic floor, sometimes involving the sphincter. On account of these lacerations, severe postpartum hemorrhage is to be feared.

Treatment.—Usually labor is over in these uncommon cases, before the obstetrician is in attendance. If labor should come on while the patient is under observation, prompt resort to inhalation anesthesia, preferably ether, will inhibit the contractions. After delivery, careful and formal attention to the maternal lacerations is of course necessary.

CHAPTER XXIX

ANOMALIES IN THE FORCES OF RESISTANCE-DYSTOCIA-DIFFICULT LABOR

PATHOLOGICAL PRESENTATIONS

ANY presentation other than that of the flexed occiput which lies in one or the other anterior quadrant of the maternal pelvis is regarded as abnormal. It is true that in many instances the occiput lies transversely or markedly posterior to the midline, eventually to rotate forward during the course of labor, thus being spontaneously converted in to a normal presentation.

In a considerable number of these cases, however, such anterior rotation does not proceed spontaneously and they are therefore to be classed as abnormal.

Errors in Flexion and Rotation.—The commonest malpresentations are those cephalic ones, in which correct and complete flexion and rotation do not occur. These are:

    (a) Posterior rotation, or persistently posterior position of the occiput.

    (b) The deflexion attitudes:

        Military presentation.

        Brow presentation.

        Face presentation.

POSTERIOR ROTATION OF THE OCCIPUT

This fairly common abnormality is found in about 5 per cent of vertex presentations and may be divided into:

(a) Primary and (b) secondary. The causes of primary occiput position are naturally those which interfere with the usual relations of the fetus to the pelvic inlet and are generally associated with some deflexion:

1. Minor degrees of pelvic contraction, especially flat pelves with asynclitism and failure of flexion.

2. Pendulous abdomen, the uterus lying so far anterior to the maternal spine that the convex surface of the fetal back may turn posterior.

3. Brachycephalus, the two lever arms of the fetal head being nearly of the same length, neither first meeting the resistance of the pelvis and flexion not occurring.

4. Negative disproportion, *i. e.,* a small child in a large pelvis, the usual forces of resistance in such circumstances being inoperative.

5. Prolapse of an arm in front of the occiput, the arm preventing forward rotation.

6. Deflexion due to tumors of the back of the child, or to fibromata in the lower uterine segment.

7. Uterine inertia.

Mechanism of Labor in Occipitoposterior Positions.—The cause of the greater frequency of primary anterior position of the occiput has already been explained, but in a considerable proportion of the cases the occiput enters the pelvic canal posterior to the midtransverse line of the brim.

Many statistics have been collected as to the position in which the head enters the pelvis but as Williams well says, they are of but

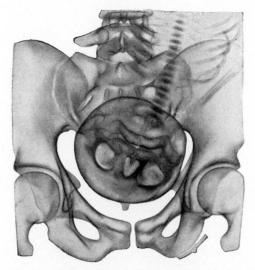

Fig. 248.—The primary position before the onset of labor (anterior view). (Caldwell, Moloy and D'Esopo in Amer. Jour. of Obstet. and Gynec., Dec., 1934, C. V. Mosby Co., Publishers.)

little value, since the conclusions reached depend so much upon the stage of labor in which the diagnosis was made.

Many observers believe that the head commonly enters the pelvis in the transverse diameter, and only after it has passed the inlet does the occiput turn toward the front or the back, almost always toward the pubis. This does not coincide with the writer's experience; examination of many women at term and in the earliest phases of labor have convinced him that engagement in an oblique diameter occurs about as often as the transverse position. Very rarely the head may enter the brim with the sagittal suture directly anteroposterior, the occiput either behind, or directly anterior, no further rotation whatever being necessary (Figs. 248, 249, 250, 251).

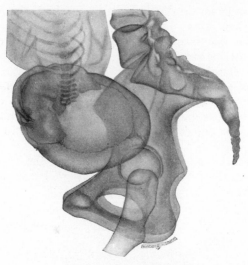

Fig. 249.—The resting primary posterior position as viewed from the lateral aspect. (Caldwell, Moloy and D'Esopo in Amer. Jour. of Obstet. and Gynec., Dec., 1934, C. V. Mosby Co., Publishers.)

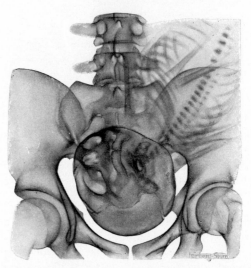

Fig. 250.—Spontaneous rotation of the case shown in Fig. 248. The head is placed transversely above the level of the ischial spines. Note that the axis of the child is inclined toward the oblique inlet and that the line of least resistance is anterior. (Caldwell, Moloy and D'Esopo in Amer. Jour. of Obstet and Gynec., Dec., 1934, C. V. Mosby Co., Publishers.)

The terminations of primary occipitoposterior positions are either arrest of the deflexed head high in the pelvis, with absolute obstruction of labor, or "deep transverse arrest" or gradual flexion under the influence of powerful labor pains, with subsequent rotation either anteriorly or posteriorly.

Secondary occipitoposterior positions develop in cases wherein the head, having entered the pelvis either in the transverse or in an oblique presentation, fails to slip forward, downward and inward along the inclined pelvic planes and rotates backward toward and sometimes into the hollow of the sacrum.

The causes of this abnormality are generally to be found in breaks in the smooth pelvic muscles and fasciae such as occur after old

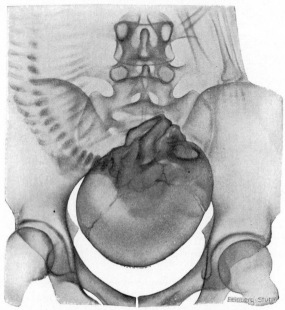

Fig. 251.—The resting primary transverse position (anterior view). Note the state of physiologic ease as illustrated by the curved spine and right-angled relationship to the long axis of the head. The head is resting across the inlet, well flexed with respect to the pelvis, the posterior parietal bone overhanging the inlet and the sagittal suture directed toward the symphysis. (Caldwell, Moloy and D'Esopo in Amer. Jour. of Obstet. and Gynec., Dec., 1934, C. V. Mosby Co., Publishers.)

lacerations and sometimes as a result of overstretching of these planes with consequent relaxation and loss of tonicity.

In some instances, however, this phenomenon develops in young and strong primiparae when the modus operandi of its occurrence has not been satisfactorily explained.

In cases of primary occipitoposterior position, there is usually much delay in engagement and the first stage of labor is prolonged. This is explained by the fact that there is usually some disproportion between the head and the inlet, and if for one of the reasons enumerated above, the head finally enters the inlet with the occiput posterior, the long biparietal diameter of the head is opposed to the inadequate sacrocotyloid diameter of the pelvis rather than to the long oblique diameter, as in occiput anterior. In order to accomplish engagement under these circumstances excessive molding of the head is necessary

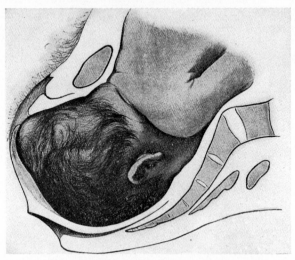

Fig. 252.—Formation of the caput succedaneum on the right parietal bone in an occipitoposterior presentation. (Bumm.)

to accommodate it to the decreased pelvic diameter, as well as long-continued and powerful uterine contractions to overcome the increased resistance (Fig. 252).

Provided the disproportion is not excessive, the head usually passes the pelvic brim and enters the cavity. The mechanism proceeds as

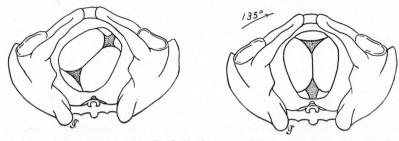

Fig. 253.—Long rotation of an R. O. P. through 135 degrees to a directly anterior position.

in anterior position with the exception that the occiput must rotate through an arc of 135 degrees or three eighths of a circle rather than 45 degrees or one eighth of a circle as in the latter. Obviously, much more time and greater force are necessary to overcome friction and resistance through the longer arc, whence the delay in rotation (Fig. 253).

Where the disproportion is marked or the uterine muscle deficient, rotation ceases when the sagittal suture lies in the transverse diameter of the pelvic cavity, the head still lying incompletely flexed—the so-called "transverse arrest." Exceptionally, labor proceeds under these conditions, the head being driven through the pelvis and born in the transverse diameter (Fig. 254), but much more commonly labor comes to a standstill, the uterus becoming exhausted. Generally, however, after a long first stage, rotation is completed and delivery is accom-

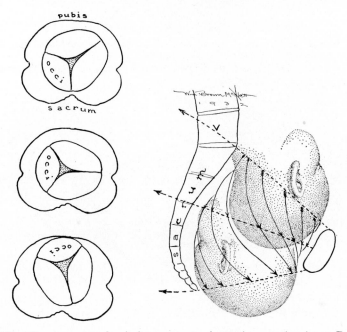

Fig. 254.—The descent and spiral movement of anterior rotation in an R. O. P. presentation.

plished by the usual mechanism of occipito-anterior position (Fig. 255). It is a moot point among obstetricians as to just at what plane of the pelvis anterior rotation occurs, some holding that this movement takes place at the upper pelvic planes and is complete when the head reaches the perineum, while others believe that the whole phenomenon of anterior rotation occurs on the pelvic floor. The truth probably lies between the two extremes, inasmuch as the movement is a spiral arc beginning as soon as the occiput meets the resistance of the upper segments of the pelvic fasciae, at the level of the ischiatic spines, and continuing until the turning has been completed at the vulvar outlet. In general, it may be stated that the greater the dis-

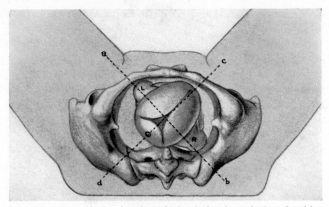

Fig. 255.—Rotation of the head and the behavior of the shoulders in the right occipitoposterior position before rotation. O, Occiput; L, left shoulder; R, right shoulder; *ab,* left oblique diameter of the pelvis; *cd,* right oblique diameter of the pelvis.

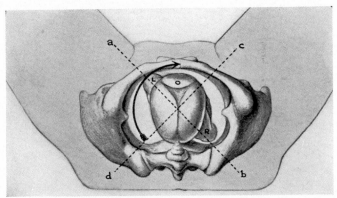

Fig. 256.—Rotation with the shoulders engaged. They do not rotate with the occiput but remain in their original position in the pelvis.

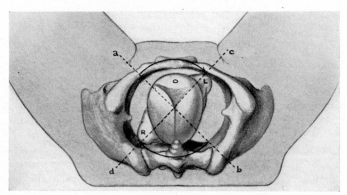

Fig. 257.—Rotation continued. With the shoulders unengaged and upon the pelvic brim they rotate with the occiput.

proportion and the more imperfect the flexion, the lower in the pelvis will rotation occur.

In a small proportion of cases the occiput, instead of rotating anteriorly, will turn in the opposite direction and finally come to

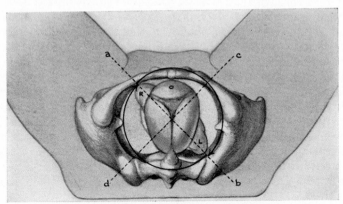

Fig. 258.—With the shoulders unengaged they rotate in an atypical mechanism overrotating and engaging in the left oblique diameter.

rest in the hollow of the sacrum (Fig. 259). The reason for this anomalous motion has not been established definitely but it does occur frequently in the presence of funnel pelves, and also when deflexion

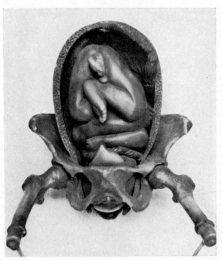

Fig. 259.—Model. Occiput directly in the hollow of the sacrum.

is a prominent factor. Under these conditions the greater fontanel occupies a lower position in the pelvis than does the small, and consequently the former first strikes the plane of the pelvic floor and is

31

directed forward, downward and inward, the occiput so being directed backward (Fig. 260).

An interesting experiment has been conducted to demonstrate the action of the inclined pelvic planes. The head of a fetus was repeatedly forced through the pelvis of a female cadaver and it was found that as long as the integrity of the pelvic floor was preserved, the occiput rotated anteriorly, but when the muscles and fasciae were stretched and torn from many repetitions of the maneuver, the occiput either failed to rotate at all or turned backward toward the sacrum.

Mechanism When the Occiput is in the Hollow of the Sacrum.— There are two methods by which delivery may take place: first, the head is thrown into extreme flexion with an enormous increase in the occipitomental diameter, the chin is pressed firmly against the neck and the fetal body becomes a rigid cylinder, which cannot accommodate itself to the sharply angulated birth canal, which latter must either stretch greatly or tear, to permit the passage of the unbendable

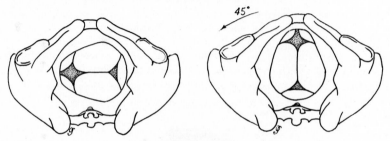

Fig. 260.—Rotation of a transverse position into occiput in the hollow of the sacrum.

fetus. Under such circumstances descent, under powerful uterine and abdominal contractions, continues until the occiput is forced either over or through the lacerated perineum, after which the brow and face appear under the symphysis, the head being born in extension.

A second mechanism may occur in the more deflexed cases. Here the forehead becomes the point of direction, descent continuing until the brow appears at the vulva, the glabella lying under the pubis. The occiput now escapes over the perineum by partial flexion, the long occipitofrontal diameter of the head usually producing extensive laceration, after which extension occurs, the brow, face, and chin successively slipping out from under the pubis. The remainder of the mechanism is that of anterior presentation.

The Diagnosis of Posterior Occipital Position.—R. O. P. is about five times more common than is L. O. P. The diagnosis is made by abdominal palpation, abdominal auscultation and vaginal palpation.

*Abdominal Palpation.—*At the onset of labor or before, the back of the child is felt away from the midline toward the right or left, and is sometimes difficult to feel. The extremities are quite prominent and may lie on either side of the midline. The head is at the pelvic brim, the breech in the fundus.

In women with firm or thick abdominal walls, abdominal palpation is often unconvincing as to the true position.

Abdominal auscultation reveals the heart sounds in the lower quadrant far out toward the flanks, and they may be faint and indistinct.

Vaginal examination before labor or during the early part of the first stage, may only reveal a poorly dilating cervix, and a head not deeply engaged. When the cervix has finally dilated, the large fontanel will be felt anteriorly, on the right or left and the small fontanel is palpated posteriorly, the sagittal suture lying in the oblique diameter. If the fontanels are nearly at the same level, imperfect flexion is present as a further complication. Inasmuch as labor is usually slow in posterior positions, a considerable caput may form and disguise the true position. If the head has passed through the cervix or the hand can be entered into the canal, palpation of an ear will confirm the diagnosis. If the finger, passing along the side of the child's head, from the front of the maternal pelvis toward the back, slips over the ear without catching in the attachment of the ear to the head, the occiput is surely posterior. Sometimes, when the patient is anesthetized the nape of the neck may be felt lying posteriorly.

Clinical Course of Labor in Occipitoposterior Position.—Labor is usually slower; the pains inefficient at the outset and engagement is delayed. Because of the poor fit of the head into the brim, cervical dilatation is delayed, effacement is often incomplete, and the membranes tend to rupture prematurely.

Whatever mechanism finally results in delivery, the uterine and abdominal effort is greatly increased in order to procure the long 135-degree rotation if this be the final position, or to force the occiput over the resisting perineum if short (45 degrees) posterior rotation occurs.

During the second stage of labor, the diagnosis can often be surmised by observing the power and length of the pain and the corresponding lack of progress.

The patient tends to become exhausted and the fetal heart tones by their alteration in rate and rhythm may denote fetal distress.

Management of Posterior Occiput.—Posterior positions of the occiput demand close individual study and the obstetrician must be prepared to deal with delayed and obstructed mechanisms as they arise. For the purpose of considering treatment, persistent posterior positions are best divided into first, those primary malpresentations where the arrest is at the pelvic brim, in which complete engagement does not occur and in which the uterine contractions, though they may be strong and active, are not followed by flexion and descent.

In these cases there is usually some disproportion and cesarean section must be thought of in the interests of the child. If no disproportion can be detected, internal version and extraction may be attempted, although the life of the fetus is apt to be endangered.

The second and far commoner type of occipitoposterior position is found when the head has entered the pelvis, is through the brim but is more or less deflexed, the occiput lying in one or the other bays of the sacrum. Here arises the question as to the time for interference, for which there is no definite rule.

However, in a general way, given a patient with the cervix fully dilated, the head in the pelvic cavity and with strong and active labor pains, if no progress in descent and anterior rotation is made in two hours, operative delivery is indicated. The various plans for managing this complication are:

1. Leaving the case to nature's efforts, apply a firm abdominal binder from costal margin to pelvic brim with or without a folded towel placed under the palpable shoulder to aid rotation.

Have the patient lie on the side to which the fetal back is turned. This tends to facilitate flexion.

A long labor is to be anticipated and the patient given opportunity for rest by the use of morphine in small doses ($\frac{1}{6}$ grain hypodermically with $\frac{1}{150}$ grain scopolamine hydrobromide).

Food must be provided at intervals, and the taking of fluids is encouraged.

The urinary bladder should be emptied by catheter at six-hour intervals if the patient is unable to void.

By this plan anterior rotation is eventually accomplished in most of the cases and spontaneous or outlet forceps delivery occurs. Sometimes the second mechanism becomes operative, the head being born with the occiput still posterior.

When the above plan has been given a fair trial, and the occiput remains posterior or transverse, or has slipped into the hollow of the sacrum, and progress comes to a standstill, it is imperative that some assistance be given to secure delivery.

2. *Manual Rotation.*—When the head has reached the cavity of the pelvis, usually at the level of the ischiatic spines or a little below them, and the occiput remains unrotated, this procedure is by far the most generally available to secure rotation.

Technic.—The patient is anesthetized with the legs in leg holders, the perineal region is scrubbed and prepared as for any vaginal operation, and the operator also prepared. A mediolateral episiotomy is performed to secure ample vaginal room for the entrance of the hand, and the perineal floor ironed out, for better relaxation. (These measures are sometimes unnecessary in multiparae with relaxed pelvic floor.)

That hand whose palmar surface when in supination will slip over the occiput is introduced into the vagina, the operator either

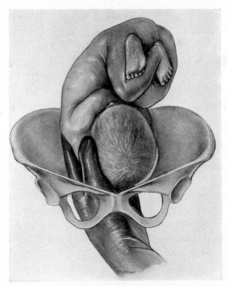

Fig. 261.—Author's method for manual rotation of the posterior occiput. The hand slips past the head which rests lightly in the palm. The first two fingers make pressure upon the anterior fetal shoulder slowly turning the body of the child. Trendelenburg posture greatly favors this procedure.

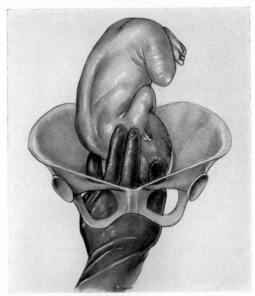

Fig. 262.—Author's method for rotation of the posterior occiput. The body of the child has been turned and the occiput is now in an anterior position.

sitting or kneeling so that the wrist is extended, the elbow being below the level of the vagina (Figs. 261, 262).

The hand is introduced, the diagnosis of position being confirmed on the way by palpating the ear. The first and second fingers slip past the head and seek the anterior shoulder. Now with the fingers in the axilla, the head of the child lying loosely in the palm of the hand, the shoulder is firmly pushed around the anterior aspect of the pelvis, until the body has been rotated almost 90 degrees. The occiput becomes dislodged from under the promontory of the sacrum, if it has gone so far, and turns with the body first into an anterior position on the same side as the occiput originally lay, and the turning being continued finally comes to rest in the opposite oblique diameter of the pelvis, *i. e.*, R. O. P., is rotated past R. O. A. until it eventuates into L. O. A.

This accomplished, the hand is withdrawn and forceps applied as to a primary L. O. A. position and delivery completed. This maneuver has the advantages of being easy and simple of performance, it is not traumatic, and is almost always successful in securing rotation, unless sufficient disproportion is present to prevent any rotation.

3. *Rotation with Forceps* (Scanzoni maneuver if the head is on the pelvic floor, Bill principle if the head is high in the cavity).—The forceps are applied as to an anterior position and traction and rotation are combined, until the necessary amount of turning has been accomplished. The blades are then withdrawn, reapplied as to an anterior position and delivery completed. (For details see Chapter XLI.)

4. *Version and Extraction.*—In some cases, when rotation of the head offers unusual difficulties, podalic version first pushing the head back out of the pelvis, and followed by extraction is the method of choice. (For technic see Chapter XLIII.)

5. *Cesarean Section.*—This procedure is only indicated when marked disproportion renders any form of vaginal delivery hazardous for the child, and dangerous to the mother.

6. *Craniotomy.*—When the child is dead and great disproportion exists, craniotomy may be required, but this only upon rare occasions.

THE DEFLEXION ATTITUDES

Occasionally, the head enters the pelvic brim in imperfect flexion, which usually is corrected spontaneously by the continuing uterine contractions, the small fontanel sinking and the large one rising until the usual flexion obtains. In other instances, happily uncommon, this desideratum does not take place, and labor continues with the head in some degree of extension.

For practical purposes, four varieties of deflexion position are distinguished, *i. e.:*

Median vertex presentation, the head being midway between flexion and extension—the so-called "military presentation."

Presentation of the forehead.

Presentation of the brow.

Presentation of the face.

Frequency.—The deflexion attitudes are uncommon, the whole comprising about 0.3 per cent of deliveries, face being the most frequent.

Etiology.—Deflexion attitudes are the result, generally, of some type of pelvic deformity, shortening of the conjugata vera being the most common. They may occur as a result of an unusually dolicocephalic head in which the occipital segment is prolonged, or there may be conditions preventing flexion as tumors of the fetal neck or thorax. Sometimes a complicating pelvic tumor may force the head into the brim in extension.

Whatever the final outcome, all of the deflexion attitudes begin as median vertex presentations from which greater extension there develop brow or face, or as a result of improved flexion, the usual vertex presentation may eventuate.

Mechanism of Labor in Median Vertex Presentation.—Engagement is delayed because the long anteroposterior diameter does not easily descend into the pelvic cavity. Either anterior or posterior asynclitism may develop to a marked degree, until one or the other parietal eminences enters the cavity, when labor becomes absolutely obstructed.

If the median vertex does pass through the brim, the mechanism may proceed in one of four ways: (1) flexion occurs, a normal position resulting. (2) Extension increases, terminating in a brow or face presentation. (3) The occiput may rotate into the hollow of the sacrum, some flexion occurring and delivery following as in posterior occiput. (4) Labor becomes obstructed with the head in the transverse position, the so-called "deep transverse arrest."

In any of the first three terminations, spontaneous delivery is possible, but the length of labor and the fatigue of the patient generally indicate some form of operative aid. When the fourth termination, "deep transverse arrest" occurs, great difficulties offer themselves to vaginal delivery.

Diagnosis of Median Vertex Presentation.—Abdominal palpation and auscultation are of no aid, the impression received being that of posterior occiput.

Vaginal examination will disclose the sagittal suture running directly across the pelvic brim, either in the midline or a little in front of or behind it. The anterior and posterior fontanels are on the same level. Dilatation of the cervix is slow and imperfect and the labor is characterized by powerful uterine contractions, which produce no progress whatever.

Treatment of Median Vertex Presentation with Deep Arrest.— *Version and Extraction.*—When the disproportion is not too great, version may be utilized but the extraction of the after-coming head is often attended by so much injury to the child that the procedure is invalidated.

Forceps Extraction.—The ordinary obstetric forceps are not well suited for this variety of dystocia because of the difficulty of accommodating their pelvic curve to an anteroposterior application; and hence the straight forceps of Kielland, or the Barton instrument are best used (Chapter XLII).

To overcome the difficulties, which even these forceps present, the author has developed a maneuver which is highly satisfactory in his hands.

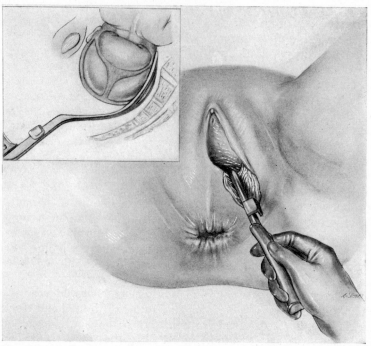

Fig. 263.—Author's maneuver for the correction of deep transverse arrest. A mediolateral episiotomy is made on the side on which the occiput lies. One blade of a Kielland forceps is passed behind the head, the handle dropping into the episiotomy wound, which in practice is protected by a gauze pad.

When the head lies in anterior asynclitism, the anterior parietal bone tightly pressed against the symphysis, it is sometimes practically impossible to insert a forceps blade, even the slender Kielland forceps, between skull and symphysis. Depressed fracture of the parietal bone and wide lacerations of the maternal bladder too often result from such attempts.

The maneuver in question involves a simultaneous use of one blade of the Kielland forceps as a lever, with the hand assisting the flexion and partial rotation of the head.

With the patient deeply anesthetized, and in moderate Trendelenburg posture, a wide mesiolateral episiotomy is made on the side toward which the occiput lies (Fig. 263).

The posterior blade of the Kielland forceps is then introduced behind the head, the major portion of the blade behind the ear if possible. The handle of the blade is now permitted to drop into the cleft of the episiotomy incision, which has previously been protected against too great pressure by a thick pad of gauze. The hand of the

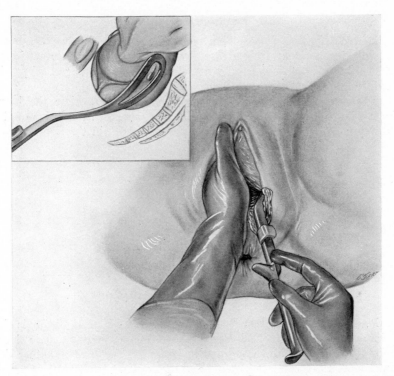

Fig. 264.—Author's maneuver for the correction of deep transverse arrest. Stage two. One hand enters the vagina, the fingers forcing the brow upward and backward, while the other makes pressure on the forceps handle downward and outward. This flexes the head until after a few moments the flexed head will occupy the oblique diameter.

operator which corresponds in position to the face of the infant is inserted into the vagina and the forehead sought with the first two fingers. Now simultaneous pressure is made, downward and outward on the forceps handle, and upward and backward with the finger on the forehead. As is readily seen, this combined pressure acts to force the occiput forward and downward while the face is thrust upward and backward (Fig. 264). Considerable force must sometimes be used to dislodge the parietal bone from behind the symphysis, but usually in a few moments the head will be felt to slip free, adequate flexion taking place and the sagittal suture moving into the oblique diameter of the pelvis. The hand is now withdrawn, the original forceps blade readjusted to a correct cephalic grasp, the anterior blade applied as in any anterior position of the occiput and delivery completed. This procedure requires a little practice for its correct performance, but once learned, it is a most satisfactory addition to the armamentarium of the obstetrician.

BROW PRESENTATION

When extension proceeds a trifle beyond median vertex, brow presentation results. It is a rare development being seen about once in 3000 labors, and is generally associated with some degree of pelvic contraction (Fig. 265).

The diagnosis is made by vaginal examination, when the large fontanel is found distinctly lower than the posterior, the bulge of the brow presenting, and the orbits are palpable high in the pelvis.

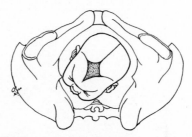

Fig. 265.—Brow presentation, the occiput posterior.

Mechanism of Labor in Brow Presentation.—Here the brow is the point of rotation, and as it meets the resistance of the pelvic floor, it rotates forward, downward and inward until the sagittal suture lies anteroposteriorly and the brow is at the vulva. Under strong pains, the brow, the vertex and the occiput pass over the perineum, the nape of the neck rests on the pelvic floor, and the face and chin appear from under the symphysis. This unusual mechanism naturally requires great uterine force, and implies serious damage to the pelvic floor, deep extensive laceration, often involving the sphincter ani, being the rule.

This mechanism of brow presentation is quite uncommon, the usual course of labor being either further extension, with a resulting face presentation, or obstruction of labor high in the pelvis.

Treatment.—When a brow presentation is firmly impacted in the pelvis it presents a formidable complication.

Sometimes, with the patient in deep anesthesia, in Trendelenburg position and possibly by the aid of lubrication with green soap after the manner of Piper (*q. v.*) the head may be pushed out of the pelvis and version performed.

It may be possible by manual efforts to flex the brow and convert it into a vertex, or even sometimes to further the extension until a face presentation results. In other instances cesarean section may be required, or even craniotomy if the child is dead or the mother in poor condition.

The prognosis for the child is grave, since the great compression leads to intracranial injuries.

FACE PRESENTATION

When extension is carried to its greatest extreme, face presentation, the most common of the deflexion attitudes, results (Fig. 266).

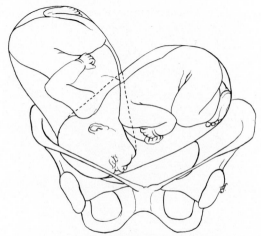

Fig. 266.—Face presentation due to lateroversion of the uterus. (Redrawn from Ahlfeld.)

Etiology.—The etiology is that of the other causes of extension. Sometimes obliquity of the uterine axis to that of the pelvic inlet, as in pendulous abdomen, is responsible. In our experience at Kensington Hospital, face presentation occurs about once in 400 deliveries.

Diagnosis.—Abdominal palpation reveals the breech in the fundus, the back to one or the other side of the midline, and usually difficult to palpate.

The small parts are easily distinguishable. The uterus seems longer than usual, because the extended head pushes the buttocks higher and causes the fundus to rise.

The head is felt at the pelvic brim, the rounded mass of the occiput to one side of the midline, with a deep cleft between it and the fetal body, marking the depression between the extended head and the back.

On abdominal auscultation the heart tones are heard in one or the other lower quadrant but higher toward the level of the umbilicus than in vertex presentation. The heart sounds are unusually loud and clear, and are heard best on the side on which the fetal extremities lie. This circumstance, together with the very apparent depression at the nape of the neck, makes the diagnosis clear.

Vaginal examination early in labor finds the presenting part high up, a large broad pouch of membranes protruding. Later in labor the structures of the face may be felt, the mouth and jaws, the nose, and orbits descending into the pelvis. Still later, the swelling of the face may obliterate these landmarks and the presentation may be

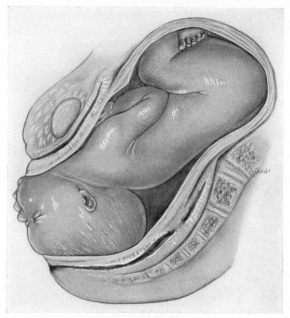

Fig. 267.—Face presentation. Chin anterior and beginning to stem under the symphysis.

confounded with that of the breech. Palpation of the hard gums or the orbits will usually clear up the question.

In face presentations the chin is the determining point, and consequently there may be, theoretically, six varieties. (L. M. A.; R. M. A.; L. M. T.; R. M. T.; L. M. P.; R. M. P.) The most common positions are left mento-anterior, left mentotransverse, and right mentoposterior (Fig. 267).

Mechanism of Labor in Face Presentations.—The steps in the mechanism are:

1. Extension and some molding. The head at the beginning of engagement is somewhere between flexion and extension, and the brow

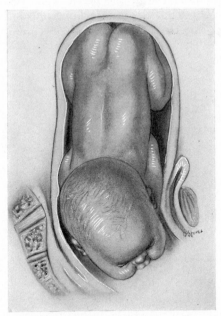

Fig. 268.—Face presentation. Chin in transverse position.

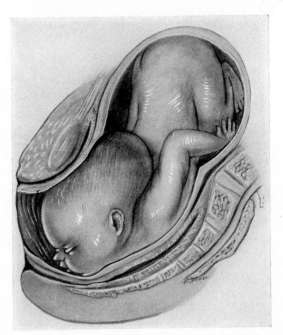

Fig. 269.—Face presentation. Chin in the hollow of the sacrum.

being held by the resistance of the pelvic walls remains stationary, while the chin slowly sinks, the head coming into full extension (Fig. 268). Molding is mostly confined to the occipital region but the face also undergoes slight pressure changes (Fig. 269).

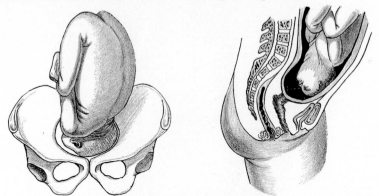

Fig. 270.—The mechanism of labor in face presentation. The head above the pelvic brim. Beginning of extension.

2. Lateral inclination of the head, one malar bone being a little deeper in the pelvis than the other—*asynclitism*.

3. Descent of the head, mostly at first by further extension (Figs. 270 and 271).

4. Anterior rotation of the chin, which is the determining point in the mechanism and, meeting the resistance of the pelvic floor, ro-

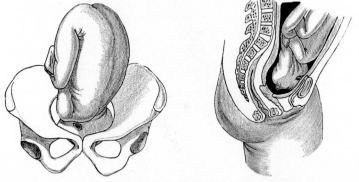

Fig. 271.—The mechanism of labor in face presentation. The head engaged and beginning descent.

tates forward, downward and inward until it comes to rest under the symphysis (Fig. 272).

5. Birth of the head by flexion, the mouth, nose, eyes, forehead and occiput sweeping over the perineum, when the chin escapes from under the arcuate ligament (Fig. 273).

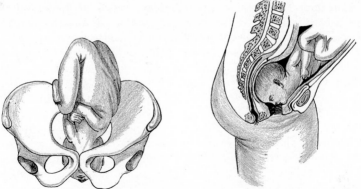

Fig. 272.—The mechanism of labor in face presentation. Anterior rotation of the chin under the symphysis.

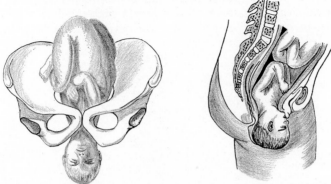

Fig. 273.—The mechanism of labor in face presentation. The head delivered by flexion.

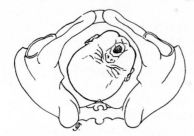

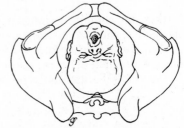

Fig. 274.—The mechanism of labor in face presentation. L. M. A.

Fig. 275.—The mechanism of labor in face presentation. Anterior rotation of the chin.

6. Restitution, the head turning in the direction from whence the chin rotated (Figs. 274, 275).

7. External rotation.

8. Birth of the shoulders.

9. Birth of the body.

These steps are identical with those of vertex mechanism.

Abnormal Mechanisms and Clinical Course of Labor.—Engagement occurs late, the parietal eminences not passing the pelvic inlet until the chin has almost reached the vulva. It must be remembered that face presentations are rarely primary, being usually due to an increase of extension by the downward thrust of the fetus in a primary median vertex or brow position. The cervix dilates slowly because the contours of the face do not accurately fill the orifice and also because of the delayed descent.

Delay in anterior rotation is usual because of the difference in the length of the lateral walls of the pelvis (8.8 cm.) and the fetal neck (3.8 cm.), the latter must therefore be enormously stretched, before the chin can impinge upon the pelvic floor and be subject to rotation.

When anterior rotation does not occur and the chin sinks into the hollow of the sacrum, labor is absolutely obstructed, because of the still greater length of the posterior aspect of the pelvic canal. The chin has no directing planes upon which to rotate, and to descend

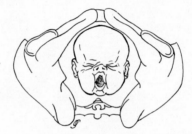

Fig. 276.—The mechanism of labor in face presentation. Posterior rotation of the chin into the hollow of the sacrum.

further, the combined diameter of head and thorax must pass through the pelvis, an obvious impossibility (Fig. 276).

When the arm becomes displaced and prolapsed behind the head or back, vaginal delivery, by any means, becomes exceedingly difficult. If the pelvis be unusually large, and the child correspondingly small and soft, birth may occur even with these aberrant mechanisms, but when both are of normal size, obstruction is the rule.

The first stage of labor is quite prolonged, but when anterior rotation has finally been completed, the second stage may be short and easy.

Prognosis.—The accepted fetal mortality is from 10 to 15 per cent; but under intelligent obstetric care, and with the exclusion of unrecognized neglected cases, the mortality should easily be reduced to from 6 to 8 per cent.

The mother runs a slightly greater risk than in vertex presentation by reason of the long duration of labor, and the occasional necessity of traumatizing operative delivery.

Treatment of Face Presentation.—Statistics show that 85 per cent of all face presentations deliver spontaneously or possibly by the use of outlet forceps. When one takes into account the comparative rarity of this abnormality, it will be seen that complications arise quite infrequently.

The treatment varies with the stage of labor and the station of the head when the diagnosis is made. *If the head be high in the pelvis* and *the cervix dilated* (a somewhat uncommon coincidence)

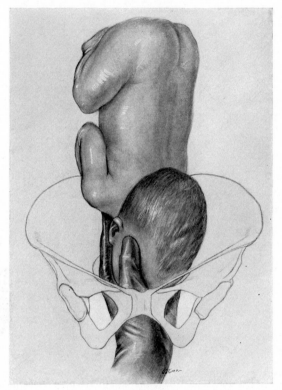

Fig. 277.—Correction of chin in hollow of sacrum. The fingers in the axilla, begin rotation of the fetal body.

version and extraction, to anticipate a possibly posterior rotation of the chin, is advisable.

When the head has descended and anterior rotation is beginning, watchful expectancy is the keynote of treatment. The usual rest for the patient by mild narcosis, and the maintenance of her resistance by the administration of food and fluids are all that is required.

When the head is in the pelvis and the chin lies posterior to the midline or is in the hollow of the sacrum, conversion of the presentation into one favorable for delivery may be attempted.

32

Baudelocque devised the procedure and Thorn and DeLee have emphasized the value of converting a face into a vertex position by manual means. The technic is to grasp the occiput and pull it down with a hand in the vagina, while the abdominal hand makes pressure upon the chest of the child, pushing it toward the side upon which the occiput lies, to straighten the spine and inaugurate flexion. When the child has become movable, the face is pushed upward with the vaginal hand, the occiput sinking into the pelvis (Figs. 277, 278).

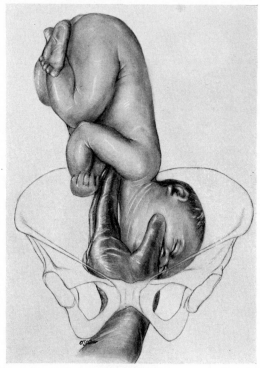

Fig. 278.—The correction of chin in hollow of sacrum. Pressure on the shoulder has rotated the fetal body, the head following and the chin coming into an anterior position.

In my hands this plan has been difficult of execution because the long, swollen caput exerts so much pressure upon the pelvic wall that flexion has been impossible.

It is much simpler to rotate the posterior chin anteriorly and permit delivery as a face presentation, chin anterior.

Details of this maneuver are as follows:

The patient being deeply anesthetized, in Trendelenburg position, the operator assumes a position in which the wrist of the operative hand is in moderate extension, that is, the arm must be below the level of the pelvis.

A generous mesiolateral episiotomy incision is then made and the well lubricated gloved hand is introduced into the vagina, palm up. The first and second fingers are slipped gently past the head, which is usually somewhat disengaged from its impacted position during the process.

The fingers seek the anterior axilla and, this found, the head is ignored altogether, simply resting on the palm of the hand, very lightly held by the thumb.

Next, firm and steady pressure is made in the axilla, freeing the shoulder from its forced position in the lower uterine segment and slowly turning it laterally either from right to left or vice versa, depending on the position of the child in relation to the median line. The shorter rotation being always chosen.

The hand of an assistant, on the abdomen, aiding the rotation externally is of great service in facilitating this act and, slowly and steadily, the hand will move from supination to almost complete pronation, the head moving with the rotating body of the infant until the shoulder has completed about a quarter circle (90°) and the chin has slipped anteriorly under the symphysis. The hand is then withdrawn, and a simple forceps extraction completes the delivery.

After a little practice it is astonishing how simple this rotation becomes, and how by its means, a formidable complication revolves itself into an easy and nontraumatic finale.

When the head is so firmly impacted that it is immovable, and the chin lies in the hollow of the sacrum, cesarean section if the child and mother are in good position, and craniotomy, if the former be dead and the latter potentially infected or exhausted, are the procedures of choice.

Effect Upon the Child.—An infant born in face presentation is often much disfigured. Tremendous swelling of the lips and tongue, a contused caput over the anterior cheek and eye and marked exophthalmus. Sometimes there are hemorrhages under the skin and the neck presents transverse lacerations from overstretching. There is also a long caput on the occiput. Nursing is impossible, sometimes for several days, and dehydration may require hypodermoclysis or the intraperitoneal injection of saline solution. The swelling usually disappears after a few days when nursing takes place normally, although the lacerations on the neck and the facial contusions may persist for several weeks.

BREECH PRESENTATIONS

When the caudal extremity of the fetus lies over the pelvic inlet, the presentation is termed breech. The lie of the child is longitudinal as in vertex presentation, but the polarity is reversed.

Frequency.—Breech presentation occurs in from 3.5 to 4 per cent of all cases, including prematures, and in about 1.5 per cent of full-term single pregnancies. It is sometimes regarded as a form of normal position, but when one takes into consideration the difficulties in delivery and the greatly increased fetal mortality, it seems proper to classify breech among the pathological presentations (Fig. 279).

Etiology.—The true reason for breech presentation is not known, but certain morphological peculiarities in the shape of the uterus, as double uterus, uterus septus, etc., are sometimes operative, as witness a patient of the writer's who possessed a double uterus, with one rudimentary horn, and had three successive breech deliveries.

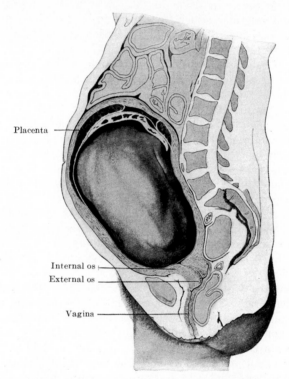

Fig. 279.—Median sagittal section of a pregnant woman at term. Fetus in breech. (Bumm, from Waldeyer "Das Becken.")

Low insertion of the placenta may turn the head upward, as may tumors in the pelvis and certain pelvic deformities, as flat pelvis.

Individual variations in shape of the normal uterus, the fundus being narrow and the lower uterine segment broad, so that the larger buttocks with the moving legs are better accommodated in breech presentation may be a factor (Fig. 280).

I am of the opinion that the position frequently develops as a pure accident. Until the twenty-fourth week of pregnancy, or even later, the child is freely movable in the uterus, and successive x-ray photographs often show marked and rapid change in position at this time. If now, while the buttocks chance to lie over the inlet of the pelvis, a series of the normal uterine contractions should occur, it is reasonable to believe that the breech might be forced well down into the lower uterine segment and not again rise out of its new position.

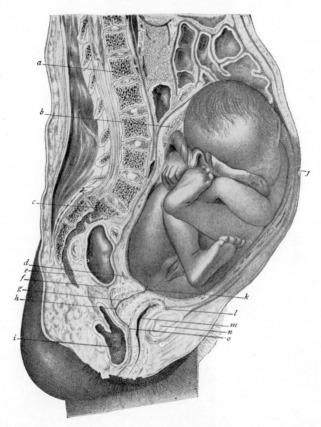

Fig. 280.—Breech presentation. Waldeyer's section of an X-para at full term, who died from hemorrhage some hours after both her legs had been cut off by a locomotive: *a*, first lumbar vertebra; *b*, placenta; *c*, fractured first sacral vertebra; *d*, coronary vein; *e*, blood extravasation; *f*, pouch of Douglas; *g*, cervical canal; *h*, os externum; *i*, rectum; *j*, umbilicus; *k*, os internum; *l*, uterovesical reflection of peritoneum; *m*, bladder; *n*, symphysis pubis; *o*, vagina. (B. C. Hirst.)

Contemplation of multiparous women who have had one or two perfectly normal vertex presentations, then a breech, then another vertex, with no peculiarities of the babies to account for the variation, gives weight to the view that accident must be a factor in the production of this abnormality.

Varieties.—Complete breech is that form in which the thighs are

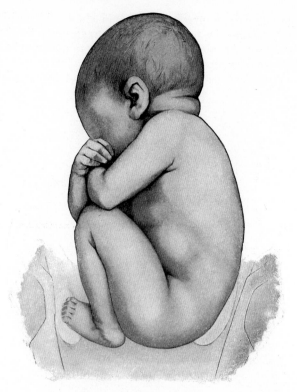

Fig. 281.—Mixed breech presentation. (From Edgar's "Practice of Obstetrics," published by P. Blakiston's Son & Co., Inc.)

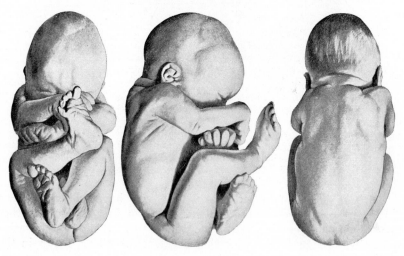

Fig. 282.—Frank breech presentation, showing attitude of the fetus. (After Chievitz from Bumm.)

flexed on the abdomen and the legs on the thighs, so that the buttocks, with the feet beside them, are at the pelvic inlet (Fig. 281).

Incomplete breech occurs when one or both legs are extended and lie in the cervix, single or double footling.

Frank breech when the thighs are flexed on the abdomen and the legs fully extended, the child being doubled up at the hips, the buttocks alone presenting (Fig. 282), is the third variety.

Diagnosis.—*Abdominal palpation* discloses the back to be on one side of the median line, the extremities on the other. Sometimes the back is almost directly anterior and the small parts difficult to find. The smooth caudal end of the fetus lies in the pelvic brim, while the

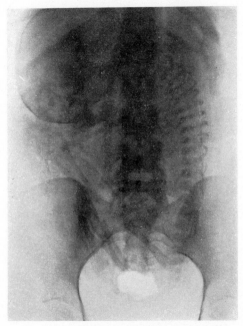

Fig. 283.—Breech presentation. L. S. A.

rounded, movable hard head can be palpated at the fundus, sometimes well off the median line.

On abdominal auscultation, the heart sounds are best heard over the fetal back, in one of the upper quadrants of the abdomen, generally well above the umbilicus (Figs. 283, 284).

Vaginal examination early in labor is notable by reason of the absence of the ovoid, large head blocking the inlet. The breech may be felt as a smooth but somewhat irregular mass.

When the cervix is dilated, the anus, the tuberosities of the ischia and the nates may be made out and confirm the diagnosis.

Mechanism of Labor.—In breech presentations the sacrum is the point of determination and accordingly there may be the usual six positions.

The only common positions are L. S. A. and R. S. P.

Engagement is very slow, the breech remaining high in the pelvis often until almost full dilatation of the cervix has been reached. This process is also slow, because the soft and wedge-shaped buttocks do not fit well into the cervix and act badly as dilators.

Descent is slow for the same reason and this inaccurate fit also tends to cause early rupture of the membranes, which feel the full pressure of the uterine contractions.

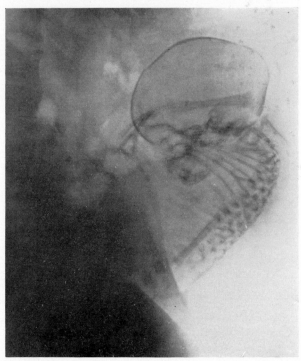

Fig. 284.—Breech presentation. R. S. T. Marked obliquity of the fetal body.

Prolapse of the cord is frequently seen, also by reason of the spaces left in the cervical ring by the irregular and poorly-fitting breech.

The mechanism of descent and birth, in breech, naturally divides itself into three phases—the movement of the breech, of the shoulders and of the head. For a description of these movements, it is convenient to use a typical position, usually the most common, L. S. A.

The Breech.—After the delayed engagement the sacrum lies in the left anterior quadrant of the pelvis, the bitrochanteric diameter occupying the left oblique.

As descent goes on *lateral flexion* occurs, the right or posterior hip sinking into the cavity of the pelvis, and being there held, while the left or anterior hip meets the resistance of the pelvic floor and undergoes *internal anterior rotation,* through an arc of 45°, finally coming to rest under the symphysis (Fig. 285).

Descent and lateral flexion continuing, the anterior hip stems under the symphysis, the posterior hip sweeps over the perineum and is born, the body straightens and the anterior hip slips under the symphysis, the pelvis of the child tilting upward toward the pubis of the mother, as soon as born. The legs follow the breech and drop down. Restitution may occur, but more often does not.

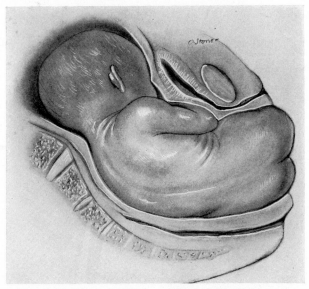

Fig. 285.—Mechanism of labor in breech. The anterior hip stemming under the symphysis, the body in lateral flexion.

The Shoulders.—The bisacromial diameter engages in the left oblique as did the bitrochanteric. Descent occurs while the arms are flexed across the chest. The anterior or left shoulder then rotates from the right anterior quadrant into the anteroposterior diameter of the pelvis and comes to rest behind the symphysis, while, by a continuance of lateral flexion, the posterior shoulder sweeps out over the perineum, to be followed by the anterior or left one (Fig. 286).

In case of a delay in the descent of the head, restitution again takes place, the back turning toward the left. This, however, occurs only occasionally.

The Head.—In the meantime the head has become engaged in the opposite oblique diameter, to that occupied by the shoulders and the breech. In L. S. A. the sagittal suture lies in the right oblique, the occiput anterior. Descent and rotation occur, the occiput coming under the symphysis, and the brow being in the hollow of the sacrum.

Further flexion of the head now occurs, the nucha is held under the symphysis, while the chin, face, forehead and brow emerge over

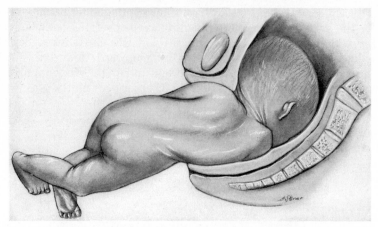

Fig. 286.—The mechanism of labor in breech. Anterior rotation and birth of the shoulders.

the perineum, the occiput finally escaping from under the pubis. The head, if well flexed, is usually delivered without difficulty, because its narrowest planes traverse the pelvis like a wedge, the broad biparietal diameter coming last (Fig. 287).

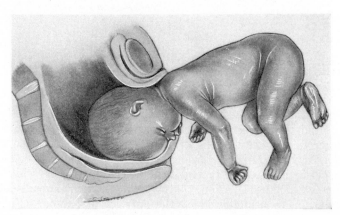

Fig. 287.—The mechanism of labor in breech. The occiput under the symphysis, the head being delivered by extension.

The various stages of the mechanism of labor in breech presentations have necessarily been described separately, but the process *in vivo* is a smooth, synchronated series of movements. Thus while

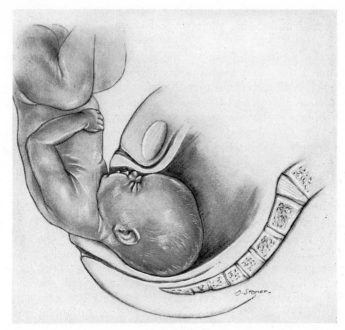

Fig. 288.—The mechanism of labor in breech. The occiput posterior, the head in extreme flexion.

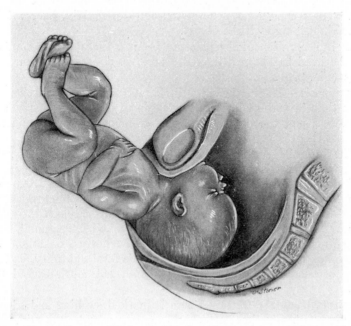

Fig. 289.—The mechanism of labor in breech. The head extracted, the chin held above the symphysis, the occiput being born by flexion.

the buttocks are rotating and being delivered, the shoulders are descending and undergoing their several changes in position, as is the head.

Posterior positions of the sacrum are uncommon and the mechanism is much the same as in anterior. For example, in R. S. P. the bitrochanteric diameter occupies the left oblique, the anterior or right hip rotates as before and the mechanism becomes identical with that of L. S. A. except that the back is on the opposite side of the pelvis.

Posterior Rotation of the Occiput in Breech.—This accident is very rare unless premature attempts at extraction have been made. When it does occur, two mechanisms are possible. If the head is well flexed, the nose catches behind the symphysis, and the occiput, vertex and brow pass over the perineum which is generally deeply lacerated during the process, the face finally appearing from under the symphysis (Fig. 288).

If the head is extended, the chin is arrested by the symphysis (Fig. 289), further extension occurs and spontaneous delivery cannot take place, unless the body of the child is lifted to more than a right angle with the mother's long axis, when the occiput may be pulled over the perineum, the forehead and face falling into complete extension. Usually manual rotation, or forceps extraction, are necessary to secure delivery under these circumstances.

Clinical Course of Labor.—The first stage is generally markedly lengthened, in breech, engagement, dilatation and descent all being slow. The second stage generally progresses rapidly, once the body of the child is through the cervix.

Early separation of the placenta because the uterus is empty before the head has been delivered occurs, as does postpartum hemorrhage (Fig. 290).

Prognosis.—The mother runs little more danger in breech presentation than in vertex although by reason of possible exhaustion from long labor, and the danger of sepsis from more frequent operative delivery, there is possibly some slight increase in the risk.

The infant, however, is in much worse case. Various statistics give a fetal mortality of from 10 to 20 per cent and even higher in rural districts. This increased mortality may be due to asphyxia from cord pressure, although the traditional four minutes between the cessation of cord pulsation and fetal death has been extended to fifteen. The chief cause of death seems to be intracranial hemorrhage from injuries inflicted during the too hasty extraction of the after-coming head. In a modern clinic, the fetal mortality, excluding prematures and macerated fetuses, should not much exceed 6 per cent.

Effects Upon the Child.—There is marked swelling and edema of the nates, with sometimes petechial hemorrhage under the skin. When the labor has been difficult with vigorous manipulation required to assist the birth of the shoulders and head, fractures of the clavicle and humerus are often seen, and the lower jaw may be injured. Brachial palsy from too strong traction upon the shoulders is noted, and as stated above, intracranial hemorrhage from rupture of the tentorium or the falx cerebri is the most frequent cause of intrapartum fetal death.

The skull shows little evidence of molding and there is no cephalic caput.

Management of Breech Presentations.—*Prophylaxis.*—When a breech presentation is discovered late in pregnancy (and it always

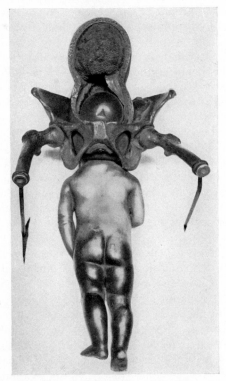

Fig. 290.—Breech presentation showing the contraction of the uterine fundus. (From the Barton Cooke Hirst Collection, University of Pennsylvania.)

should be) the malpresentation may be converted into a cephalic one by external version, a procedure which consists in reversing the polarity of the fetus by abdominal taxis alone. This principle has the enthusiastic approval of many clinics and is widely practiced.

If it be true that breech presentation is frequently an accidental event, external version would simply void the results of such error, and convert the position into a normal vertex. On the other hand, if the breech is the result of a peculiarly shaped uterus, or infant, it would seem that this position was the one best adapted to the accommodation of the fetus in the uterus, and therefore the one following which the best mechanism for delivery might be expected to develop. There is always the possibility that when the final cephalic presentation has been attained, there may be more or less deflexion of the head with a resulting dystocia on this account.

Entangling of the cord about the limbs of the fetus has also been noted and very rarely premature separation of the placenta. Not infrequently, the converted breech resumes its original position even after several attempts at external version, although in general the cephalic presentation is retained. External version should never be attempted when the breech is engaged, nor may it be utilized when there is appreciable disproportion. The technic is described in Chapter XLIV.

Management of Labor in Breech Presentation.—There are two schools of thought regarding the conduct of breech labor; one of which advocates aggressive methods, breaking up or as it is termed, decomposing the breech as soon as the buttocks reach the pelvic outlet, and following this by extraction of the infant. The other school, to which the writer subscribes, advises expectant treatment, waiting for spontaneous delivery and only interfering when signs of fetal or maternal danger become evident. The latter plan seems to offer the best results for mother and child.

The first stage of labor is conducted as in a vertex presentation, the patient and her family informed of the position and of the probability that labor will be long. Rest and fluid intake for the patient are essential.

Attention has been called previously to the necessity of continual information as to the condition of the fetus during labor, by the determination of the rate and quality of its heart sounds.

Because occult prolapse of the cord may complicate any breech delivery, the information is doubly important in this situation and the accoucheur must listen very frequently to the fetal heart.

When the breech reaches the vulva, preparations are made for extraction if this becomes necessary. The patient should be placed upon a table, but if in a home where none is available, she may be placed across the bed, never lengthwise. Inhalation anesthesia is withheld, if possible, since voluntary bearing down efforts are so requisite for spontaneous delivery. Analgesia by the barbiturates, morphine, and scopolamine or a combination of the two is very satisfactory in this connection. The bladder is to be emptied at six-hour intervals and if the first stage has been much protracted a second enema may be needed to insure an empty sigmoid and rectum.

The cord may prolapse with the breech, and if so, a loop of it must be pulled down so that it may be palpated almost continuously and any change in the rate or character of its pulsations noted.

As labor progresses, the hips are successively born and then the body is supported while the rotation and descent of the shoulders is completed. The infant should be wrapped in a warm sterile towel to protect it from cold.

The obstetrician, or better, an assistant, now makes pressure on the fundus over the head, firmly but not roughly, in order to aid the descent. Presently the shoulders rotate and are born and then the problem of the after-coming head arises. In a spontaneous delivery, the body is held upward almost at right angles to the long axis of the mother, while the face, brow and forehead slip over the perineum. If the infant be inclined too sharply inward, injuries to the neck may occur.

Sometimes when the head is large, the nose and mouth may be delivered, the trachea gently milked to force out any inspired blood or liquor amnii, and the child allowed to breathe, while the perineum is distending sufficiently to permit the completion of extrusion.

The third stage of labor is conducted in the usual manner.

When the baby is large and the cervix resistant to dilatation, it is good practice to insert a large-sized metreurynter into the canal, as soon as there is sufficient dilatation to admit the folded bag. This tends to conserve the continuity of the membranes and to aid dilatation. *The indications for interference* in breech labor are, a cessation of progress in the second stage, lasting two hours or more, and especially any sign of fetal distress as denoted by a failure of cord pulsation or a marked alteration of its rate or rhythm. If the cord is not palpable, abdominal auscultation of the fetal heart sounds must be utilized.

Obviously, any untoward change in the condition of the mother should predicate prompt delivery.

Recapitulation.—The extent to which flexion is maintained determines the ease of breech delivery. When the fetal ellipse is intact, smooth descent and rotation follow; when flexion is broken up, and extension of head and arms develops, difficulties are inevitable.

Hence, the less traction from below, and the more pressure on the fundus uteri, the better the maintenance of flexion.

The infant is in such momentary peril of asphyxia that the obstetrician must have constant knowledge of its condition as determined by abdominal auscultation or cord palpation.

Attempt at extraction before the cervix is sufficiently dilated to permit the free passage of the largest part of the fetal body, the head, usually spells disaster.

On the other hand all preparations for possible immediate extraction must be made when the breech appears in the vulva.

The technical details as to breech extraction will be found in Chapter XLIII.

TRANSVERSE PRESENTATION OR LIE

Definition.—Transverse lie is that in which the long axis of the fetus lies at right angles, or nearly so, to the long axis of the mother. The fetal poles occupy the lateral areas of the uterus, the fundus being empty. Oblique lie is when the long axis of the fetus is diagonal to that of the mother, and is a transitory phenomenon, the oblique being converted into a longitudinal or a transverse one with the first uterine contractions.

Transverse lies most commonly eventuate in shoulder presentation, or its technical equivalent, acromial presentation. However, the back may present as may the umbilicus. The back in shoulder presentation may be directed either anteriorly or posteriorly, and accordingly one speaks of dorso-anterior and dorsoposterior positions (Fig. 291).

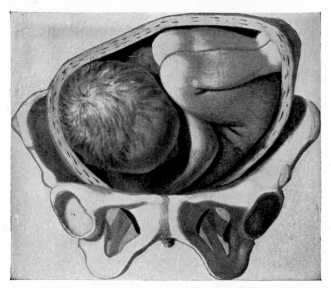

Fig. 291.—Shoulder presentation. (Hirst's "Text-book of Obstetrics.")

Frequency.—If premature, multiple and macerated fetuses be excluded, transverse lie occurs in about once in 2000 labors.

Etiology.—Anything which interferes with the forces instituting longitudinal lie may be operative in causing the transverse position, hence hydramnios with a small baby, twin pregnancy, very premature labors, macerated fetus, and monsters are responsible. When the infant is mature and well-developed, the causes are deformities of the pelvis, and sometimes the relaxed uterus and pendulous abdomen of multiparae. Tumors distorting the lower uterine segment may be a factor.

Diagnosis.—The diagnosis of transverse lie is simple. On inspection the uterus is broad and short, and the head of the child may be seen distending one or the other flank.

On abdominal palpation, utilizing the maneuvers of Leopold, the fundus is found to be empty. The ovoid head occupies one side of the lower aspect of the uterus, the breech the other (Fig. 292).

The pelvic brim may reveal the shoulders, but may be negative to palpation.

Abdominal auscultation reveals the heart sounds low down in the abdomen near the midline on the side on which the head lies.

Vaginal examination is negative unless the shoulder has become impacted in the brim, when the acromion process may be felt. The "washboard" sensation imparted to the finger when it is passed over the ribs of the fetus is characteristic.

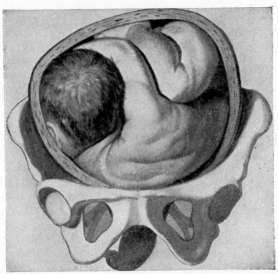

Fig. 292.—Shoulder presentation. (Hirst's "Text-book of Obstetrics.")

Mechanism of Labor.—There is no mechanism of labor in true transverse lie, the shoulder finally becoming firmly wedged in the inlet, when all progress ceases, the neck being much stretched, and the lower uterine segment thinned out to the point of rupture. In very premature, or macerated fetuses, two terminations are possible.

Spontaneous evolution, in which the neck is enormously stretched out and the shoulders descend, followed by the thorax and body, the head coming last as in breech, second, con duplicatio corpore, in which the body of the child is delivered bent double at the waist. These mechanisms only involve dead or tiny infants and are of little practical importance.

Prognosis.—When recognized before labor, transverse lie may be corrected easily. If the membranes are long ruptured and the

33

shoulder firmly impacted, the arm protruding from the vulva, the situation becomes very dangerous for mother and child. The former may die of exhaustion and shock, rupture of the uterus is an ever present peril, and sepsis a lurking foe. For the child, pressure injuries and asphyxia constitute lesions of the utmost gravity.

Treatment.—Before labor, the alteration of a transverse lie into a longitudinal one, either cephalic or caudal, is an easy matter, by the use of external version. The same procedure may be attempted very early in labor, but is more hazardous and offers less hope of success.

When labor is well established, internal podalic version is the classical plan of management, though possessing the ever specific danger of uterine rupture (*q. v.* version).

If marked disproportion exists, cesarean section, here the low cervical section, or cesarean with hysterectomy, if infection is feared, is the procedure of choice. When the infant is dead, embryotomy may solve the problem, although in some cases of advanced impaction it is a very difficult procedure.

COMPOUND PRESENTATION

Sometimes a head and arm, rarely a head and foot occupy the pelvic inlet. These malpresentations are due to pelvic deformity, small infants, very oblique lie of the uterus or pendulous abdomen. The diagnosis rests upon the discovery of a hand or foot lying alongside of the head, which may remain high in the pelvis because descent and rotation are impeded by the presence of the prolapsed limb.

Treatment.—In well-formed pelves, the arm and head may descend together, and birth be spontaneous.

Again it may be possible to displace the arm or leg, and manipulating it around the promontory of the sacrum, replace it in the uterine cavity.

In general, however, podalic version and extraction is the procedure of choice. Forceps may be utilized, but great care must be taken to exclude the prolapsed limb from the grasp of the blades.

FUNIC PRESENTATION

Presentation of the umbilicus (Fig. 293) with primary prolapse of the umbilical cord may occur but is very rare. The diagnosis makes itself, if one follows the prolapsed cord to its insertion into the umbilicus in the middle of the superior strait. The treatment is immediate version and extraction, or embryotomy, if the child be dead.

DYSTOCIA DUE TO EXCESSIVE FETAL SIZE

A fully developed mature fetus measures 50 cm. in length and 3400 Gm. or 7 to 7½ pounds in weight.

Postmaturity relatively increases both weight and length, the fontanels grow smaller, the cranial bones do not overlap easily, hence molding is difficult. The increased width of the shoulders sometimes makes their delivery a formidable procedure. Giant fetuses are infrequently reported in the literature, though in 1897 Du Bois found 28 instances in which the baby weighed 5600 Gm. or more.

In 1917 Davis reported that the largest baby born in the New York Lying-in Hospital, among more than 100,000 births, weighed 15 pounds. The greatly oversized babies on record are those of Belcher, 25 pounds; Moss, 24.12 pounds; Ortega, 24.82 pounds; Beach, 22.75 pounds; Robbins, 17.5 pounds; Brechin 18.37 pounds; Turnbull, 18.25 pounds; Gordon, 18 pounds; Hobbs and Scrivener, 16.94 pounds.

The cause of postmaturity is not known though there is a strong

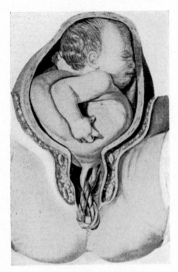

Fig. 293.—Presentation of the umbilicus.   (B. C. Hirst.)

probability of endocrine influence and possibly an excessive amount of protein and calcium in the diet may have some effect.

Overgrowth of the baby may be suspected during pregnancy by the great size of the abdomen, without hydramnion and the prolongation of the period of gestation far beyond the date of expected confinement. Measurement of the fetal length *in utero* by MacDonald's or Ahlfeld's method, together with cephalometry by the *x*-ray and Perret's procedure may aid in the diagnosis.

Prognosis.—Postmaturity and overgrowth are dangerous for the child. Birth injuries and asphyxia all are potential causes for mortality.

For the mother, labor is apt to be long and difficult and serious injuries may develop during delivery.

Treatment.—In a primipara, postmaturity with definite and recognizable oversize of the infant should cause elective cesarean section to be considered as the most conservative method of delivery. This is especially true if there is no engagement of the fetal head, which may remain floating above the pelvic brim.

Conviction that postmaturity exists should lead to the induction of labor by one of the approved methods (rupture of the membranes will usually suffice) if there be no obstructive contraindication.

During labor, forceps extraction may be necessary, but because of the distention of the uterus by the large child version is dangerous. The delivery of the shoulders may be quite difficult, one or both clavicles not infrequently being fractured during the process.

It may be necessary to rotate the shoulders into an oblique diameter of the pelvis and thus aid delivery by traction with a finger in either the anterior or posterior axilla, depending upon which one is lower.

If labor becomes absolutely obstructed, cesarean section, with hysterectomy if necessary, is the procedure of choice.

CHAPTER XXX

ANOMALIES OF THE BIRTH CANAL; CONTRACTED PELVIS

A PELVIS is regarded as contracted when any of its essential diameters are so shortened as to affect materially the normal mechanism of labor, whether or not the ultimate delivery of the child is impeded. Pelvic contraction or deformation may be congenital, or may follow certain disease processes as rachitis.

Historical Note.—The presence of pelvic deformity as an obstetrical entity was unknown or disregarded by the ancients, possibly because the bony pelvis was not considered in relation to the birth processes.

Arantius (1530–89) first recorded a pelvic deformity, but his work was not followed, and the great obstetricians of the seventeenth century, Mauriceau, Clement, Portal and others make little mention of the condition. The rachitic dwarf, patient of Mauriceau, who perished while Hugh Chamberlain was endeavoring to demonstrate his forceps with a view to selling the device to Mauriceau, was one of the few cases noted by that authority.

Deventer in 1701 gave the first detailed description of the more common varieties, with a keen insight into their effect upon the mechanism of labor, and from his time on, the subject began to receive general attention.

William Smellie followed with a more detailed study of pelvic deformities, as did Baudelocque in France and Stein in Germany. It is to these latter two men that we owe the pelvimeter.

Michaelis, and his successor, Litzmann, in the middle of the nineteenth century, measured and studied several thousand pelves from the obstetric standpoint, proposed regular classification of the various forms, and laid the foundations for modern studies of the question.

In America, Hugh L. Hodge made important contributions, describing and defining the parallel plans of the pelvic canal. Since then the subject of pelvic deformities has been a leading matter for observation and discussion throughout the obstetrical clinics of the world.

Frequency.—If the definition be applied literally, pelvic contraction occurs in from 15 to 24 per cent of all obstetric patients, but if a more practical standard be taken, namely, the limitation of the term contracted to those pelves in which there is absolute obstruction to vaginal delivery, the ratio is well under 1 per cent.

Etiology.—Deformation of the pelvis may be due to (a) congenital variation in size and shape; (b) deformation due to diseases or injury of the pelvic bones or joints; (c) disease of the skeleton of the trunk or legs.

Grouping of contracted pelves with regard to the effect upon labor:

1. Absolutely contracted pelves are those in which the vaginal delivery of a full-term living infant is impossible. Here the true conjugate is 5½ cm. in length or less, the oblique and transverse diameters being not considered.

2. Relatively contracted pelves are those in which spontaneous delivery of a full-time living infant of average size is impossible, but where operative vaginal delivery may sometimes succeed, though usually with a dead or gravely injured baby. In these, the true conjugate is from 5½ to 8½ cm. in length.

3. Moderately contracted pelves are those in which vaginal delivery is possible, but in which malpresentation, long labor, abnormal mechanism and danger of fetal injury may be anticipated. Here the conjugate varies from 8½ to 9½ cm.

4. Borderline or slightly contracted pelves are those in which delivery may be spontaneous or where operative measures may result in a successful outcome. Conjugate varies 9½ to 10½ cm.

5. Outlet contraction, where the bisischial diameter is less than 9 cm. and the posterior sagittal less than 6 cm.

Contracted pelves are of many forms and types. Sometimes the whole bony structure is simply too small, although all the diameters bear a normal relation to each other. The true conjugate may be shortened, converting the inlet into a flat, narrow ellipse, whereas the pelvic cavity and the outlet may be of normal size, or the conjugate may be of normal or greater than normal length, while the transverse diameter of the inlet is sharply decreased, converting this apparatus into a narrow, long ellipse.

In certain asymmetrical developments, the inlet is flat on one side with a normal form on the other, or it may be enormously flattened on both lateral aspects. On the other hand, the inlet may be of the correct size and shape, and the outlet extremely narrowed, by the close approximation of the tuberosities of the ischia.

The architecture of the pelvis in the abstract is not of obstetric importance, since the accoucheur is concerned only with the question as to whether the pelvis is apt for spontaneous delivery, or whether some anomaly in its structure or variation of size may impede the normal mechanism of labor, or even completely obstruct birth.

Such obstetric variations appear in certain portions of the pelvic girdle which portion should receive the chief attention of the obstetrician who is preparing to prognosticate the probable type of delivery in a given case.

The gross size of the entire pelvis is important, of course, since a dwarf pelvis will not permit the disengagement of a full-term child. In pelves not grossly diminished in size, the shape of the pelvic inlet is of prime importance, the nearly round form representing the best configuration for easy engagement. If the inlet be elliptical, the largest diameter is usually the transverse, but as the line of greater width is nearer the sacrum than the symphysis, it is not available to admit of the entrance of the long diameter of the fetal head because the sacrum in contact with the side of the head thrusts this much further forward. The *available transverse* diameter, then, is a line bisecting the true conjugate midway between sacrum and symphysis, and is 11.5 cm. in length in a normal pelvis, rather than the 13 cm. of the widest transverse diameter measurable (Figs. 294, 295).

If this be true, it follows that the shape of the horizontal rami of the pubes is of the greatest importance, for if these be sharply angulated, the anterior side of the head will impinge upon them, reducing the available anteroposterior diameter of the inlet even though the true conjugate be of normal length. The available anteroposterior diameter is also greatly altered by the degree to which the promontory of the sacrum is thrust forward, making the shape of the inlet more or less cordiform.

If the curve of the horizontal rami of the pubes be too flat, a diminution of the true conjugate follows giving rise to the flat pelvis.

The next factor of importance in the obstetric formation of the obstetric pelvis is its inclination or the angle between the promontory

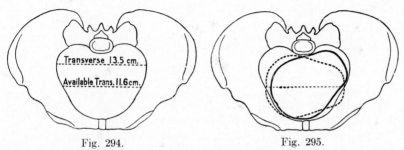

Fig. 294.   Fig. 295.

Figs. 294 and 295.—Diagrams showing why the head does not engage in the transverse diameter of the superior strait. (Williams, "Obstetrics," D. Appleton-Century Co., Publishers.)

of the sacrum and the tip of the symphysis. This, in the normal women, in the erect position is 55 degrees.

If one conceive a pelvis utterly within inclination, i. e., the symphysis on the same level as the promontory, it is obvious that a fetal head could only pass through the bony ring if it were less in diameter than the true conjugate. However, if the same pelvis bore a much exaggerated inclination, say 70 degrees, the head could pass the promontory without opposition from the symphysis, and then slipping into the capacious cavity of the hollow of the sacrum, later pass the symphysis, without difficulty, even though its diameter were appreciably greater than that of the conjugate (see Fig. 111).

For the same reason, the length of the symphysis, its thickness, and the angle which it bears to the promontory are also of importance. Thus, a long symphysis, in effect, lessens the pelvic inclination, whereas a short one increases it. A symphysis which lies vertically placed produces a shorter true conjugate than the same bone lying at a divergent angle to the promontory (see Fig. 112).

When we come to the pelvic excavation, the principal differences lie in the degree of curvature of the sacrum and the length and direction of the ischiatic spines. Variations in this portion of the pelvis, while important, play a much lesser part in the mechanism of labor than do variations in the inlet or outlet.

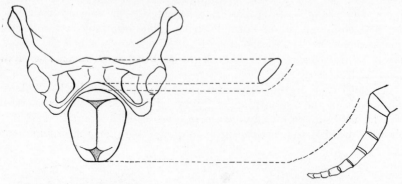

Fig. 296.—Showing effect of a wide pubic arch. There is ample room for the descending head between the descending rami of the pubes, with no tendency to outlet dystocia.

Important factors in the pelvic outlet are the width of the subpubic angle, the relation of the tuberosities of the ischia to each other, and the form and rigidity of the coccyx (Figs. 296, 297).

A narrow subpubic angle draws together the ischiatic tuberosities and narrows the outlet laterally, whereas a wide angle produces the

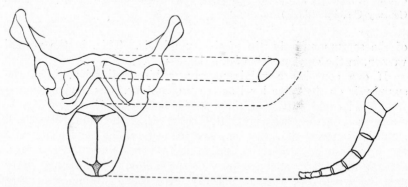

Fig. 297.—Showing effect of a narrow pubic arch. The head is forced far backward in the pelvic cavity and outlet dystocia results.

reverse effect. Thick, heavy tuberosities encroach upon the lateral width of the outlet, and a strong, sharply curved and rigid coccyx may greatly lessen the anteroposterior exit of the pelvis. The form of the subpubic angle bears no relation to the form of the inlet.

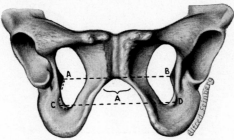

Fig. 298.—A, Narrow subpubic arch similar in size to Fig. 300. Note wide interspinous (AB) and intertuberous diameters (CD).

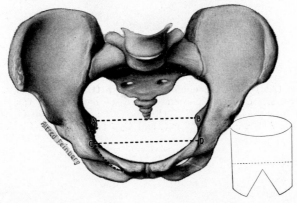

Fig. 299.—Inlet view of pelvis in Fig. 298. Typical android type. Observe that the interspinous (AB) and intertuberous diameters (CD) are long and the side walls converge in front of the latter to form a narrow subpubic arch. As a result, the entire forepelvis is well formed in spite of the narrow subpubic arch (Fig. 298). (Figures 298 and 299 from Caldwell, Moloy and D'Esopo, Amer. Jour. of Obstet. and Gynec., Dec., 1935, C. V. Mosby Co., Publishers.)

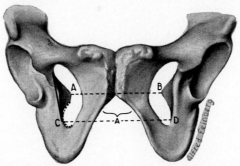

Fig. 300.—Front view of narrow subpubic arch comparable in size to Fig. 298. Note narrow interspinous (AB) and intertuberous diameters (CD).

The shape of the side walls, the general thickness of the bones and the length of the sacrum also contribute toward variation in pelvic architecture of obstetric significance (Figs. 298, 299, 300, 301).

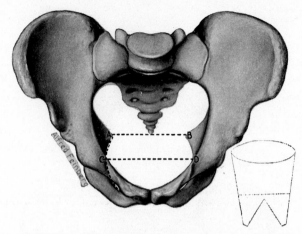

Fig. 301.—Inlet view of pelvis in Fig. 300. Typical anthropoid type. The lateral pelvic walls converge to the narrow arch, causing a decrease in both the interspinous (AD) and intertuberous diameters (CD). Thus, Figs. 298 to 301 show that the size of the subpubic arch gives no indication of the type of pelvis which may be associated with it. (Figures 300 and 301 from Caldwell, Moloy and D'Esopo, Amer. Jour. of Obstet. and Gynec., Dec., 1935, C. V. Mosby Co., Publishers.)

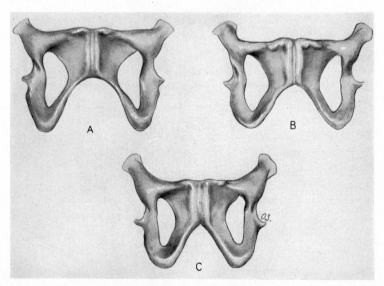

Fig. 302.—Variations in the pubic arch. A, Normal angle in female pelvis; B, excessively obtuse angle with great width between the tuberosities of the ischia; C, very narrow angle, in male type pelvis. When associated with short posterior sagittal diameter, this type arch gives rise to outlet dystocia.

Classification of Contracted Pelves.—Since the time of Deventer, who grouped pelves into too large, too small and too flat types, there have been many attempts to arrive at a complete classification of these anomalies but from the nature of the case, none is wholly satisfactory. The two methods of classifying pelves are that based upon the structural characterization which was first suggested by Michaelis, and elaborated by Litzmann. Later Siebold, Busch and others based a grouping upon the more scientific ground of the etiology of the deformities. This plan was elaborated by Schauta, Tarnier and Budin, while still later Breus and Kolisko modified both systems. The most recent work along these lines is that of Caldwell and Moloy, who divide female pelves into four major groups according to architectural characteristics. They call attention to the anterior and posterior segments of the inlet, with the widest transverse measurement as the dividing line, the variation in the subpubic angle,

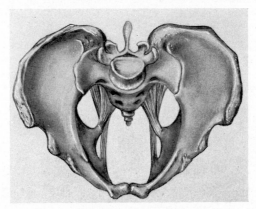

Fig. 303.—Congenitally transversely contracted pelvis. The anthropoid pelvis of Caldwell and Moloy.

the anterior and posterior segments of the outlet, and the size and shape of the sacrosciatic notch.

Based upon these fundamentals, the authors divide pelves into: A. *The Gynecoid Type* (G. *gyne,* woman).—This is the normal pelvis of other classifications and possesses the well-known anatomical characteristics attributed to the female pelvis. These features have been described under "the average female pelvis." All groups are subdivided on the basis of variations in size of the subpubic angle: (1) With a narrow outlet; (2) with a moderate outlet; (3) with a wide outlet; (4) large or small.

B. *The Android Type* (G. *andro-,* man).—These female pelves bear a resemblance to the male sex of man, particularly in the posterior segment of the inlet and the extreme forms simulate the characters described above for the average male pelvis. (1) With a narrow outlet; (2) with a moderate outlet; (3) with a wide outlet; (4) large or small.

C. *The Anthropoid Type* (G. *anthropos,* man).—These forms bear a resemblance to the pelvis of the anthropoid apes. This resemblance will be discussed in greater detail below. (1) With narrow outlet; (2) with moderate outlet; (3) with a wide outlet; (4) large or small (Fig. 303).

D. *The Platypelloid Type* (G. *platy,* flat; *pellis,* pelvis).—These pelves are broad and flat, are rare types, and bear no resemblance to the pelvic form of lower mammals. (1) With a narrow outlet; (2) with a moderate outlet; (3) with a wide outlet; (4) large or small.

E. *Asymmetrical Pelves.*—(1) With a narrow outlet; (2) with a moderate outlet; (3) with a wide outlet; (4) large or small.

In addition to the asymmetry, the general pelvic shape usually conforms to any one of the four types listed above.

This grouping is valuable and throws new light upon the structure of the pelvis and will greatly clarify the mechanism of labor in the various forms.

The writer believes, however, that a modification of the old classification of Schauta, based upon etiological factors, offers a more complete picture of the many varieties of contracted pelves and accordingly it is used here.

CLASSIFICATION OF CONTRACTED PELVIS (MODIFIED FROM SCHAUTA)

I. *Contraction due to congenital defects:*

Common
1. Justo-minor pelvis—generally equally contracted.
2. Simple, flat pelvis.
3. Justo-minor flat pelvis (1 and 2).
4. Male pelvis.
5. Assimilation pelvis.
6. Funnel pelvis.

Rare
7. Split pelvis.
8. Naegele pelvis—improper development of one sacral ala.
9. Robert pelvis—improper development of both sacral alae.
10. Justo-major pelvis—generally too large.

II. *Deformities due to disease of pelvic bones:*

Common—1. Rachitis—commonest cause of all pelvic contractions.

Rare
2. Osteomalacia.
3. Caries and necrosis.
4. Fractures.
5. Neoplasms.

III. *Deformities due to diseases of pelvic joints:*

Rare
1. Synostosis (softening of one or more joints).
2. Ankylosis of one or more pelvic joints.
(Neither of any clinical importance.)

IV. *Deformities due to diseases of the trunk:*

Common
1. Kyphosis.
2. Scoliosis.
3. Lordosis.
4. Spondylolisthesis.

V. *Deformities due to diseases of the legs:*

Uncommon
{
1. Coxitis—*e. g.,* tuberculosis of hip.
2. Congenital dislocation of the hip.
3. Clubfoot.
4. Absence of one or both legs.
5. Atrophy following anterior poliomyelitis.
}

CONTRACTION DUE TO CONGENITAL DEFECTS

The Generally Equally Contracted Pelvis (Justo-minor).—In this variety the pelvis is of normal form, except that the true conjugate may be decreased a trifle relatively. Otherwise the diameters bear a normal relation to one another, but the whole structure is too small (Fig. 304).

This form of pelvis is very common, especially in urban communities, and is thought to be due to the comparative absence of vigorous exercise among city-bred women and their forebears.

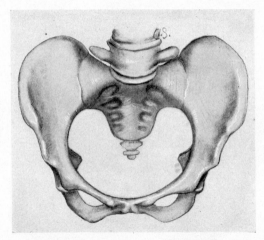

Fig. 304.—A very delicately boned, generally equally contracted pelvis.

In detail, the bones are slender and delicate, the sacrum long and narrow, the subpubic arch usually wide and the horizontal rami of the pubis flat. The rhomboid of Michaelis is short and narrow.

Justo-minor pelves are usually found in women of small stature, with slender bony formation, narrow feet and delicate features.

When similar pelvic measurements are obtained in large women with heavy bones, it is probable that the pelvis is of the male type, not truly justo-minor.

The *diagnosis* of generally contracted pelvis is easily made. The general morphology of the woman should excite suspicion, which is confirmed by pelvimetry, and especially upon finding the pelvic bones thin and small upon palpation. The average diameters of a justo-minor pelvis are:

Interspinous .... 24.0 cm.
Intercristal .... 26.5 cm.
Intertrochanteric .... 29.0 cm.
External conjugate .... 17.5 cm.
Diagonal conjugate .... 11.0 cm.
Conjugata vera .... 9.5 cm.
Bisischial .... 9.5 cm.

When the true conjugate is under 9 cm. one is probably dealing with a rachitic pelvis not a generally equally contracted one.

Effect upon Labor.—Women with too small pelves commonly have small babies, and the mechanism of labor proceeds along normal lines, except that molding is more marked, and flexion occurs early and is extreme.

These women often have but little resistance to fatigue and pain, so that the second stage may be prolonged, by reason of lack of the

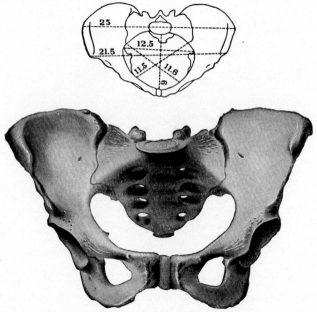

Fig. 305.—Simple flat pelvis. (From Williams, "Obstetrics," D. Appleton-Century Co., Publishers.)

secondary propulsive efforts of the abdominal muscles. Forceps delivery is often required, when the head has passed the spines of the ischia. If the infant be relatively larger than the maternal pelvis, even excessive molding may not overcome the obstacle of the narrowed lateral diameters and consequently anterior rotation is impaired and deep transverse arrest occurs, the sagittal suture lying just a trifle off the transverse diameter of the inlet and the head firmly fixed at about the level of the ischiatic spine.

Here the necessary forceps extraction offers great difficulty and the Kielland or Barton instruments are often requisite to secure proper application and delivery (*q. v.*).

The Simple Flat Pelvis (Pelvis Plana, Platypelloid Pelvis).—In this form of pelvis the only departure from the normal is a shortening of the anteroposterior diameter of the inlet (conjugata vera) brought about by an excessive straightness of the horizontal rami of the pubes and the fact that the sacrum lies lower in relation to the symphysis and further forward. The inlet thus is a broad, kidney-shaped aperture. There is no difference from the normal in the relation of the other diameters to each other, nor is there any contraction of the outlet (Fig. 305).

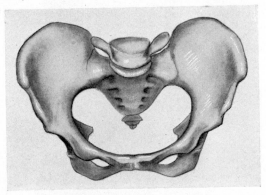

Fig. 306.—Simple flat pelvis.

The simple flat pelvis is quite uncommon, most flat pelves being of the rachitic type. The *etiology* is unknown, many more or less fanciful causes being assigned to it, but in all probability the flat pelvis is a distinctly congenital type (Fig. 306).

Typical measurements of a flat pelvis are:

Intercristal	25.0 cm.
Interspinous	28.0 cm.
Bitrochanteric	31.0 cm.
External conjugate	18.0 cm.
Diagonal conjugate	10.5 cm.
Conjugata vera	9.0 cm.
Bisischial	10.0 cm.

Diagnosis.—Sometimes well formed women possess flat pelves, although the condition may be suspected if there be a distinct flattening of the pelvic curve on inspection of the standing patient in profile. The rhomboid of Michaelis is shortened superiorly so that it approaches a triangular form. Pelvimetry will usually disclose the true state of affairs.

Mechanism of Labor.—Because of the shortness of the anteroposterior diameter of the pelvis, the head engages in the transverse, and for the same reason the wide biparietal diameter cannot enter in the midline and hence slips to one side, finally lying in the lateral aspect of the brim close to the side wall. The narrow bitemporal diameter then enters the conjugate and as descent goes on, deflexion occurs and the forehead descends because the broad occiput meets with greater resistance.

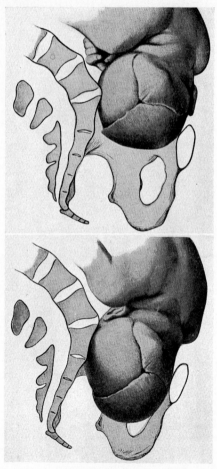

Fig. 307.—Upper, anterior parietal bone presentation. Head being molded into a flat pelvis. Lower, molding continued. The posterior parietal bone slips over the promontory. (Bumm.)

Now either anterior or posterior asynclitism takes place, depending upon whether the flattening of the pelvis is due to a thrusting forward of the promontory, or to excessive straightness of the pubic rami. In the former case, the posterior parietal bone is held by the promontory, the sagittal suture moves nearer this point and the anterior parietal bone passes the symphysis, with marked lateral flexion of the head. The symphysis passed, the lateral flexion is corrected by the posterior parietal bone slipping past the promontory the sagittal suture moving forward.

If the pelvic flattening be due to the shape of the pubic rami the reverse or posterior asynclitism occurs (Litzmann's obliquity). The posterior parietal eminence passes the promontory, the sagittal suture moves forward, until sometimes the posterior ear may be palpated beneath the promontory. This point passed, the anterior parietal bone descends past the symphysis where the lateral flexion is corrected as before.

There being no deformity of the pelvic excavation or outlet, labor proceeds along the lines of normal mechanism once the inlet is traversed.

It is obvious that for such mechanism to be successful, marked overlapping of the parietal bones is a requisite, hence labor is often obstructed in postmature infants, even though they be of moderate size.

Great pressure is exerted upon the side of the head and depressed fractures of the parietal region are not uncommon results (Fig. 307).

The Generally Equally Contracted Flat Pelvis.—This form is a combination of the two foregoing types and may be described as a too small pelvis with excessive diminution of the true conjugate. The diagnosis is made by pelvimetry and the mechanism of labor follows that taking place in flat pelves.

The Male Pelvis (Android Pelvis).—In this form the bones are heavier and thicker, the pelvis is deeper and more conical; the sacrum is long and narrow, the sacrosciatic notch quite narrow, and the space between the spines of the ischia and the sacrum very short. The arch of the pubis is angular, and not gently curved as in the female type, and the subpubic angle is narrow. The bisischiatic diameter is usually contracted, but owing to the length of the descending rami of the pubes, may be fairly wide. The male pelvis is often found in large, massive women, of masculine build; and offers obstruction to delivery both at the inlet and the outlet. The degree of contraction is usually moderate, but labor is delayed because of the great depth of the pelvis and the straight line of the sacrum which impedes rotation.

The Funnel Pelvis.—The late J. Whitridge Williams laid great stress upon funnel pelves which he defined as those in which the usual external measurements are perfectly normal, while the transverse of the outlet is 8 cm. or less.

It is now generally agreed that funnel pelvis is not an entity in itself, but that any form of pelvic architecture may be distorted by a narrowing of the outlet. Thus we may properly speak of a funnel pelvis with normal inlet, a flat pelvis with funneling of the outlet, etc. The difficulty in labor in these pelves occurs at the outlet, where serious dystocia often imperils the child.

34

Detailed measurement of the outlet should always be done, and a marked contraction calls for abdominal delivery.

The Assimilation Pelvis.—In certain women there exist developmental anomalies of the spinal column in which the transverse processes of the last lumbar vertebra may assume the characteristics of the sacral vertebrae and become fused with them. Under these circumstances, the sacrum consists of six segments rather than five, and the resulting structure is termed a high assimilation pelvis. In other examples, the reverse is true, the first sacral vertebra simulating a lumbar one so that the sacrum consists of only four segments, these forming the low assimilation pelvis. The assimilation pelvis is very common, and because there is usually little abnormality in the measurements it is often overlooked. In the high form, the posterior portion of the pelvis is quite high, and the transverse diameter of the inlet may equal or be less than the anteroposterior, the result being closely akin to the anthropoid form of Caldwell and Moloy. Such pelves give rise to errors in rotation, and frequently explain persistent posterior occiput.

The low assimilation pelvis is quite short posteriorly, and generally is of no obstetric significance.

THE RARE FORMS OF CONGENITALLY DEFORMED PELVES

The Split Pelvis.—This is the result of a congenital failure of development of the pubic bones and the symphysis, resulting in a pelvis with a missing anterior portion. This defect is very rare and being almost always associated with exstrophy of the bladder and defective development of the anterior abdominal wall, such individuals rarely survive to maturity. The split pelvis is of little or no obstetric significance.

The Naegele Pelvis; Imperfect Development of One Ala of Sacrum. —In this very rare congenital defect, one wing of the sacrum is either entirely absent or presents a defective development. Consequently the ilium on the affected side is ankylosed with the sacrum, resulting in an almost complete flattening of one side of the pelvis. The innominate bone on the affected side is pushed upward and backward, and the iliopectineal line is almost straight. The symphysis is displaced toward the healthy side of the pelvis, the ischiatic spines are pushed closer together and the consequent transverse narrowing of the pelvis extends throughout its entire depth, both inlet and outlet being diminished laterally.

This type of pelvis while usually congenital may also follow inflammatory lesions of the sacrum in childhood (Fig. 308).

Diagnosis is made by inspection, pelvimetry and vaginal palpation. Labor is usually completely obstructed though with a small infant the head may be forced into the wide side of the pelvis and eventually be delivered with extreme molding.

The Robert Pelvis; Defective Development of Both Sacral Alae.— In this very rare deformity, both wings of the sacrum are lacking and the ilia are fused with the body of that bone, resulting in excessive narrowing of all transverse diameters with little or no alteration of the anteroposterior ones (Fig. 309).

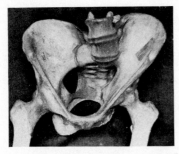

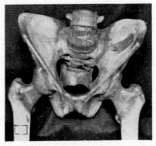

Fig. 308.—Obliquely contracted (Naegele) pelvis. (Mütter Museum, College of Physicians, Philadelphia.)

Fig. 309.—Transversely contracted pelvis; *c.v.*, 9¼ cm., trans. of outlet 5 cm. Transverse of inlet 8 cm. (Mütter Museum, College of Physicians, Philadelphia.)

Delivery through such a pelvis is impossible.

Though much discussed in the older obstetric literature, both these varieties of pelvis are extremely rare, and if discovered, should lead to elective cesarean section.

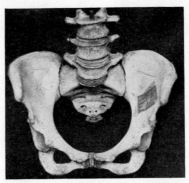

Fig. 310.—Justo-major pelvis. (Mütter Museum, College of Physicians, Phila.)

The Generally Too Large Pelvis (Justo-major).—Just as small women may have small pelves, so very large women may possess structures whose measurements are all in excess of the normal, but the diameters bear a correct relation to each other. This variety of pelvis has no bearing upon the course of labor, except that sometimes its very capacity inhibits the normal mechanism, and results in precipitate delivery with possibly severe laceration of the pelvic floor (Fig. 310).

PELVIC DEFORMITIES DUE TO DISEASE OF THE PELVIC BONES

The Rachitic Pelvis.—Rachitis, with its peculiar bone changes, eventuating (in a recovered case) in some atrophy of the osseous structure, with increased porosity and often considerable thickening, is one of the very common diseases of childhood.

Inasmuch as its earlier stages involve increased vascularity and marked softening of the bones, the tendency to produce distortions of the pelvis in growing girls is self-evident.

Many authorities consider some form of rachitic deformity to be by far the most common cause of pelvic contraction, this being notably so in the colored race. Four subdivisions of the rachitic pelvis are generally described:

Flat rachitic.

Generally contracted rachitic.

Generally contracted flat rachitic.

Pseudo-osteomalacic rachitic.

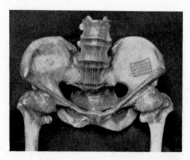 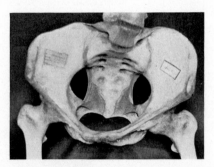

Fig. 311.—Very marked degree of flat rachitic pelvis. (Mütter Museum, College of Physicians, Philadelphia.)

Fig. 312.—Rachitic pelvis with double promontory. (Mütter Museum, College of Physicians, Philadelphia.)

The *flat rachitic pelvis* presents certain typical differences from the norm (Fig. 311). The sacrum is broad, thin, and its usual lateral concavity is either flattened, or the bone may be actually convex from side to side. The vertical concavity is markedly accentuated, a sharp bend being often found at the third sacral vertebra. Sometimes, however, the vertical concavity may be lost, the bone being almost straight. The promontory sinks forward and downward, encroaching upon the true conjugate, and the inclination of the pelvis is thereby decreased. Occasionally the body of the first sacral vertebra is displaced far forward and projects into the pelvic brim as a false or double promontory, this additional projection sometimes greatly reducing the already diminished conjugata vera (Fig. 312).

Because the sacrum has sunk forward and downward, the posterior portions of the ilia are drawn together, their anterior extremities flaring apart in consequence, so that commonly the distance between their anterior superior spines is as great as or greater than the intercristal length. The outlet is not affected.

The obliquity of the symphysis is decreased and as a result the conjugate-symphysial angle is increased.

Typical measurements of a flat rachitic pelvis are:

Interspinous	24 cm.
Intercristal	23 cm.
Intertrochanteric	28 cm.
External conjugate	16 cm.
Diagonal conjugate	9 cm.
Bisischial	10 cm.

The *generally contracted rachitic pelvis* is represented by a too small pelvis possessing rachitic characteristics, consequently all the diameters of the inlet are reduced, the anteroposterior more markedly so.

The outlet is correspondingly contracted, but not to an excessive degree.

The Generally Contracted Flat Pelvis (Rachitic).—This is simply a very small rachitic pelvis with great shortening of the true conju-

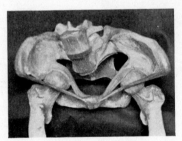

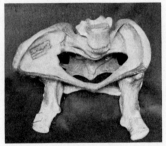

Fig. 313.—Pseudo-osteomalacic pelvis probably of rachitic origin. (Mütter Museum, College of Physicians, Philadelphia.)

Fig. 314.—Scoliotic-rachitic pelvis. (Mütter Museum, College of Physicians, Philadelphia.)

gate. Pelves conforming to this type usually present anteroposterior diameters of the brim of 7 cm. or less and are mostly to be included in the group of absolute contractions.

The Pseudo-osteomalacic Pelvis.—This term is used to describe the advanced form of pelvic distortion, following upon severe and long-continued active manifestation of rachitic disease (Fig. 313, 314). The pubic rami may be so sharply bent as to lie almost parallel to each other, creating a beaklike anterior pelvic aspect. The sacrum may project so far into the inlet as to leave practically no space between the promontory and the pubes. There may be also oblique contractions and the spine is often involved in the deformation. The pseudo-osteomalacic pelvis is very rare.

The Mechanism of Labor in Rachitic Pelves.—In the more notable form of rachitic deformity engagement of the head is generally impossible and labor becomes obstructed while the presenting part is above the brim, cesarean section being necessary to effect delivery.

In the very common flat rachitic form, the mechanism follows that described for the simple flat pelvis, with abnormal molding and danger of fetal skull fracture from the protruding promontory.

Once the inlet is safely passed, labor proceeds as usual, since outlet contraction is not common in this form of pelvic anomaly.

Osteomalacia.—This disease is so rare in America that no examples of its effect on the pelvis are seen, except as rare importations from Europe. Most instances of pelves approximating the osteomalacic form are of rachitic origin. The disease is characterized by excessive softening of the bones so that the pelvis is distorted out of all resemblance to a normal structure (Fig. 315). Because of the flexibility of the bones, these patients cannot walk and should pregnancy occur the only treatment is cesarean section, although some European case

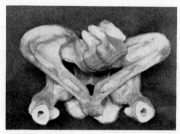

Fig. 315.—Advanced osteomalacic pelvis. (Mütter Museum, College of Physicians, Philadelphia.)

histories recite delivery by the spreading apart of the extremely soft bony tissues.

Caries and necrosis of the pelvic bones occurring in childhood, may give rise to irregular deformities in the mature structure which may produce any form of distortion (Figs. 316, 317).

Such pelves are usually recognized by their asymmetrical outline and the diagnosis may be proved by *x*-ray examination.

The effect upon labor is determined by the nature and extent of the deformity.

Neoplasms of the Pelvic Bones.—Tumors of the pelvis may be enchondromata, fibromata, sarcomata, or bone cysts. If nonmalignant, they usually lead to multiform exostoses, of no obstetric importance except when they encroach upon the pelvic cavity, when the decision as to the manner of delivery depends upon their size and the degree of obstruction they offer.

Fracture of the Pelvis.—The increasing frequency of automobile accidents has brought fracture of the pelvis into considerable prominence from the obstetric standpoint.

Within the past two years the writer has observed three patients who had suffered from this traumatism in one of whom, the consequent deformity and callus formation necessitated cesarean section, in another, a medico-legal case, the resulting pelvic contraction was such that expert testimony proved the necessity for cesarean section, should pregnancy occur, while in the third, although there was con-siderable distortion of the pubic rami, spontaneous delivery took place.

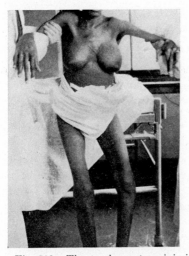

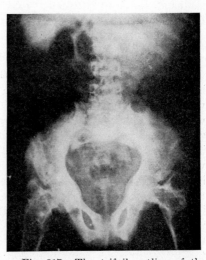

Fig. 316.—The tendency to minimize weight-bearing upon the lower extremi-ties is shown. The triangular head and the sharply angulated sternum are seen, as well as the relative elongation of the arms and hands with clubbing of the fingers. The bowed and sharp tibiae, with flattened ends are notice-able. The spine showed a left dorsal scoliosis of mild degree and a slight lumbar kyphosis. The scoliosis is sug-gested in the photograph. (From Stone in Surg., Gynec., and Obstet., vol. 39, Nov., 1924.)

Fig. 317.—The trifoil outline of the superior strait is clearly shown with the transverse contraction from inward trochanteric pressure. The beaked symphysis is demonstrated while the narrowing of the pubic arch is less evident upon the plate. The bone substance is characterized chiefly by generalized halisteresis best seen in the vertebral bodies and the upper extremi-ties of the femora. A medium size cyst is present near the posterior spine of the left ilium. (From Stone in Surg., Gynec., and Obstet., vol. 39, Nov., 1924.)

The important clinical point in this connection is that a history of fracture of the pelvis should always demand careful roentgenological study of the pelvis during pregnancy.

DEFORMITIES DUE TO DISEASES OF THE PELVIC JOINTS

Ankylosis: There is always a certain amount of play in the nor-mal sacro-iliac articulature, of which the obstetrician takes advantage in employing the Walcher position.

It has been shown that there is usually a slight separation of the symphysis during labor, with a subsequent trifling widening of the joint. The sacrococcygeal joint may also become ankylosed, sometimes resulting in a fracture at the point with subsequent distressing disability. One of the stated causes of dystocia in elderly primiparae is the complete rigidity of the pelvic girdle.

Relaxation of the pelvic joints is rare. There may be congenitally loose articulation or there may be fluid in the joints. When present, the condition is usually noted by the difficulty in walking experienced by the patient, a wabbling, insecure gait being characteristic.

DEFORMITIES DUE TO DISEASES OF THE TRUNK

Spondylolisthesis.—This term (literally a sliding of the vertebrae) is applied to a peculiar condition in which the body of the last lumbar vertebra becomes dislocated anteriorly, sliding over the sacrum, forward and downward into the pelvic brim, necessarily carrying the superimposed spinal column with it. The etiology is either a severe injury to the spine, or some defect in the ossification of the lumbar vertebrae. There is some dispute as to whether the condition is a true luxation in the beginning or whether it is due to changes in the interarticular position of the bone itself. This academic dispute, while interesting, is of no special significance to the obstetrician. The resulting deformity is well marked. On inspection of the patient, there is definite lumbar lordosis, and a distinct shortening of the torso, the rib edges being almost in contact with the crests of the ilia. The hips are notably prominent and there is usually pendulous abdomen. The gait of the woman is a characteristic rolling motion, the entire pelvis rotating with each step.

On vaginal examination, the lumbar vertebrae overlying the inlet may be clearly felt and sometimes the bifurcation of the aorta presents to the examining finger. The sacrum may be differentiated from the lumbar vertebrae, the angle between them being quite acute.

Lateral x-ray photographs will confirm the diagnosis. The effect upon labor, is, of course, due to the anteroposterior shortening of the inlet, and the disappearance of pelvic inclination, the pelvic brim lying practically parallel to the horizon.

In cases where the lumbosymphysial distance is 8 cm. or more, vaginal delivery is possible, but in most instances elective cesarean section is the rule.

Kyphosis.—The effect of kyphosis, the end-result of arrested Pott's disease, upon the pelvis varies with the location of the hump or gibbus. If this is in the dorsal region, the compensatory lordosis of the lower spine directs the force of the body weight normally upon the sacrum and little or no alteration is observed in the pelvis.

If the spinal deformity is in the lumbar spine, however, the effect is very marked. The backward direction of the body weight tends to rotate the sacrum on its transverse axis, the promontory being directed downward and backward, while the coccyx is thrown upward and forward. The rotation of the wedge-like sacrum forces the posterior portions of the ilia far apart, so that the intercristal diameter is often longer than the intertrochanteric one. By the same motion the ischia are pushed together with a sharp diminution in the bisichiatic diameter.

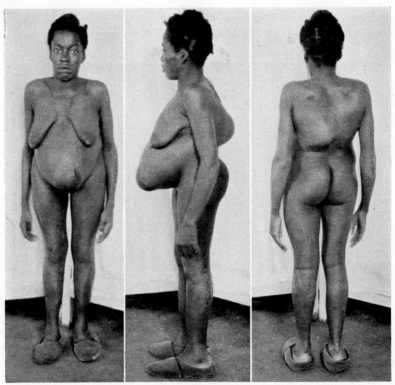

Fig. 318.   Fig. 319.   Fig. 320.

Fig. 318.—Kyphosis. Anterior view. This patient's mother is strikingly similar in stature having a dorsolumbar kyphosis due to Pott's disease.

Fig. 319.—Same patient in profile. Showing pendulous abdomen and ventral hernia from a previous section.

Fig. 320.—Kyphosis. Three cesarean sections. (Author's case, Philadelphia General Hospital.)

The result of these movements is a pelvis of large inlet, the true conjugate considerably longer than normal, with a rapid conical narrowing as the outlet is approached, the tuberosities of the ischia being close together, while the jutting coccyx decreases the anteroposterior diameter of the inferior strait.

In the unusual cases of lumbo-sacral kyphosis, the angulation of the spine covers the brim of the pelvis, so that while the inlet may be amply large, the head cannot enter by reason of the projecting vertebrae. This is the so-called "pelvis obtecta."

Kyphosis in the sense of an obstruction to labor is uncommon among child-bearing women, the generally quoted statistics giving a ratio of 1 in 6000 labors. In my own experience, the condition is much less common than these figures would indicate.

The diagnosis of kyphotic pelvis is made by observation of the spinal curvature, but careful mensuration supplemented by x-ray measurements must be made in order to determine the degree of contraction present. It is surprising how many women with very

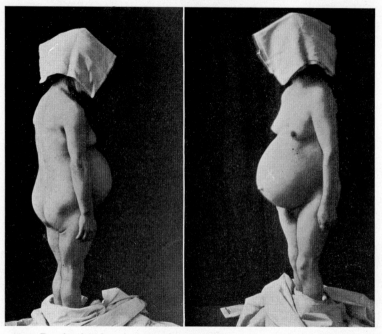

Fig. 321.—Poorly developed cretin dwarf delivered by celiohysterectomy. (Edward P. Davis.)

prominent "hump back" deliver easily and spontaneously (Figs. 318, 319, 320).

Effect upon Pregnancy and Labor.—Because of the angulation of the spine, annoying dyspnea may complicate pregnancy. For the same reason, the uterus is forced forward with exaggerated pendulous abdomen. The head of the fetus being directed backward toward the promontory rather than into the pelvic brim may bring about various deflexion attitudes. If the head can enter the pelvis there is no delay at the brim, but obstruction occurs when the narrowed outlet is approached; and this may be absolute if the bisischiatic diameter is less than 8 cm.

In all marked outlet contractions cesarean section offers the best hope of success.

Scoliosis.—Lateral curvature of the spine is obstetrically unimportant, unless of rachitic origin, when the oblique contraction of the pelvis which follows, may be a source of dystocia. In this lesion the sacrum is forced toward the side opposite the convexity of the spine and is rotated upon itself while one side is shortened and the other correspondingly elongated.

As a result the pelvis becomes obliquely contracted, the flattening being upon the same side as the lumbar convexity. The inlet only is affected, the outlet remaining normal.

In rachitic cases, the other pelvic deformities commonly associated with this disease are present and dystocia is due not to the scoliosis alone but to the other rachitic factors (Fig. 321).

DEFORMITIES DUE TO DISEASES OF THE LEGS

Unilateral lameness whether due to an old coxalgia, the atrophy following poliomyelitis or other cause, usually produces an oblique deformity of the pelvis, the affected side being flattened and lower than the healthy one.

Inasmuch as these diseases usually attack children and are very chronic, failure in bony development is a common accompaniment, so that one deals with a justo-minor pelvis in addition to the oblique contraction. If the malformation be the result of coxalgia, ankylosis of the hip may add to the difficulty.

The diagnosis depends upon observation of the lameness, history and pelvic measurement. Dystocia is to be expected in these patients, for they are usually of poor physique and resistance to fatigue, in addition to their pelvic difficulties.

Long tests of labor are inadvisable and early resort to hysterotomy is the procedure of choice if serious dystocia seems imminent.

Bilateral lameness, from congenital dislocation of the hips, clubfeet, etc., generally results in a pelvis wider than ordinary. Funnel pelvis has been reported in clubfoot. Ordinarily one expects little difficulty in parturition other than that induced by the systemic physical inferiority of the patient.

THE CLINICAL COURSE OF PREGNANCY AND LABOR IN CONTRACTED PELVES

The course of pregnancy in women who possess contracted pelves depends upon the degree and nature of the deformity. In many cases where labor is extremely difficult, the pregnancy may be entirely normal with nothing to arouse suspicion of any impending complication until the onset of labor reveals the difficulty. In the more extreme degrees of contraction, pendulous belly may be much in evidence, and it has been well said that such condition in a primipara presumes advanced pelvic deformity to exist. In multiparae, relaxation of the abdominal walls may be solely responsible.

When, in a primipara, the head cannot engage and the abdominal muscles are too tense to permit the falling forward of the gravid uterus, the organ is held high in the abdomen with consequent embarrassment of respiration during the later months of pregnancy.

Malpresentations are four times more often seen in contracted pelves than in those of normal size and indeed, transverse presentation is almost an indication that a marked deformity is at fault.

Labor in Contracted Pelves.—Because of the general constitutional inferiority of many women who have pelvic defects, the premature onset of labor is said to occur often, although my personal experience does not tend to corroborate this statement.

Premature rupture of the membranes is frequently noted, a short time before term, for since the presenting part cannot properly enter the brim, and does not fit its walls accurately, there are wide spaces wherein the preparturient uterine contractions may force a pouch of membranes filled with liquor amnii, through the brim, until they give way under the pressure.

It is probably due to the fact that such premature rupture often occurs in pelvic contractions that dry labor is so often considered a complication. When the membranes are deliberately ruptured, in normal cases, in order to induce labor, these difficulties are not met.

Delay in Dilatation of the Cervix.—When the head does not engage well, it fails to offer an area of counterpressure, over which the retraction of the powerful muscles of the uterine fundus may pull the cervix and so compel its dilatation. Consequently both effacement and dilatation are slow and unsatisfactory and the woman may experience hours of powerful pains, with but little or no gain in either.

Uterine Inertia.—Primary inertia may occur because, as before mentioned, many women with contracted pelvis have little general power, and a lowered threshold of fatigue.

Uterine exhaustion or secondary inertia is far more common, the uterus expending its power in a vain effort to drive the fetus through an impassable barrier. It is in this type of case that the obstetrician must be on his guard to differentiate between primary and secondary inertia, so that he may not make the error of attempting further to stimulate a worn-out uterine musculature.

Prolapse of the Cord.—Imperfect fit of head to pelvic brim, premature rupture of membranes and malpresentations are the three most common causes for prolapse of the cord and since all three are characteristic of contracted pelvis, it follows that this complication is most often met with when such deformities are present. Indeed, prolapse of the cord at or near term may be utilized as an affirmation of probable distortion of the pelvic brim.

Complications of the Second Stage.—It has been shown above that in several varieties of pelvic abnormality the difficulty lies not in the inlet, but in the outlet of the pelvis. Hence, engagement and the first stage of labor may progress without untoward symptoms, but delay and even complete obstruction may supervene when the head is on the perineum. Some of the greatest and at times insuperable difficulties arise at this time. In other types of contraction, the dystocia may occur when the head has passed the inlet and lies in the cavity of the pelvis, deep transverse arrest and the like.

Rupture of the Uterus.—The effort of the uterus to force the presenting part past an obstruction may produce a rise in the contraction ring and ultimately a spontaneous rupture in the segment between its fundus and the attenuated lower uterine segment. This advent of this contingency is accompanied by definite symptoms which have been described already.

Pressure Necrosis and Fistulae.—Long labors, with the continual strong pressure of the head upon the soft parts, may lead to pressure necrosis and subsequent sloughing of the cervix or the vaginal walls.

Vesicovaginal and rectovaginal fistulas may follow such necrosis, although they are more often due directly to the added trauma of difficult instrumental delivery.

Rupture of the Pelvic Joints and Fracture of the Pelvis.—Rarely, spontaneously, and uncommonly during forceps delivery, the pubic bones may be fractured, the injury being attended by a loud report. The sides of the pelvis separate at once, and delivery is usually easy thereafter, although the recovery of the mother is much delayed, by the slow union of the fractured margins, and may be further complicated by injuries to the bladder occurring as a part of the accident.

Fracture of the Coccyx.—The coccyx or sacrococcygeal joint may be fractured, especially in elderly primiparae when their joints are ankylosed. The accident may occur during spontaneous labor, but is more frequent during forceps extraction, as the head passes through the pelvic outlet.

The accident is often not recognized until well on in the puerperium, when a dull and constant backache occurs, aggravated by sitting and defecation, and to be diagnosed by the painful motility of the coccyx upon pressure with a vaginal finger.

This condition is known as coccygodynia and is treated by the excision of the fractured portion of the bone.

Puerperal Infection.—Premature rupture of membranes, frequent vaginal examinations to determine the cause of the delay, difficult operative deliveries and severe laceration of the birth canal, all attend labor in contracted pelves and all are sovereign causes for puerperal infection which is accordingly much increased. The most meticulous care in the maintenance of asepsis, the minimizing of blood loss, and the avoidance of undue trauma, are the essentials in preventing this unfortunate sequel.

Effects upon the Child.—With every centimeter of pelvic contraction the fetal mortality rises, except in the cases of absolute contraction where early recognition leads to elective cesarean section and a consequent salvage of the babies. Asphyxia, from prolonged pressure or cord prolapse, intracranial hemorrhage or pressure from fracture of

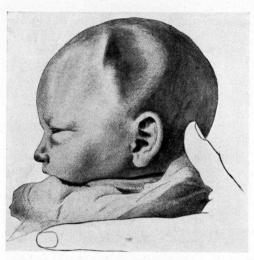

Fig. 322.—Spoon-shaped depression in skull after spontaneous delivery through a flat pelvis. (Bumm.)

the skull and fractures and dislocations of the long bones during traumatic deliveries make up the account. The remedy lies as always in the early recognition of pelvic deformities and the utilization of the proper means to overcome their ill effects (Fig. 322).

THE DIAGNOSIS OF PELVIC DEFORMITIES

The determination of the existence and extent of pelvic deformity constitutes one of the major duties of the obstetrician, and I am of the opinion that the whole subject must be revised in the light of more recent additions to our knowledge.

Every obstetrician of experience has been disappointed to find that the most painstaking pelvic mensuration, plus efforts to ascertain the relative size of the fetal head, ends in difficult labor. This because some alteration in the pelvic form which eludes pelvimetry has caused a sometimes formidable dystocia.

The advent of accurate roentgenograms of the pelvis has shown clearly that moderate transverse narrowing of the brim, thickening of the bones, an unreached, false promontory, a narrow subpubic angle, all of these tend to defeat the accoucheur's hope of a spontaneous delivery and are generally unrecognized until the inevitable obstruction has occurred. Indeed, it is more probable that the generally accepted and classical idea of the shape of the ideal pelvis is erroneous. The work of those enthusiastic students, Thoms, Caldwell and Moloy and Jarcho has demonstrated that the most useful pelvic inlet is round in outline rather than oval as usually thought. In my own clinic we have been routinely making direct measurements of the pelvic inlet in all laparotomies on the gynecological service and have found a preponderance of the round form in women who relate good obstetric histories.

The workers mentioned above have also shown that the type pelvis in which primary occipitoposterior positions may be expected, can be definitely demonstrated by roentgenological study, prior to labor. The conclusion is inevitable that instrumental and digital pelvimetry is not adequate to satisfy the demands of modern obstetrical practice, and it is my considered opinion that an x-ray measurement and description of every primiparous pelvis is an integral part of a well managed obstetrical clinic. In private practice, physicians should refer primiparae to roentgenologists for a report upon the pelvis, early in pregnancy. On their part more roentgenologists should learn the comparatively simple technic requisite to enable them to report authoritatively upon the shape and size of a given pelvis. As a teacher, I feel so strongly upon this subject, that it is with some reluctance that I continue to emphasize pelvimetry to my students, since I am convinced of its inadequacy except in cases of gross deformity.

However, we are not yet ready for the widespread use of this advance, and pelvimetry still remains the most efficient method of prognosticating the nature of the impending labor, for most physicians. All too often the pregnant woman is fortunate indeed, if she be given the advantage of even this attempt at a precise diagnosis.

The diagnosis of the form and capacity of the pelvis, then, is made upon:

Inspection of the woman.

Pelvimetry, external and internal.

Roentgenological examination.

Inspection of the Woman

Lameness is noted, difference in the level of the two sides of the pelvis when the patient is erect; spinal curvature, a peculiar gait together with the general bodily contours, give valuable information.

The best obstetrical pelves are generally found in women of medium size, with the classically feminine figure, i. e., sloping shoulders, the hips broader than the shoulders, well arched feet and columnar neck. Women with long torsos have better pelves than those who are, to use a turf term, "short coupled." Marked knock knees or bowlegs make one suspect pelvic deformation.

Very large women should theoretically possess equally large pelves but this is not necessarily true, as so many of these patients have heavy, stout bones and pelves which are largely masculine in type. Brunhilde did not produce a brood of supermen.

The stigmata of rachitis should be sought in the square-shaped head, and the rachitic rosary on the costosternal articulations.

The *history* will determine the outcome of previous pregnancies, if any, and also record any accidents involving the pelvis, or debilitating disease of long standing; especially if these occurred during the period of adolescence.

All the information so gained indicates the possibility only of pelvic contraction and accurate information must be obtained by pelvimetry or better x-ray measurement.

At the onset of labor in primiparae the head is normally engaged. If it be not, and lies free above the brim it is said to be floating and this is almost certain evidence of marked disproportion of some type and vaginal delivery must be approached with the greatest care if engagement does not occur.

PELVIMETRY

Ever since Baudelocque insisted upon the value of direct external pelvimetry and Stein devised his original internal pelvimeter, the importance of obtaining accurate information as to the pelvis, by this means, has been emphasized by obstetricians.

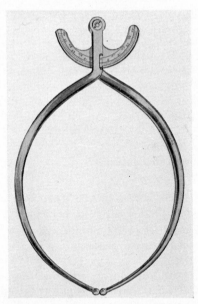

Fig. 323.—Baudelocque-Breisky pelvimeter. Very slightly modified by DeLee. (From DeLee, "Principles and Practice of Obstetrics.")

Pelvic measurements should be made early in pregnancy and the probable outcome of labor predicted upon the findings. The measurements should be rechecked near term.

For external pelvimetry a simple pair of calipers, well curved and long enough to span the pregnant abdomen are utilized. The arms of the instrument terminate in small rounded knobs and the distance between them is read upon a scale affixed near the hinge joint.

The pelvimeters of Breisky, Martin and Collyer are simple and well suffice for the purpose (Fig. 323).

For internal pelvimetry many devices have been invented, some of them most complex, some simple and ingenious, but none of them satisfactory. The procedure is too involved and too painful for practical use, so that the method has been rather generally abandoned.

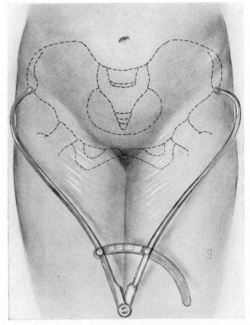

Fig. 324.—Measuring the distance between the spines of the ilia.

No instrument can supplant the trained hand in estimating the form of the pelvic cavity.

The outlet is measured by one of several excellent instruments, those of Williams, DeLee and Thoms being the simplest and best.

External Pelvimetry.—For this purpose the patient should lie on her back on a couch or table, the abdomen and pelvis bared or covered by a thin sheet.

The measurements to be taken are:

The distance between the spines of the ilia; the *interspinous diameter*—26 cm. (Fig. 324).

The distance between the crests of the ilia, the *intercristal diameter*—29 cm. (Fig. 325).

35

The distance between the trochanters (the feet together) the *inter-trochanteric diameter*—31 cm.

The distance from the depression beneath the last lumbar verte-bra to the anterior surface of the symphysis, the *external conjugate diameter* or the diameter of Baudelocque—20.25 cm. (Fig. 326).

Two oblique diameters—the *right oblique,* from the posterior supe-rior spine of the right ilium to the anterior superior spine of the left ilium—22 cm.

The *left oblique* from the posterior superior spine of the left ilium to the anterior superior spine of the right ilium—21.5 cm. (Fig. 327).

The oblique diameters are of value only when the pelvis is asym-metrically deformed. The circumference of the pelvis—measured with

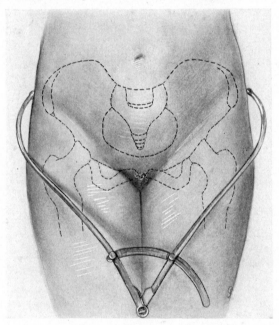

Fig. 325.—Measuring the distance between the crests of the ilia.

a tape line, between the crests of the ilia and the trochanters—90 cm. This distance varies so greatly that it is of little value, and has been discarded in my practice.

In making these measurements, the physician stands facing the patient, and first outlining the bony prominences to be utilized, he places the balls of the pelvimeter over each pair in turn, reading the distances upon the scale of the instrument. The external conjugate may be measured with the woman in the erect posture, or lying on her side, her back toward the examiner.

The spine of the last lumbar vertebra is quite prominent and may be located by lightly running the finger down the spinous prominences. Just beneath this spine is a palpable depression into which one end of the pelvimeter is placed, while the other is firmly pressed against the top of the symphysis.

Baudelocque felt that if **8 to 8.5 cm.** were deducted from the external conjugate, the length of the conjugata vera would be closely approximate but this has been found to be erroneous.

The oblique diameters are also measured with the patient on her side, having her turn over for the estimation of the opposite oblique. It must be remembered that the crests of the ilia are 1 or 1.5 cm. thick, and that as the measurements are made from the external surface, this distance is by so much greater that of the space between the inner margin of the bones.

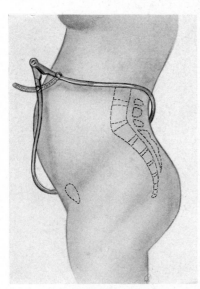

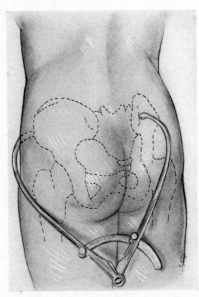

Fig. 326.—Measuring the external con-   Fig. 327.—Measuring the oblique diam-
jugate or diameter of Baudelocque.   eter of the inlet.

The Rhomboid of Michaelis.—During the course of pelvimetry, there may be noted upon the back of the patient a geometrical rhomboid, formed by the dimples marking the sites of the posterior spines of the ilia, laterally, the top of the gluteal fold, below, and the depression beneath the spine of the last lumbar vertebra above (Fig. 328).

If these points be connected by imaginary lines, a kite-shaped figure results, the upper triangle being shorter than the lower. If the rhomboid be symmetrical, the line drawn between the lateral angles, horizontal, the pelvis is presumably not obliquely deformed. If one posterior superior spine lies at a higher level than the other, some pelvic asymmetry is probable.

The Measurement of the Pelvic Outlet.—Here two external dimensions are of importance. The distance between the tuberosities of the ischia, the bisischiatic diameter—10 cm. The distance between a transverse line connecting the tuberosities of the ischia and the top of the sacrum, the posterior sagittal diameter or diameter of Klein—8 cm.

TECHNIC.—For the measurement of the outlet, the patient may lie across a bed with the legs flexed, but it is better to have her on a

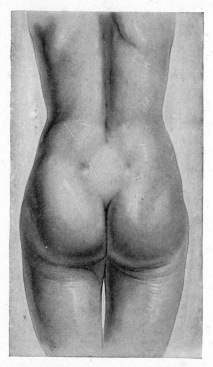

Fig. 328.—This lozenge-shaped space marked by four dimples and which the Greek sculptor shows so clearly in his Venus de Milo, is called the rhomboid of Michaelis. The upper dimple is the one from which the external conjugate is measured. The beautiful rhomboid is distorted when the woman has a contracted pelvis. It becomes squat with a flat pelvis and irregular if the woman is asymmetrically built. (DeLee.)

table in the lithotomy position, the feet in stirrups. The examiner then locates the tuberosities of the ischia and places the terminals of an outlet pelvimeter in contact with their inner margin, reading the scale (Fig. 329).

To measure the posterior sagittal diameter, the Thoms pelvimeter is best but one may utilize a wooden tongue depressor or any straight edge, which is placed from one ischial tuberosity to the other, and the distance from the midpoint of this line to the top of the sacrum, measured with a pelvimeter (Fig. 330).

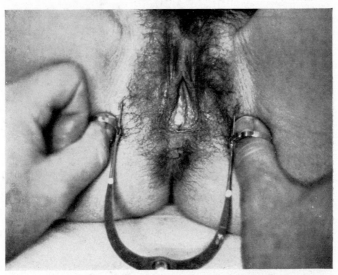

Fig. 329.—Measuring the transverse diameter of the outlet with Williams' pelvimeter.

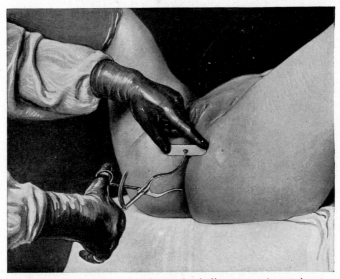

Fig. 330.—Measuring the posterior sagittal diameter. A wooden tongue depressor is cut to fit between the tuberosities, and the distance from its center to the end of the sacrum measured with any pelvimeter. (DeLee.)

This posterior sagittal diameter is of great importance in pelves contracted at the outlet, because the narrowing of the pubic arch, in such pelves, so reduces the available anteroposterior of the outlet that delivery depends upon the space between the tuberosities and the sacrum. A convenient rule for practice is that when the sum of the bisischial and the posterior sagittal diameters is 15 cm. or more, vaginal delivery is possible in outlet contractions, whereas if this figure is below 15 cm., vaginal delivery is questionable or impossible (Fig. 331). A crude but fairly practicable method of measuring the outlet is to place the closed fist between the tuberosities of the ischia. If the fist enters easily, between them, the lateral length of the outlet is probably adequate (Fig. 332).

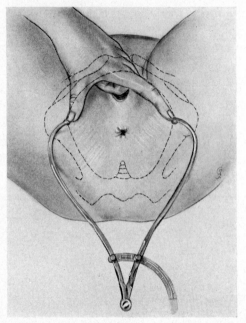

Fig. 331.—Measuring the transverse diameter of the outlet.

The Significance of External Pelvimetry.—Comparison of external measurements with the actual size of the pelvis reveals the fact that great differences appear.

The error possible in estimating the true conjugate from the length of external conjugate has already been mentioned. The thickness of the symphysis, the inclination of the pelvis and the length of the promontory cannot be determined by external pelvimetry.

However, the external conjugate gives valuable information, because if it be decreased to below 19, there is always great probability of pelvic contraction. A short external conjugate then offers fairly definite evidence of pelvic difficulty, but one of normal length does not preclude the possibility of contraction. The same statements apply to the transverse external measurements.

Internal Pelvimetry.—It has been well said that the best pelvimeter is the skilled hand, and the obstetrician of experience can determine the availability of the pelvis from the viewpoint of spontaneous delivery with almost unfailing accuracy. The only gross error made by such men is their inability to reach a false promontory.

I urge upon students the painstaking manual examination of women whenever practicable, in order to educate the sense of touch and to translate the sensation so received into a mental conception of the size and shape of the pelvic cavity.

This is not a scientific method of approach but it is obstetric art in the highest sense and is all too much neglected.

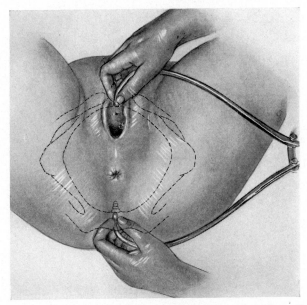

Fig. 332.—Measuring the anteroposterior diameter of the outlet.

Personally I should prefer the opinion of a Hirst, DeLee or Williams as to the outcome of labor, after simple bimanual examination, to the most careful set of figures obtained by pelvimetry with any instrument ever invented.

The most important diameter of the pelvis is the true conjugate, whose direct measurement is only possible with elaborate instruments, the use of which is often extremely painful, and whose accuracy is questionable.

Happily it is possible to approximate this diameter closely by estimating the distance between the promontory of the sacrum and the lower border of the symphysis, the diagonal conjugate, and making certain deductions from it.

Technic.—With the patient on an examining table, the feet in stirrups, or across the bed with the legs flexed, the examiner, wearing sterile gloves, inserts two fingers between the labia (Fig. 333). The pelvis is now digitally explored, the tone and elasticity of the levator ani noted, the direction and length of the spines of the ischia, and the curve of the side walls of the pelvis are determined. The sacrum is carefully palpated to discover the extent of its concavity, or whether it possibly is flat or even convex. The height and thickness of the symphysis are estimated as is the nature of the subpubic angle and the degree of curvature of the rami of the pubes, and the cervix is carefully palpated to discover old lacerations or other lesions. If the examination is made late in pregnancy, the position and presentation of the fetus is made out.

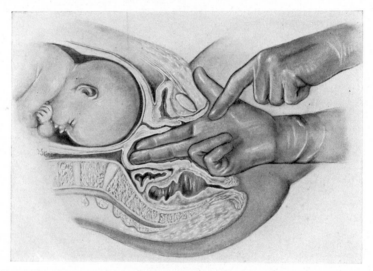

Fig. 333.—Measuring the diagonal conjugate by direct vaginal palpation.

Then the examiner proceeds to measure the diagonal conjugate. By firmly but gently inverting the perineum with the knuckles of the fourth and fifth fingers, the top of the third finger may be made to reach the promontory. This is facilitated by resting the foot upon a stool so as to use the knee as a support for the elbow. When the promontory is reached, the hand is raised until the arcuate ligament on the lower border of the symphysis rests upon it. This point is marked by the index finger of the other hand, and the vaginal finger being withdrawn, the distance from third finger top to the point of contact with the arcuate ligament is measured by the pelvimeter, the distance (12½ cm.) being the diagonal conjugate.

This line is one side of a triangle, the other two being the height of the symphysis and the true conjugate, so that by simple triangulation the length of the latter may be estimated. The usual deduction

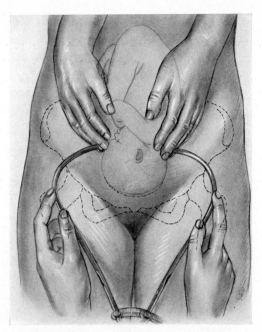

Fig. 334.—Measuring the fetal head.

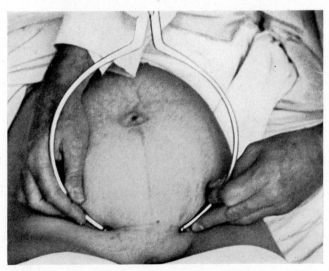

Fig. 335.—Direct measurement of the occipitofrontal diameter of the fetal head.

is from 1½ to 2 cm. The height and inclination of the symphysis may make considerable variation in this estimation as does the position of the promontory, the diagonal conjugate being lower when the former is high, and shorter when it is low (Figs. 334, 335). (See Chapter XI.)

Estimation of the relative capacity of the pelvic inlet by using the fetal head as an index is a simple and fairly effective procedure. It is best carried out during the last two weeks of pregnancy and consists in locating the spines of the ischia with the vaginal finger (patient and examiner being aseptically prepared), and then having the patient exhale deeply, upon which the fetal head is grasped through the abdominal wall and firmly pushed into the pelvis, the vaginal hand determining whether it can be advanced to the level of the spines.

This method is not available in very obese or unduly sensitive women, but ordinarily is easy of performance and furnishes valuable

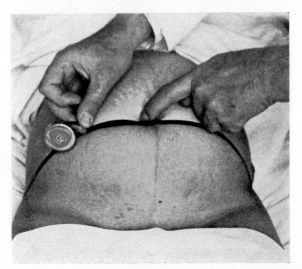

Fig. 336.—Measuring the circumference of the pelvis.

information as to the outcome of labor in so far as the inlet is concerned.

Roentgen Pelvimetry.—This is the most nearly accurate method of determining the size and shape of the pelvis now at our command. From the groping efforts of Pinard and Tarnier in 1897, there has been an enormous advance to attain the precision and simplicity of modern technic. Several methods of photographing and calculating the size of the pelvic inlet are in common use, the two most widely known being those developed by Johnson and Thoms. The method of the latter is so satisfactory that his instructions for its employment are quoted here in toto:

Centimeter Grid Method (Thoms).—1. The patient is placed on the roentgenographic table in the semirecumbent position.

2. The level of the superior strait above the sensitized film is established.

3. The tube target is centered about 5 cm. posterior to the symphysis, at 32 inches from the sensitized film. The exposure is made.

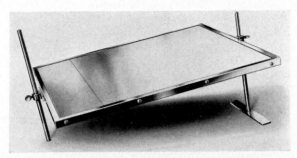

Fig. 337.—The centimeter grid. Under the thin aluminum protective sheet is the lead grid with perforations exactly 1 cm. apart. By means of the supports, the grid may be raised and lowered to any position. (Thoms in "Radiology," August, 1933.)

4. The patient is removed from the table, the tube target and sensitized film remaining *in situ*.

5. A lead plate, or centimeter grid (Fig. 337), with perforations exactly 1 cm. apart, is introduced into the same plane as that previously occupied by the superior strait and a second (flash) exposure

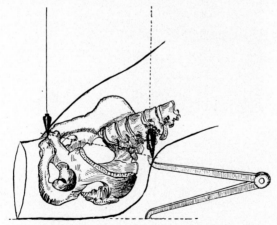

Fig. 338.—Measuring the distance of the superior strait above the sensitive plate by means of calipers and plumb lines. (Thoms in "Radiology," August, 1933.)

is made on the same sensitized film as was used in the previous exposure.

6. Development of the film shows the outline of the superior strait and the shadows of the perforations, the distance between which

represents centimeters in the plane of the superior strait. The anteroposterior and transverse diameters of the superior strait may be read directly. In addition, a pelvigram of the superior strait in its true proportions may be drawn on centimeter-squared paper by following the course of the shadow of the superior strait and transcribing it (Fig. 338).

Points in Detail.—1. Two points on the external body of the patient must be identified, namely, a point on the anterior surface about

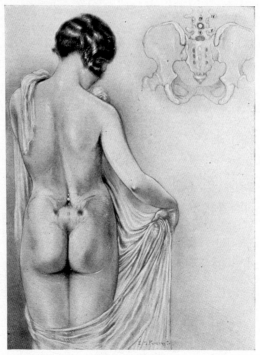

Fig. 339.—Anteroposterior diameter of pelvic inlet is determined by imaginary line extending from upper and anterior border of symphysis pubic to interspace between fourth and fifth lumbar vertebrae. A small adhesive tab is placed in latter location for identification. This can be located in well-formed women immediately above apex of Michaelis' rhomboid. Insert shows relation of this tab to bony structures. (Jarcho in Amer. Jour. of Surg., November, 1931.)

1 cm. below the upper and anterior border of the symphysis pubis, and a point on the back at the interspace between the fourth and fifth lumbar vertebrae. For purposes of identification, this is usually marked with a small adhesive tab. An imaginary line between these two traverses the anteroposterior diameter of the superior strait. The accuracy of this imaginary line, for all obstetric purposes, is entirely adequate (Fig. 339).

2. The patient is placed in a comfortable position on the roent-

genographic table. The back is supported by means of a back rest, and the patient assumes the semirecumbent position. A foot board at the end of the table serves to steady the patient. The lower 6 inches of the back are uncovered and the surface of the body over the symphysis and lower abdomen are made ready for palpation (Fig. 340).

3. The distance of the posterior adhesive tab above the table is measured with calipers and the point at which the lower arm comes

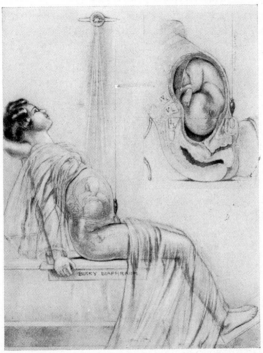

Fig. 340.—Position of patient on table for roentgen pelvimetry. Lower spine is arched so as to bring anteroposterior diameter of pelvic inlet, measured from anterior superior border of symphysis to identifying adhesive tab on back, on horizontal plane, that is parallel with sensitive film in Potter-Bucky diaphragm. Calipers measure distance from adhesive tab to sensitive film, and plumb-bob locates distance of symphysis pubis. Insert is a sagittal section showing relation of various parts to anteroposterior diameter of inlet. (Jarcho in Amer. Jour. of Surg., November, 1931.)

in contact with the table is marked. The level of the anterior point at the symphysis is fixed by a plumb bob.

4. The target of the tube is centered at a point about 5 cm. posterior to the upper border of the symphysis, from 30 to 36 inches above the sensitized film. Usually we use a 32-inch distance. The exposure is made. We have not felt that it is essential for the patient to hold her breath. The technic of exposure, etc., is essentially that

of taking the usual anteroposterior pelvic roentgenograms. The exposure is varied, of course, with the individual patient, thickness of tissues, etc.

5. With the tube and sensitized film still in position, the patient is removed from the table. The centimeter grid is placed in the same plane as that occupied by the superior strait. This is accomplished by bringing the anterior portion of the grid under the anterior plumb bob, and, for the posterior point, bringing another plumb bob down to the point of the upper arm of the posterior caliper measurement. The anterior and posterior portions of the grid touch, on the upper surface of the grid, the points of the plumb bobs. With the grid in

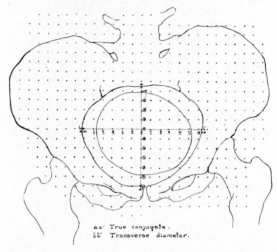

Fig. 341.—How true conjugate and transverse diameter may be measured by simply counting spaces between perforations and expressing in centimeters. Although these spaces are actually more than 1 cm. apart on film, they have been distorted to exactly the same extent as the pelvic inlet. (Jarcho in Amer. Jour. of Surg., November, 1931.)

position, a second (flash) exposure is made on the previously exposed plate.

6. The plate is developed and viewed (Fig. 341).

7. The centimeter grid must be very carefully calibrated.

This method has been found to be accurate, within 0.2 to 0.3 cm. a negligible error.

Roentgen Cephalometry.—To accurately learn the size of the fetal head has long been an obstetric goal. The x-ray seems to offer a reasonable assurance of the head size, the method in use being similar in principle to that described in measuring the pelvis. For details of technic, the reader is referred to the papers of Thoms and Jarcho (see bibliography).

THE TREATMENT OF CONTRACTED PELVIS

The intelligent management of this complication of pregnancy and labor epitomizes the whole philosophy of obstetric therapy, and an obstetrician is competent or not as he measures up to the solution of the problems presented by the various phases of disproportion. To be intelligently presented, the treatment must be discussed under two headings. First: management of contracted pelves in a proper hospital and with every facility for various operative procedures at hand. Second: the management of those cases in homes, and inadequately equipped institutions, without the aid of special skill and knowledge.

As has been emphasized often in this book, I consider a case of dystocia a major surgical problem, to be referred to a specialist's hands, in hospital, whenever this is humanly possible, and not to be managed under unsatisfactory conditions or by untrained men, unless circumstances absolutely forbid the obtaining of more favorable conditions for a successful outcome.

The Management of Labor in Pelves Contracted at the Inlet.— This is best approached by dividing the pelves according to the length of the anteroposterior diameter.

Conjugata vera of 7.5 cm., or less, constitutes an absolute indication for cesarean section, since a living child of normal size cannot be delivered through such a pelvis.

When discovered during pregnancy, the complication should be explained to the family, and the patient prepared for elective cesarean section shortly before term. Test of labor, in such cases, is of no value, and only imperils the success of the inevitable section.

If, unhappily, the condition is not known until the patient is well advanced in labor the treatment offers great difficulties. The child being still living, and the mother in fairly good condition, the low cervical section or the Latzko operation are the procedures of choice, although in both there is a considerable risk of postoperative sepsis, especially when many vaginal examinations and perhaps attempts at forceps delivery have been made. When the patient is definitely infected as shown by febrile temperature, and the child is dead or dying, craniotomy is the wiser course, provided the pelvis is not too small. A true conjugate of 6 cm. or less is a definite contraindication to craniotomy, as even the crushed skull and the body of the child cannot be extracted through such a canal. Under these circumstances, therefore, the cesarean section of necessity must be invoked, whether the child is dead or not and here hysterectomy or perhaps the Portes operation should be chosen. It is unsafe to attempt a conservative hysterotomy in the presence of known infection.

Conjugata vera of from 7.5 to 9 cm. constitutes relative pelvic contraction and here the treatment varies with the experience and skill of the obstetrician and the facilities for adequate surgical procedure. If the patient be a multipara, the outcome of previous labors will prove a valuable guide, it being always remembered that multiparity presupposes children successively larger at birth, so that a woman who has undergone several traumatic forceps deliveries may present a totally obstructive labor because of the large size of later babies. Colored women with small pelves have better fortune in deliveries than their white sisters, because of the greater elasticity of the tissues and the tendency to smaller headed babies. If the patient is in her home, and surgical skill and facilities are not available, she may be given a trial labor.

Test of Labor.—This term is applied to labors of varying duration and force of uterine contractions, the progress being carefully studied meanwhile in an attempt to evaluate the probable outcome. No generally accepted definition of a test of labor has been reached, some authorities depending upon the time element alone, others upon the frequency and force of the labor pains, while Tweedy states a rule to the effect that as long as the mother's temperature and pulse rate remain under 100, while the fetal heart tones remain over 100, neither is in danger and labor may be permitted to continue until some variation in one of the factors betokens impending catastrophe. During the progress of the test of labor all examinations are carried out with meticulous regard for asepsis, and no attempts are made at operative delivery.

Upon the completion of the test period, to the satisfaction of the obstetrician, the patient is either subjected to cesarean section, if progress be unsatisfactory, or delivery is allowed to proceed to a spontaneous termination, forceps extraction or version being utilized if the normal outcome is too greatly delayed.

Where opportunities for cesarean section are lacking, obstructed labor after a fruitless test is terminated by the use of "high forceps." An instrument of the Tarnier type is preferable because of its power and the small cephalic curve which aids in the necessary but unfortunate compression of the head. The forceps having been applied as nearly in a cephalic application as may be, traction is made, in order to determine whether extraction by this means is practicable.

If the head remains immovable, the forceps are to be removed and craniotomy performed, since mutilating injury to the mother and almost certain fetal death follow brutal forceps extraction. Before abandoning forceps delivery, the Barton or Kielland instrument may be tried, sometimes with surprisingly good results. If these prove ineffectual craniotomy should be done unless religious objections prevent. In the latter case, forceps extraction may be persisted in, or if the patient can be gotten into hospital, or arrangements made for acceptable preparation in the home, some form of cesarean section may be performed.

It is in the above type patient, namely, a woman with a true conjugate of 7.5 to 9 cm., that elective cesarean section, done by a trained specialist, under proper conditions, offers such excellent results as compared with any other plan of delivery. Under such circumstances, the operation carries a negligible mortality, certainly not greater than that of interval appendectomy, while the subsequent morbidity of the mother, from the laceration and detachment of the deep fascial slings of the vagina, is enormously decreased.

The outlook for the child is immeasurably improved, it being spared the ever-present dangers of asphyxia and intracranial hemorrhage. By elective cesarean section in this connection I refer to operation performed deliberately, before the onset of labor, after a

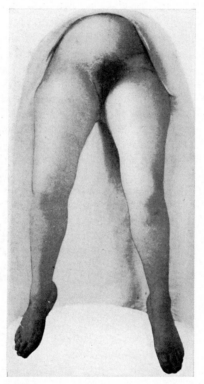

Fig. 342.—The Walcher position. (Kerr.)

painstaking examination to determine the relative size of fetal presenting part and maternal pelvis. The test of labor, while invaluable where conditions are adverse to cesarean section, has many inherent faults, since in the first place it is impossible to set up a standard. The utilization of the time factor or the severity of the uterine contraction is unsatisfactory, since both elements vary so greatly among different women. Furthermore, all too often, while one is observing a test of labor, the golden moment of election for hysterotomy is lost. The membranes rupture, or the woman becomes suddenly ex-

36

hausted, is no longer a justifiable risk for section and labor must be terminated by some form of operative vaginal delivery with more or less disastrous consequences to mother and child.

Conjugata Vera of 9 to 10 cm.—Such pelves constitute the large group of minor contractions and are best managed by vaginal delivery, unless there is a strong element of fetal disproportion.

In these women malpresentations, posterior rotation of the occiput, face, etc., are common and must be diagnosed. Here a test of labor becomes the rule and the completion of engagement may be aided by the employment of the Walcher position.

The Walcher position consists in bringing the buttocks of the patient to the edge of the delivery table and allowing the legs to hang free, their weight dragging the fore part of the pelvis downward and appreciably lengthening the true conjugate.

I have found the Walcher position difficult to maintain, most uncomfortable for the patient and of little practical utility. If labor is unduly delayed, delivery is accomplished by the use of the obstetric forceps which here come into their own (Fig. 342).

Should transverse arrest occur, the Barton or Kielland instrument is of the greatest value.

The Place of Version in Contracted Pelvis.—When any real disproportion is present, version is an unsatisfactory procedure. Either the membranes have long been ruptured, and the uterus being closely applied to the body of the child renders the operation difficult and dangerous, or if it be resorted to early, the head has not been given time to mold and becomes an obstacle to easy delivery. When the disproportion is but slight, and the uterine contractions are not strong, version may be attempted.

The Induction of Premature Labor in Contracted Pelvis.—It has been thought that a small child, with a more malleable head, could pass a contracted pelvis with better hope of success and hence induction at the thirty-fourth or thirty-sixth week would prove a solution of the problem. The premature child, however, has less chance for life than a mature one, and the very softness of the skull makes the probability of intracranial injury all the greater, so that all in all, the infant mortality is increased by this practice, which has been abandoned in most clinics.

The Management of Outlet Contractions.—Absolute outlet contraction, that is, when the sum of the bisischial diameter and the posterior sagittal is under 15 cm., is an indication for elective cesarean section, since the probabilities of a living mature fetus being delivered through such an outlet are very slight.

If the condition is not discovered until late in labor, section may still be performed if there is no infection or if this be impossible, forceps delivery may be effectual, although with a dead or injured baby, a craniotomy may be necessary.

The assumption of the squatting position which widens the outlet, may offer some hope, but like the Walcher position, it is not usually of much avail.

Summary of the Treatment of Contracted Pelvis.—Conjugata vera of 7.5 cm. or less constitutes an absolute indication for cesarean section if a living child is to be obtained. Section is imperative to secure delivery of even a dead child if the conjugate is 5.5 cm. or less, as no other method of delivery is possible. Craniotomy may be performed if the conjugate is between 5.5 and 7.5 cm.

Conjugata vera of 7.5 to 9 cm. constitutes an indication for cesarean section. If this is impossible high forceps delivery with craniotomy when the child is dead is the treatment, after a test of labor.

Conjugata vera of 9 to 10 cm. should have a test of labor, with operative delivery to terminate, if necessary.

CHAPTER XXXI

DYSTOCIA DUE TO ANOMALIES OF THE BIRTH CANAL

Stricture of the Cervix.—Syphilis sometimes produces a dense, undilatable stricture of the cervix, which is most resistant. Scar tissue from inflammatory lesions, amputation and trachelorrhaphy, or old lacerations may cause constriction at any level of the cervical canal, their significances in obstruction depending upon the site of the stricture.

If the stenosis is at or near the external os, the cervix may become effaced, and simple dilatation with the fingers, perhaps aided by a shallow incision or two will permit the attainment of dilatation.

If, however, the constriction be high in the cervix, the entire mechanism of effacement is disturbed and the long, canalized cervix may be forced down toward the vulva, the head greatly distending the lower uterine segment in the effort to force it into the cervix. Deep incisions (Dührssen) in the four quarters of the cervix, or even abdominal delivery may become necessary under these conditions.

Rigidity of the Cervix.—Sometimes for no known reason, the apparently healthy cervix is resistant to dilatation and offers a serious obstacle to delivery. Generally the failure to dilate may be ascribed to an abnormal presentation, or pelvic contraction, when the head does not fit the pelvic brim and does not enter the cervix in the manner of the normal ovoid. The only forces involved in producing dilatation in these cases are the pouch of membranes and the pull of the retracting upper uterine segment, neither of which are competent, if the head does not fit.

After a period of imperfect effacement or dilatation, the cervix becomes swollen and edematous, its surface dry and glazed. The anterior lip may be compressed between head and symphysis even to the point of necrosis. This rigidity is sometimes observed in elderly primiparae.

Treatment.—The first thing in treatment is to give the patient rest with morphine, and wait for time to soften and dilate the cervix. Two old devices are of value in combating cervical rigidity. One is to pack the vagina with gauze soaked in boroglyceride solution, taking care to make firm pressure against the cervix. After a few hours the packing is removed, when the cervix will be found soft and moist.

Another plan is to expose the cervix with a bivalve speculum and play a stream of very hot (110°–112°), sterile water against it with considerable force, the irrigating can being hung as high as may be. I have seen a tough cervix literally melt away under the influence of the hot stream. Should both of these measures fail, the cervix may be incised, an incision being made on each side, one in the midline anteriorly and one posteriorly. Care must be taken that the bladder is not injured by the anterior incision and that the lateral ones are not deep enough to sever the circular artery. The use of the metreurynter in selected cases may prove efficacious.

Cesarean section is rarely required to terminate labor in cervical rigidity.

A vaginal septum, or tense pelvic floor may delay labor, but are of little clinical importance since simple incision eliminates the septum, and unilateral or even bilateral episiotomy will sufficiently enlarge the vaginal outlet to permit the expulsion of the child.

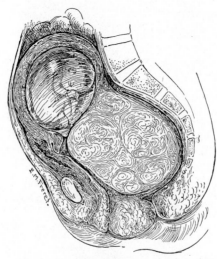

Fig. 343.—Impacted tumor blocking delivery. Treated by section and hysterectomy. (Polak in Surg., Gynec., and Obstet., vol. 46, 1928.)

Very rarely vaginal cysts may impede delivery, but as the force of the uterine contraction increases, the cysts usually rupture and present no further barrier to descent.

Labor Complicated by Fibroid Tumors of the Uterus.—The obstetric importance of fibroid tumors varies with their location, more than their size. A comparatively small growth situated in the lower uterine segment may block the birth canal, whereas a huge tumor above the fetus may exert little or no effect upon labor (Fig. 343).

Any traumatism to a fibroid during delivery must be avoided as pressure necrosis with subsequent gangrene of the tumor may readily result, with peritonitis as a sequel (Fig. 344).

In the event of a woman going into labor, with a previously undiscovered fibroid, careful palpation will usually determine its potentiality for causing trouble (Fig. 345).

If the tumor lies above the fetus, all is well. If it occupy the pelvic brim, gentle pressure upon it from the vagina, with traction by the abdominal hand, may dislodge it and permit the head to slip

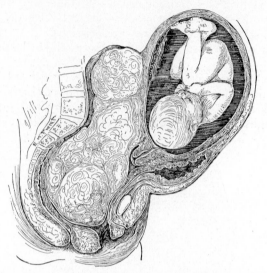

Fig. 344.—Immense impacted tumor necessitating section and hysterectomy. (Polak in Surg., Gynec., and Obstet., vol. 46, 1928.)

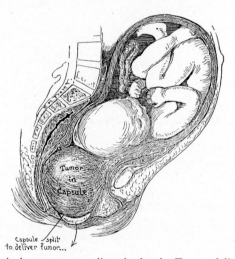

Fig. 345.—Cervical myoma preceding the head. Tumor delivered by vaginal myomectomy followed by spontaneous birth. (Polak in Surg., Gynec., and Obstet., vol. 46, 1928.)

past it, anesthesia being used for the furtherance of this maneuver, if necessary. Should the tumor resist dislodgment, cesarean section is indicated, preferably leaving the tumor undisturbed, though if it shows signs of degeneration, or undue pressure as marked by areas of hemorrhagic infiltration, myomectomy or hysterectomy is to be done.   If the obstructing tumor is recognized only late in labor,

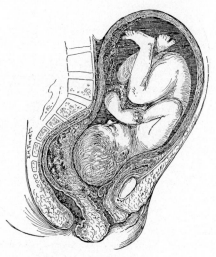

Fig. 346.—Necrotic fibroid causing fatal sepsis.   Fetus delivered by forceps traumatizing growths in passage.   (Polak in Surg., Gynec., and Obstet., vol. 46, 1928.)

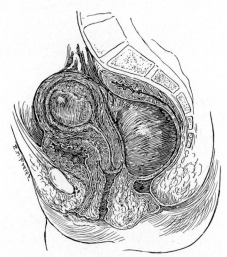

Fig. 347.—Twisted pedunculated subserous tumor incarcerated; cesarean followed by myomectomy.   (Polak in Surg., Gynec., and Obstet., vol. 46, 1928.)

hysterectomy is generally advised by reason of the danger of secondary peritonitis, if the injured neoplasm is not removed (Figs. 346, 347).

In actual practice, fibroids rarely complicate delivery, as they are usually drawn above the fetal body by the upward growth of the uterus. During the third stage, and immediately after, the presence

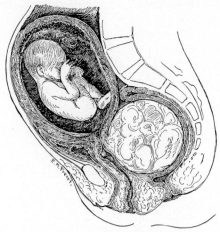

Fig. 348.—Incarcerated myoma of lower segment, posterior wall, making intra-vaginal delivery impossible. (Polak in Surg., Gynec., and Obstet., vol. 46, 1928.)

of fibroid nodules in and about the muscle bundles may interfere with the normal rhythm of contraction and retraction, and so delay the expulsion of the placenta as well as predisposing toward postpartum

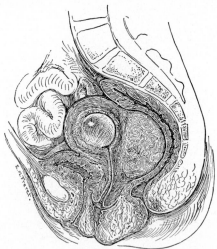

Fig. 349.—Incarcerated interstitial growth raised out of the pelvis by the developing uterus. (Polak in Surg., Gynec., and Obstet., vol. 46, 1928.)

hemorrhage. The accoucheur, apprised of the presence of uterine fibromata, should be well equipped with material for packing the uterus (Figs. 348, 349).

Ovarian Cysts Complicating Labor.—As in fibroids, if the cyst is above the fetus no difficulty need be feared, but if it obstructs delivery, an attempt should be made to dislodge it by vaginal pressure, the head being first pushed out of the pelvis, anesthesia being employed if the patient is sensitive.

This procedure failing, cesarean section should be done and the tumor removed or not, depending upon the condition of the patient.

If the cyst ruptures during labor, delivery should be completed per vaginam, followed by immediate laparotomy and oophorectomy.

Labor in Elderly Primiparae.—The profession has long held that after the age of twenty-five years, first labors become progressively more pathological.

During pregnancy there is some increased tendency to toxemias of various forms, and premature labors seem to be more common.

During labor there may be rigidity of the cervix, uterine inertia, and lack of power of the abdominal muscles.

My own experience coincides with that of Quigley, namely, that any of the complications of labor may occur in elderly primiparae, but that they are not appreciably more frequent than among younger women. The conduct of labor in older primigravidae does not differ from the usual procedure except in one particular.

The first child of a woman in her late thirties is very apt to be the last, and hence is more important than the first fruit of a young girl who may readily engage in a number of pregnancies.

Therefore in the presence of any obstacle to spontaneous delivery, cesarean section is invoked upon a much slighter indication than in a young woman in order to insure the patient a living and well baby.

Dry Labor, Premature Rupture of Membranes.—Dry labor has an unsavory reputation, it being said to have a longer duration, be more often followed by infection, and be complicated by malpresentation.

This is true if the membranes rupture spontaneously before the onset of labor, because the accident is due, in the great majority of cases, to maladaption of the presenting part to the pelvic brim, a pouch of membranes being forced past the head and undergoing the full force of the early uterine contractions.

Sometimes, an abnormal delicacy of the membranes tends toward early rupture, but not commonly. When the accident is due to malpresentation, the labor is complicated not only by the absence of amniotic fluid, but by the mechanical fault as well.

The renewed interest in deliberate rupture of the membranes as a means of inducing labor (this procedure was mentioned by Denman in 1796 as having been practiced for years before his time), has shown definitely that early rupture *per se*, rather aids the progress of labor than the contrary. Statistics involving large groups of cases have been adduced, which prove that rupture of the membranes artificially, before the onset of labor, results in a shortened first stage, a percentage of spontaneous deliveries which compares very closely with control cases, and a morbidity and mortality rate for both mother and child, which is even slightly better than in the controls. It is probable that our conception of the mechanism of cervical dilatation will be much changed by the acquisition of these new facts.

Dry labor resulting from malpresentations and consequent early rupture of the membranes remains a somewhat annoying complication.

From several hours to several days may intervene between the rupture and the onset of labor, and in the interval, infection of the open amniotic cavity is a constant menace.

During this interval, the patient must be cautioned to avoid coitus, tub baths, vaginal douches, in short anything which might lead to the carrying of infectious bacteria into the reproductive tract.

She should not go about, but remain quietly at home or in hospital, awaiting the onset of labor.

When uterine contractions do come on they are often irregular and weak, and there is very slow progress in labor. Meanwhile the uterus molds itself to the irregular contour of the child's body and undue compression is exerted, especially upon the umbilical cord with the accompanying peril of intra-uterine asphyxia.

It may be necessary to aid cervical dilatation and stimulate uterine contraction by the use of a dilating bag, and forceps delivery is rather the rule. Version is dangerous when the membranes have long been ruptured, by reason of the great contraction of the uterus and the probability of introducing infection.

CHAPTER XXXII

DYSTOCIA DUE TO ABNORMALITIES OF THE FETUS

DISEASES OF THE FETUS COMPLICATING LABOR

ENLARGEMENT of the fetal body may be caused by general edema, urinary retention with enormously distended bladder, congenital cystic kidneys, tumor of the liver and so on. All of these conditions are rare, and usually remain undiagnosed until obstruction to the delivery of the fetal body leads to a recognition of its increase in bulk.

When discovered, the dystocia can only be overcome by opening the body of the child, allowing the ascitic fluid to drain away, or by removing a portion of a visceral tumor if such be the source of the dystocia.

The child need not be considered as none of the conditions described are compatible with extra-uterine life.

MALFORMATION OF THE CHILD

Hydrocephalus.—This fairly common malformation (Fig. 350) is due to sometimes enormous distention of the cerebral ventricles by

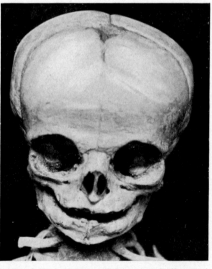

Fig. 350.—Hydrocephalic skull. (Mütter Museum, College of Physicians, Phila.)

centrospinal fluid, as a result of the obliteration of the foramen of Magendie.

571

The heads of such children become greatly increased in size, often to several times the normal dimensions, while the brain has been stretched and compressed to form a thin layer lining the skull, or it

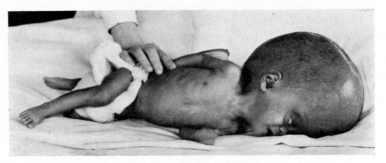

Fig. 351.—Hydrocephalus.

may have disappeared almost completely, only a few scattered fragments remaining about the base of the skull. The cranial bones are usually badly developed, the sutures wide, the fontanels large (Fig. 351).

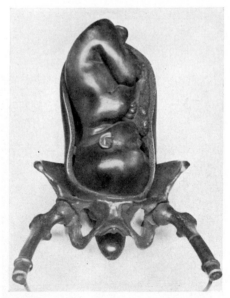

Fig. 352.—Hydrocephalic head impacted at the brim. (From the Barton Cooke Hirst Collection, University of Pennsylvania.)

Diagnosis.—Under expert obstetrical care, the presence of hydrocephalus should be suspected before the onset of labor, abdominal palpation disclosing a head out of all proportion to the size of the body of the fetus, while by vaginal touch, the fluctuating character of the head may be made out even through the thickness of the lower uterine segment. If there is doubt, *x*-ray examination will settle the matter (Fig. 352).

Clinical Course of Labor.—In cephalic presentation, labor is obstructed from the outset. The huge head cannot enter the pelvis, the membranes rupture early, the cervix undergoes partial dilatation and progress ceases.

In the event of breech presentation, the buttocks of the child may be delivered easily but when the after-coming head reaches the pelvic brim it cannot pass and again labor comes to a standstill.

The outcome of labor in advanced degrees of hydrocephalus is rupture of the uterus, from violent efforts to expel the child. Ex-

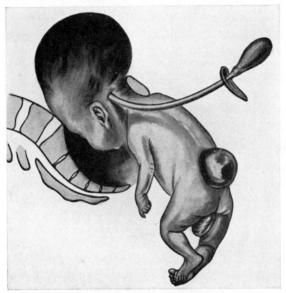

Fig. 353.—Puncture of hydrocephalus with trocar. Note spina bifida. (DeLee.)

cessive molding of the skull when the distention is not a tense one, may lead to spontaneous delivery, but this is rare. Still more so is spontaneous rupture of a fontanel, with evacuation of the fluid and delivery.

Prognosis.—The child need not be considered since most hydrocephalics are stillborn, most of the remaining few die in a few weeks and only rarely does an infant with this anomaly survive, usually in the form of low-grade idiot.

Treatment.—Labor should be allowed to proceed until the cervix is fully dilated or easily dilatable. The hydrocephalic head is then perforated, with a perforator or sharp-pointed scissors, the points being passed in a suture or fontanel under the guidance of vaginal fingers. With the gush of released cerebrospinal fluid the head collapses and delivery is completed by extraction with forceps or by version. In perforating the skull it is important that the vital centers at the base of the brain be destroyed, since because the thinned-out cerebrum is so spread out on the inner surface of the skull, mere perforation does not necessarily inflict enough injury to cause death; which is obviously essential.

In the event of a breech presentation, the perforation may be much more difficult and must be carried out with great care, the scissors being introduced along the back of the infant and so into the base of the skull. A trocar is less liable to cause injury to the maternal soft parts and is an excellent instrument in this situation (Fig. 353).

DYSTOCIA DUE TO MONSTERS

The occurrence of monstrous infants has long been a source of wonder and dismay to mankind. From the viewpoint of the obstetrician, there are two phases of the subject which have weight, first, of course, the effect of teratomatous infants upon pregnancy and labor, and second, the possibilities of prophylaxis against their development. There is, as yet, no answer to the second question, but a recent study by Murphy shows conclusively that monster bearing is familial, that is, women who have borne one deformed infant are very likely to suffer the identical misfortune once, or often more than once, in succeeding pregnancies.

These findings should change the attitude of the obstetrician with regard to his statements to women and their husbands who have been the parents of a monster. They should be apprised of the fact that there is a greater liability to more deformed fetuses in their case, than had a monster not been born to them, but that there is a fair probability that healthy children may follow. One must remember that syphilis plays little or no part in the production of monsters.

The Influence of Monsters Upon Pregnancy.—Deformed embryos are frequently aborted, and the investigation of Mall showed that a great proportion of all aborted fetuses submitted to him for examination were teratological.

Hydramnion and aggravation of the toxemia of early pregnancy is a common concomitant to deformed fetuses, indeed so often is this the case, that the presence of hydramnion constitutes an important diagnostic point.

Any suspicion of such development should lead the accoucheur to insist upon roentgenological examination, which will generally determine the question, if done during the last two months of pregnancy.

Effect Upon Labor.—Single monsters usually do not cause dystocia, and the most common variety, the anencephalic form, are usually easily delivered by reason of the absence of cranium (Figs. 354, 355, 356).

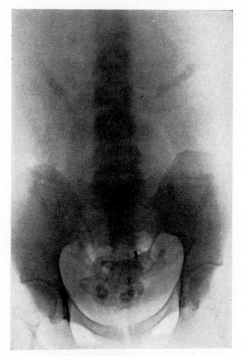

Fig. 354.—x-Ray photograph of an anencephalic monster diagnosed during eighth month of pregnancy. (Kensington Hospital for Women.)

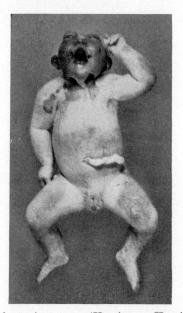

Fig. 355.—Fetus shown in x-ray. (Kensington Hospital for Women.)

During labor the diagnosis may be made by the frequency of face presentation, the bulging prominent eyes, and the fact that no occiput can be palpated.

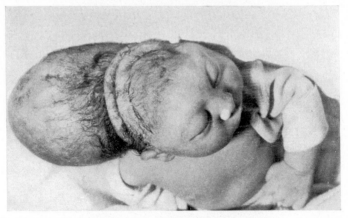

Fig. 356.—Anencephalus with hernia cerebri. This infant lived and gained weight for twelve days. (Kensington Hospital for Women.)

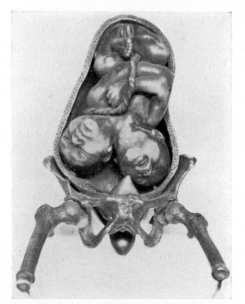

Fig. 357.—Dicephalus. Neither head engaged.

Double monsters or united twins may take various forms, as:
Dicephalus, single body with two heads (Fig. 357).
Thoracopagus, two bodies and heads, the union being at the thorax.
Pyopagus, two infants united at the sacrum.

Ischiopagus, two infants united at the buttocks.

Craniopagus, two infants with the heads joined (Fig. 358).

Rachiopagus, two infants with union of the spines.

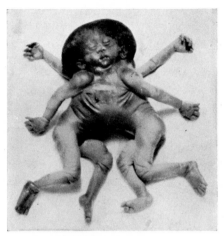

Fig. 358.—Prosopothoracopagus.

Parasitic monsters are those in which a trunk of one infant grows out of the body of the other and is dependent upon it for existence.

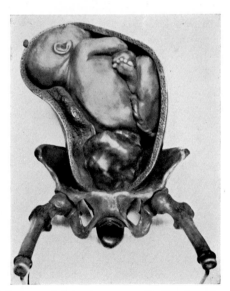

Fig. 359.—A huge caudal teratoma complicating breech presentation.

Of the many single forms, few are of obstetric significance from the standpoint of delivery, and most of them perish immediately,

37

though those due to defective fusion may survive and if the defect is not too extensive may reach adult life (spina bifida, exstrophy of the bladder, cleft palate, etc.) (Figs. 359, 360).

Treatment During Labor.—Cesarean section is contraindicated in the presence of a monster, although it may be preferable to a mutilating operation upon the fetus which by its very difficult character may more endanger the mother than section.

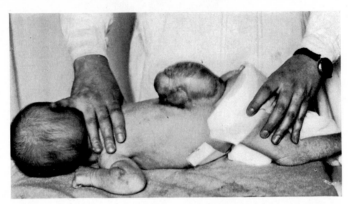

Fig. 360.—Enormous spina bifida.   (Philadelphia General Hospital.)

Destructive operations are the rule in these cases, and no definite rules may be laid down, each one being managed as required by the individual presentation.   Sometimes joined twins are spontaneously delivered as witness the Siamese twins and other forms so often seen on exhibit.

VI. THE ACCIDENTS OF LABOR

CHAPTER XXXIII

RUPTURE OF THE UTERUS

THIS dreadful calamity may take place during pregnancy or more commonly, intrapartum. In either case it may be spontaneous or traumatic.

During Pregnancy.—Uterine rupture or better, perforation, may occur in the early months from attempts at abortion or other instrumentation, the walls of the uterus being perforated by the curette, catheter or whatever is used.

At this time the clinical picture is not usually that of hemorrhage, but a peritonitis or pelvic cellulitis may develop, with its attendant symptoms. Very rarely, the ovum may escape through the opening in the uterine wall, become reimplanted somewhere upon the peritoneum and go on to a secondary abdominal pregnancy.

Spontaneous rupture of the uterus never occurs during the early months of normal pregnancy, but the syncytial cells in hydatidiform mole may perforate the muscle, sometimes in several separate areas.

There were four fatal cases of uterine perforation in early pregnancy found during the Philadelphia County Medical Society survey of maternal deaths in that city, all of which had followed perforation by the curette or placental forceps.

Rupture in the later months of pregnancy is more often spontaneous than traumatic. Here it follows previous weakening of the uterine wall or anomalies of that organ.

The scar of previous cesarean section provides the most frequent occasion for rupture, and less common but definite factors are scars from old curette perforations, and of myomectomy wounds; thinning and fibrosis of the uterus from adherent placenta or placenta accreta in previous pregnancies, or possibly areas of adenomyomatosis or even fibroid tumors in the uterine wall. Sometimes anterior or posterior sacculation after ventrofixation, or incarcerated retroversion may be responsible.

Among the congenital anomalies in which rupture of the uterus is found, may be listed pregnancy in one horn of a double uterus, uterus septus, congenital hypoplasia of the uterine wall.

When spontaneous rupture occurs during late pregnancy, the injury is almost always in the upper portion of the uterus and the solution of continuity is complete, all coats of the uterus being torn through.

Symptoms and Clinical Course.—At the moment of spontaneous rupture, the woman may experience a sharp abdominal pain, or she may simply note a slight discomfort. Later there may develop the evidence of massive intraperitoneal hemorrhage or peritonitis. In some instances the fetus escapes through the rent and goes on developing among the intestines, either to be delivered by laparotomy or continue to lithopedion formation.

In one of my cases, a woman who had had a cesarean section walked into the hospital complaining of not feeling well. Physical and laboratory examination showed nothing remarkable, but being cognizant of the previous cesarean, the abdomen was opened, the living fetus (about eight months) found free in the abdominal cavity, the uterus well contracted about the still-functioning placenta. The scar of the previous section had separated along its entire length, the cord protruding through the opening. There was practically no free blood in the abdomen and removal of the fetus, cutting the cord and supravaginal hysterectomy was followed by uneventful recovery.

Diagnosis.—The diagnosis sometimes offers great difficulty since the symptoms are often negligible. Finding the uterus contracted, with a large extra-uterine fetus is conclusive, but often the entire fetal body has not escaped from the uterine cavity and no sign of rupture can be elicited by palpation.

However, there is usually considerable internal hemorrhage, which gives its physical signs and suggests laparotomy which is the sole treatment.

Rupture of the uterus during labor is by far the more common finding, when as before, the accident may be spontaneous or traumatic. The *causes for spontaneous rupture are:*

1. Separation of scars of the uterine wall from previous cesarean section, myomectomy, placenta accreta and the like.

2. Overstretching of the lower uterine segment in transverse presentation, contracted pelvis, neglected impossible presentation as face with the chin posterior, gross oversize of the child, pelvic tumors or indeed any obstacle to vaginal delivery.

3. Congenital defects as double uterus, etc.

The causes for traumatic rupture are: rough and unskilled attempts at operative delivery, the addition of the hand into the already overstretched uterus, being often sufficient insult to bring about rupture. Direct perforation with a forceps blade may also occur, and after embryotomy the jagged ends of splintered fetal bones may penetrate the uterus.

Frequency.—In urban communities where patients suffering from dystocia are commonly referred to obstetric specialists in hospitals, rupture of the uterus is uncommon. I have seen one case in the last 6000 deliveries, and that was a traumatic rupture inflicted by the hand of a junior obstetrician while he was engaged in performing a version. Prompt recognition of the accident and immediate hysterectomy avoided any unfavorable consequences.

In remote districts where medical care is difficult to obtain, rupture occurs more frequently, possibly once in 800 or 900 labors. A few years ago when the furore for pituitrin was at its height, this accident was far more frequent than it is now, since physicians generally have been imbued with a knowledge of the danger of this oxytocic drug.

In the survey of maternal deaths in Philadelphia before referred to 24 of the 717 fatalities followed upon rupture of the uterus during labor. Since there were, during the same period, about 95,000 births in the city, deaths from uterine rupture occurred in 0.036 per cent, or

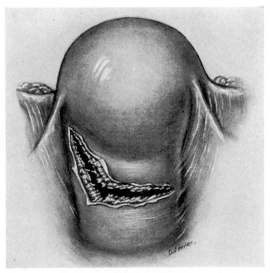

Fig. 361.—Traumatic rupture of the uterus. Bandl's contraction ring may be seen running transversely, just above the rent.

1 in about 3600 deliveries. This, of course, accounts for the fatal cases only, so that the number might have to be doubled, to include all cases, resulting in a frequency of about 0.07 per cent.

Multiparae suffer from the accident much more frequently than do primiparae, the ratio being about 12:1.

Mode of Production of Rupture.—The classical work of Bandl in 1875, made clear the mechanisms involving the lower uterine segment in labor and showed definitely how this accident develops. Under the influence of the uterine contractions, the uterus becomes differentiated into two portions, an upper, powerful, contractile segment and a lower, weaker, dilating segment. Between the two lies a circular ring of muscular tissue which is called the *contraction ring,* or *Bandl's ring* (Fig. 361).

As the upper segment contracts strongly, it tends to stretch and dilate the lower segment and to propel the fetus through it. Under normal conditions this is the course of labor, but when an obstacle is present to prevent descent of the fetus, the mechanism becomes pathological.

The cervix is fixed by the attachments of the uterosacral ligaments behind, the cardinal portions of the broad ligaments laterally and the uterovesical ligaments in front. Therefore it cannot be pulled up over the fetus and into the abdomen, but the strain falls upon its upper portion. The fixation is increased if the anterior lip of the cervix becomes imprisoned between the fetal head and the symphysis.

Now under continued contraction of the upper segment, the lower is pulled more and more away from the fixed cervix so that it be-

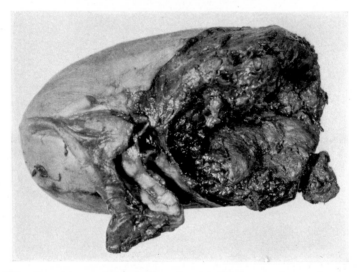

Fig. 362.—Complete rupture of the uterus following version and extraction. (Kensington Hospital for Women.)

comes thinned out to the point of rupture. This thinning is usually asymmetrical, being most pronounced in the side to which the head lies. Synchronously, the contraction ring rises until it may be felt and sometimes seen as a tense band running transversely or obliquely across the abdomen, until at length it may lie nearly at the level of the umbilicus. The round ligaments which act as counterforces preventing the fundus uteri from rising in the abdomen may be noted as tense bands running from this uterine attachment to the inguinal canals. The uterus, violently contracting to overcome the obstruction, finally becomes tetanic, and remains in almost continuous tonic contraction.

Usually the membranes have long been ruptured before this situation occurs but cases have been reported in which oligohydramnios and a rigid cervix caused rupture with membranes intact.

When the uterus finally ruptures the tear may involve the entire thickness of the uterine wall, *complete rupture* (Fig. 362), or the serosa may remain unbroken, *incomplete rupture*.

The rent may be anywhere in the lower uterine segment, but is usually oblique, and may run under the bladder reflexion, sometimes involving that organ, may extend into either broad ligament or may extend upward toward the fundus, reaching to and beyond the retraction ring. Sometimes the tear runs downward through the lateral wall of the cervix and into the vagina.

Spontaneous rupture through a defective area in the fundus uteri occurs much earlier in labor, often when there is no other obstruction than the normal forces of resistance. The mechanism here is simply a tear through a previously weakened muscle. It is not associated with tetanic contractions nor with a rise of the contracting ring.

Traumatic Ruptures.—These occur when an already overstretched or weakened uterus is further distended by the hand during version, or directly perforated by a forceps blade. Sometimes during the performance of a version the uterus will be felt to give way, the tension is immediately reduced and one knows that the uterus has been torn.

Pathology.—The pathology of uterine rupture varies with the site of the laceration. If the fundus be involved, there is a long tear usually longitudinal or slightly oblique, the great sinuses are open, the uterus cannot contract until the fetus is expelled into the abdomen and hemorrhage is furious though there may be no vaginal bleeding whatever. When the rupture lies in the lower uterine segment, the same conditions exist, if it be complete, but if incomplete there may be a stripping of the uterine peritoneum by blood and the formation of a large subperitoneal hematoma. When the rent extends into the broad ligament, the tension created by the hemorrhage into the primary tissues of this structure may give rise to slow percolation of blood from under the parietal peritoneum at the sides of the pelvis.

External hemorrhage is sometimes massive in lower segment tears, especially when the placenta and its site are involved. The fetus may escape into the abdomen, or it may remain in the uterus, which does not contract regularly once rupture has occurred.

Symptomatology.—The symptoms of uterine rupture may be divided into those of *impending rupture* and those of *actual rupture*.

In impending rupture, the uterine contractions are tumultuous and violent. The contraction ring may be palpated, well above the symphysis and rising steadily. Obstetrical examination will disclose some form of obstruction to delivery. The patient complains of extreme pain, is anxious and restless and the pulse rate rises.

Actual rupture is marked by a sudden violent tearing pain, described by women as entirely different from the labor pains from which they have been suffering. Uterine effort promptly ceases, the patient experiencing marked relief. At this time there may be a gush of blood from the vagina. On vaginal examination the presenting part no longer crowds the pelvic inlet and indeed, may not be palpable at all. In a short time signs of internal hemorrhage become apparent. The patient feels weak, becomes restless and anxious, the skin is leaky, the lips pale, and the respiration rapid. The pulse rapidly increases in rate and the volume becomes less, dichrotism sometimes occurring. The blood pressure drops, rapidly, in a word the picture is one of rapid and profuse internal hemorrhage.

When the rupture is incomplete, these symptoms may be delayed, but suddenly become very acute should a large subperitoneal hematoma undergo secondary rupture.

Occasionally, in an incomplete rupture, the symptoms may be slight, and if the child has been delivered (as in rupture occurring during version), they may be unrecognized until peritonitis develops or possibly the rent may heal without ever having been known to exist.

The diagnosis of rupture during labor is usually self-evident. The violence of the labor, the fact of a known obstacle to delivery, and the symptoms described above should clear up the question.

If on vaginal examination, the presenting part no longer lies in the brim, and if the uterus may be felt, firm and contracted, with no fetus in it, the diagnosis is obvious.

Diagnosis of Impending Rupture.—One should always fear rupture of the uterus in obstructed labor, when the uterine contractions are excessive, and when the contraction ring becomes palpable well above the symphysis. Also when there is a history of previous incision of the uterus, one should be prepared for rupture. Sometimes the scar of a previous cesarean section can be felt through the abdominal wall, as a groove on the anterior surface of the uterus. This finding should at once demand laparotomy. When rupture impends, the obstetrician must always be prepared for section, and if in a home, the woman should be sent to a hospital at once, if one is available.

Prognosis.—Very few children survive the accident, unless delivery was almost a fact before it occurred, as in version or forceps extraction.

Sometimes the child may escape into the abdomen, its placenta continuing to be attached to the uterine wall, when prompt laparotomy may preserve it. Generally speaking, however, the infants perish.

The mother dies in most instances when prompt laparotomy is not possible. In hospitals, where immediate operation can be done, the mortality falls to some 10 per cent, but otherwise it may reach 60 per cent.

Treatment.—a. *Prophylaxis.*—With adequate prenatal care, rupture of the uterus becomes a rare accident. Careful anamnesis brings out the past experience of the patient as regards wounds or injuries to the uterus, and proper pelvimetry determines the presence or abscence of disproportion. If there is a history of previous cesarean section, myomectomy, or adherent placenta, the obstetrician should be on his guard and be prepared to intervene at any time. Marked disproportion indicates either a carefully observed test of labor, or purely elective cesarean section. Transverse presentation discovered early in labor should be treated by version and extraction before rupture is imminent. Needless to say all intra-uterine manipulation must be carried out with the utmost gentleness.

Impending rupture during labor as shown by the rising contraction ring, malpresentations or other obstructions and tumultuous pain should be met by the administration of morphine in generous doses (¼ grain hypodermically and repeated if necessary). Adrenalin in doses of 1 cc. of a 1:1000 solution also acts well to relax a tetanically contracted uterus.

The temporary respite so secured gives time for the decision as to whether immediate hysterotomy should be performed or whether the obstruction may be overcome by some form of vaginal operative delivery. Craniotomy or other varieties of embryotomy are often of great value here, whereas version is dangerous, and likely to cause the very accident it is designed to prevent.

Treatment of Active Rupture.—Laparotomy, usually resulting in supravaginal hysterectomy, is the wisest plan to pursue. If the child is alive and in the abdominal cavity, this procedure is always indicated. If the child is still within the uterus, living or dead, section offers the best hope for the mother, and I cannot agree with those who advocate the delivery of the child per vaginam, either as the entire treatment or preliminary to an abdominal section.

Where no facilities are available for section, it is proper to attempt the vaginal delivery of the child, and then after manual exploration of the uterus, packing it firmly in the hope that firm contraction may tend to obliterate the bleeding vessels.

Ergot given after the packing further maintains uterine contraction. The packing may be removed in forty-eight hours, and if no untoward symptoms develop, no additional treatment is necessary.

Peritonitis may not set in for several days, and must always be watched for.

CHAPTER XXXIV

INJURIES OF THE BIRTH CANAL

THERE is some degree of laceration of the parturient canal in all primiparae and in many multiparae. Depending upon the elasticity of the tissues and the character of the delivery, these wounds may vary from negligible nicks in the mucosa to multiple, wide and extensive lacerations. Sometimes the deep fascial slings of both anterior and posterior divisions of the pelvic fasciae are torn or stripped off from their attachments, leaving mutilating injuries which result in hernia of the bladder or rectum, cystocele or rectocele, later on.

The Vulva.—Lacerations of the vulva often follow forceps delivery and may involve any portion of this structure. They are rarely deep, and require but little attention other than superficial suture. This, however, should not be neglected since these wounds are prone to infection and sometimes resistant ulceration follows. If the crura of the clitoris be torn, severe hemorrhage may occur and here careful suture and ligature is requisite.

THE PERINEUM AND PELVIC FLOOR

Lacerations of the perineum are very varied in their anatomical aspects. The lower fibers of the levator may be extensively lacerated, even torn from their pelvic insertions. Sometimes the tear runs up one sulcus of the vagina, sometimes both sides are injured. The recto-vaginal septum is not infrequently split, and when the sphincter ani is involved, the vagina and rectum may be converted into a single cloaca.

Etiology.—Injuries to the birth canal are the result of overstretching of the tissues, and hence they are most common in disproportion, malpresentation and contracted pelvis. A narrow pubic arch which decreases the available anteroposterior diameter of the outlet, thus forcing the head backward against the perineum is often responsible. Forceps delivery and version are followed frequently by extensive lacerations, and sometimes disease or abnormalities of the tissues themselves has considerable bearing. Scarred peroneii from condylomata or previous Bartholin abscess give way easily and there is a marked variation in the elasticity of the structures comprising the pelvic floor in different women.

Clinical Course.—For practical purposes lacerations of the perineum are divided into three types:

First-degree tears in which the tissues composing the posterior commissure of the vagina are separated in the midline, the sphincter ani not being involved (Fig. 363).

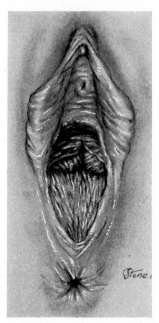

Fig. 363.—An extensive first-degree laceration, extending well down the perineum but not involving the sulci.

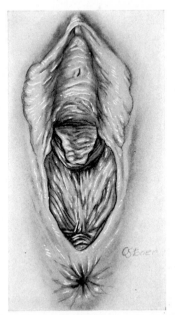

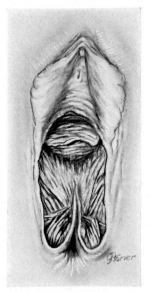

Fig. 364.—A second-degree laceration of the perineum involving both vaginal sulci.

Fig. 365.—A third-degree laceration involving the sphincter ani and the rectovaginal septum.

Second-degree tears, in which the foregoing injury may be added to a laceration extending up one or both sulci of the vagina (Fig. 364).

Third-degree tears in which the sphincter ani is torn through and possibly the rectovaginal septum also (Fig. 365).

These groupings are at best inaccurate, because the depth and extent of the solution of continuity cannot be described so briefly, but it is at least a workable classification.

Central laceration of the perineum is a rare type of injury in which the child is delivered through the tear which may lie between the vulva and anus or at one side of the former.

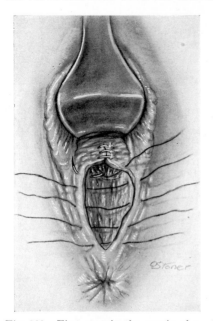

Fig. 366.—First step in the repair of a first-degree laceration.

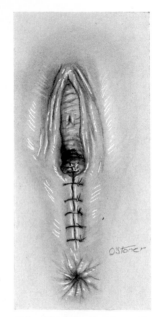

Fig. 367.—First-degree laceration repaired.

Such tear may be found when the perineum is very long anteroposteriorly, and a small child with occiput posterior is driven downward through the tissues by the force of the labor pains.

These tears are exceedingly rare.

Treatment of Laceration of the Perineum and Floor.—*Prophylaxis.*—Careful reinforcement of the perineum by the hand as described in the conduct of labor, will often curtail the extent of a laceration, as well as sometimes prevent its occurrence. Episiotomy, properly performed, is also quite efficacious. A careful ironing out of the pelvic floor before operative delivery as well as in spontaneous cases when the tissues seem to lie in danger, is a valuable measure. It is done by first instilling a lubricant, sterile green soap is excellent, into the vagina, and then using the palmar surface of at first two, then three and finally all four fingers, gently but firmly pressing downward on the perineum, with a side to side movement of the hand. It is surprising to note how much relaxation can be secured by a five-minute ironing.

Forceps deliveries should be conducted slowly, the head allowed to recede between efforts at traction, to permit a return of blood supply, and the blades being removed before the head is wholly delivered (*q. v.*).

Repair of Lacerations.—It is wise to repair lacerations immediately after the completion of the third stage of labor, and when the cervix is uninjured the work may be done before the expulsion of the placenta, when the field is less bloody, and the patient may be spared some minutes of anesthesia (Figs. 366, 367).

The instruments necessary to repair these wounds are:

Needleholder.

Full-curved Martin needles of various sizes, the smallest, thinnest needle which will suffice being always the best.

Tissue forceps.

Hemostats.

Scissors.

4 Allis forceps.

Gelpi retractor.

Forty-day chromic catgut No. 2.

Silkworm-gut.

If the cervix is involved, there should be added 2 ring forceps for grasping the cervix.

1 narrow-bladed abdominal retractor of the Deaver type.

Technic.—If the delivery has been at home, the patient should be drawn across the bed, the feet placed upon chair or the legs held by attendants.

The vulvar outlet is recleansed and draped. A large tampon of gauze is placed deep in the vagina, to prevent blood from obscuring the field of operation, and good exposure is obtained with a Gelpi retractor. Surgical asepsis, of course, is maintained. Lacerations vary so much that each is a problem in itself and only general directions for these repairs can be enunciated (Figs. 368, 369, 370).

It is always wise to attempt as accurate approximation of tissue as possible, and the layer plan of closure is much the best. By this means the deeper muscular bundles are first brought together by interrupted catgut sutures, then their overlying fasciae and finally the mucosa. When the skin is involved, the final superficial suture should either be subcuticular, or the gaping wound should be closed by interrupted silkworm-gut, the ends left long and tied together.

The old plan of shotting these sutures with perforated shot, squeezed shut, is practiced by the writer who feels his best ultimate results are so obtained.

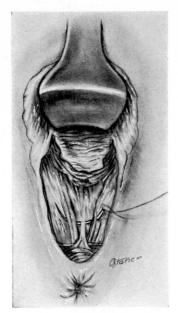

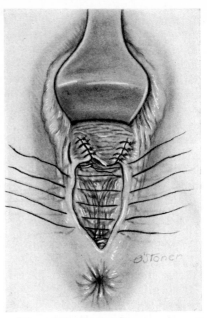

Fig. 368.—Second-degree laceration. The deep structures of the
perineum being approximated.

Fig. 369.—Second-degree laceration.
The sulci repaired. Stitches placed in the
perineum.

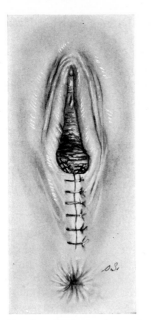

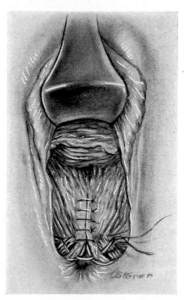

Fig. 370.—Second-degree laceration repaired.

Fig. 371.—Third-degree laceration.
The rectovaginal septum has been sutured. Repair of the sphincter.

Interrupted catgut on the skin surface is absorbed too quickly, and often results in open wound surfaces, which heal slowly by granulation.

In third-degree tears when the sphincter is torn, the ends of these muscles must be carefully isolated, held in Allis forceps and united by one or two catgut sutures. The opening in the rectovaginal septum is then closed and the sphincter repair reinforced with one or two silkworm-gut sutures (Figs. 371, 372, 373).

The details are set forth in the legends of the accompanying illustrations.

Intermediate Repair of Laceration.—Some years ago B. C. Hirst and others warmly advocated delay in repairing perineal tears until six days after delivery. This plan had the advantage that swelling and

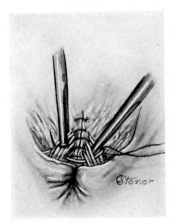

Fig. 372.—The end of the severed sphincter head in forceps and sutured.

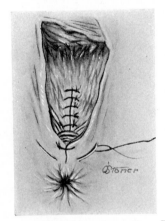

Fig. 373.—Third-degree laceration. The completion of the repair.

bleeding had ceased, the separated tissues were easy to identify and the repair was more anatomic and gave better results.

The disadvantages were a second anesthesia and a prolonged period of hospitalization or confinement to bed if at home. Intermediate repair is useful when the patient is in poor condition after a traumatic and long operative delivery and when the parts are much distorted by edema and hemorrhage into the tissues, otherwise it is not advised.

Bubis and his followers seize the opportunity of a recent laceration to perform a formal repair, correcting the lesions left by previous deliveries at this time. Though highly lauded by a number of obstetricians, this procedure has never appealed to the writer, for many reasons.

LACERATION OF THE CERVIX

Like the pelvic floor, the cervix is invariably torn to some degree in primiparae, and often in multiparae.

The tear may be a simple slit at the external os, a deep laceration running laterally up the cervical wall to the broad ligament or even a series of tears, the so-called "stellate laceration."

The injury is due to the overstretching of the cervical musculature by the fetus, or its too rapid and forcible dilatation as in precipitate labor. Severe laceration of the cervix may lead to profuse, even fatal, hemorrhage. Indeed, in some of the unusual accidents when the entire cervix is torn off from the lower uterine segment, the bleeding may be tremendous in amount. Small tears, especially those near the external os, usually heal spontaneously, and require no treatment.

Treatment.—*Prophylaxis.*—The less interference with physiological dilatation and effacement of the cervix, the fewer the tears. Hence, manual dilatation, accouchement forcé, attempts at version and forceps extraction before full dilatation has been attained are decried.

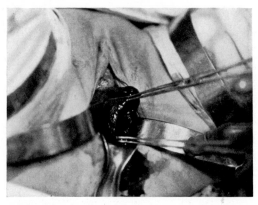

Fig. 374.—Inspection of the cervix, preparatory to repair. (Goff.)

As to the repair of cervical injuries, theoretically all cervices should be inspected after delivery, but in practice this may be omitted in multiparae who have had easy labors. All primiparae should be subjected to this examination when surgical asepsis is attainable and provided the patient is in good condition (Fig. 374).

With the patient across the bed, or in stirrups on the delivery table, the cervix is inspected as a preliminary to the repair of the perineum. The long anterior lip is seized with a ring forceps and easily drawn to the vulva. The posterior lip is much shorter and more nearly obliterated and sometimes is found only after some difficulty.

A Deaver retractor, applied to the lateral wall of the vagina, greatly facilitates the exposure.

If the tear (worse usually on the side to which the occiput lay) is immaterial, the cervix is released, and allowed to retract. If the tear be of moment, it is repaired by interrupted sutures of forty-day chromic catgut No. 2 (Fig. 375).

It is sometimes much easier to place the lowest suture first, carefully coapting the lower margin of the laceration, leaving this suture long as a traction rod and then "climbing up the tear," drawing the cervix further and further down with successive sutures until the upper angle of the laceration has been secured. The sutures are then cut short.

In the event of postpartum hemorrhage, especially if the uterus be firmly contracted, the cervix must always be inspected, since severe hemorrhage may follow laceration of the circular artery. Immediate ligation in such case is naturally obligatory. Inasmuch as carcinoma of the cervix is infinitely more common in parous than in nullip-

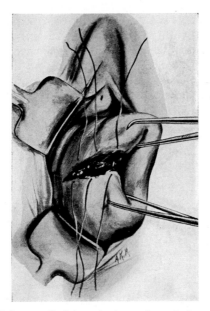

Fig. 375.—Stitches applied in suturing a lacerated cervix. (Kerr.)

arous women, conservative obstetrics requires that extensive laceration of this organ be repaired at the time of delivery and that remaining erosions and eversions be corrected by the cautery at the close of the puerperium.

HEMATOMA OF THE VULVA AND VAGINA

This unusual accident may be the result of a traumatic delivery, or as occurred in one of the two cases observed by the author, may follow an apparently uncomplicated spontaneous birth.

Any of the pelvic vessels may rupture, and the blood extravasates along the lines of cleavage of the muscles and fascia, forming sometimes enormous hematomata either wholly within the vagina, or more

38

commonly distending the paravulvar tissues and the perirectal space. The symptoms are intense pain, with pressure upon bladder or rectum, evidences of acute anemia, and if external, the formation of a subcutaneous hematoma.

These cases are very grave, the death rate from subsequent infection, or immediate blood loss being quite high.

Treatment.—If large, the tumor is incised and packed, and the bleeding vessel ligated if it can be reached. Small hematomata are treated expectantly.

THE AFTERCARE OF LACERATION

Simple cleansing is the only treatment necessary after the repair of injuries to the birth canal. Irrigation with a mild antiseptic after urination or defecation, and then drying the areas by gentle pressure with a cotton ball is advised. No dusting powder should be used nor meddlesome dressing done. Active movements of the patient's legs are forbidden for ten days at the end of which time nonabsorbable sutures are to be removed, with no further treatment.

CHAPTER XXXV

POSTPARTUM HEMORRHAGE

Excessive bleeding from the genital tract which appears between the birth of the child and the end of the puerperium is termed "postpartum hemorrhage."

The amount of blood lost may vary, from only a few hundred cubic centimeters above the average physiological bleeding to a hemorrhage of such volume that death results in a short time. The average blood loss in normal labor has been calculated to be about 250 cc. and if the amount increases to over 600 cc. the case is regarded as one of hemorrhage.

Frequency.—Postpartum hemorrhage occurs about once in 100 cases, though slight hemorrhages are more frequent and very large ones less so.

The incidence is less in well organized maternities than in home practice, largely because the accident is anticipated and active treatment is begun before the anemia becomes dangerous.

Prognosis.—In the Philadelphia survey of maternal deaths there were 33 of the total 717 in which postpartum hemorrhage was the primary cause in 27 and the contributory cause in 6. Thus 4.4 per cent of all the deaths were due to this accident.

If the 95,000 births reported for the period of the survey be considered, fatal postpartum hemorrhage occurred in 0.0347 per cent or one in about 2900 deliveries. In experienced hands, DeLee thinks the mortality is about 1 in 11,000 deliveries.

Etiology.—Hemorrhage after childbirth may originate in the uterine blood spaces, *atonic hemorrhage.*

It may develop from faulty placental separation—*placental site hemorrhage;* or it may follow laceration of the birth canal—*traumatic hemorrhage.*

When the bleeding arises from the uterine wall, its etiology becomes quite complex. Among the generally recognized causes are:

Uterine inertia, an inherent lack of contractile power in the uterine muscle (*q. v.*). This in turn may be essential or idiopathic (which means simply cause unknown), may follow overstretching of the muscle, in hydramnios, multiple pregnancy, very large child, long exhausting labor, etc.

Tumors of the uterus, notably fibromata, may break the rhythm of the contracting muscle bundles.

Constitutional Inferiority.—Women with profound anemia, syphilis, persistent hypotension and other debilitating conditions seem to have an increased tendency to atony of the uterus.

Blood Dyscrasia.—Hemophilia is given as a cause but must be very rare. Normally the pregnant woman is possessed of an excess of fibrin in the blood, as well as a definite plethora. She is therefore fitted to withstand considerable blood loss, but when there is definite alteration in the quality of the blood, this advantage is overcome. Blood dyscrasias are rare in parturient women and their influence upon the production of postpartum bleeding is slight.

Bleeding from the placental site may be due to imperfect separation of the placenta, a portion of the organ being attached while another part is detached, permitting free bleeding from the underlying blood spaces.

Improper management of the third stage of labor, with forced separation of the placenta before the uterus has had time for contraction, retraction and the rearrangement of the muscle bundles, is often responsible. Retention of a cotyledon of the placenta or even fragments of this organ may cause the bleeding.

Placenta praevia, with laceration of the cervix and the aberrant placental site sometimes is a potent factor in this accident as is the premature separation of the normally situated placenta.

The placenta may have separated and become incarcerated in the lower uterine segment, when if the uterus be atonic a quantity of blood may accumulate in its cavity, without external evidences of bleeding.

Traumatic hemorrhage from laceration requires but little discussion. When the uterus is hard and firmly contracted, and the bleeding persists, inspection by speculum of the cervix and vagina will disclose a laceration with a bleeding vessel. The deeper tears of the cervix involving the circular artery are potent causes. Primiparae are slightly more susceptible to postpartum hemorrhage than are multiparae.

Symptoms and Diagnosis.—Excessive bleeding with its subsequent constitutional reactions constitute the symptomatology. The hemorrhage may take the form of a continued dribble of blood, which fails to abate after the discharge of the placenta, or there may be a massive bleeding, sometimes unbelievably violent. All obstetricians of experience have observed cases in which the hemorrhage was so rapid and profuse that the patient became exsanguinated and in imminent peril of her life within a few minutes.

Concealed hemorrhage sometimes is overlooked until the systemic evidences of anemia calls attention to its existence, when palpation of the fundus will find a soft, distended uterus, sometimes extending upward beyond the umbilicus. Massage of this dilated uterus will release a great quantity of free blood and clots.

Constitutional symptoms soon develop, if the hemorrhage is profuse. Pallor, air hunger, thirst, a rapid and thready pulse, leaking skin, falling blood pressure and temperature and shallow rapid respiration are signs of grave import.

Treatment.—*Prophylaxis.*—Adequate prenatal care will enable the obstetrician to segregate women who are potential victims of postpartum hemorrhage. Malnutrition, anemia, systemic disease, a history of bleeding after previous deliveries and overdistention of the uterus are predisposing causes, and should receive their appropriate treatment during pregnancy.

During labor, the prophylaxis consists largely in the proper conduct of that process, chiefly directed to the management of the third stage. Enforced, rapid separation and expulsion of the placenta are to be avoided.

The time required for uterine contraction and retraction varies in different women and in different labors in the same woman and no time rule is possible to determine attempts at Credé expression; vigorous massage and so on should not be made for at least thirty minutes after delivery unless persistent bleeding renders such action imperative.

It is the practice of the author to give 1 cc. of pituitrin and an ampule of ergot, or ergotrate, intramuscularly, immediately after the birth of the child. Theoretically, this may cause retention of the separated placenta from cervical contraction but practically it does not seem to occur, the time required for ergot to act as an oxytocic being sufficiently great for the placenta to have been expelled.

While waiting for the separation of the placenta, the fundus uteri is watched and frequently lightly palpated to ascertain whether or not it is filling with blood, but no massage is practiced, nor is the uterus held. Placental separation is a purely physiologic process and should not be interfered with. The abdominal binder must not be applied until some time, fifteen to thirty minutes, after the placenta is expelled, so that the state of the fundus may be continually known.

Treatment of Postpartum Hemorrhage.—If the uterus be well contracted, lacerations should be sought by exposure of the parts with a speculum, the bleeding vessel ligated and the accompanying laceration repaired, when the bleeding will cease at once.

If the uterus be soft and relaxed after the placenta has escaped it is stimulated to contraction by pressure and massage. One hand inverts the lax abdominal wall behind the uterus, the other makes pressure just above the symphysis and the uterus is firmly squeezed between the two, and at the same time is pulled upward, thus making anteroposterior pressure and putting the uterine arteries on the stretch. If the placenta remains attached, with free bleeding, the Credé mode of expression may be utilized. As described by Credé in 1853 (but known and practiced at the Rotunda Hospital a century before) the method consists in the obstetrician grasping the uterus through the abdominal wall, the thumb in front and the fingers behind, and after waiting from five to ten minutes, gently kneading it, thus facilitating contraction and separation. Then when a contraction occurs firm and steady pressure downward is made. If the placenta fails to separate by this maneuver, it is probably adherent, or rarely a placenta accreta may exist. In such cases, hemorrhage is usually slight and time may be given before manual removal is attempted. If the bleeding is severe, removal must be done at once (Chapter XXI).

Most really dangerous postpartum hemorrhages occur after the expulsion of the placenta and if simple massage, pituitrin, etc., do not *promptly* control the bleeding, the uterus is to be firmly packed with sterile gauze packing, an abundant supply of which should be in every obstetric bag and delivery room.

The author's pack consists of a folded strip of gauze of four thicknesses, 3 inches wide and 6 yards long, the free edges turned in. These packs are kept sterile in large glass tubes or ordinary jars, one pack to the tube.

Technic.—While an assistant makes light pressure on the fundus, through the abdominal wall, the operator introduces the folded hand into the uterus and removes clots, at the same time searching for retained fragments of placenta. The hand is then quickly withdrawn and the packing introduced *with the hand,* no packing, dressing forceps or other instrument being employed. The assistant notes when the packing gauze reached the top of the uterine cavity as felt by the impulse given to his hand. Gauze is introduced until the uterus is full, fundus, lower segment and cervix being firmly packed.

A separate tampon then fills the vagina. In dangerous cases, the packing becomes saturated with blood in an hour or sometimes less, and under such circumstances the gauze is removed *at once* and the entire process repeated, with due attention to the maintenance of asepsis. If the bleeding still continues, the situation is grave indeed, and heroic measures are requisite.

The cervix may be sewn shut over the packing to retain the blood in the uterus in the hope that clotting will occur.

Long Péan clamps may be placed on the uterine arteries, through the vagina. The uterine arteries may be exposed and ligated per vaginam. Finally abdominal hysterectomy may be necessary.

These are desperate measures for desperate conditions and if they are required, the prognosis is most unpromising. I have never found it necessary to employ any of them except hysterectomy which must be done sometimes, but not frequently.

Some authorities advise compression of the aorta by strong pressure with the fist through the abdominal wall, over the lower lumbar vertebrae, and Momberg's belt is literally a tourniquet fastened around the abdomen so tightly as to compress the aorta. These devices are so brutal that the cure is worse than the disease, and except in the absence of any equipment for gentler measures, are strongly condemned.

General Treatment.—While the above local efforts at combating the hemorrhage are in progress, systemic measures to combat the anemia should be inaugurated. The failing heart is temporarily stimulated by caffeine benzoate or digitalis. Most important is blood transfusion, 500 cc. or more, as quickly given as suitable donors can be assembled.

In the meantime, the intravenous administration of glucose solution 10 per cent or gum acacia or, lacking that, normal saline, will supply the fluid lacking in the circulatory system. As soon as the uterine manipulations are completed, the patient is returned to bed, the foot of which has been elevated, and external heat is applied by wrapping her in blankets, with hot water bottles or electric heating pads.

Ice-caps over the uterus are inadvisable because they only add to the dispersion of the necessary body heat.

Blood transfusion may be repeated frequently in severe cases, and the patient is encouraged to partake of hot liquid nourishment, and abundant fluids.

The personal experience of the writer leads him to formulate the following generalities.

Parturient women are less able to withstand repeated hemorrhage of moderate amount than one massive bleeding.

. A woman who has slowly lost considerable blood may show no evidence of constitutional reaction, until collapse suddenly occurs after only a little additional bleeding. A common mistake is to delay too long before resorting to packing, in the hope that the hemorrhage will cease.

In hospital or home where asepsis may be secured by a conscientious medical attendant, there is little reason to fear infection from packing the uterus, and I have never had occasion to regret having done this, but have often wished it had been done earlier.

Next to actual control of bleeding, the most vitally important phase of treatment is immediate blood transfusion, and any maternity not equipped with available blood donors is derelict in its duty to its clientele.

Failing blood, the intravenous administration of any suitable fluid should not be delayed.

Interference with the normal mechanism of the third stage of labor and rough handling of the uterus at this time invites hemorrhage.

Late Puerperal Hemorrhages.—Any uterine bleeding occurring after twenty-four hours after labor and before the completion of the puerperium is termed a delayed, postpartum hemorrhage.

Etiology.—Retained fragments of placenta, or accessory placenta form the most common causes, while sometimes a retained, organized clot may be responsible.

Subinvolution of the uterus, with bleeding upon any unwonted exercise is a cause, as are degenerated submucous myomata, ulcerations of the cervix involving a vessel of more or less magnitude, placental polyp, and a number of rare causes which have been reported once or twice each.

Treatment.—Stimulation of the uterus to contract by the exhibition of ergot or pituitrin, with the use of a hot vaginal douche and possibly gentle massage of the uterus are the local measures available.

Intrauterine manipulations are to be avoided, until late in the puerperium when most danger of infection has passed. Blood transfusions, if the hemorrhage has been severe, or hematinics to stimulate the blood-making tissues are the general procedures to be used.

CHAPTER XXXVI

INVERSION OF THE UTERUS AND PROLAPSE OF THE CORD

INVERSION OF THE UTERUS

This uncommon accident consists in the literal turning inside out of the uterus. It may be *partial,* when the fundus only is involved, and occupies the lower uterine segment, or *complete* when the entire organ is inverted (Fig. 376).

Sometimes the inversion may occur spontaneously, as in two of my cases, but it usually follows undue traction on the umbilical cord, or too vigorous attempts at placental expression.

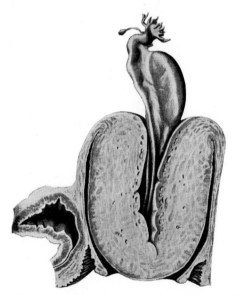

Fig. 376.—Sagittal section through an inverted uterus. (Zangemeister.)

In one case seen in consultation, during a breech extraction an assistant made pressure upon the uterus with his fist to facilitate the expulsion of the after-coming head. The head was suddenly delivered and the fundus literally pushed down into complete inversion by the abdominal pressure.

Symptoms.—Occasionally the symptoms are slight and if the inverted fundus does not protrude through the vulva, the condition may escape notice for some time.

Generally, however, there is profuse bleeding and the woman promptly goes into profound shock.

Inversio uteri is a very dangerous complication, death in an hour or two often occurring, or subsequent sepsis later closes the scene.

Diagnosis.—A purplish-red tumor protruding from the vagina, its surface covered with ragged, bleeding decidua, with the placenta sometimes still attached makes the diagnosis simple.

In complete inversion, the routine inspection of the field will reveal the state of affairs.

The diagnosis is confirmed by feeling a crater where the fundus should be, upon abdominal palpation.

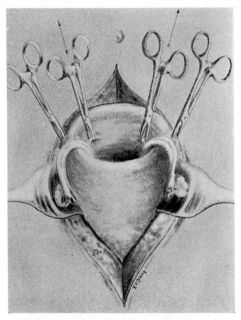

Fig. 377.—Correction of inversio uteri by abdominal reposition. First step. (Huntington, Irving and Kellogg in Amer. Jour. Obstet. and Gynec., vol. 15, 1928, C. V. Mosby Co., Publishers.)

Treatment.—Proper management of the third stage of labor avoiding cord traction and undue uterine massage will prevent most cases.

When the inversion is present, the simplest means of reposition is manual taxis. Two fingers make firm pressure upon the most prominent portion of the protrusion, and as it begins to yield to the pressure, a third and fourth are added, until the organ will be felt to slowly slip right side out. The placenta must always be detached prior to reposition as its added bulk often defeats the successful outcome. After the uterus is replaced, it is firmly packed with sterile gauze to prevent a repetition of the accident. If taxis fails after a few minutes of intelligent manipulation, the protruding mass is covered by gauze dressings held in place by a **T**-binder, and the patient treated for shock in the usual manner, not neglecting the high elevation of the foot of the bed.

In a day or two taxis may be repeated and, if unsuccessful, laparotomy is performed, the inverted fundus seized with Jacob forceps after the manner of Huntington *et al.*, or better, one or two mattress sutures of strong silk are placed in the depth of the muscle of the inverted fundus and slow strong traction made. The traction is assisted by pressure upon the uterus made from the vagina, when

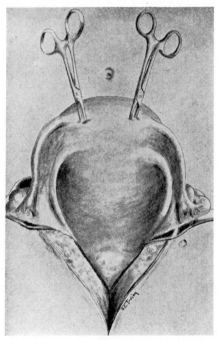

Fig. 378.—Correction of inversio uteri. The reposition completed. (Huntington, Irving and Kellogg in Amer. Jour. Obstet. and Gynec., vol. 15, 1928, C. V. Mosby Co., Publishers.)

in most instances the reposition may be accomplished. The replaced uterus is then packed from below (Figs. 377, 378).

In chronic inversion, the Spinelli operation is the classical procedure. By the vaginal route the bladder is separated from the anterior uterine wall, the constricting cervical ring and the body of the uterus are divided in the midline, the uterus replaced and the incision closed by interrupted suture after which the bladder is allowed to fall into place and the vaginal wound closed.

In one case, which I observed, an ignorant accoucheur was about to ligate and cut off the inverted uterus, believing it to be a submucosal fibroid tumor. Happily he was prevented from completing his plan before any damage was done.

PROLAPSE OF THE UMBILICAL CORD

True prolapse of the cord occurs when the membranes have been ruptured and the cord escapes past the fetus into the vagina and often descends out of the vulva.

Forelying cord is the condition found when a loop of this structure lies beside or lower than the presenting part, but still within the intact bag of membranes.

Occult prolapse of the cord is a term applied to a low position of the cord, a loop descending to a point between the presenting part

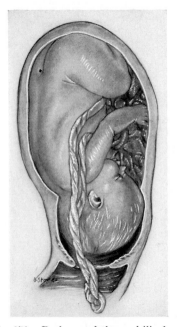

Fig. 379.—Prolapse of the umbilical cord.

and the contraction ring at the lower uterine segment, but not palpable through the cervix.

Prolapsed cord must not be confused with the very rare anomaly of umbilical presentation, when the funis is not prolapsed at all, but is merely the most dependent portion of the presenting part of the fetus.

Forelying cord and occult prolapse may develop during pregnancy but true prolapse is only possible after the rupture of the membranes and therefore usually occurs during labor.

Frequency.—Cord prolapse is not a particularly common accident, being observed about once in 300 labors in my experience, though statistics vary from 1 in 180 to 1 in 400.

Etiology.—Anything which produces an imperfect fit between fetus and pelvic brim may be responsible for funic prolapse, and it follows that it is rarely seen in vertex presentations or frank breech in normal pelves, whereas in transverse, footling or face positions it occurs fairly frequently.

In contracted pelves, where engagement is imperfect and spaces are left between head and pelvis, the cord may easily slip down, and if in such cases the membranes rupture during a contraction, it may be swept down with the rush of fluid.

Prognosis.—The mother suffers no ill except possibly from a traumatic delivery hurriedly done before dilatation is complete in an effort to save the child.

The infant mortality is high, 50 to 60 per cent of babies being lost as a result of pressure upon the umbilical vessels and consequent asphyxia. The mortality varies greatly with the stage of labor at the time of the prolapse. The lower the fetus in the pelvis and the more nearly complete the dilatation and effacement of the cervix, the better the prognosis, since delivery may be quickly effected under such circumstances.

Diagnosis.—The recognition of true prolapse when a loop of the cord lies in the vagina or protrudes from the vulva is so obvious as to require no comment.

Forelying Cord.—This unusual condition may only be determined by painstaking vaginal examination, when the cervix is sufficiently dilated to admit the finger. The loop of cord may then be felt under the membranes alongside the presenting part.

Occult Prolapse.—When the cord has been incarcerated between the head and the contraction ring, direct diagnosis is impossible but the condition may be suspected, when the fetal heart slows markedly at each uterine contraction. Sometimes the rate increases, but retardation is the rule. When this happens, it is well nigh impossible to differentiate between occult prolapse and short cord, except possibly by the fact that in the latter condition the progress of labor is slow, the advance of the head being checked by the pull of the taut cord.

Treatment.—In *forelying cord* it is essential that the integrity of the membranes be maintained until the dilatation of the cervix has reached a stage when rapid delivery is possible.

The patient is placed with the head lowered and a Barnes or Voorhees bag is placed in the cervix to hasten dilatation and hold back the cord should the membranes rupture.

Cesarean section must always be considered in these cases as the safety of the baby is much enhanced by abdominal delivery before the rupture of the membranes.

When occult prolapse is suspected, dilatation may be hastened by the use of the dilating bag, and here again the advantage to the baby of elective cesarean section must not be forgotten.

True Prolapse of the Cord.—Here the management is based upon two phases of the situation: first, whether the child is living or dead, and second, the degree of cervical dilatation and effacement.

1. Child living, cervix not fully dilated or easily dilated.

Here reposition of the cord is indicated. After washing the cord with tincture of green soap and water, it is painted with an antiseptic as 3 per cent solution iodine, or 4 per cent mercurochrome solution, and the asepsis of physician and patient having been attended to, the operator attempts to replace the cord with the finger. If the patient be cooperative, the knee-chest position is best, otherwise the Trendelenburg posture is employed. A loop of the cord, lightly held in the finger is reintroduced through the cervix and looped about a projecting part of the fetus, a shoulder, hip or knee. When all of the slack of the cord is again within the uterus, the hand is withdrawn and a previously sterilized dilating bag is immediately placed in the cervix against the presenting part, to retain the cord in position (Figs. 380, 381).

If the cervix will not admit the fingers, a repositor is necessary. Many ingenious instruments for this purpose have been invented but usually none is at hand when needed. A classical method is the use of a stiff catheter, with a fillet of tape threaded through its eye, but this is open to the same objection, *i. e.*, not present. All that is really necessary is a foot or two of sterile 2-inch gauze bandage and a pair of uterine dressing forceps or long thumb forceps which form part of every obstetrical kit. A single turn of the middle of the piece of bandage is taken about the most dependent portion of the cord, and the bandage grasped about ½ inch from the cord by the dressing forceps. Under guidance of the finger, the cord is replaced and hooked over the fetus as before described, the forceps withdrawn, with the bandage left in place, the ends hanging from the vagina. The metreurynter is now introduced to prevent a repetition of the prolapse, and the accoucheur awaits the completion of dilatation before attempting delivery.

Careful attention to the fetal heart sounds will disclose kinking and obstruction to the blood interchange, when more active steps must be taken.

2. Child alive, cervix fully dilated or easily dilatable. Here the best treatment is version or extraction, or if the head is well engaged, forceps delivery, great care being taken to exclude the cord from the grip of the forceps.

3. Child dead. Cervix not well dilated. In such cases it is best to carefully wrap the prolapsed cord in a sterile towel or gauze, and await the issue of labor.

If no progress is made, the procedure of choice is craniotomy, after sufficient dilatation has been attained by the use of a bag if necessary. A small baby may be delivered by forceps or version, but in general, this is not good practice in the event of a dead child. Cesarean section is sometimes indicated in prolapsed cord, as, for example, when there is a contracted pelvis, a fetal disproportion or

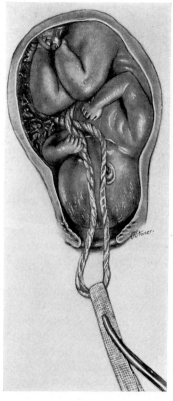

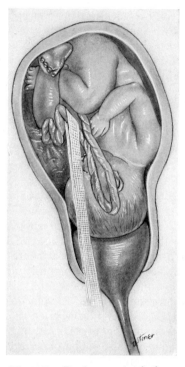

Fig. 380.—Replacement of prolapsed cord. A strip of sterile gauze is passed round the loop of cord and grasped in dressing forceps.

Fig. 381.—Replacement of the prolapsed cord. The loop of cord has been carried into the uterus and hooked over an extremity of the infant. Further prolapse is prevented by the insertion of a dilating bag.

where the securing of a living child is of vital importance, in elderly primiparae and the like.

When abdominal hysterotomy is determined upon, great care must be taken not to drag the soiled cord through the uterine incision, but this organ should be clamped and cut close to the child, then the placental end clamped and cut close to the placenta after which the freed cord is pulled out of the vagina by an assistant.

DYSTOCIA DUE TO SHORT UMBILICAL CORD

Short umbilical cord may give rise to severe dystocia and constitutes a very definite peril to the infant intrapartum. From the clinical standpoint, short cords are divided into the absolutely short, 32 cm. or less in length, and the relatively short, 35 cm. in length. To these must be added the shortened cord, which, originally of normal or even greater length, has been shortened by looping or coiling about parts of the fetal body.

Gardiner who has deeply studied this subject states that in a vertex presentation the placental insertion of the cord must not be farther than 5 cm. above the superior strait in order that the fetus may be born without traction, and the cord must be 32 cm. in length. In a breech presentation, in order that the fetus may be born without cord traction, the cord must be 55 cm. in length. In a vertex presentation with a loop of cord about the neck, the cord must be 76.5 cm. in length, if birth is to occur without traction. In a vertex presentation with a coil of cord about the neck, a length of 93.5 cm. is required. In a breech presentation with a loop of cord about the neck, the cord becomes a spiral and very little needs to be added to its length. In a breech presentation with a coil of cord about the neck, a length of 101.5 cm. in necessary if undue traction is to be avoided.

Etiology.—The etiology of coiling or looping of the cord about the fetus is not clear, but it seems reasonable that fetal movements in the presence of an abundant supply of liquor amnii plus the spiral vermicular movement of the cord itself are chiefly responsible.

Symptoms and Treatment.—Clinically, the short cord is important because traction upon it may cause prolonged delay in the second stage, may cause fetal asphyxia, or, rarely, may produce either premature separation of the placenta or spontaneous intra-uterine rupture of the cord itself, several cases of which appear in the literature. Inversion of the uterus and umbilical hernia of the fetus may also develop. False labor pains are also attributed to short cord, as are malposition of the fetus, notably transverse positions.

The chief symptoms of insufficient length of the cord are delayed second stage and a slowing of the fetal heart tones. Treatment consists in prompt delivery by the best available means, with regard to the degree of descent and the character of the cervix as to effacement and dilatation.

CHAPTER XXXVII

PUERPERAL SEPSIS

Definition.—Puerperal sepsis is an infection of the parturient canal, arising just prior to, during, or shortly after labor. It is in fact a wound infection and may remain localized, may become widespread and may lead to bacteremia and pyemia.

Etiology.—In most cases puerperal sepsis is a result of inoculation of the tissues with pyogenic bacteria from without, *i. e.*, the hand or instruments of the accoucheur, or nurse, the utensils used in the care of the patient, coitus or douches just before or during labor, or organism carried from the infected respiratory tract of someone in contact with the patient. It is undoubtedly true that a definite proportion of cases of puerperal sepsis are traceable to an autogenous infection. A remote focus, an abscessed tooth, tonsils, diseased gallbladder or fallopian tubes may be responsible.

Also the vagina itself may harbor pathogenic bacteria which grow luxuriantly upon the blood clots both in and about the many small wounds in the cervix and uterus and so cause the sepsis, especially if they have been spread about by careless examinations and manipulations.

From the standpoint of good obstetrics, it is well for the physician to minimize autogenous infection and to concentrate his efforts upon the reduction of introduced organisms to the least possible number and to perfect the technic of the conduct of labor.

Any pyogenic bacteria may be causative but those most frequently noted are Streptococcus pyogenes, hemolyticus and viridans, Staphylococcus aureus, albus and citreus, gonococcus, bacillus of diphtheria and colon bacillus.

There are certain cases wherein severe puerperal sepsis follows easy, spontaneous labor which has been conducted with every safeguard against infection and entirely without vaginal or even rectal manipulation or examination. It is probable that the infective agents in these baffling cases are anaerobic bacteria, inhabiting the vagina and uterus and not demonstrable by ordinary culture methods. The work of Schottmüller which has since been confirmed by Schwartz and others is extremely suggestive and further study may prove conclusively that anaerobic forms of the pyogenic bacteria play an important rôle in the production of septic infection following delivery.

Frequency.—Though two thirds of the women in a lying-in hospital no longer die of puerperal sepsis, as occurred in the Hôtel Dieu in Mauriceau's time, still the ravages of the disease are appalling. It is a matter of the gravest concern to obstetricians that its incidence has not been reduced materially during the past two decades, even though the attention of the profession has been most intensely concentrated upon staying its frequency.

In the survey of maternal deaths in Philadelphia during the years 1931, 1932, and 1933, 119 women died of puerperal sepsis, which number constituted 18 per cent of all women dying during pregnancy or the puerperium, and 28 per cent of the deaths in women who were over twenty-eight weeks pregnant.

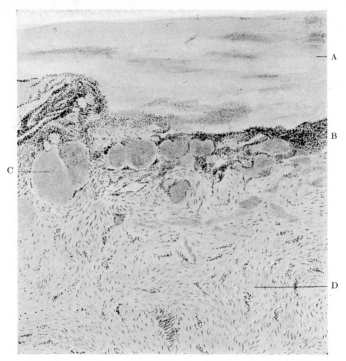

Fig. 382.—Uterine mucosa third day after normal delivery, showing: A, adherent blood clot; B, slight zone of leukocytic infiltration; C, thrombi; D, uterine muscle. × 25. (Lea, "Puerperal Infection," Oxford University Press, Publishers.)

Sepsis is then the greatest single cause of death in the child-bearing women, outnumbering all other causes, and accounting in its own right for over one fourth of all obstetric fatalities.

Pathology.—It has been stated above that puerperal sepsis is a wound infection generally carried to the tissues from without. In addition the vagina always harbors saprophytic bacteria, which may include the streptococcus in a saprophytic phase. These organisms may become pyogenic if they grow on fresh wound surfaces and they tend to complicate by their putrefactive qualities, infection by the ordinary pyogenic bacteria. Puerperal infections are usually localized at first (Fig. 382) and they remain so, or become diffuse, according to the degree of resistance of the patient as evidenced by the rapid formation of a protective zone of leukocytes, fibrin, etc., beneath the area of sepsis; if the initial infection be within the uterus as in the common puerperal endometritis, the spread of the infection depends also upon the relaxation or contraction of the uterus. A firmly contracted uterus will close the lymphatics and blood vessels, and will empty itself of superficial necrotic tissues in a short time, whereas if the uterus be relaxed and retroverted the blood and lymph spaces are open portals to carry infective materials to deeper tissues; the mass of necrotic endometrium is not expelled, and the relaxed and open cervix affords an avenue of entrance to pyogenic bacteria whose advent may inaugurate a mixed infection of greatly increased virulence.

The tendency for a primary local infection to remain so or not, depends then, upon:

(a) The nature of the infective organisms—whether highly virulent or not, and their power of diffusibility, whether they possess the power to pass rapidly through superficial tissues without evoking much local reaction, and enter the blood or lymph streams, or whether they tend to mass in these superficial tissues with more or less massive local reaction.

(b) The breaking down of the protective zone of lymphocytes and fibrin which separates the area of infection from healthy tissue. This may occur spontaneously but is usually due to misdirected efforts at the removal of necrotic material by the obstetrician.

Puerperal sepsis may be limited to purely local infections of vagina or vulva, it may involve the endometrium in one or two forms, putrid (or saprophytic) endometritis or septic endometritis, it may involve the tubes, ovaries, pelvic cellular tissues, and the veins of the pelvis, may eventuate in a generalized or localized peritonitis, or may either primarily or secondarily become a systemic infection of the blood or lymph stream.

Puerperal Vaginitis and Vulvitis.—A preexisting inflammation of Bartholin's glands may light up after delivery giving rise to a localized abscess, with its attendant swelling, induration and rise of temperature. Simply evacuation of the pus usually terminates the symptoms promptly, systemic involvement occurring but rarely.

Vaginitis.—May disclose itself as a purulent inflammation of the mucosa, which becomes reddened, thick and may present local shallow ulcers. The perineum, if repaired, usually breaks down, with free purulent discharge. Occasionally the vagina may show a grayish, necrotic membrane, pseudodiphtheritic in character.

Here again, surgical cleanliness, the use of antiseptic solutions to the vagina and free drainage usually prevents any serious consequences. The vulva and vagina being resistant tissues are not commonly involved.

Puerperal Endometritis.—The most common manifestation of puerperal sepsis is endometritis, due to the fact that the inner surface of the uterus after labor is a raw surface presenting innumerable small wound areas.

The portal of entry is usually the cervix, which itself is the seat of many wounds of more less size. Shreds of decidua, adherent to the

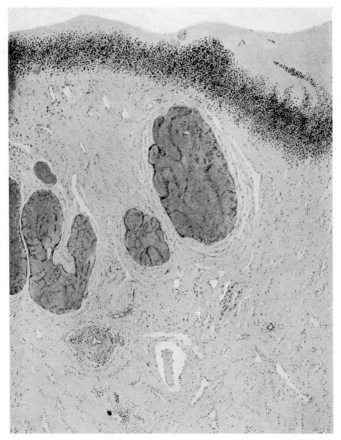

Fig. 383.—Acute infective endometritis with well-developed leukocytic protective zone, thrombi in decidua. × 150. (Lea, "Puerperal Infection," Oxford University Press, Publishers.)

uterine wall, together with retained blood clots make the uterine cavity a fertile field for bacterial growth.

Puerperal endometritis assumes one of two forms, according to the nature and virulence of the causative microogranisms.

Putrefactive Endometritis.—When the infection is due to streptococcus of low virulence, possibly associated with colon bacilli or other saprophytic forms, the innner surface of the uterus becomes an area of sloughing necrotic tissue, separated from the underlying healthy muscle by a well-defined protective zone of leukocytes. The lesion manifests itself usually on the third day after labor, when there may be a slight chill followed by a moderate elevation of temperature and considerable leukocytosis (15,000 to 20,000), with an increased rapidity of the pulse. The patient complains of painful uterine contractions, with the occasional expulsion of a foul blood clot (Fig. 383).

The lochia is bloody, excessive and fetid, and on bacteriological examination, streptococci and saprophytes are found in large numbers. Sometimes, too early contraction of the cervix, its occlusion by a blood

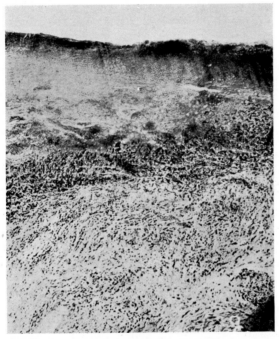

Fig. 384.—Acute streptococcic endometritis. Layer of coagulative necrosis on surface. Leukocytic invasion of uterine wall. × 200. (Lea, "Puerperal Infection," Oxford University Press, Publishers.)

clot, or an angulation at the cervical uterine juncture, causes a suppression of the lochia, with an intensification of the local and general symptoms. This condition is termed "lochial block."

The systemic reaction is due to the absorption of toxins from the invading bacteria, hence the term toxic endometritis or sapremia. Microscopic section of the uterine wall shows a layer of necrotic decidua, laden with bacteria, then a thick limiting wall of leukocytes and fibrin and under this the healthy uterine muscle, all layers being well defined.

Examination reveals the uterus, large, subinvoluted, soft and tender, and the cervix may be patulous or, in case of lochial block, may be closed and swollen.

Pyogenic, Septic or Coccal Endometritis.—If the endometrium be invaded by streptococci or staphylococci of high diffusibility and marked virulence, there develops pyogenic endometritis (Fig. 384).

Here there is but little local reaction in the uterine mucosa, the surface being smooth, and bathed with a thin purulent discharge, which is odorless. Microscopically the granulation zone is either entirely absent or thin and poorly developed. The uterus is not materially enlarged, nor is it tender and boggy, but is apparently well involuted. Septic endometritis is the most formidable manifestation of the disease, since the virulent nature of the infecting organisms and the lack of a restraining protective zone of granulation, tend toward the rapid penetration of the uterine muscles by the bacteria, the blood stream becoming infected with a resultant bacteremia, and extension by way of the lymph and blood leading to parametritis, peritonitis, etc.

The sequelae of septic endometritis are:

Bacteremia or pyemia.

Parametritis.

Pelvic thrombophlebitis.

Peritonitis.

Salpingitis and oophoritis.

THE MECHANISM OF THE EXTENSION OF SEPSIS FROM THE UTERUS

It has been stated that this extension usually follows endometritis but bacteria may invade the deeper tissues via the lymphatic supply of the cervix, which is so common a portal of entry of infection, or may even follow infection of the perineum.

I believe, however, that most systemic sepsis is secondary to a primary endometritis.

Extension by the Blood Stream.—*Thrombophlebitis, with Bacteremia or Pyemia.*—Bacteria of high virulence, invading a uterus in which the inhibiting granulation layer is deficient, rapidly penetrate to the blood spaces in the uterine wall, notably at the placental site. Here, and in the veins of the broad ligament, phlebitis occurs, either primarily or as a result of vein blocking by infected thrombi, and from these original sites, thrombi are carried into the iliac veins and so on to the lungs where infection may occur, thence through the pulmonary veins to the heart and so into the general circulation. As some of the thrombi soften and liquefy, their bacterial contents are discharged freely into the blood stream, to set up multiple abscesses, possibly, acute bacterial endocarditis, cloudy swelling of kidney, liver and spleen, in short the typical picture of pyemia (Fig. 385).

Generally, however, death closes the scene before there is time for secondary abscess formation, and in other cases, recovery from septicemia takes place without the development of pyemia.

The bacteria most apt to be responsible are the Streptococcus pyogenes in one of its forms and the Staphylococcus albus or aureus. These organisms may be recovered from the blood by culture of a specimen taken at the time of the chill.

Thrombophlebitis of the Veins of the Broad Ligament.—The distended veins occupying the broad ligament may become occluded by infected thrombi when a localized phlebitis follows. The veins become converted into varicose masses, the infection spreading by transudation into the surrounding cellular tissues, until the entire broad ligament becomes a tense, hard, fixed and extremely painful mass. This may remain localized or eventuate in a generalized blood infection. Resorption is the rule after many days of septic temperature.

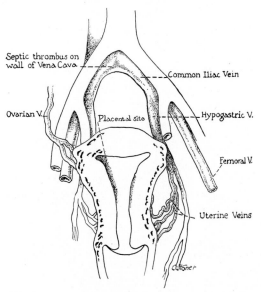

Fig. 385.—Puerperal sepsis. The spread of infection via the blood stream. (Redrawn from Bumm.)

Extension by the Lymph Stream.—The lymphatics may carry septic material to distant points of the body, and this form of extension is generally more dangerous to life than is the hematogenous dissemination. It must be remembered that lymphatic and hematogenic extension may occur simultaneously, an extremely grave expression of puerperal sepsis (Fig. 386).

Lymphatic extension is generally from a primary endometritis, but any portal of infection, even a comparatively insignificant wound of the perineum or cervix may suffice.

The route is via the uterine lymphatics, to the broad ligament, to the pelvic cellular tissue, to the peritoneum, which may become generally involved; to the subdiaphragmatic lymph glands and so eventually to the pleura and endocardium. There may be retroperitoneal extension with massive abscess. Widespread lymphangitis may secondarily cause blood stream infection with its consequences as described above.

Parametritis; Pelvic Cellulitis.—The loose celluar tissue surrounding the base of the uterus, lies under the peritoneum, and radiates from the uterus in all directions to the pelvic wall (Fig. 387). It makes up the bulk of the material between the layers of the broad ligaments. This cellular tissue is much increased during pregnancy,

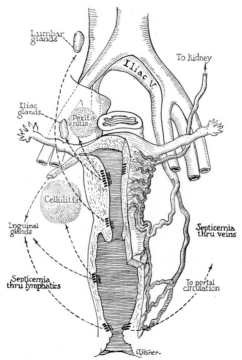

Fig. 386.—Puerperal sepsis. The spread of infection via the lymphatics.

and is very rich in its vascular and lymph supply. When infected lymph reaches this tissue, a hyperemia is produced, followed by the formation of an exudate which soon becomes swollen and begins to extend along the cleavage lines of the parametrium, forming a hard, dense mass irregular in outline and which may be unilateral, bilateral, or may entirely surround the uterus, involving the pararectal tissues and may extend anteriorly to the bladder.

The pelvic peritoneum soon becomes involved by contiguity and there develops a perimetritis which may involve the fallopian tubes. On examination parametritis presents itself as a hard, dense, irregular mass filling the vaginal vault, in which the cervix is fixed as though set in cement. The mass is hot, tender and very painful (Fig. 388).

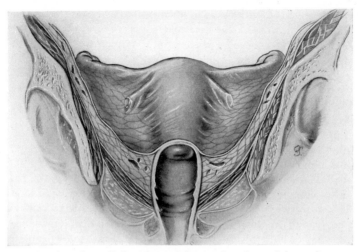

Fig. 387.—Showing the cellular tissue lying under the pelvic peritoneum and above the levatores ani muscles. (Redrawn after Polak.)

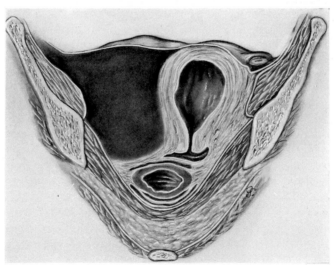

Fig. 388.—Puerperal sepsis. Exudate into the lateral parametrial tissues, displacing the uterus and obliterating the fornices and vaginal portio. (Redrawn after Polak.)

The end-results are either slow resorption of the exudate, a process requiring weeks and even months, or the tissues break down into a pelvic abscess, which may point into the rectum or vagina, but which generally is recognized and evacuated per vaginum.

Peritonitis.—Localized pelvic peritonitis accompanies many forms of puerperal sepsis and may continue without involvement of the general peritoneal cavity if the organisms be of low virulence and diffusibility and the patient have strong resistance.

Too often, however, the peritonitis becomes a spreading one of great severity and generally with a fatal outcome.

Peritonitis may follow either blood or lymph extension and may be the first clinical manifestation of puerperal sepsis, there being many cases in which there is no evidence of sepsis other than a rapid, fulminating peritonitis.

The *pathology* is that of peritonitis in general, a lusterless, hyperemic appearance, followed by paralytic ileus and the formation of intestinal adhesions, with pus pockets between the folds and possibly localized hemorrhages.

Cornual Abscess of the Uterus.—Extension of a septic endometritis into the uterine wall, may cause the formation of a small abscess in the muscle, along the lumen of the uterine cavity leading to the tube. Such abscesses may be recognized by the presence of a dense, rounded, circumscribed mass, palpable at the cornua of the uterus and giving rise to the usual symptoms of intense pain and temperature elevation.

Salpingitis.—Except as a part of a general or pelvic peritonitis, salpingitis is uncommon in puerperal sepsis unless the gonococcus is the offending organism when the tubes are often involved.

Gonococcal infection is not common in the puerperium and when it occurs, it is usually of low grade, and involves the mucosa of the uterus and tubes, with their underlying layers, but does not often become widespread or give rise to systemic infection.

The development of acute salpingitis, with its enlargement and increased density of the tubes, a small pelvic peritonitis from the escape of pus through the fimbriated extremity of the tubes, and the definite localization to these structures, should lead to the suspicion of gonorrheal origin. The occurrence of fever and pelvic pain within a few hours after delivery also suggests gonorrhea.

CLINICAL COURSE AND SYMPTOMATOLOGY

The development of puerperal sepsis, no matter what proportion of the reproductive tract is first attacked, is always heralded by systemic symptoms. From one to six days after delivery, depending upon the location and bacteriologic nature of the infection, the patient experiences a sense of chilliness, or a distinct rigor, followed by a rise of temperature. This is true of all cases except very mild infections where the febrile reaction may be slight, and after a few days the temperature returns to normal. Occasionally an initial rise of temperature of but a degree or so may persist, gradually showing daily increments until a typical septic fever curve develops. The initial chill and sharp fever, however, is characteristic of the disease and anemia becoming progressively worse is a usual accompaniment.

Four out of five patients suffering from puerperal sepsis are completely symptom-free except for the fever and rapid pulse, and at this time one cannot predict what form the sepsis may finally assume. The specific clinical characteristics of these phases are as follows: it being remembered that there are all possible gradations of the disease, that one form may be overlaid by another at any time and that the picture changes markedly from day to day.

In putrefactive or saprophytic endometritis (sapremia) there is a sharp chill accompanied by a rise of temperature to 101° to 103° F. usually on the third day after delivery. The uterus is subinvoluted and tender, the lochia very fetid, and may be scant or quite profuse, with shreds of necrotic decidua and organized clots. There is a moderate leukocytosis and the fever is subject to daily remissions.

Putrefactive endometritis is generally a mild form of puerperal sepsis and if the protective zone be not disturbed, usually runs its course within a few days, the temperature falling by lysis and the lochia becoming normal. There is an old axiom among obstetricians, that the more pain and the more fetid the discharge, the lower the virulence of puerperal sepsis.

The *temperature* depends upon the maintenance of drainage, and the securing of continued uterine contraction.

The former is attained by very gently introducing the finger through the occluded cervical canal, dislodging a possible blood clot, or straightening a flexion. *No attempt should be made to remove the necrotic material either by finger or instrument,* since it has been shown abundantly that any sort of trauma to the delicate zone of granulation tissue, opens passageways for extension and that parametritis or even blood stream infection is a constant sequel to digital or instrumental interference. I subscribe freely to the terse statement of DeLee that "it is about as reasonable to curette the nose and throat in diphtheria as to curette the uterus for sepsis." Intrauterine douches and in fact all forms of local intervention are strongly condemned.

Contraction of the uterus is an essential factor and is best maintained by the administration of fluid extract of ergot, either by mouth, in doses of 1 drachm three times daily, or hypodermically in the form of one of the preparations of the drug made for the purpose.

In septic endometritis the only symptoms usually found are systemic, there being no local tenderness or pain or change in the lochia although the discharge may be pale and scant.

On the second or third day after delivery, the patient suffers a severe chill, with a sharp elevation of temperature which may rise to 105° or 106° F. There is usually a sense of well being except during the chill and these patients are apt to emphasize the fact that they feel perfectly well and wonder at their daily or diurnal rigors. Pelvic examination discloses nothing but a moderate degree of subinvolution. The pulse rate is rapid, the leukocytosis high, and the Schilling index may deviate sharply to the left.

The chills are usually repeated once or twice daily and succeeding the cold spell, the temperature rises to a very high level, dropping to subnormal within a few hours, until the chart presents the typical septic temperature curve.

In from five to seven days there develops evidence of one or more of the sequelae of septic endometritis.

Parametritis, Pelvic Cellulitis.—Five or six days after the initial chill, the temperature curve assumes a quotidian form, the afternoon temperature rising to 103° to 104° F. and falling to normal in the morning, the pulse rate bearing a correct ratio to the temperature. There is a sharp leukocytosis of 18,000 to 25,000 and profuse sweating occurs. Severe pain begins in the pelvis, the abdomen is tender and rigid, especially below the umbilicus and movement, defecation and coughing or sneezing are painful. Nausea and restlessness are disturbing accompaniments. On vaginal examination a dense mass is felt in one or both vaginal fornices. The masses are irregular, the uterus is fixed and vaginal palpation excites severe pain, and usually is followed by an exacerbation of the fever, as bacteria are forced into surrounding tissues by the examining finger.

These symptoms persist for from two weeks to two months and the condition terminates in one of these ways:

(a) The exudate slowly undergoes resorption, the pain and tenderness decreasing, the fever gradually falling by lysis, appetite and strength returning until recovery is complete.

This form of parametritis is managed by absolute rest, heat to the pelvis and, after absorption has begun, local heat to the parametrium, by the Elliott machine, or by mild diathermy. The constitutional treatment is that of puerperal sepsis in general.

(b) The parametritis leads to suppuration (pelvic abscess), the pus usually accumulating in the cul-de-sac of Douglas, where it presents as a bulging, fluctuant tender mass. The pus may spread laterally, may dissect upward anterior to the bladder and may completely fill the pelvis.

Spontaneous rupture into the rectum is not uncommon, into the bladder less frequent and into the general peritoneum quite rare.

Pelvic abscess may be suspected when the patient complains of throbbing pain, almost intolerable upon defecation and the temperature curve shows a marked fluctuation. The doughy mass in the cul-de-sac found on vaginal examination, will confirm the diagnosis.

The treatment is vaginal evacuation of the pus by posterior colpotomy, the vaginal incision always being made in the midline, and drainage being secured by means of a large rubber tube inserted into the colpotomy wound.

After a week or two, the drainage ceases, the temperature reaches normal and the case is terminated.

(c) The symptoms continue day after day, unabated, the temperature continues elevated with septic remission, severe anemia develops, the Schilling index shifts to the left, and death from septic absorption closes the scene.

Thrombophlebitis of the Pelvic Veins.—The usual precursor of thrombophlebitis is an endometritis. Within a few days after the initial rise of temperature, the patient complains of severe pain in the pelvis, the temperature continues high, is of the remittent form, the pulse rate is rapid, leukocytosis rises and pelvic examination discloses tense and very tender masses running from the uterus to the pelvic wall, without the massive generalized exudate which characterizes parametritis. The course is extremely slow, complete resorption requiring weeks or months and at any time, small emboli may separate and give rise to a generalized septicemia.

The treatment is that of sepsis in general, heat to the pelvis being the only local measure available.

General Peritonitis.—The peritoneum may become infected either via the blood or lymphatic transmission from a uterine focus and when this occurs the usual evidence of peritonitis becomes evident. A septic temperature, a rapid pulse soon becoming thready, high leukocytosis and an anxious, restless facies, soon becoming "Hippocratic," form the picture. Tympanites, intestinal paresis and vomiting soon becoming almost continuous with sordes on the lips from the irritating vomitus are additional symptoms, and these unfortunate women usually succumb in four or five days from the overwhelming toxemia.

Treatment—Peritonitis may be treated by laparotomy and attempts at drainage or by expectancy, the patient's resistance being built up by general measures. The latter plan is favored in my clinic, though the prognosis is most grave in any case, the mortality being over 80 per cent.

Bacteremia; Septicemia or Pyemia.—The presence of bacteria in the blood stream may be demonstrated by blood culture, but I am convinced that this condition exists in many cases where the blood cultures remain persistently negative. The Streptococcus pyogenes is a common causal agent, but Staphylococcus aureus and albus, Bacillus pyocyaneus, the gonococcus and the Bacillus aerogenes capsulatus may be found.

The blood stream may become infected by lymphatic transmission but usually the origin lies in thrombophlebitis of the placental site or pelvic veins.

The pathology is that of a generalized septic invasion. There may be septic endometritis, parametritis, peritonitis, etc. Pericarditis and pleuritis, localized cerebral abscesses, meningitis, acute bacterial endocarditis, cloudy swelling of liver, spleen and kidney are all characteristic.

Rapid hemolysis takes place, with profound anemia and a mottling of the skin about the superficial veins.

The disease is marked by a rapid and severe onset; the temperature reaching 104° to 106° F. and the chill being long and violent. The pulse is very rapid and soon becomes thready. Because of the hemolysis, respiration becomes rapid and shallow, a high leukocytosis is noted and as stated before, the offending organism may be shown in blood culture.

Scattered abscesses may develop—superficial, cerebral, pulmonary or hepatic—and a scarlatiniform eruption may appear on the skin, followed by a general pustular dermatitis.

In other cases the symptoms are less severe, consisting only of the intensely septic temperature, rapid pulse, hemolysis and rapid failure of the patient's resistance. It is my conviction that bacteremia plays a greater rôle in puerperal sepsis than is generally recognized, and that many patients without localized evidence of septic foci, but with the general reactions of severe infection suffer from it.

Gonococcal Puerperal Sepsis.—Infection by the gonococcus must be discussed apart from puerperal sepsis in general, because this organism acts differently from its fellow pyogenic bacteria. Gonorrheal infections travel by continuity, along mucous pathways, the foci rarely are metastatic and generalized involvement is uncommon.

The gonococcus moves from its cervical or endometrial point of origin, and attacks the entire endometrium, then the mucosa of the tubes, where suppuration ensues, pus dripping from the fimbriated ends, affecting the surrounding peritoneum and giving rise to a local pelvic peritonitis.

It follows that gonococcal infections are rarely as dangerous or severe as those arising from the streptococcus or staphylococcus. The symptoms are a moderate rise of temperature, a short chill, possibly a fairly sharp leukocytosis, followed in a few days by pelvic pain and shortly thereafter by the development of painful masses in the adnexa; gonorrheal salpingitis.

Localized peritonitis may reveal itself by pain, rigidity of the lower abdomen and possibly vomiting and tympanites.

Under rest and general treatment the symptoms subside in one or two weeks, although a residual salpingitis may remain.

THE PROGNOSIS OF PUERPERAL SEPSIS

In localized infection of the vulva and vagina, the prognosis is good, a moderate morbidity being the only result.

In putrefactive endometritis, recovery within a few days is the rule, but one of the sequelae above described may occur at any time.

Parametritis involves a long illness with possible colpotomy and prolonged drainage, but fatalities are few.

Thrombophlebitis, peritonitis and bacteremia are extremely serious conditions and the mortality is very high. In the two latter, about 75 per cent of patients perish, the outlook being somewhat better in thrombophlebitis.

The diagnosis of puerperal sepsis rarely offers difficulties, the rise of temperature and the chill telling the story. There may be a totally extraneous infection in which these symptoms occur, as a tonsillitis, acute bronchitis, etc., but these may be easily excluded.

A skin rash may suggest scarlatina which may be coincident, but generally such rashes are of streptococcal origin and only serve to confirm the diagnosis of sepsis. Later, typhoid fever may confuse the issue; but its presence is more apt to be based upon the hope of the accoucheur than upon actuality. The Widal reaction and the course of the disease will make the differentiation.

For scientific purposes a knowledge of what bacteria have invaded the uterus is of value, and many devices have been utilized to obtain the uterine contents.

One of the simplest is Little's modification of Döderlein's tube (Fig. 389), a simple bent glass tube being threaded with silk to the

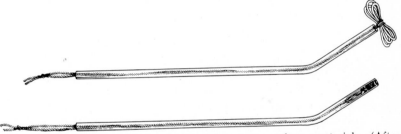

Fig. 389.—Little's apparatus for taking intra-uterine culture material. (After Williams.)

end of which a folded rubber band is tied, to act as a plunger. The folded band is pulled into one end of the tube, which, being sterilized, is introduced into the uterine cavity, the cervix having been exposed with a speculum and its intravaginal portion cleansed. When the tube end is in the uterine cavity, the thread is pulled and the rubber band acts as a piston to draw some of the lochia into the tube, which is then carefully withdrawn and its contents cultured. This plan is valuable for the first four days after delivery, but subsequent to this time it is useless, because bacteria generally are found in the lochia after a few days, and because the original cause of the infection will be obscured by the number of varieties of organisms found.

Defense Mechanisms to Puerperal Infection.—It is rather a source of wonder, not that so many women suffer from puerperal sepsis, but that more do not acquire the disease.

There are certain mechanisms which serve to prevent the invasion of bacteria into the uterus and to inhibit those growths when they do gain entrance.

The gush of amniotic fluid serves to wash away infected blood clots and bacteria when the membranes rupture.

Blood itself is mildly bactericidal and serves to destroy some of the organisms. Hofbauer has shown that toward the end of pregnancy there is an increase in the number of leukocytes and clasmatocytes in the parametrium adjacent to the uterus, which act as phagocytes.

It is believed that a previous attack of scarlet fever acts in some measure as an immunizing factor against streptococcal infection.

CHAPTER XXXVIII

THE TREATMENT OF PUERPERAL SEPSIS

PUERPERAL sepsis develops as a result of the introduction of pyogenic bacteria into the birth canal, before, during, or after labor. The tendency toward infection is enhanced by exhaustion, long labors, traumatism, and blood loss.

When infection has occurred, the cause of the disease is more or less severe as the patient does or does not possess the vital forces of resistance required to combat its ravages. In women of good resistance, who have undergone well-conducted labors, without the introduction of infective material, the danger of sepsis is slight.

The most important aspect of treatment, therefore, is prevention.

PROPHYLAXIS AGAINST PUERPERAL SEPSIS

During pregnancy the health of the patient should be closely guarded, respiratory infection treated, foci of infection or diseased teeth removed, anemia sought for and appropriately managed, the emunctories kept active; in short, the woman should approach her confinement in as good health as medical science can afford her.

During late pregnancy the entrance of organisms into the vagina should be minimized as much as possible. Sexual intercourse is prohibited during the last two months, and especially great stress laid upon its avoidance in the last month.

Vaginal douches are contraindicated during pregnancy, especially from the seventh month on.

Shower baths are substituted for tub bathing during the last two months if this is practicable, but if not, the patient should be warned of the possible danger (which in my opinion is quite remote if the membranes are intact).

Vaginal examinations from the seventh month are to be conducted with strict asepsis.

A knowledge of the capacity of the pelvis, the position and presentation of the child and the probable course of labor, is essential in order that pathologic delivery may be anticipated.

During Labor.—This is the critical time for the development of sepsis and here the responsibility for the introduction of infective material rests squarely upon the shoulders of the obstetrician.

Premature rupture of the membranes always carries with it increased danger of infection and patients should be instructed to report such event at once, in order that appropriate advice may be given. If the woman is to be delivered in a hospital she should be admitted without delay, there to await the onset of labor. If at home, she must be strongly cautioned as to the great danger of coitus, douches, baths or self-examination of any kind.

The Vaginal Examination.—It is probable that most cases of sepsis originate in unsterile manipulation during labor, and too great emphasis cannot be laid upon care at this time. In many clinics rectal examination has entirely supplanted vaginal touch, with a view to lessening the possibility.

I cannot agree with this, because it is so often necessary to execute some vaginal manipulation during the course of delivery and it would seem wise that the obstetrician so train himself that he is safe to perform such manipulations. The technic of vaginal examination has been given in Chapter XIV, but for purposes of emphasis it is repeated here.

Technic of the Vaginal Examination.—The patient is draped with the knees flexed, and if very corpulent, is drawn across the bed, the buttocks at its edge, and the legs held by attendants who sit on either side of the woman.

The physician then rolls up his cuffs and scrubs with brush, soap and running water as for an operation. The hands are dried on a sterile towel, a sterile gown is donned and sterile gloves drawn on. The entire perineal area is then carefully scrubbed with soap and water and sterile cotton sponges, care being taken not to enter the vulvar orifice. The labia and the pudenda are then painted with an antiseptic—diluted tincture iodine, 4 per cent mercurochrome, metaphen or whatever solution best suits the individual practitioner. The gloves are now changed and with the finger of one hand separating the labia, the first and second fingers of the examining hand are introduced into the vagina, under the eye, and if possible not touching the external surfaces. By sweeping the finger about the pelvic cavity, its capacity may be ascertained, the resistance of the pelvic floor estimated, the amount of cervical effacement and dilatation discovered; whether or not the membranes have ruptured, the status of the head, the position of the fontanels and of the sagittal and other sutures. Should a labor pain come on while the fingers are in the vagina, the movement of the head may be learned as well as the progress of molding.

It is emphasized that one careful vaginal examination is sufficient in all cases, except when the development of dystocia renders further investigation imperative.

Technic of the Rectal Examination.—The patient being draped as above and, the physician having scrubbed, a glove preferably but not necessarily sterile is drawn on, anointed with petroleum or other lubricating jelly and one finger gently introduced into the rectum. With practice one can determine the effacement and dilation of the cervix, the position of the head, with its sutures and the station of the presenting part. The presence or absence of intact membranes is difficult to determine by this method, and the capacity of the pelvic cavity cannot be estimated.

Should labor be unexpectedly prolonged rectal examination may be repeated to ascertain the cause of the dystocia.

During long labors the tendency to frequently repeat the examination should be curbed, a very occasional and gentle rectal examination sufficing.

The question of introducing antiseptics into the vagina during labor has given rise to considerable discussion, and has many adherents. It is not practiced in my services, except when the patient is known to suffer from active gonorrhea when a silver solution is used.

During labor nothing is permitted to touch the genital tract of the patient, unless it is absolutely sterile, and this rule admits of no exceptions.

Rough and traumatic deliveries are avoided as much as possible, and all wounds of the birth canal must be repaired immediately after labor, in an aseptic manner.

Excessive hemorrhage is met by blood transfusion or the administration of 10 per cent glucose solution by vein.

Since it has been shown that puerperal infection may be carried from the respiratory tract of attendants upon delivery, it is essential that all occupants of the delivery room should be masked at all times, the nose as well as the mouth being covered.

During the Puerperium.—Too much attention to the genital tract during the puerperium may have an opposite effect to that intended, and may indeed favor septic invasion. The ubiquitous vulvar pad probably tends to retain material which would otherwise drain away and is better left off. However, this results in much soiling of the bed and patients grow rebellious at the discomfort of lying in vaginal secretion. The pad may therefore be retained, for forty-eight hours at least, when it may be dispensed with.

Cleansing the perineum by the nurse is often overdone. Simple irrigation, by pouring a mild antiseptic such as lysol solution over the tissues after urination and defecation is all that is required, no sponging or other manipulation being countenanced.

The uterus is to be kept well contracted by small doses of ergot (20 minims three times a day) for the first six days after labor.

CURATIVE TREATMENT

Local treatment has but little place in the management of puerperal sepsis. If the lochia becomes scant, with elevation of temperature, the finger may very gently be introduced through the cervix to dislodge a clot, or correct a temporary angulation of the canal.

Whenever and wherever a localized collection of pus makes its appearance, it should be evacuated and drainage instituted, whether it be in the pelvic floor, the parametrium or the uterine cornua.

Otherwise local interference is ill advised.

The practice of ligation and exercise of the pelvic veins for thrombophlebitis had quite a vogue for a time, but its usefulness has not been demonstrated and it has been generally abandoned.

General Treatment.—This may be considered under two heads. Maintenance and improvement of the vital forces of the patient. Measures to combat the septic process.

Under the first grouping comes general hygienic care.

Abundance of fresh air and sunshine are extremely valuable. If in a home, the bed should be moved so that the woman lies in the sun, and she being well covered, the windows should be kept open.

In hospitals, sun rooms are often available for this purpose and should be freely used.

Food, light and easily digestible food with abundant fluids are essential. When there is no peritoneal involvement, the diet should be generous, including the free use of fruit juices.

If peritonitis develops, food by mouth should be withheld, and the administration of glucose by vein substituted for a few days. The bowels are kept active by enemata and possibly the use of mineral oil by mouth. Cathartics are contraindicated. An ice-bag over the uterus favors involution, though if there be much pain, heat locally is often better borne.

Pain should be combated by the free use of morphine, and hypnotics as barbiturates may allay restlessness and insomnia.

The child should be removed from the breast at once, and the latter emptied as occasion arises by the use of a breast pump. The Fowler position favors drainage and may be used, provided the patient is comfortable in this posture.

Blood Tranfusion.—The great ally of the physician in treating puerperal sepsis is the frequent use of blood transfusion, from 250 to 300 cc. being given every fourth or fifth day.

The use of properly typed and matched blood is the best single method of treatment available. Not only does it maintain the oxygen-carrying properties of the patient's blood at a high level but it introduces an ever-renewed supply of phagocytes and antibodies.

If peritonitis has developed, the accompanying dehydration may be combated by the intravenous use of glucose in doses of 500 cc. of 10 per cent solution daily. In cases of long duration the heart may require stimulation by digitalis carefully administered, preferable by the hypodermic route.

Whisky in milk acts as a food and also as a stimulant.

Specific Treatment.—It has been stated before that in my opinion bacteremia, even though not demonstrable, is common in puerperal sepsis, and therefore any means of destroying the organism in the blood stream is of the greatest value.

Many agents have been employed for this purpose, none of them completely satisfactory.

Chemical sterilization of the blood stream has a long history. Mercurials have been used to considerable extent, the work of the late Dr. Piper with mercurochrome being noteworthy. Recently another mercury-bearing drug, metaphen, has been employed with considerable success.

Metaphen is an organic mercury compound which possesses a low affinity for the blood proteins and does not easily form a precipitate.

It has a very high bacterial coefficient, inhibiting the growth of staphylococci in a dilution as high as 1:2,000,000. This drug exerts very little untoward effect upon the kidney, the usual drawback to the intravenous use of mercury compounds, and is relatively of low toxicity.

It is used intravenously in doses of 10 cc. of a 1:1000 solution, and may be given at two-day intervals for five or six doses.

If the drug has a beneficial effect, the temperature drops promptly and may remain normal or thereabout or may rise again in one or two days, when injection is repeated.

Reactions are uncommon, and in several instances I have been impressed by the usefulness of the drug. It has been utilized extensively by Bernstein, who reports an impressive group of cases.

Immunotransfusion.—The use of nonspecific immunotransfusion was first suggested by the work of Wright and others, and has since been developed by Crocker and his associates at the Philadelphia General Hospital.

It consists in the injection of blood from a donor who is suffering a profound reaction from the administration of killed typhoid bacilli.

The donor having been typed and matched is given intravenously 50,000,000 killed typhoid bacilli in the form of the ordinary commercial antigen either typhoid or typhoid and paratyphoid A and B.

Within an hour there is a severe reaction with headache, chills and fever, the temperature often reaching 104°. At the height of this reaction the required amount of blood, usually 200 to 300 cc., is withdrawn and immediately transfused into the patient, who experiences little or no reaction herself. Immunotransfusion may be repeated daily if required.

The donor's symptoms rapidly subside and his condition returns to normal within twenty-four hours.

The transfusions are controlled by hemography which implies the study of the Schilling index and its shift to left or right.

Nonspecific immunotransfusion therapy is based upon the principle of increasing the formation of nonspecific antibodies or opsonins in the blood of the donor and their immediate transference to the blood stream of the patient. This treatment is still sub judice, but it has been used with considerable success at the Philadelphia General Hospital. Antistreptococcic serum is of doubtful value, although some observers report success, in known streptococcic blood infection, by the use of massive doses, 50 to 100 cc. daily.

Surgical treatment, hysterectomy, etc., has not proved of great value.

The whole treatment of puerperal sepsis may be summed up by preventing its development and if it should occur in spite of all possible prophylaxis, local manipulation should be avoided and only general supportive measures utilized.

PHLEGMASIA ALBA DOLENS (MILK LEG)

Thrombophlebitis of the femoral and long saphenous veins may be an extension of a similar process in the pelvic veins and may then form part of a serious puerperal sepsis.

More often, however, there is little or no indication of pelvic-vein involvement and the evidences of inflammation in the veins of the leg do not appear until late in the puerperium, often between the eighth and the fifteenth days.

The patient complains of pain in the groin and in the calf of the leg, and on examination the limb is found swollen, with a dense ligneous quality to palpation. The skin is pale and opalescent and the swelling may be intense. Sometimes the hard and thrombosed veins may be felt in the groin and in the popliteal space. There is irregular fever, some increase in the pulse rate and the patient may be quite ill, the legs sometimes being extremely painful.

Owing to pressure upon the lymphatics there may be great lymph-edema, especially noteworthy in the upper leg.

Phlegmasia is a disease of long duration, requiring weeks of bed rest usually, and the affected leg rarely ever regains its normal contour and is apt to swell on exertion for years after the acute onset. The pathology is a thrombophlebitis, with periphlebitis, which may extend upward to the pelvic veins.

Cases are recorded where the thrombosis was complete and the arteries were also involved, resulting in gangrene and death.

Treatment.—Thrombophlebitis is practically always an expression of infection, so that the general measures designed to prevent puerperal infection apply with equal force to this condition.

When present, the treatment consists of rest in bed, elevating the affected leg upon pillows, preventing sore heel by a pad under the tendo achillis, and elevating the bed clothes with a cradle, to prevent irritating pressure. The leg should be wrapped in cotton wool, saturated with lead water and laudanum (liquor opii et plumbi acetatis). Heat in the form of an electrically lighted cradle is very beneficial.

When the swelling has subsided, the leg may be lowered and the patient permitted to sit up with immediate return to bed upon the recurrence of pain and marked swelling. A rubber stocking or elastic bandage may be required for months afterward.

Varicose ulcers are an annoying sequel. During the acute stage, the treatment applicable to puerperal sepsis in general is practiced.

CHAPTER XXXIX

PUERPERAL DISEASES AND ANOMALIES OF THE BREASTS

THE BREASTS

Engorgement of the Breasts.—Very often the first three days after delivery are accompanied by marked swelling, heat, and pain in the breasts. This is due to the pressure of excessive lymph stasis and not to too much milk. Indeed it often occurs before lactation has been established. The breasts may be edematous and are quite tender.

Management.—The treatment consists in supporting the breasts by a firm binder, the application of heat in the form of hot-water bags or better the electric heating pad and by avoiding massage and other manipulation. If the pain is excessive a small dose of morphine with phenacetin (5 grains) may be required. Saline laxatives and restriction of fluid intake aid in giving relief. The engorgement almost invariably disappears after one or two days, when "the milk comes in."

Polygalactia is an abnormally great secretion of milk. It has no obstetric significance but in maternity hospitals the excess supply may be collected by the breast pump and utilized for feeding premature infants, etc. The mother should be known to be Wassermann negative before such use is made of her milk.

Galactorrhea.—This term is used to define the continuous flow of milk, after nursing has ceased, and it may persist for months. The cause is unknown, and the treatment is unsatisfactory.

Camphor, 3 grains in oil, injected hypodermically twice daily for several days may give relief. Atropine, theelin and a tight binder are sometimes successful. The excess flow usually ceases upon the return of menstruation.

Agalactia.—Absence or scarcity of milk is a very common complaint. It occurs in the highly sensitive society girl, and in the stolid ward type patient with almost equal frequency, and if one eliminates profound systemic disorders, or diseases of the nipples, the cause seems to lie in a congenital deficiency of gland tissue. This is especially noticeable in those large, heavy breasts which contain an excess of fat.

Emotional disturbances play a part and ofttimes a woman, who is worried about domestic conditions or finances while in hospital, experiences a marked increase in secretion upon her return to her home.

Treatment.—Except for general good hygienic care, abundant food and fluids, rich in vitamin A and B, I know of no treatment which offers any success and it is a common experience that women who are unable to nurse one child never succeed in subsequent pregnancies.

Drying up the Breasts.—If the child is dead, or the milk unsuited to it, or for some other reason it may become necessary to stop the secretion of milk. This is best done by leaving the breasts absolutely alone, supporting them with a firm binder and using no pumping or massage.

If pain becomes severe, opium may be necessary to relieve it.

Restriction of fluids, a light diet and frequent saline laxatives serve to dehydrate the patient and her breasts.

The only drug of value is camphor in oil 3 grains hypodermically twice daily for seven days.

The usual application of ointments to the breast is a useless procedure.

DISEASES AND ANOMALIES OF THE NIPPLES

The nipples vary greatly in size and form in different women. The only important deviations from the normal from a clinical standpoint are infantile and inverted nipples.

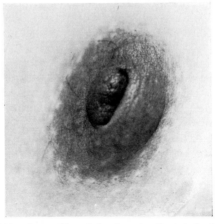

Fig. 390.—Anomalies of the breast. Inverted nipple.

The former present flattened, conical structures which scarcely rise above the surrounding areolar tissue and offer no hold for the infant to suckle. When such nipples are discovered during pregnancy, daily traction upon them may stimulate growth but even this is not commonly successful.

A nipple shield may be tried but if this fails, it is best to dry up the breasts as nursing will never prove satisfactory as such nipples are usually associated with a deficient milk secretion.

Inverted nipples are those in which the surface of the nipple lies below the surface of the breast, being inverted into a little crater in the areolar tissue. The treatment is that described for the infantile variety (Fig. 390).

Fissures and Cracks of the Nipples.—Painful nipples constitute a very common and an extremely painful complication of the puerperium.

About one fourth of all lactating women suffer from this cause, and in many instances the pain on nursing is so intense that the mothers anticipate with the greatest dread the approach of their infant to the breast. Many women have told me that sore nipples caused them more distress than all the pain of labor plus the discomfort of pregnancy. Often the pain is so severe that lactation cannot be continued and the cracks and fissures not infrequently lead to infection and the formation of mammary abscess.

Infantile or inverted nipples are prone to develop fissures and exfoliation of the epithelium and are especially susceptible to deeper infection.

Painful nipples may be due to fissures, erosions or small blisters, sometimes developing into ulcers.

These lesions are the result of the traumatism and maceration of the skin caused by the child's efforts at suckling, and readily become infected.

Sometimes superficial vessels are involved when bleeding may be quite free.

Treatment.—*Prophylaxis.*—During pregnancy the nipples should be anointed with cocoa butter or lanolin and light traction made upon them for a few minutes daily to stimulate the erectile fibers and to accustom the skin to handling.

After Delivery.—There being no milk present for the first two or three days, the nipples should not be subjected to the violent suckling efforts of the infant, who should be placed to the breast at eight-hour intervals for five minutes only, until the flow of milk is established.

During nursing the mother should lie on her side, with the baby's head so held by pillows that it may nurse comfortably and the nipples be maintained in a straight line, so that the ducts are not shut off by angulation.

Immediately before and immediately after each nursing the nipples should be lightly washed with cotton (not gauze), saturated with boric acid solution or a mild astringent as sodium perborate solution. After nursing the area should be gently dried and preferably left exposed to the air until completely dry, when they may be covered by a sterile pad, or the lead nipple shields known as Wansbrough's nipple shields.

The drier the nipples between nursings, the less likely is maceration of the epithelium and exposure of the sensitive subepithelial tissues to occur.

When nursing becomes painful, close inspection of the nipples should be made to disclose incipient cracks or erosions.

All such abrasions should be touched with a solution of silver nitrate 5 per cent, by means of a tiny cotton applicator, made by winding a few wisps of cotton on a tooth pick and sterilized.

The silver is not permitted to cover the nipple but should be applied only to the eroded area.

The entire nipple may then be painted with tincture of benzoin compound and covered with a sterile pad.

If a scab forms it may be softened with warm sterile water, and the underlying raw surface again touched with silver nitrate.

It is well to omit a nursing if the lesion be excessively painful, emptying the breast either with a hand pump or better, the electrically driven pump. At the next nursing a nipple shield is used to prevent contact of the lips of the infant with the abraded area. In

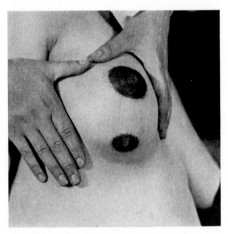

Fig. 391.—Supernumerary nipple.

resistant cases, nursing should be stopped until healing is complete or if the patient is a sensitive woman, the child may be weaned.

Greasy and oily unguents are worthless and only predispose to infection. It is to be remembered that mastitis generally develops via an eroded or fissured nipple, hence the most painstaking asepsis is a sine qua non.

MAMMARY ABSCESS

Mastitis.—Puerperal mastitis is an important complication of the puerperium. Productive of great pain and disability, it interferes with nursing and renders the puerperal woman a complete invalid, sometimes for weeks, as well as usually requiring surgical interference of some type.

Mastitis may be of two general varieties.

Parenchymatous inflammation, in which the infective bacteria pass from a nipple abrasion along the lacteal tubes and so gain access to the parenchyma of the gland. In this form, the Staphylo-coccus albus or aureus is commonly found.

Interstitial or phlegmonous mastitis in which the bacteria are lymph-borne and find their way along the connective tissue trabeculae and around and between the lobes in the mammary fat, producing a widespread cellulitis.

In addition there are found small superficial abscesses involving the tubercles of Montgomery which are not of especial significance, and occasionally the pus dissects its way under the breast, even penetrating the fascia of the pectoralis muscle—submammary abscess.

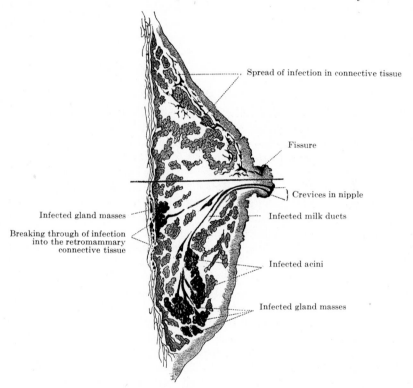

Fig. 392.—The spread of infection of the breast. (Bumm.)

Etiology.—Mastitis almost always originates in an erosion or fis-sure of the nipple and even in cases where such lesions are not ap-parent close examination with a hand lens will disclose perhaps a minute area of exposed subepithelial tissue (Fig. 392).

Very rarely the pyogenic organisms may be transmitted from a distant focus by the blood stream.

Symptoms and Diagnosis.—In parenchymatous mastitis the symp-toms usually develop after the sixth day and from then on to any time during the continuance of lactation. The condition is usually unilateral, though it may involve both breasts, but very seldom simultaneously.

The patient complains of localized pain usually in the lower or upper outer quadrant, although any part of the breast may be affected.

The temperature rises abruptly to 103° to 104° and there may be a chill. Leukocytosis is moderately high.

On inspection the inflamed area of the breast is red, a trifle swollen and on palpation a distinct area of induration may be felt which is very tender. In some instances the extent of the inflammation is seemingly out of all proportion to the degree of constitutional reaction, this being due to the high tension of tightly confined pus. Under treatment by heat and support, the symptoms may subside rapidly, or the inflammatory reaction may go on to suppuration, in which case the fever continues, the pain becomes more marked and a dull red area, indurated, but usually with some overlying edema appearing on the breast.

The abscess may point on the skin surface, but usually unless incision and drainage is done, the pus burrows in and about the gland tissue involving one lobule after another until the entire breast is honeycombed with abscesses and their communicating sinuses.

The phlegmenous form of mastitis presents the same onset, the symptoms rapidly become more severe, the whole breast is the seat of a brawny swelling and the adjacent lymph glands are enlarged.

Treatment.—At the onset, rest and heat are the important items of treatment. The child should not be permitted to nurse from the diseased breast, which may be gently emptied by the breast pump at four-hour intervals. A firm but not tight binder elevates the organ and prevents passive congestion. Heat may be applied in a number of ways but I prefer a thick dressing of hot clay in glycerine. The cataplasma kaolini compound of the pharmacopeia, or one of the more elegant proprietary preparations may be used. The paste is heated and spread generously upon a square of lint in which a hole to admit the nipple has been cut. The dressing is applied as hot as the patient can bear it and allowed to remain for twenty-four hours, heat being maintained by hot-water bag or electric heating pad. In my experience cold has not produced satisfactory results in these cases.

The presence of suppuration is marked by redness, fluctuation, or if deep, edema of the surface skin. Once these signs appear, no further time should be lost but free drainage must be instituted. Under local or a light nitrous oxide anesthesia, a free incision is made over the point of greatest swelling or redness.

The incision is made radially to the nipple in order to avoid cutting the lactic ducts transversely.

A hemostatic forceps is introduced into the wound and withdrawn opened to separate the deeper tissues without dividing the vessels. If the abscess has burrowed, the finger may explore the cavity, opening into communicating channels, until complete drainage is assured. Several radial incisions may be necessary. Drainage tubes for the larger abscesses and folded rubber dam for the smaller, are pushed into place, and the breast covered with a wet dressing of saturated solution of magnesium sulphate which is kept hot by the use of hot-water bags and moistened from time to time by pouring more of the solution over the dressing pad.

In slow, resistant cases, the use of an autogenous vaccine and the ultraviolet lamp sometimes hastens resolution.

ANOMALIES IN THE INVOLUTION OF THE UTERUS

Subinvolution of the uterus implies a retardation of the autolytic processes by which the uterus normally retrogresses to its nonpregnant size within six to eight weeks after delivery. Subinvolution is due to deficiency in the contractile power of the uterine muscle and follows inertia uteri quite frequently.

It is also caused by the retention of fragments of placenta and shreds of decidua, and the subsequent detachment of these masses may give rise to delayed puerperal hemorrhage, sometimes a sharp bleeding occurring several weeks postpartum. Endometritis also is a productive factor as are fibroid nodules in the uterine wall.

Symptoms.—In subinvolution, the lochial discharge may persist for several weeks and then be replaced by a profuse and continuous leukorrhea. There may be hemorrhage as above. The patient complains of lassitude, a dull heavy feeling in the pelvis, backache and constipation. On examination, the uterus is found soft and boggy, considerably enlarged and usually retroverted. The cervix is soft and is covered with mucous leukorrhea.

Treatment.—Tonics as iron, quinine and strychnine, regulation of bowel function, very hot vaginal douches of sterile water at 110°, and reposition of the retroverted uterus with an appropriate pessary (the Smith-Hodge is best), together with small doses of ergot (½ drachm fluidextract) daily for a week, usually suffice to restore tone to the uterus and to stimulate complete involution. These measures failing, curettement should be done to remove any remaining decidual fragments.

Hyperinvolution of the Uterus (Lactation Atrophy).—Sometimes after prolonged nursing, the involution of the uterus proceeds to an abnormal degree, until the organ may be reduced to a tiny infantile nodule and permanent amenorrhea with sterility results.

The condition is attributed to reflex irritation from the breasts in long-continued lactation, and after weaning the child, the uterus generally returns to normal. I am disposed to regard hyperinvolution as an endocrine phenomenon, the details of whose mechanism are not yet clear. In one of my patients who nursed her child only ten months, the uterus continued to involute until after a year it could scarcely be palpated by vaginal touch. She suffered from total amenorrhea and sterility for six years, after which she again became pregnant, and had her baby with no return of the trouble.

Treatment.—Lactation atrophy is treated by weaning the child at once, and later attempting stimulation of the uterus by the administration of folliculin and by the bipolar intra-uterine galvanic current.

CHAPTER XL

INJURIES AND ACCIDENTS OF THE INFANT

BALLANTYNE once sagely defined delivery as the traumatic transition from an intra-uterine to an extra-uterine existence.

The traumatism consists first in the effects produced by pressure upon the fetus, especially upon the head, and second upon the disturbance of its oxygen supply with resulting asphyxia.

Viable infants perish during labor or shortly thereafter from many causes but those most commonly observed are, in the order of their frequency:

Birth traumatisms.

Asphyxia.

Toxemia.

Prematurity.

Congenital deformities of a degree incompatible with extra-uterine existence.

The premature infant has less chance of life than its mature fellow, because of imperfections of digestive function, immaturity of the heat-regulating mechanism, atelectasis, and failure of the circulatory system to function in an extra-uterine environment. It is also much more susceptible to birth trauma.

Infants born of toxemic mothers suffer from a transmitted toxemia as well as being underdeveloped and -nourished as a result of abnormalities of the uteroplacental circulation induced by the toxemic state.

Neither of these conditions is directly ascribable to the exigencies of delivery, nor are deformed infants to be grouped in this category.

Birth traumatism accounts for nearly 40 per cent of immediate infant deaths.

INTRACRANIAL INJURY

Intracranial injury, which practically implies intracranial hemorrhage, is a direct result of excessive pressure, from the maternal birth canal.

Such injuries are more often seen after prolonged and difficult labor, forceps delivery, version and breech extraction, precipitate labor and the like, but they may also occur after easy, spontaneous deliveries and have been reported in infants delivered by elective cesarean section. They may result from the pressure of the contracting uterus but more commonly are due to a difficult passage through a resistant pelvic girdle.

The lesions to which the cranial contents are subjected are caused by the abnormal cranial stress brought about by molding of the head. The changes in shape and the irregular compression to which the head is subjected cause variable tensions upon the dural membranes and their lacerations with injury to the neighboring vessels. The common sites of injury are the falx, and its junction with the tentorium, and when these structures are torn, the adjacent vein of Galen and its tributaries are easily lacerated (Fig. 393).

Depressed fractures of the skull and forceps compression also lead to brain injury with or without hemorrhage.

It has been shown that nearly 10 per cent of all infants disclose blood in the spinal fluid as evidenced by lumbar puncture shortly after birth, no matter whether the labor was easy or difficult.

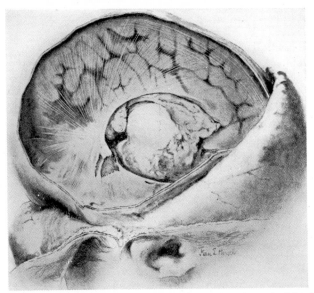

Fig. 393.—Birth trauma. Intracranial damage. Laceration of right tentorium resulting from version and extraction. (Adair and Schumann.)

Symptoms.—Intracranial injuries vary in degree from those of sufficient gravity to cause stillbirth, to very minor lesions which may cause only localized edema.

In severe cases, especially in tentorium laceration, asphyxia is the most prominent manifestation, and often these children never breathe. If they are resuscitated, there is lack of muscle tone, the infant remaining flaccid, the cry is a continuous moan or whine, the respirations are irregular and there may be convulsive movements. Heart action is slow and may be irregular.

If the injury is less severe, there may be spasticity, and great restlessness, with muscle twitchings and convulsions.

The symptoms may be immediate, or, if hemorrhage is slow, they may not appear for a day or two.

Diagnosis.—Accurate diagnosis as to the nature and extent of intracranial injury cannot be made, but the general aspect of the infant, plus the recovery of blood by lumbar puncture (made by one skilled in the technic to obviate bleeding from the puncture) will usually suffice.

Prognosis.—The shorter the duration of symptoms, the better the hope of recovery, since death usually occurs in the first twenty-four hours after birth.

Duration of symptoms for more than a week or ten days predicates a serious lesion with grave danger of death or at best permanent cerebral damage.

Treatment.—The management of cerebral injuries and hemorrhage is largely expectant.

The infant should be handled as little as possible, placed at rest in a warm crib, and not exposed to noisy surroundings.

If there are evidences of intracranial pressure as shown by spasmodic movements and great restlessness, lumbar puncture and withdrawal of from 1 to 5 cc. of cerebrospinal fluid may be of value.

Should the infant survive, the first few hours after delivery, dehydration may be met by the intramuscular or intraperitoneal administration of normal saline, 20 to 40 cc.

If one is suspicious that bleeding is continuing, the intramuscular injection of from 10 to 20 cc. of maternal blood may cause coagulation.

Occasionally, depressed fractures of the skull occur and these may often be reduced by the simple expedient of inserting the point of a heavy straight surgical needle through the scalp into the periosteum at the center of the depression and then levering the bone back into line.

INJURIES TO THE ABDOMINAL VISCERA

The liver, spleen, kidneys and intestines may suffer from pressure during delivery, or from rough handling and squeezing in breech extraction. To avoid the latter, no pressure should be used upon the abdomen during extraction, the brim of the pelvis being grasped for this purpose. In one of the author's recent cases at Kensington Hospital, a mature, apparently healthy baby was born after a normal spontaneous labor. The infant did well for about four days, then suddenly refused food, went into shock and died. On autopsy there was found a huge subcapsular hematoma of the liver which had evidently developed during labor, and bleeding continuing had eventually ruptured into the peritoneal cavity, with massive intra-abdominal hemorrhage (Fig. 394).

41

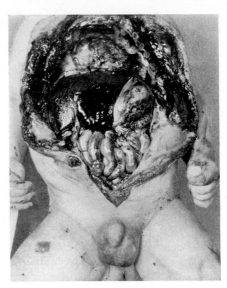

Fig. 394.—Massive subcapsular hemorrhage of the liver developing during a spontaneous delivery. (Kensington Hospital for Women.)

INJURIES TO THE PERIPHERAL NERVES

Any of the peripheral nerves may be hurt during delivery, but the ones most commonly involved are the facial nerve and the brachial plexus.

Facial paralysis or Bell's palsy results when the facial nerve has been compressed or torn, an accident which is usually noted after forceps delivery, the end of the forceps blade making pressure upon the nerve as it passes through the parotid gland. It may however follow spontaneous delivery when it is due to pressure of the bony pelvis.

Facial paralysis is apparent at once, the muscles on the affected side remaining smooth, when those of the opposite side are contracted by crying. The eye on the paralyzed side remains open, while the angle of the mouth is drawn to the nonparalyzed side.

Prognosis and Treatment.—Facial palsy is usually transitory, disappearing in from a few days to six weeks. Cases have been recorded in which the paralysis was permanent. The only treatment is the possible necessity for nursing through a Breck's feeder, if the child is unable to suck.

Injury to the Brachial Plexus (Obstetrical Palsy).—This serious injury is usually the result of ill-advised traction upon the head of the child in difficult shoulder extraction and may follow the delivery of the shoulder or of the after-coming head in version or breech extraction.

Any portion or all of the plexus may be injured, although the fifth and sixth motor nerves (Erb's paralysis) are probably the most commonly involved. It is still a moot point whether the nerves are actually torn, or whether laceration of the deep cervical fascia with injury to the perineurium causes the paralysis. Some observers believe that a subluxation of the humerus with resulting pressure palsy is responsible. The clinical picture is characteristic—the arm hangs flaccid, the hand rotated inward. Muscular atrophy is rapid and there is often a permanent disability of the affected arm.

Treatment.—Prophylaxis is the keynote. Excessive traction upon the head should not be made, especially if it lie obliquely or transverse to the axis of the birth canal. When the head lies directly anteroposterior, there is much less danger of compressing or lacerating the plexus.

It is most important not to twist the head upon the shoulders and in breech extraction strong traction upon the clavicle is dangerous, delivery being best completed by expressing the head by pressure from above (Wiegands method).

The active treatment consists in expectancy with a neuroplastic repair, if the paralysis continues.

FRACTURES OF THE LONG BONES

Difficult labors are often accompanied by fracture of the humerus or clavicle in shoulder delivery, and of the femur in version or breech extraction (Fig. 395).

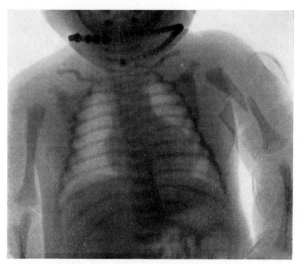

Fig. 395.—Fracture of the humerus in the newborn. (Kensington Hospital for Women.)

The fracture is usually evident at once and is managed by appropriate splinting. It is my invariable practice to subject to x-ray

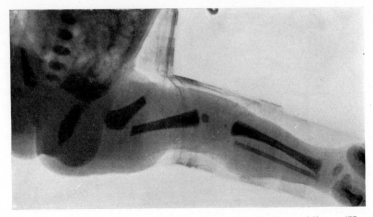

Fig. 396.—Fracture of the femur of the newborn. Marked overriding. (Kensington Hospital for Women.)

examination every baby who has undergone difficult delivery, and quite a few unsuspected fractures have turned up as a result of this rule (Fig. 396).

LESSER INJURIES OF THE HEAD AND NECK

Cephalhematoma.—There may be found subperiosteal hematoma of the cranial bones, usually the parietal, which may be unilateral or bilateral, and is confined by the attachment of the periosteum to the margin of the bone, so that a circumscribed, rounded, doughy elevation results.

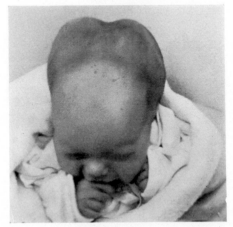

Fig. 397.—Bilateral cephalhematoma. (Chestnut Hill Hospital.)

Cephalhematoma may be due to a birth traumatism, although Ballantyne maintains that it is frequently an expression of congenital maldevelopment of the vessel walls of the cranium, which rupture under the slightest trauma, the accident occurring even before the onset of labor. The recognition of cephalhematoma offers no difficulties, and the important point in treatment is to avoid incision and drainage which so frequently leads to infection (Fig. 397).

The swellings slowly subside and have usually disappeared entirely within six to eight weeks after birth. Lesser injuries of the head, scalp wounds, laceration and contusions of the face from forceps application and lesions of the jaws after breech extraction are sometimes unavoidable, but may be minimized by a consideration of the delicacy of the infant's tissues.

The treatment is expectant, with ordinary surgical dressing if necessary.

INJURY OF THE STERNOCLEIDOMASTOID MUSCLE

This accident occurs as a result of overtwisting the neck and sometimes from direct traction. It has been ascribed to a congenital weakness and defect of the blood vessel walls, making them exceedingly susceptible to rupture (Ballantyne).

There is usually hematoma of greater or less degree with a distinct swelling, and disabilities on the part of the child to turn the head toward the affected side. Spontaneous recovery is the rule, although sometimes infection and permanent shortening of the muscle, with wryneck, results.

Treatment is based upon care in delivery and rest for the infant in whom the lesion is present with a minimum of handling.

ASPHYXIA

This, the second cause of infant death in point of numbers may occcur during pregnancy, intrapartum and postpartum.

During pregnancy asphyxia may be due to coiling of the cord about the neck and limbs of the fetus or prolapse of the cord, partial placental detachment, placenta praevia, the presenting part making pressure enough upon the placenta to derange the circulation, narcosis from drugs, etc.

During labor asphyxia is due to the same causes plus compression of the brain from pressure, with vagus paralysis, or a secondary asphyxia due to slowing of the heart, or the respiratory center may be directly compressed.

Postpartum asphyxia may be due to the above causes, plus continued atelectasis and occlusion of the respiratory passages by inspired blood, mucus, etc., or a veil of membranes covering the face (caul).

The normal baby starts to breathe under essentially the same stimulus that causes an adult to breathe again after holding his breath.

In utero, the fetal blood is so well arterialized that the rather insensitive neurorespiration of the infant is not stimulated.

Henderson believes that if intrauterine respiration does occur, the efforts of the thoracic muscles are so feeble that only a small amount of liquor amnii is inspired and this is quickly absorbed into the blood. At birth the cutaneous stimulus of the cold air causes the baby to catch its breath in a deep and prolonged respiration which serves to partially expand the lungs, and the vagi carry impulses to the respiratory centers to initiate the Hering-Breuer reflexes which control the regular alternation of inspiration and expiration.

If the respiratory center is compressed by external pressure or intracranial hemorrhage, the blood supply to the center is lessened, and if the cord be compressed the entire body becomes asphyxiated.

There is a formation of lactic acid, the pH and alkali of the blood are reduced and the carbon dioxide, which at first is increased, is later diminished.

To whatever extent the sensitivity of the respiratory center has been diminished by lack of oxygen, a stronger stimulus in the form of increased pressure of carbon dioxide is needed to excite the neuro-respiratory system to activity.

Clinically, asphyxia presents itself in one of two phases:

Asphyxia livida when the asphyxia has been brief is marked by a deep bluish or purple color of the skin, veins distended, muscle tone good, heart slow and strong.

Asphyxia pallida occurs when the lack of oxygen is more profound. The infant is flaccid and white, muscle tone is very poor, the heart beats feeble, irregular and may be either slow or rapid, usually the former.

The two conditions are simply degrees of asphyxia and the prognosis is necessarily much better in the livid type than in the advanced pallid form.

Symptoms and Diagnosis.—During pregnancy and labor the diagnosis of impending asphyxia may be made from the alteration in the heart sounds. Sudden retardation is a sign of danger, and when the normal rate of 136 to 146 is reduced to below 100 beats per minute the fetus is surely in peril. Great increase in rate is also evidence of some difficulty in oxygenation as are irregularities in rhythm, and in the intensity of the sounds.

When the membranes have ruptured, the passage of liquor amnii stained with fresh meconium gives evidence that the fetus is becoming asphyxiated.

Sometimes there are sudden violent fetal movements almost spasmodic in character. During labor, the fetus may make attempts at respiration and may even cry while still in utero (vagitus uterinus). Marked alteration of the heart rate during labor is an indication for immediate delivery if this be possible, an indication which is strengthened by the appearance of meconium in the vaginal discharge. Frequent auscultation of the heart sounds in the course of delivery and prompt action upon the information of impending asphyxia so gained will save many infants. The condition of the asphyxiated baby when born has already been described.

Resuscitation of Asphyxiated Infants.—No time should be lost in beginning efforts to encourage respiration in a child which does not breathe at birth; but the usual rough and traumatic passive movements are mentioned only to be condemned.

The first essential is to make certain that the respiratory passages are not obstructed and for this purpose the child is first held suspended by the feet while the trachea is gently stroked toward the mouth in order to milk out secretion which may be blocking it.

After a few moments of this, the pharynx and nostrils are cleared by suction with an Arnold tube (Fig. 398).

In many cases the cleansing of the airways and the irritation of the Arnold tube will provoke a respiratory reflex and breathing will begin.

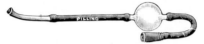

Fig. 398.—Arnold aspirator.

If not, the inhalation of a 5 to 7 per cent carbon dioxide, administered with an ordinary infant face mask, if there is any respiratory excursion or by the intratracheal catheter, at regular and rhythmic intervals by means of an appliance such as the Flagg apparatus should be begun. The tracheal catheter may also be utilized for mouth to lung insufflation, if no apparatus is at hand.

Mouth to Mouth Insufflation.—This time honored method of resuscitation has been widely condemned because it is said to rupture the alveoli by too great pressure, and because the air enters the stomach rather than the bronchi and causes dilatation of that organ, even with rupture.

My own experience has been that properly employed, this simple procedure has probably more merit than any other except the rhythmic injection of carbon dioxide via the intratracheal catheter by an apparatus.

One or two light breaths from the mouth of the obstetrician held in contact with that of the infant whose air passages have been cleared previously, will increase the heart rate from 20 to 40 beats per minute, and distinctly improve its quality. Cyanosis clears temporarily, even though the child does not at once begin to breathe; but after a few insufflations, respiration often begins and continues unimpaired. Great gentleness is required and the air pressure applied is just sufficient to lightly expand the lungs.

The respiratory impulse may sometimes be initiated by a light, rapid, staccato percussion along the spine, with the fingertips, the child being held suspended by the feet.

The maintenance of bodily heat is of equal importance to any other measures in the resuscitation of the newborn. Immediately after the cord is cut, the child should be well wrapped in warm blankets and all manipulations are to be carried out with the body well covered. In hospital, the electrically warmed crib is an excellent device, or a warm bath may be used.

External irritants to stimulate respiration, bending and compressing the thorax and swinging the child over the shoulder of the obstetrician are usually productive of much more damage than their improbable advantages warrant. In mild cases, spanking the buttocks may be tried but no other traumatic procedure. The use of alternate

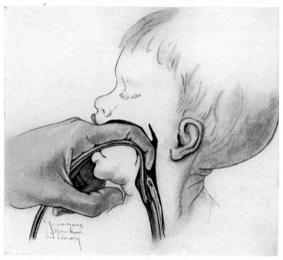

Fig. 399.—Tracheal catheter in position for artificial respiration. The left index finger is introduced over the base of the tongue and the epiglottis located. A tracheal catheter No. 14 or 15 F is passed along the palmar surface of the hand and finger and its tip is guided forward past the epiglottis into the larynx and trachea. (Baer.)

hot and cold plunges adds to the shock and does no other good. The various respirators on the market would seem to be physiologically correct, but their actual operation is quite disappointing and I have abandoned their use.

The technic of the introduction of the tracheal catheter is as follows (quoted from DeLee's excellent description, see Fig. 399).

The index finger of the left hand pulls the epiglottis forward and comes to touch the arytenoid cartilages. At the same time the catheter is passed along this finger until it lies over the rima, just behind the epiglottis. Now the inside index finger pulls the very tip of the catheter sharply forward, while the right hand, giving the tube a slight twisting motion, pushes it down into the trachea. The lips are applied to the glass mouthpiece and a light suck draws the contents of the trachea into the catheter, which is then removed and its contents forcibly blown out on a towel for inspection. Sometimes the sucking on the catheter is continued as it is withdrawn to clear the whole tract. It may be necessary to repeat this procedure several times. It is wise also to compress the chest between the thumb and four fingers to force the material out of the smaller bronchi, to gain the advantages claimed for Schultze's swingings. By pushing the catheter deeply into the chest and turning the head and neck of the child sharply to either side, the right and then the left bronchus may be emptied.

OPERATIVE OBSTETRICS

THE PREPARATION OF THE PATIENT

ABSOLUTE asepsis is a sine qua non for success in any operative procedure, doubly so in the parturient woman because of the added danger of infection presented by the pregnant uterus.

The operator and assistants must be scrubbed, gowned and gloved according to approved surgical principles.

For vaginal operation, the patient must be shaved as to the pubic hair, the bladder and rectum emptied. She is then placed upon a table (in the home a kitchen table equipped with a Glover crutch or adjustable stirrup is satisfactory) in the lithotomy position.

The entire pudendal region and the inner side of the thigh should then be painstakingly scrubbed with soap and water, followed by painting with tincture of iodine 5 per cent, mercurochome 4 per cent, metaphen, or in fact any antiseptic favored by the operator, after which the field is to be draped with sterile drapes.

Anesthesia of some type is indicated in all obstetric operations, whether it be local or an inhalation anesthesia with ether, nitrous oxide, ethylene or others.

For abdominal operation, the same general rules hold, although nowadays with the number of hospitals available throughout the country, transfer of the patient to such an institution is advised if at all practicable.

THE INDUCTION OF ABORTION

The performance of abortion must always be hedged about with the most rigid safeguards. It may never be done except for the absolute indication of preserving the life of the mother and then only after careful consultation with another physician who should express his concurring opinion in writing. The indications for therapeutic abortion have been considered in the several chapters devoted to the pathology of pregnancy.

Technic During the First Eight Weeks of Pregnancy.—At this time the uterus may be emptied by dilatation and curettage. Under anesthesia (nitrous oxide, ethylene, etc.) and with proper asepsis and draping, the cervix is grasped with tenaculum forceps and slowly dilated, either with the branched Goodell dilator or Hegar's graduated bougies. When the cervical canal has reached at least 2 cm. diameter, a large sharp curet is introduced to the fundus, taking the greatest care to avoid perforation of the soft uterus by allowing the curet to enter by its own weight and without any pushing. After gentle curettage when the uterus is felt to be practically empty it is lightly packed with sterile gauze, both to prevent hemorrhage and because upon its removal twenty-four hours later, any shreds of decidua or ovum which have remained in the cavity are withdrawn with the gauze. After the end of the third month of gestation, dilatation and curettage becomes an unsatisfactory method for inducing abortion, because the fetus has attained such bulk that it is difficult to draw it through the

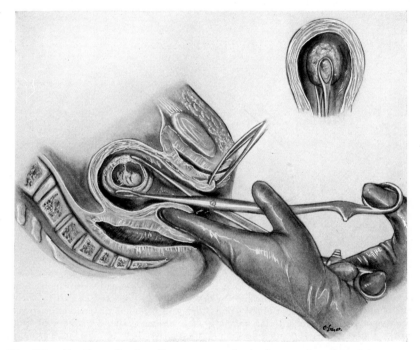

Fig. 400.—Abortion, showing the proper method of removing placental masses.

imperfectly dilated cervix, and if dismembered in the process, there is danger of leaving a portion of the fetal body behind to become infected. Also the bleeding during attempts at extraction may be alarming (Fig. 400).

A two-stage operation is much better at this time. With conditions as before, the cervix is dilated, the ovum broken up with ovum forceps, making sure that the membranes are ruptured, and a gauze pack inserted into the cervix. Labor usually comes on within twenty-four hours and the products of conception are expelled with the gauze.

It may be necessary to curet the uterus a few days later to remove any residual débris, or the ovum and decidua may be discharged in toto without subsequent symptoms. If bleeding is free, during the progress of the abortion, it may be necessary to repack the uterus.

After the fifth month, the induction of abortion is practically identical with that of premature labor. The cervix should be dilated and a firm pack or better a small metreurynter introduced. Labor usually comes on within twelve hours.

Anterior Vaginal Hysterotomy.—If haste is indicated, anterior vaginal hysterotomy may be done.

This operation is applicable up to the end of the seventh month, after which time the fetus is too large, and delivery should be secured by the induction of labor.

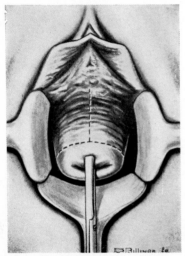 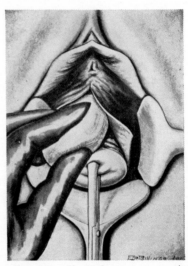

Fig. 401.—Vaginal cesarean section: cervix drawn forcibly downward by volsella forceps. Longitudinal and transverse incisions in anterior vaginal wall. Lateral retractors used for purposes of illustration not necessary for operation. (Peterson.)

Fig. 402.—Vaginal cesarean section: vaginal wall dissected away from bladder wall for short distance on each side of incisions. Bladder dissected from uterus by few strokes with sponge. (Peterson.)

Technic.—With the patient in the lithotomy position, aseptically prepared and anesthetized, the anterior lip of the cervix is exposed by the use of a weighted speculum, and grasped on either side of the midline with tenaculum forceps (Fig. 401, 402, 403).

A short transverse incision is then made at the vaginocervical juncture just below the inferior border of the bladder. By combined blunt and sharp dissection the bladder and anterior vaginal wall are pushed upward off the uterus until the lower segment is denuded. The bladder is retracted upward with a narrow-bladed retractor and anterior wall of the cervix divided vertically in the midline through its entire length. The fetus is then delivered either by manual trac-

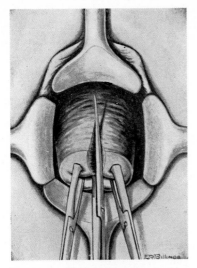

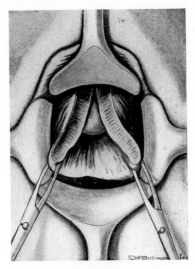

Fig. 403.—Vaginal cesarean section: cervix grasped at each side of median line by volsella forceps. Cervix split upward in median line by stout scissors. Bladder held up behind pubes by retractor or sponge. (Peterson.)

Fig. 404.—Vaginal cesarean section: anterior cervical wall split upward. Membranes bulging downward. Through this opening child can be delivered by version or forceps. (Peterson.)

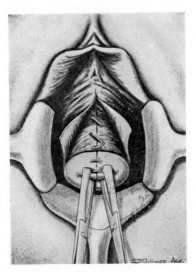

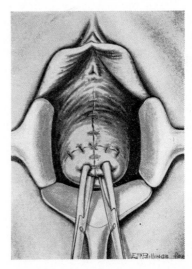

Fig. 405.—Vaginal cesarean section: suture of cervical incision completed. (Peterson.)

Fig. 406.—Vaginal cesarean section: the vaginal mucosa can be united by continuous or interrupted suture. Care should be taken not to have too accurate coaptation, for fear of oozing under flap. (Peterson.)

tion on the head if it be small, forceps extraction or version. After the expulsion of the placenta the wound in the cervix is closed by interrupted sutures of catgut and the bladder and vagina fastened in place by a few sutures.

This operation has been proposed in full-term pregnancy as an alternative to abdominal hysterotomy, but the child at this time is so large that the procedure becomes bloody, difficult, and dangerous and is not advised (Figs. 404, 405, 406).

THE INDUCTION OF LABOR

The induction of labor, before, at or after term, may often be accomplished by medical means alone, but these frequently fail, when manual or instrumental measures must be utilized.

The indications for the induction of labor are:

Before term but after the child is viable (thirtieth to thirty-eighth week).

Preeclampsia, which does not improve under the usual treatment.

Marginal or lateral placenta praevia.

Any illness of the mother which renders termination of pregnancy desirable.

Hydramnios, with roentgenological diagnosis of deformed fetus.

Contracted pelvis (rarely).

The indications for induction at term are as above with the exception of contracted pelvis.

When pregnancy is unduly prolonged, as shown by a knowledge of the correct date of estimated confinement together with overgrowth of the fetus, labor should be induced.

The medical induction of labor causes no risks to mother or child, but there is distinct danger in surgical induction. For the mother the possibility of infection following the unusual complication of hemorrhage from complete or partial detachment of the placenta during the operation and most of all the fact that if, in a given case, attempts at induction must be followed by cesarean section, the latter is rendered unduly dangerous by reason of the previous invasion of the uterus by bag or bougie. For the child, the dangers are premature rupture of the membrane and prolapse of the cord.

The Medical Induction of Labor.—While this does not properly belong in the domain of operative obstetrics it will be considered here.

The method in common use is generally ascribed to Watson, and consists in the administration of 2 ounces of castor oil followed by a hot soap suds enema when the oil begins to act. After the enema, pituitrin in doses of 2 minims, subcutaneously, every twenty minutes until pain begins to recur regularly or until a maximum of eight doses has been given.

In women at term this simple expedient inaugurates labor in from 40 to 50 per cent of the cases but in the remainder it has no perceptible effect.

The Surgical Induction of Labor.—Simple Rupture of the Membranes.—This old method has recently been revived by Slemons, and is enjoying great popularity. It consists in a preliminary medical induction, without pituitrin, and after the enema has been expelled, the patient is shaved, scrubbed and draped as for delivery, the operator having also prepared himself in an aseptic manner. With the legs in stirrups or held by attendants two fingers are inserted into the vagina and the external os sought. This usually admits the finger easily and the pouch of membranes may be palpated over the fetal head. The membranes are then ruptured with toothed forceps or better, the amniotome, after which a sterile pad is placed over the vulva and the patient returned to bed (Fig. 407).

Pituitrin is now administered either by divided doses, as before described, or by the intranasal use of a cotton applicator saturated with 0.5 cc. of the solution. There is usually a latent period which may last several hours after which labor comes on.

This method of induction has been carefully studied and the accumulated statistics serve to prove that the duration of labor runs parallel to that of spontaneous onset, there is no increased danger of

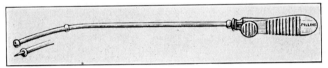

Fig. 407.—Amniotic trocar.

cervical or perineal laceration and that the fetal and maternal morbidity and mortality are not increased, provided proper precautions are taken to insure freedom from infection.

Induction by Bougie or Tube.—For this purpose either a stiff woven bougie, or better a new, sterile rectal tube are used. Under the same preparatory technic the finger is inserted into the cervix and the membranes gently stripped off the posterior surface. With the finger as a guide, the tube is then introduced and gently pushed in until most of it lies coiled in the lower uterine segment.

If a bougie is used this is introduced in the same manner, but instead of coiling in the lower portion of the uterus, the bougie passes between the uterine wall and the membranes until the fundus is reached. Two bougies lying side by side are often used. If there is any obstruction to the passage of tube or bougie, the instrument should be removed and reinserted in a different direction.

Occasionally a sharp gush of blood indicates perforation of the placenta by the bougie, in which case prompt withdrawal causes the hemorrhage to cease, after which the bougie may be again inserted. When the membranes are ruptured accidentally during this type of induction it is well to remove the tube and proceed with pituitrin as in simple rupture.

When the bougies or tubes are in position a light pack of gauze is placed in the vagina and the onset of labor awaited.

Induction by Dilating Bag (Metreurynter).—This method of induction carries with it definite danger as to complication. The bulk of the bag may displace the presenting part and lead to malpresentation or prolapse of the cord. Further, the initial dilatation of the long cervix by a bag is difficult. The method is of much more value for completing the dilatation of an already partially effaced and dilated cervix than when used to inaugurate the dilatation.

Technic.—The Pomeroy, or Voorhees bag is most commonly chosen, there being four sizes generally available ranging from $2\frac{1}{2}$

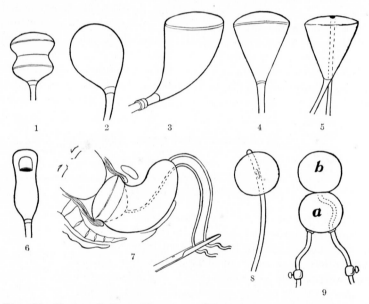

Fig. 408.—Various balloon dilators. 1, Hirst; 2, Braun's; 3, Champetier de Ribes'; 4, Voorhees'; 5, Stowe's; 6, Barnes'; 7, Pomeroy's; 8, Tarnier's; 9, Chassagny's. (From DeLee, "Principles and Practice of Obstetrics.")

to 10 cm. in diameter when distended. It is good practice to use the largest bag that can be entered into the cervix (Fig. 408).

The patient is prepared as before and, the finger having stripped the membranes from the posterior aspect of the cervix, the bag, folded longitudinally, is inserted in the grasp of long dressing forceps and held in place by a finger, while it is being filled with a sterile solution, by means of a syringe manipulated by an assistant. It is important that the bag be tested for leakage before use and that the quantity of fluid required to distend it be accurately known.

When the bag is filled the end of its tube is tied off or clamped in a hemostat. A weight of $\frac{1}{2}$ pound may be attached to the end of the tube by a cord and hung over the foot of the bed to hasten dilatation.

In an hour or two labor begins in most cases and the bag may be expelled in from four to six hours.

Sometimes labor pains cease after the expulsion of the bag, when one may either rupture the membranes or proceed to the insertion of a larger bag.

Many operators prefer to introduce an antiseptic solution into the vagina before any attempt at surgical induction. Mercurochrome 4 per cent, metaphen 1:1000, a weak lysol solution or other bactericide may be employed, about 10 cc. of solution being inserted by means of a syringe.

Dilatation and Incision of the Cervix.—Manual dilatation of the cervix was a common maneuver in the obstetrics of the past, but improvements in cesarean section, in the employment of dilating bags and a better understanding of the principles underlying labor, have relegated this procedure to a very insignificant place and it is rarely used nowadays.

It consists in slowly dilating the cervix with first one finger, then two, next the thumb and first two fingers, until all five may be inserted and spread apart to complete the dilatation. It is a traumatic act, involving great possibility of infection and has been properly abandoned except upon some unusual indication for rapid vaginal delivery.

Instrumental dilatation of the cervix with such weapons as the Bossi dilator belongs to obstetrical history alone.

Incision of the Cervix.—In uncommon instances the partially dilated cervix resists all efforts at further stretching and it must be cut in order that labor may continue.

The cervix must be dilated to at least 4 cm. and partially effaced before incision may be done. This condition being fulfilled, the patient is prepared, the cervix grasped with tenacula and deep incisions made with scissors, one on each side just anterior to a transverse line drawn through the center of the os, and one in the midline posteriorly.

Bleeding may require vaginal packing. After the completion of the third stage of labor the wounds in the cervix are carefully coapted and united by suture.

SYMPHYSIOTOMY AND PUBIOTOMY

To enlarge the pelvis and permit delivery from below is the object of both of these operations.

Symphysiotomy involves the division of the pubic joint, either subcutaneously with a blunt-pointed bistoury or openly with a heavy scalpel.

Pubiotomy involves the sawing through of the pubis to the side of the symphysis, either by open dissection or subcutaneously with a Gigli saw.

42

Both operations are indicated in contracted pelvis when the true conjugate is 7½ cm., and by their use, this diameter may be increased up to 3 cm. With the improvement in the technic of cesarean section, both procedures have become more or less obsolete, and the writer confesses that not only has he never performed either of these operations but has never seen them done by others.

CHAPTER XLII

THE OBSTETRICAL FORCEPS

THE invention of this instrument, one of the epoch-making developments of medicine, is a fascinating story and the writer regrets the necessity for conserving space in a textbook and omitting this chapter of medical history. The reader who is interested in this phase of the obstetric art should consult the excellent memoirs of Aveling and Das, upon this very important subject (see Figs. 409, 410).

The obstetric forceps is an instrument designed to facilitate delivery in head presentation although it is sometimes used on the breech.

Description: The forceps consists of two separable blades with handles, the blades possessing two curves, one made to conform to

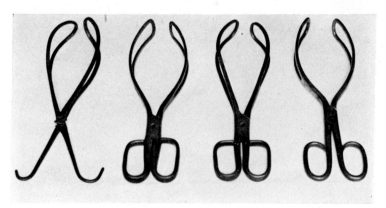

Fig. 409.—The four forceps found in the famous Chamberlen chest. (From the Barton Cooke Hirst Collection, University of Pennsylvania.)

the rotundity of the fetal head and called the "cephalic curve," and one corresponding to the concavity of the sacrum and termed the "pelvic curve."

The blades may be solid as in the Tucker-McLane forceps, or fenestrated as in the Simpson model.

The two portions of the instrument articulate at the lock of which two varieties are in general use.

(a) The English lock which consists of a socket upon each branch into which fits the shank of the opposite half of the instrument. This arrangement permits of ready articulation but does not hold the blades firmly together.

(b) The French lock in which a pivot is screwed into the shank of

659

the left branch, while the right presents an opening which can be adjusted to it, the screw being tightened after articulation.

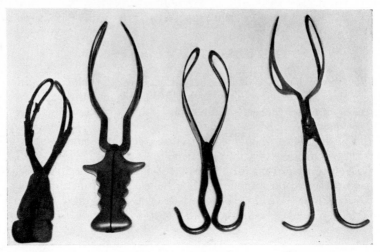

Fig. 410.—The evolution of the obstetric forceps. From left to right: Smellie's original instrument and its successor the Simpson forceps. Levret's original and the Hodge forceps. (From the Barton Cooke Hirst Collection, University of Pennsylvania.)

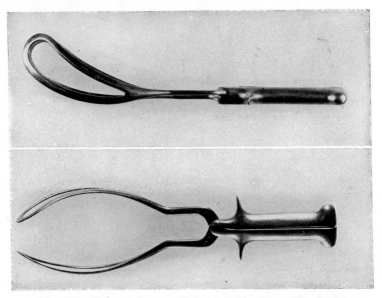

Fig. 411.—Simpson forceps, DeLee modification. (Danforth.)

There are many types of obstetric forceps in common use, those most favored in America being the Simpson and the Tucker-McLane, together with an instrument possessing the axis-tractor principle as exemplified in the Tarnier or Dewees forceps (Fig. 411).

To meet special indications, the forceps of Kielland and Barton are of great value and should be included in every well-equipped armamentarium.

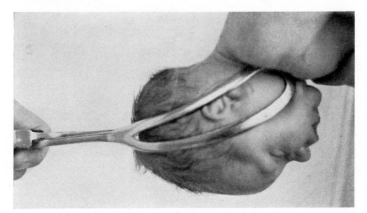

Fig. 412.—Correct cephalic application of forceps to an anteriorly placed occiput.

The branches of the forceps are named left and right. The left branch is that one in which the cephalic curve corresponds to the

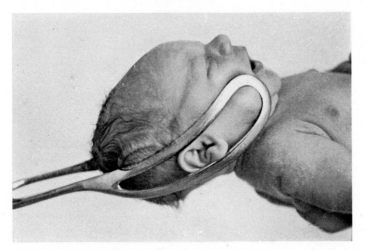

Fig. 413.—Correct application of forceps when the occiput is posterior.

curved left side of the maternal pelvis, the right one being that which fits the right side of the maternal pelvis. Incidentally the left blade is held in the left hand of the operator during introduction, the right in the right hand.

A *cephalic application* of the forceps is obtained when the cephalic curve of the instrument approximates the sides of the infant's head (Fig. 412).

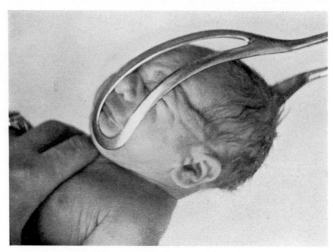

Fig. 414.—Faulty application of forceps.

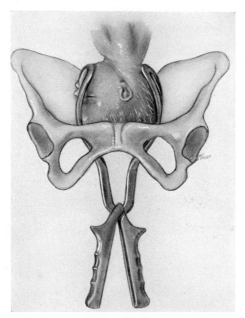

Fig. 415.—Forceps extraction. Faulty application, one blade over face, one over occiput.

A *pelvic application* is secured when the pelvic curve of the forceps corresponds to the concavity of the maternal sacrum. Thus when the sagittal suture is in the anteroposterior diameter of the pelvis, application of the forceps will be both cephalic and pelvic (Fig. 413). When the sagittal suture lies in an oblique diameter of the pelvis the application will be cephalic but not pelvic. When the sagittal suture lies in the transverse diameter of the pelvis and one blade of the forceps lies over the infant's face, the other over the occiput, the application will be pelvic but not cephalic (Figs. 414, 415).

In the use of the forceps, cephalic applications are always a desideratum, but pelvic application need not be considered as this develops during rotation of the descending head.

THE FUNCTIONS OF THE OBSTETRIC FORCEPS

1. *As Tractors.*—This is the common use for which the instrument was designed, namely, to reinforce or supplant the natural forces of labor in cases of dystocia.

2. *As Rotators.*—In certain malpresentations as occiput in the hollow of the sacrum, the forceps may be utilized to turn the presenting part into a favorable position for extraction or possibly spontaneous delivery.

3. *As Levers.*—This is a dangerous and uncommonly used procedure, as it greatly endangers the maternal soft parts.

4. *As Compressors.*—It is inevitable that some measure of compression will accompany every forceps extraction, but it is the interest of the accoucheur to reduce this force to a minimum.

In difficult labor, when the child is dead, the forceps may be properly used as compressors, to reduce the width of the head and so facilitate delivery.

THE INDICATIONS FOR THE EMPLOYMENT OF THE FORCEPS

1. To reinforce the expulsive powers in (a) Slight or moderate disproportion between fetal head and maternal pelvis.

(b) In uterine inertia or exhaustion, if there be no insuperable obstacle to delivery.

(c) In faulty presentation of the head as posterior rotation of the occiput, defective flexion, etc.

(d) In unyielding pelvic floor, when delivery may be expedited by episiotomy and some assistance to the natural forces.

(e) In undue delay in the second stage, when the head has passed the ischial spines and further progress ceases, even though there may be no tangible reason for the obstruction.

Here the time element is an important factor since nothing is to be gained by allowing the mother to go on in labor for hours, after the head is well through the pelvic brim and the cervix widely dilated, whereas there is active danger to the child from prolonged compression of the head in the pelvis, and the body in the uterine cavity. One cannot definitely determine when to apply forceps under these conditions but if the pains are strong, the cervix fully dilated and the head well in the pelvis, below the spine, one hour's labor without progress is a sufficient indication.

2. To insure rapid delivery when systemic disease in the mother, such as grave cardiac lesions, advanced phthisis, acute illness as pneumonia, forbid the exhausting effects of a long spontaneous labor.

3. In the interests of the fetus, when its distress is shown by irregularity of the heart sounds, excessive slowness or great rapidity of the heart beat or the passage of meconium.

Of those, irregularity in rhythm betokens the most grave danger to the child, marked bradycardia follows, while tachycardia and the passage of meconium are signs of less moment.

CONDITIONS WHICH MUST BE FULFILLED BEFORE THE FORCEPS CAN BE APPLIED WITH SAFETY

1. *The head must be engaged.* The use of forceps upon a head which has not yet entered the pelvic inlet (floating head) is fraught with great danger, since it is probable that such great disproportion exists that the attempt will end in disaster, and also because a correct application of the blades cannot be insured.

One should be certain that the broad biparietal diameter has actually descended into the inlet as sometimes a long caput succedaneum may descend below the level of the ischiac spine and give the impression that the head is fully engaged. The same is true of excessive molding with overlapping of the parietal bones and exaggerated asynclitism, so that the anterior parietal descends deeply into the pelvis, while its fellow is still above the promontory.

2. *The membranes must be ruptured.* This condition is necessary, because the presence of the membranes and the contained liquor amnii militate against a proper application of the blades, and because of the danger of separation of the placenta by traction, before the delivery of the child has been accomplished.

3. *The cervix must be effaced and fully dilated or easily dilatable.* The use of forceps as cervical dilators is not permissible, since not only do dangerous lacerations of the cervix develop as a result of such effort, but the child is put in great jeopardy by compression of the head.

In certain instances of great fetal distress, forceps extraction is sometimes attempted in the face of an only partially effaced and dilated cervix. Inasmuch as such measures only accentuate the trauma to the fetus they are almost always inadvisable.

4. *The position and presentation must be clearly recognized.* Accurate diagnosis by detailed vaginal examination should precede every forceps delivery, because lack of the knowledge so obtained often leads to attempts at delivery of impossible positions as face with chin in the hollow of the sacrum, etc.

5. *The disproportion must not be too great.*

CONTRAINDICATIONS TO THE USE OF FORCEPS

1. Marked disproportion between fetal head and maternal pelvis.
2. Failure of the head to engage (floating head).
3. Nondilatation and effacement of the cervix.
4. Face presentation with the chin arrested in the hollow of the sacrum.
5. Hydrocephalus.

PREPARATION FOR FORCEPS APPLICATION

1. The patient must be anesthetized. (In extraordinary cases, when delivery is imperative and anesthesia cannot be obtained, it is sometimes, though rarely, permissible to use forceps without anesthesia.)

2. The bladder and rectum must be empty.

3. The operative field, the operator's hands and arm and the instruments must be aseptic.

4. Permission for the operation must be obtained from the patient (over twenty-one years of age), her husband, or guardian.

TYPES OF FORCEPS OPERATIONS (Fig. 416)

1. Low or *outlet* forceps, when the head is on the perineum, the scalp at the vulva.

2. Midforceps, or midplane, when the parietal bosses lie in the bispinous line.

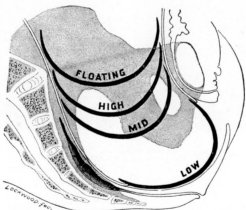

Fig. 416.—Diagram showing position of head in various forceps operations. (Williams, "Obstetrics," D. Appleton-Century Co., Publishers.)

3. High or *inlet* forceps, when the parietal bosses lie in the plane of the inlet but have not yet completely passed through it. The use of the high forceps operation is not to be employed in the presence of a living baby, unless such complications as prolonged labor with potential or actual infection of the uterus, or advanced exhaustion of the mother, render cesarean section impracticable.

THE FORCEPS OPERATION

Conditions necessary and indications as above being fulfilled, the patient is placed upon a table in a semilithotomy position. It is important that the thighs be not abducted to too great an extent, nor too much flexed, since the integrity of the pelvic floor is menaced by overstretching if this be done. The Piper leg holders are admirably suited for forceps deliveries, although any other form may be used.

If in a home, a kitchen table may be used, with a Glover crutch, or a sling passing from one popliteal space over one shoulder, behind the other and so to the opposite knee, or best of all, when available,

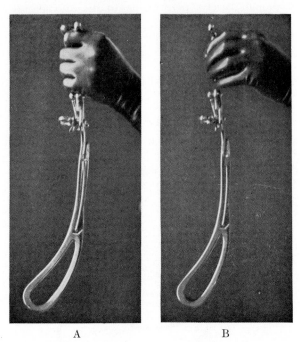

A   B

Fig. 417.—A, Incorrect method of holding the forceps blade during introduction; B, correct method of holding the forceps blade during the introduction. Only the tips of the fingers are used. (Shears, "Obstetrics," J. B. Lippincott Co., Publishers.)

the legs may be held by appropriately gowned attendants. If delivery is to be in a bed, the buttocks should be drawn to the edge of the bed and the legs supported by a sling or by attendants sitting on the sides of the bed.

The patient being anesthetized, scrubbed and draped, the soft parts are stretched and relaxed by a maneuver known as ironing out the perineum. Anointed with a sterile lubricant, at first two, then three, then four fingers are introduced into the vagina, palmar surface downward, and with a firm but gentle semicircular side-to-side movement of the hand, the perineum is gradually relaxed and presently stretched to a considerable extent. The ironing-out process usually consumes five or six minutes and well repays the effort, in the minimizing of laceration. If it be deemed necessary, episiotomy is then done, before the perineum has become so tense from distention by the head, that the anatomic relations are disturbed, and the correct line of incision made difficult to determine. The actual operation consists of four steps, application, locking, extraction and removal. The procedures are described as being used in the L. O. A. position of the occiput.

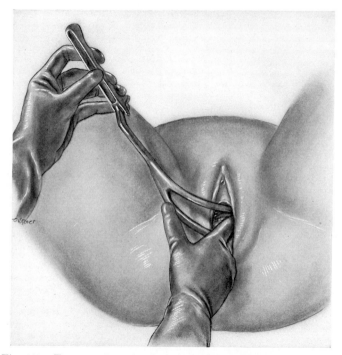

Fig. 418.—Forceps. Introduction of the left blade of the forceps.

First Step. Application (Fig. 417).—The operator stands or sits between the thighs of the patient. The left blade of the forceps is always applied first. Having introduced two fingers of the right hand into the vagina, the left blade, grasped at the lock by the left hand, as a pen, is held perpendicularly to the woman's body, with the tip of the blade opposite the vulva. The tip of the blade is inserted into the vagina, and is pressed backward along the pelvic floor toward the sacrum (Fig. 418). The blade is then rotated outward on its long axis to bring it in apposition with the posterior inclined plane of the pelvis, and to escape the promontory of the sacrum; the handle is depressed and the tip of the blade is thus elevated, the fingers of the right hand in the vagina guiding the blade and protecting the soft parts. Finally, the handle is carried to the left side in order to engage the tip of the blade over the curve of the child's head.

The right blade is now introduced (Fig. 419), the protruding handle of the left one being supported by an assistant, or pushed out of the way by the left hand, two fingers of which are in the vagina, guiding the forceps.

When both blades are in the vagina it is impossible to lock them, since both of them have been pushed upward along the posterior

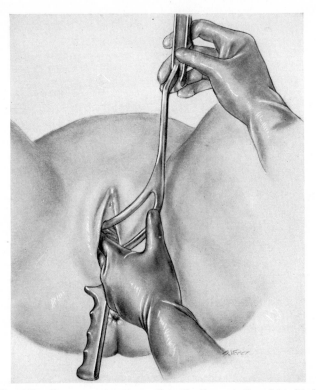

Fig. 419.—Forceps extraction. Introduction of the right blade.

inclined planes of the pelvis after being rotated outward on their long axis. It is thus necessary to rotate one blade around the head of the child to permit locking. The rule for this rotation is that that blade is rotated which, in name, corresponds to the oblique diameter of the pelvis in which the sagittal suture lies. Therefore, since in L. O. A. the sagittal suture occupies the right oblique diameter of the pelvis, the right blade must be rotated. This is accomplished by depressing the handle and elevating the right blade of the forceps until it is felt to slip over the side of the child's face and fall into position, directly opposite its fellow. Or the handle is lightly sup-

ported by the fingers of the right hand, while the first two fingers
of the left hand are inserted under and to the outer side of the heel
of the blade and gently pry it upward, outward, and then inward.
If the operator finds it more convenient, he may reverse the hands.

Second Step. Locking (Fig. 420).—If the head closely fits the
pelvic walls, there may be some difficulty in securing rotation, the
tendency being to make the blades lock by moving the unrotated
blade. This will cause a failure of cephalic application and should
be avoided whenever possible. In the usual operation of forceps the
head is low down, and the small fontanel has rotated all the way or
nearly all the way to the front, and the blades, after being inserted,

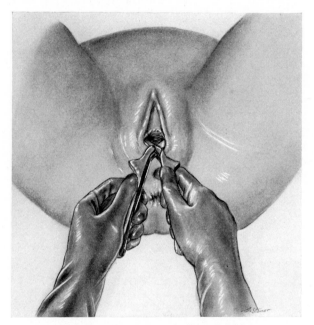

Fig. 420.—Forceps extraction. Locking.

fit naturally to the sides of the head. Often, however, they need a
little adjusting before it is possible to lock them without using undue
force. A downward movement of the blades toward the perineum
often facilitates their conjunction, though it may be necessary to
twist or rotate each blade a little to secure apposition. If these
manipulations do not result in easy locking, the blades must be removed and again applied, since it is evident that proper position has
not been obtained. It is dangerous to use force in closing the blades
of the forceps, because serious injury to the child or maternal soft
parts may ensue. The fetal heart tones should be auscultated before
the forceps are locked and again after the blades are closed. If irregularity or marked slowing of the heart occurs, it indicates that a

loop of cord is caught and is being compressed and the forceps should again be removed and reapplied, after examination to locate a possible occult prolapse of the cord.

Third Step. Extraction.—The forceps being locked, a tentative traction is made to determine whether their position is correct and that the instrument does not slip. This fact being established, extraction is begun. The forceps when locked will be found to lie with the concavity of their pelvic curve directly upward, or somewhat obliquely, depending upon the degree of anterior rotation of the head which has taken place. If the latter, the application is not a true pelvic one, but this is of no importance provided a correct cephalic application (*i. e.*, to the sides of the head) has been secured.

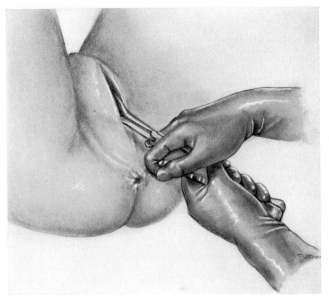

Fig. 421.—Forceps extraction. The correct grasp for traction.

As successive tractions are made, the forceps will be observed to rotate with the descent of the head, and on no account should this movement be impeded by the operator, since it is a definite indication that the normal mechanism of rotation and descent is being accomplished.

The operator takes the grip on the forceps shown in Fig. 421. The forefinger of the left hand being extended and in contact with the scalp of the child, to note any slipping of the blades. A folded towel between the handles of the forceps tends to prevent too great compression of the head.

The tractions are made in the direction of the birth canal, at first downward and outward. The old maneuver of Pajot (Fig. 422), in which one hand depresses the upper portion of the forceps handle while the other elevates the end of the handle, may be used. By this means the axis-traction principle is utilized, the blades being made to sweep around the curve of the birth canal, rather than being drawn straight through it. Traction should be intermittent, lasting for about one minute, with an interval of two minutes, during which time the blades are unlocked to permit a free return of circulation in the uncompressed fetal head. It is advised to make the tractions with the uterine contractions, an important matter when the patient is conscious or very lightly anesthetized, but meaning very little when deep surgical anesthesia has been induced, as is the case in most forceps deliveries.

The tractions should be made with the arm and shoulder of the operator; brutal dragging, by bracing the feet and utilizing the

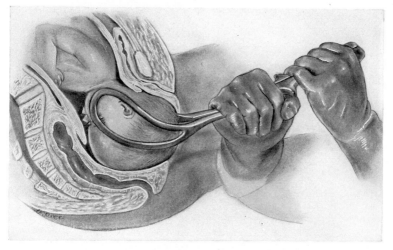

Fig. 422.—Forceps extraction. Pajot grasp, the right hand making downward pressure while the left hand pulls.

muscles of the back being unspeakably bad practice. (I once had a student do this on a summer day in a small home, the result being that the forceps slipped and he fell backward out of an opened window, to the street below, fracturing his skull, while the patient remained undelivered.)

The force permissible in forceps extraction is variable. Obviously it must be sufficient to accomplish the purpose of delivery, but it may not be so great as to injure the child or severely lacerate the maternal tissue by precipitate delivery (Fig. 423).

The most important point is the avoidance of haste. Unless some urgent condition of mother or child demands rapid delivery, the forceps operation should require from thirty minutes to an hour, the traction being always intermittent and of a strength only sufficient to produce slow progress in the natural mechanism of labor.

When the head is well in the vulvar outlet, about one third of its surface visible, the direction of the forceps pull is altered, to conform with the normal mechanism of labor. The operator changes his grip upon the forceps, holding the handles in his right hand, and very slowly and intermittently raises them directly upward toward the symphysis, thus bringing about extension of the head, the forehead, brow and face rolling successively over the perineum. At the same time, the head is lightly pulled upward, maintaining the nucha in contact with the lower border of the symphysis.

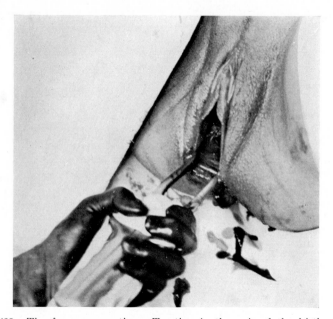

Fig. 423.—The forceps operation. Traction in the axis of the birth canal.

The left hand, meantime, protected by sponge or towel, protects the perineum from injury by firm pressure against it. It is better practice not to deliver the head with forceps, but to remove them when the head is extending at the outlet, and complete the delivery by manual means.

Fourth Step. Removal.—When the head is about to emerge from the vulva the forceps should be removed, by first unlocking the blades and then gently slipping them around the child's head, first the right, then the left, care and gentleness being used to avoid injury of the pelvic floor and laceration of the ear of the infant. After removal of the forceps, the delivery of the head may be completed by gently pushing the vulvar ring backward over the prominent parietal eminence, or by pushing forward and upward from behind the anus (Ritgen's maneuver).

FORCEPS EXTRACTION IN ABNORMAL PRESENTATION AND POSITION

Forceps on Posterior Position of the Occiput.—It has been stated that manual rotation is the most effective method of securing anterior rotation of a persistently posterior occiput, but should this fail, rotation by forceps may be utilized. This operation has for years been called the Scanzoni maneuver although this is in fact a misnomer.

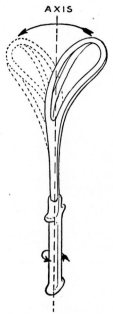

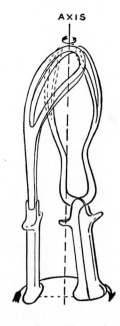

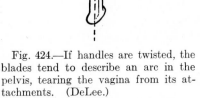

Fig. 424.—If handles are twisted, the blades tend to describe an arc in the pelvis, tearing the vagina from its attachments. (DeLee.)

Fig. 425.—If we wish to give a rotatory movement to the blades, the handles should be made to describe an arc. (DeLee.)

The method consists in an application of the forceps to the side of the child's head as in anterior position, the rotation of the blades through an arc of 135° followed by the removal of the forceps, which now have their pelvic concavity opposite to that of the pelvic cavity and then reapplication to the now anterior occiput, with extraction in the usual manner.

In the initial application, it is sometimes difficult to secure a true cephalic application and in such cases the blades perforce grasp the head diagonally, one being over the malar bone. The danger of serious injury to the child under these circumstances must be taken

43

into account, and rotation very gently done, *without traction.* As soon as may be the blades are unlocked and a true cephalic application obtained when, and only when, traction may be made.

The rotation must be done by sweeping the handles of the forceps through a wide circle, rather than simply twisting them around, in order to avoid extensive laceration of the vagina by the tips of the blades, which occurs by reason of their pelvic curve in the latter event (Figs. 424, 425).

When the occiput has been fully rotated, gentle traction is made, not to deliver but to fix the head in its new position and then the blades are withdrawn. They are immediately reinserted, the posterior one first (in R. O. P. converted to R. O. A. the right blade) in order to prevent the head slipping back into its original position, and then the extraction is carried out as in primary anterior position of the occiput.

The plane of the pelvis in which the head should lie, in order to obtain an optimum result in forceps rotation has given rise to much controversy.

The original Scanzoni technic contemplates drawing the head down to the pelvic floor and there rotating it, whereas Bill and his followers believe that rotation should generally be done as soon as the cervix is fully dilated and while the head is still in the pelvic cavity.

The truth probably lies between the two extremes, and rotation should be done when it is apparent that labor is delayed and progress has ceased, be the head where it may, always provided the cervix is fully dilated and effaced.

Forceps extraction of occiput in the hollow of the sacrum, without rotation, is occasionally necessary because of impaction or lack of room to effect rotation. Under these circumstances, the blades are applied as in an anterior occipital position, cephalic application being secured. Traction is then made in the axis of the birth canal, the forceps handles being elevated after each traction, to keep the presenting part as far anterior as possible. When the head has almost escaped from the vulva, the handles of the forceps are moved backward, slowly turning the brow and face out from under the symphysis, the perineum being strongly supported by the hand during the process. Serious and extensive laceration of the perineum often involving the sphincter ani is a common sequel in forceps extraction of a posterior occiput as such. This is due to the enormous strain to which the perineum is exposed by the rigid head and body of the fetus in this position. Hence, generous episiotomy should be a preliminary step, and indeed, the entire operation is to be avoided, if it is at all possible to rotate the head.

Application of the Forceps in Deep Transverse Arrest.—Sometimes labor becomes obstructed with the head in the pelvic brim, the sagittal suture lying transverse or nearly transverse, and being in some degree deflexed so that the fontanels lie in the same plane. The application of the ordinary type of forceps is very difficult in this situation, since by reason of the pelvic curve of the instrument a true cephalic application cannot be secured, and it becomes necessary to apply one blade over the occiput, the other over the face of the child. To avoid injury, traction must be very light and gentle and every attempt should be made to rotate the head, in order that a better application becomes possible.

The Kielland or Barton forceps (*q. v.*) are infinitely better adapted for dealing with such position, and should be employed whenever available.

Application of Forceps in Face Presentation (Fig. 426).—In face presentation, delivery may be aided by forceps only when the chin is well forward of the transverse diameter of the pelvis. When the

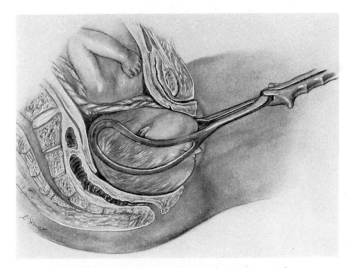

Fig. 426.—Forceps extraction in face presentation.

chin is posterior to this line, extraction by forceps is generally impossible except when the child is very small and immature.

When the chin is anterior, the forceps are applied as to an anterior occiput position, except that by reason of the position of the head, the handle must be higher than usual thus depressing the blades into the hollow of the sacrum, where they will fit better over the biparietal diameter of the fetal head.

After locking, the handles are moved downward, which further increases extension, and the tractions are at first downward to continue the extension and when the chin slips out from under the symphysis, the handles are raised, permitting the face, brow and occiput successively to slip over the perineum (Fig. 427).

Inlet or High Forceps Operation.—This term is used to describe cases in which the broadest diameter of the fetal head has not yet passed through the pelvic inlet, and the indications for such operations are very few, version or cesarean section being much preferable. When the child is dead or dying, and sometimes when the mother is a bad risk for section because of exhaustion or hemorrhage, high forceps extraction may be attempted, but only after a most scrupulous investigation as to other and safer methods. High forceps operations demand that an instrument made upon the principle of axis traction be used, because the high head must traverse a sharp curve, and if a straight pull as with ordinary forceps be employed, most of the effort

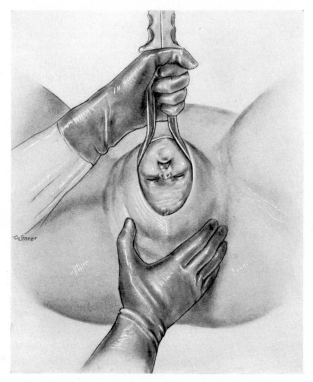

Fig. 427.—Extraction with forceps in face presentation, the chin anterior.

will be wasted in forcing the head of the child against the symphysis, rather than around the curves of the pelvic canal.

The axis-traction principle provides that the forceps be equipped with a device for transmitting the force of the pull to the beginning of the pelvic curve of the instrument, and imparting to the blades a motion in the arc of a circle, thus parelleling the axis of the birth canal (Fig. 428).

Levret was the first to appreciate this principle but its most important advocate was Tarnier who constructed an instrument upon which most recent modifications are based. It is essential in any axis-traction forceps that an oblique application of the blades, together with a direct sagittal traction must be possible. Such an instrument is the Tarnier, and the Dewees forceps, a great favorite of the writer.

In performing high forceps extraction, one should endeavor to secure a cephalic application but this is often impossible and the blades must be placed in the best position available.

The first tractions should be gentle, in order to learn whether the forceps are firmly seated, or whether slipping will occur, after which

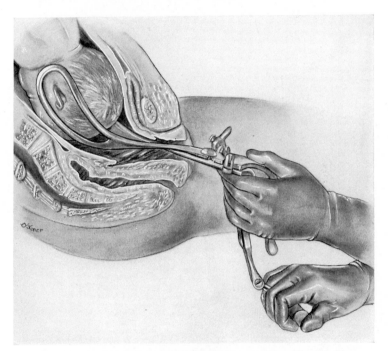

Fig. 428.—Forceps extraction with Dewees axis-traction forceps.

a few powerful attempts at delivery may be made. If there is no progress, the operator should desist from his efforts and proceed with the extraction, either by cesarean section, version or embryotomy. Version and forceps are not complementary operations, as DeLee wisely observes, rather where version is indicated, the forceps are contraindicated. Sometimes, however, especially if the obstruction be due to a malpresentation, version will succeed where forceps have failed.

It is bad obstetrics to continue attempts at high forceps extraction against insuperable obstructions, and indeed, ordinarily, high forceps is at best a make-shift and dangerous procedure, and should

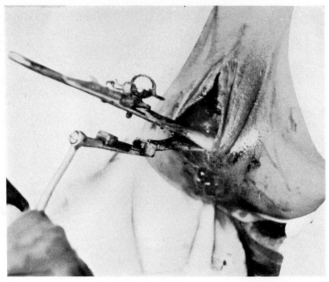

Fig. 429.—The forceps operation. Traction with Tarnier's axis-traction instrument.

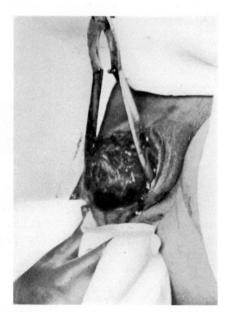

Fig. 430.—The forceps operation. Delivery with Tarnier's forceps almost completed.

not be performed unless there is no other safer way out of the difficulty (Figs. 429, 430, 431).

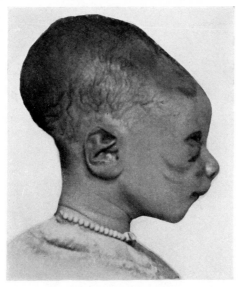

Fig. 431.—Marked molding of the head with superficial injuries of the face, from forceps extraction.

SPECIAL TYPES OF FORCEPS

The Kielland Forceps and Their Use.—In 1915 Kielland of Norway, realizing that the pelvic curve of the forceps was not only valueless but a positive detriment in cases where the sagittal suture remained markedly oblique or in the transverse diameter of the pelvis, devised an instrument in which the pelvic curve is largely eliminated, as in the early models of Smellie. The original purpose of the instrument was to permit the anterior blade to be introduced into the pelvis between fetal head and symphysis, concave side of the cephalic curve upward. When entered into the pelvis, the blades may be rotated and the cephalic curve brought into contact with the side of the fetal skull (Fig. 432).

The great advantages of these instruments is that their blades may be applied in the sagittal diameter of the pelvis without injury to the maternal tissues, and with a correct cephalic grasp of the fetus.

The Kielland forceps vary from the classical form in that they lack almost entirely a pelvic curve, being shaped like a bayonet; they have a sliding lock, which permits the blades to be approximated, even when one is higher in the pelvis than the other, as in marked asynclitism; third, the forceps are very light in construction.

For application in a deep transverse arrest, the anterior blade is introduced first, the concavity of the cephalic curve upward, its slight pelvic concavity toward the leading point of the head, usually the occiput (the chin in face presentation) (Figs. 433, 434, 435).

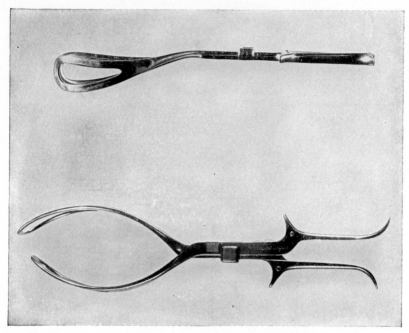

Fig. 432.—Kielland forceps. In the lower figure the blades are joined asymmetrically to illustrate the sliding block. Upper figure shows absent pelvic curve. (Danforth.)

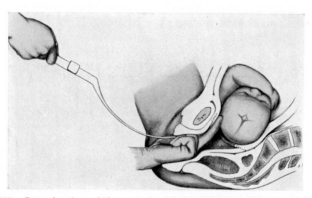

Fig. 433.—Introduction of the anterior blade of Kielland forceps in transverse arrest. Concavity is upward. (Jarcho in Amer. Jour. of Obstet. and Gynec., vol. 10, 1925, C. V. Mosby Co., Publishers.)

The anterior blade is then slipped between symphysis and head, under the guidance of two vaginal fingers, the concavity upward. The blade will be felt to pass up over the head, after which it is ro-

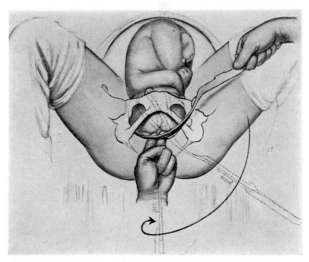

Fig. 434.—Second method of introducing the anterior blade by slipping it over the occiput. (Jarcho in Amer. Jour. of Obstet. and Gynec., vol. 10, 1925, C. V. Mosby Co., Publishers.)

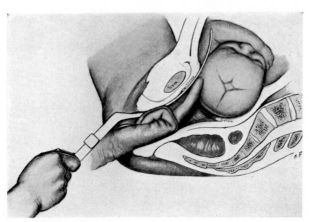

Fig. 435.—Further insertion of the anterior blade. (Jarcho in Amer. Jour. of Obstet. and Gynec., vol. 10, 1925, C. V. Mosby Co., Publishers.)

tated within the pelvis so that the concavity of the pelvic curve is directed toward the occiput (Fig. 436).

The posterior blade is then introduced, its cephalic concavity upward, between head and promontory, after which the blades are locked, with a little twisting motion if necessary. Traction is made downward and in favorable cases the head will be felt to rotate and slip into an oblique diameter of the pelvis, after which traction may be continued as in any forceps delivery until completely anterior rotation and descent has occurred (Fig. 437).

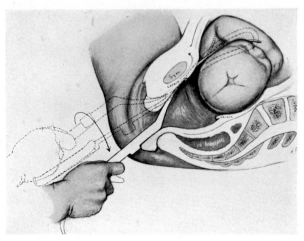

Fig. 436.—Rotating the anterior blade within the uterine cavity, in order to secure a cephalic application. (Jarcho in Amer. Jour. of Obstet. and Gynec., vol. 10, 1925, C. V. Mosby Co., Publishers.)

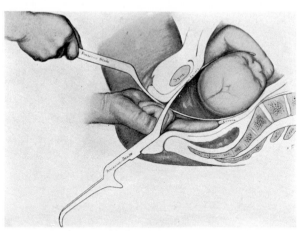

Fig. 437.—Introduction of the posterior blade between the head and the promontory. (Jarcho in Amer. Jour. of Obstet. and Gynec., vol. 10, 1925, C. V. Mosby Co., Publishers.)

Rotation is much aided by the use of these forceps which are of special advantage in the unrotated and deflexed head, delayed high in the pelvic cavity. Their proper use demands some practice on the mannikin (Figs. 438, 439, 440).

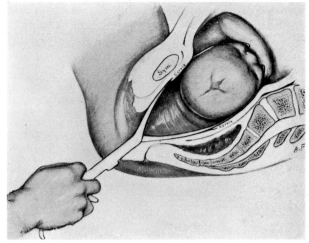

Fig. 438.—Beginning traction and rotation of the head. (Jarcho in Amer. Jour. of Obstet. and Gynec., vol. 10, 1925, C. V. Mosby Co., Publishers.)

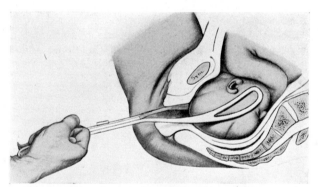

Fig. 439.—Rotation completed, head drawn into pelvic cavity. (Jarcho in Amer. Jour. of Obstet. and Gynec., vol. 10, 1925, C. V. Mosby Co., Publishers.)

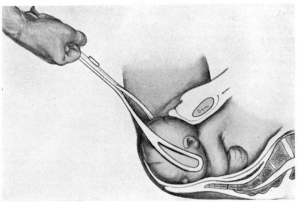

Fig. 440.—Completion of extraction. (Jarcho in Amer. Jour. of Obstet. and Gynec., vol. 10, 1925, C. V. Mosby Co., Publishers.)

The Barton Forceps.—A most ingenious and valuable forceps is that designed by Dr. Barton which differs from the usual type in that the blades join the shanks at an angle as shown in Fig. 441.

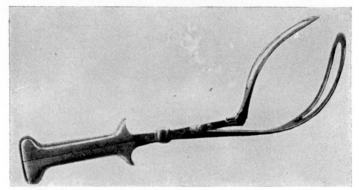

Fig. 441.—Barton forceps assembled. (Barton, Caldwell and Studdiford in Amer. Jour. of Obstet. and Gynec., vol. 15, 1928, C. V. Mosby Co., Publishers.)

This angle corresponds to the angle between the axis of the pelvic inlet and the outlet. The anterior blade has a hinge at the juncture of the blade and shank. The lock is a sliding one, and the whole instrument is slight and delicately made.

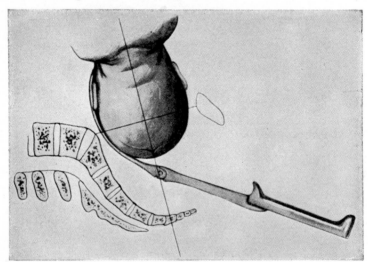

Fig. 442.—Introduction of anterior blade in midline posteriorly. (Barton, Caldwell and Studdiford in Amer. Jour. of Obstet. and Gynec., vol. 15, 1928, C. V. Mosby Co., Publishers.)

There is an axis-traction attachment, to be attached to the middle of the shank. In using the instrument the hinged anterior blade is slipped between symphysis and head until it rests over the parietal

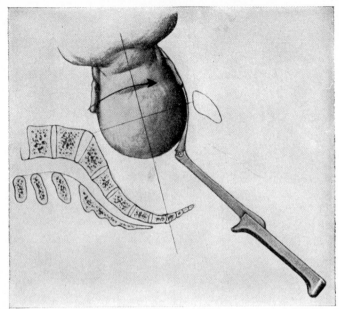

Fig. 443.—Anterior blade rotated to position in front of head. (Barton, Caldwell and Studdiford in Amer. Jour. of Obstet. and Gynec., vol. 15, 1928, C. V. Mosby Co., Publishers.)

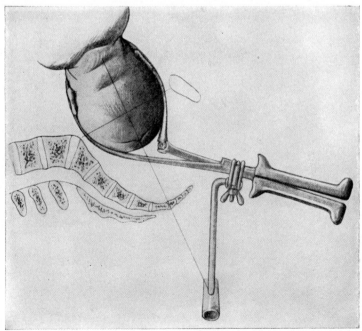

Fig. 444.—Posterior blade introduced, forceps locked, axis-traction rod attached. Note normal relation of head to pelvic axis and handle of axis-traction attachment in line with the axis of the superior strait. (Barton, Caldwell and Studdiford in Amer. Jour. of Obstet. and Gynec., vol. 15, 1928, C. V. Mosby Co., Publishers.)

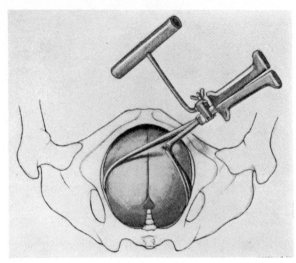

Fig. 445.—Rotation of head completed. (Barton, Caldwell and Studdiford in Amer. Jour. of Obstet. and Gynec., vol. 15, 1928, C. V. Mosby Co., Publishers.)

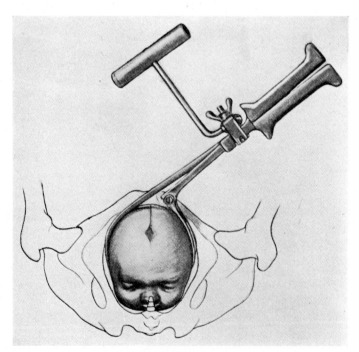

Fig. 446.—Delivery by extension of the head. (Barton, Caldwell and Studdiford in Amer. Jour. of Obstet. and Gynec., vol. 15, 1928, C. V. Mosby Co., Publishers.)

eminence. If this proves difficult, the blade may be directed to the lateral pelvic wall and then rotated around the occiput, until it reaches the correct position over the side of the head. The posterior blade is now introduced between head and promontory, the cephalic curve of the locked blades being directly anteroposterior in most cases of deep transverse arrest (Figs. 442, 443, 444, 445, 446).

Traction is made downward and backward directing the sagittal suture back toward the sacrum, and then with a levering motion the head is rotated into an anterior occipital position.

Delivery may be completed by these forceps, but it is often easier to remove them, when correct rotation has been effaced, and to complete the extraction with the ordinary type instrument.

COMPLICATIONS OF THE FORCEPS OPERATION

Laceration of the pelvic tissues is an ever-present danger. The blades of the forceps are sharp, and should their tips be misdirected, very deep incised wounds may follow, while lacerations through the sphincter ani are common sequelae of too enthusiastic effort upon the part of an athletic obstetrician. Slipping of the forceps from the child's head is dangerous because of the tendency to skull fracture of the fetus and the very severe injuries to the maternal tissues.

Even if these accidents do not occur, forceps extraction (other than outlet forceps) too often result in fetal damage, from compression of the brain, pinching of the cord between blade and head, injury to the eye and orbital plates and facial paralysis from pressure on the facial nerve.

By reason of the traumatism and the invasion of the pelvis by the forceps, infection is prone to follow this operation, which, hence, should always be performed with the most meticulous regard for asepsis.

THE ROUTINE DELIVERY OF PRIMIPARAE BY OUTLET FORCEPS AND EPISIOTOMY

In several of America's finest clinics most primiparous labors are terminated by episiotomy and forceps extraction, when the head has reached the outlet and is beginning to separate the pillars of the vulva.

Under ideal surroundings and in the hands of skilled specialists, such procedure has much to recommend it, indeed there are statistics on record comprising large series of cases, wherein it is clearly shown that fetal and maternal morbidity and mortality have actually been reduced by it, as compared to equally large series of spontaneous deliveries.

In general, however, it is much better practice to employ forceps only on indication, and to substitute for their use intelligent expectancy combined with analgesia and allow all labors to terminate spontaneously unless direct cause for intervention presents itself.

CHAPTER XLIII

BREECH EXTRACTION

THE dangers of breech presentation revolve mostly about the child, which is in peril from (a) compression of the cord between pelvis and body, (b) the malpresentation of a nuchal arm, (c) difficulty in the extraction of the after-coming head.

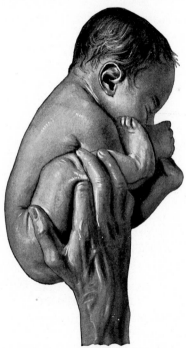

Fig. 447.—Bringing down foot. Pinard's maneuver. Passing the hand high up into the uterus, avoiding the cord, which is kept on the back of the hand, the index finger is pressed into the popliteal space. This shortens the hamstring muscles and flexes the leg, upon which the three fingers slip over the knee to the ankle, the foot now being wiped along the other thigh posteriorly into the pelvis and out. During the pains no move may be made—the hand should lie passive until the uterus relaxes. (DeLee.)

It is wiser to allow breech presentation to proceed spontaneously, at least until the buttocks are born, after which delivery may be manually completed if there should be delay.

The indications for extraction before the birth of the buttocks are prolonged delay in the second stage of labor, elevation of temperature, signs of exhaustion in the mother, and irregularities or abnormal slowing of the fetal heart.

Technic.—The patient must be anesthetized, bladder and rectum emptied and aseptically prepared. Extraction should never be attempted until the cervix is fully dilated, or so soft and yielding that the dilatation may be completed with the finger, without undue trauma. The woman is placed upon a table, the thighs elevated and slightly raised, but not too high.

The perineum is then ironed out as before described and when indicated an episiotomy is performed.

Breech extraction should not be carried out by traction alone, but there should always be synchronous suprapubic pressure upon the head.

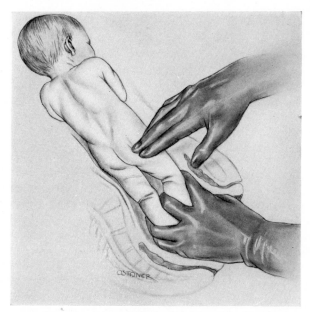

Fig. 448.—Breech extraction. Bringing down the feet.

The maintenance of flexion is one of the most important factors in successful extraction, and since traction has a constant tendency to break up flexion and favor extension, this must be met by the compensating pressure from above, which neutralizes the extensor force.

The operator then inserts his hand in the vagina and endeavors to secure both feet. If one foot is difficult to bring down, Pinard's maneuver is often successful (Fig. 447). This consists in pressing the index finger into the popliteal space which flexes the leg on the thigh. The fingers then slip along the leg, from the knee to the ankle, and the foot is passed along the other thigh, posteriorly into

44

the pelvis, the thigh being pushed outward and backward during the movement (Fig. 448).

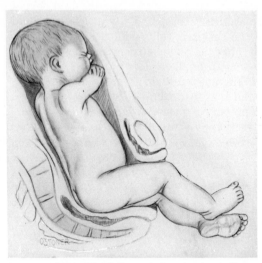

Fig. 449.—Breech extraction. The infant sitting in the hollow of the sacrum.

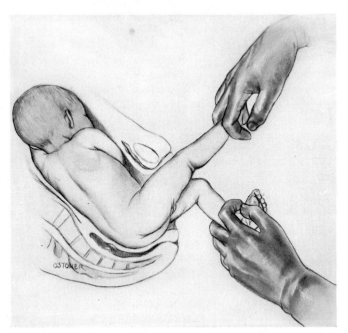

Fig. 450.—Breech extraction. Beginning the turning of the child.

The breech having thus been converted into a double footling, traction is made upon the posterior leg, to rotate the fetal back pos-

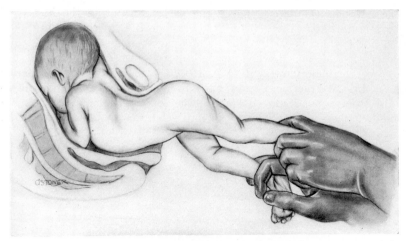

Fig. 451.—Breech extraction. Turning the body of the child in order to bring the back anterior.

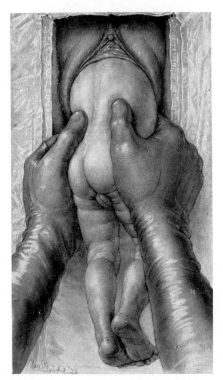

Fig. 452.—Breech extraction; extraction of body, thumbs over sacrum (Williams, "Obstetrics," D. Appleton-Century Co., Publishers.)

teriorly, so bringing the buttocks into the hollow of the sacrum. The buttocks should not be on the perineum, but in the hollow of the sacrum itself (Fig. 449). *Step two* consists in rotating the back anteriorly which is easily done by crossing the legs of the fetus, when by gentle traction downward, pulling the feet slightly apart, the fetus is completely rotated (Fig. 450), the back being now anterior (Fig. 451). Traction is continued in a direction somewhat downward from a horizontal line, until the scapulae appear. When the umbilicus has been delivered, the cord should be pulled down a little,

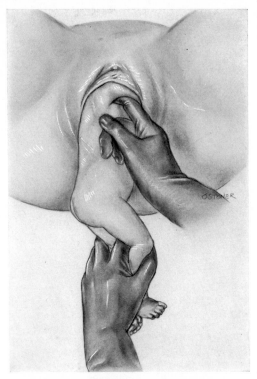

Fig. 453.—Breech extraction—delivery of the anterior arm by a finger in the axilla making backward pressure against the scapula.

and slipped away from a point of pressure. Its pulsations are noted, and if these be vigorous, no great haste is required. If, however, they be feeble or absent, the child is in great peril of asphyxia, and the delivery must be completed in as short a time as possible (Fig. 452).

The body is now rotated until one shoulder stems under the symphysis.

Step Three.—Then by placing the finger in the axilla, and pressing the scapula firmly backward and upward (Fig. 453), the arm slips out over the thorax and may be delivered by hooking a finger in the elbow joint, when the forearm and hand will slip out. If the child is small, the body may be raised and the posterior shoulder and arm delivered over the perineum, but if the fit is a tight one, the fetus should be again rotated, until the remaining shoulder is anterior, when it is brought out by the same manipulation as was used for the first shoulder.

Step Four.—For the delivery of the after-coming head. The methods in the order of their value are:

1. *Forceps.*—When the shoulders have been born, the back being anterior, the body of the child is carried upward toward the symphysis (not too high, to avoid undue angulation of the neck) and held by an assistant.

The Piper after-coming head forceps, or lacking these, a standard model, are applied to the sides of the child's head, and with moderate

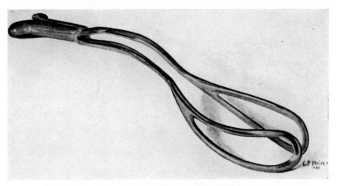

Fig. 454.—The Piper after-coming head forceps.

traction, and elevation of the handles, the chin, face and brow are swept over the perineum by extension (Fig. 454).

The Piper forceps, by far the best instrument for use on the after-coming head, in my opinion, embodies the following features:

A blade having a somewhat flattened pelvic curve for high application; a lengthened shank which permits an unusual amount of spring between the blades and thus prevents compression of the head and depressed handles for greater ease of manipulation and application in the presence of the delivered fetal body (Figs. 455, 456).

2. *Wiegand's Method.*—The first three fingers of the supinated hand are inserted into the vagina that hand being used whose palm corresponds to the abdomen of the child, whose body rests astride the forearm, a leg and arm hanging on each side.

The middle finger of the vaginal hand is inserted into the child's mouth, and the head brought into complete flexion by very gentle traction upon the jaw (Fig. 457).

The free hand of the operator, or better, that of an assistant, now seeks the fetal head through the abdominal wall and makes firm and continuous pressure downward upon it. The operator meanwhile,

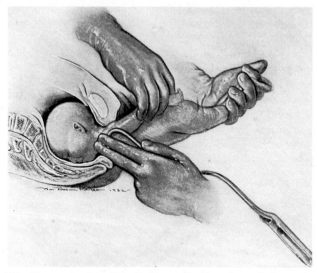

Fig. 455.—Demonstrating the direct application, from below, of the after-coming head forceps to the sides of the fetal head while an assistant holds the child's arms and legs out of the way. (Piper.)

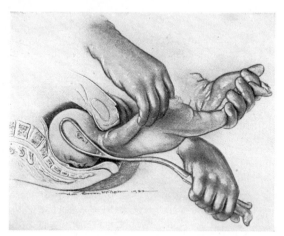

Fig. 456.—Both blades applied; ready for the extraction. (Piper.)

guides the head in the axis of the birth canal, making no traction other than the slight amount required to maintain flexion, and the chin, face, brow and occiput successively pass over the perineum, the whole head being literally pushed out of the parturient canal.

3. *The Mauriceau-Smellie-Veit Method.*—Here the hand is inserted in the vagina as described above, the middle finger in the

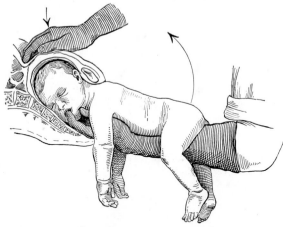

Fig. 457.—Delivery of the after-coming head in flexion by seizure of lower jaw, and extrusion by means of pressure in axis of brim (Wiegand's method). (B. C. Hirst.)

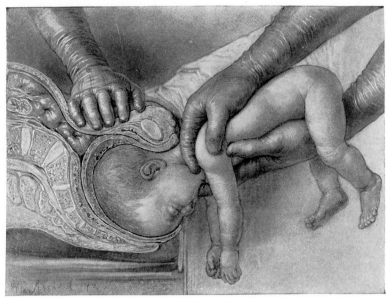

Fig. 458.—Mauriceau's maneuver, upward traction. (Williams, "Obstetrics," D. Appleton-Century Co., Publishers.)

child's mouth, the body resting astride the forearm as before. The middle finger of the other hand is now placed against the occiput of

the fetus, the forefinger and three fingers are flexed over its clavicles
and traction is made by this hand, the head being maintained in
flexion by the combined pressure of the finger on the occiput, and
the pull upon the jaw. As the head descends to the outlet, the body
is carried upward, delivery being effected by extension (Fig. 458).

A combination of this and the foregoing method of Wiegand is
often very valuable in cases of difficult extraction.

4. *The Deventer Method.*—This consists in grasping the legs of
the child and making strong traction downward and outward. The
arms usually extend along the sides of the head and when the
shoulders appear at the vulva, traction is continued, the child's body

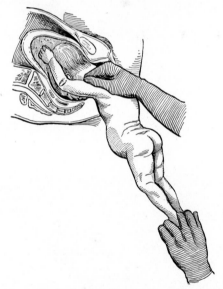

Fig. 459.—Deventer's method of extraction of the after-coming head and arms.
(B. C. Hirst.)

being depressed toward the buttocks of the mother, when the head
rolls out from between the arms, which rapidly follow. This is a
traumatic procedure, only employed when the child is small and premature, and is no longer in common use (Fig. 459).

THE DIFFICULTIES AND DANGERS OF BREECH EXTRACTION

Difficulty in reaching the feet may be experienced when the breech
is high in the pelvis. To bring the buttocks to the outlet, the forefinger may be hooked into the groin, or a forefinger may be introduced into each groin, when traction brings the body down.

If this is impracticable, forceps may be applied to the breech,
the blades resting over the crests of the ilia, the pull being downward
in the axis of the birth canal until the buttocks appear at the vulva.

This method is dangerous, first by reason of the tendency of the forceps to slip from their poor application and second because the end of the blade may cause injury to the liver or spleen of the child.

The blunt hook of the older accoucheurs has almost disappeared from the obstetrical armamentarium.

The arms may offer great obstruction to delivery, if they become extended, and especially should one or both come to lie behind the occiput; the so-called "nuchal" arm. This faulty position is often induced by rapid traction upon the body of the child, without pressure from above, and its occurrence may be recognized by a strong resistance to further descent, after the body of the child is born. The scapulae do not come down to the outlet, except under influence of vigorous traction.

The management consists in having the patient fully anesthetized, then pushing the child back into the pelvis until the shoulders become disengaged at the brim, when by rotating the body, so that the back is fully anterior, the arms are released and drop into their natural position of flexion.

If this does not serve, it may be necessary to insert the hand into the vagina, after pushing the fetus well up, as before, and then by finding the elbow joint, the arm is gently brought down, the hand passing over the face of the fetus, until it is again folded over the chest. The same procedure may be necessary for the release of the other arm.

Sometimes the shoulders are so broad that they cannot pass the outlet, in which case serious laceration of the pelvic floor with possible fracture of the clavicles of the child often follows. The situation can sometimes be remedied by extracting one arm and making traction upon it as well as upon the legs, though there is danger of brachial plexus injury if this be necessary.

Persistent posterior position, the head coming down with the chin anterior, and finally coming to rest under the symphysis, presents an awkward complication.

Whenever possible, the accident should be avoided, the body being turned back anterior during extraction.

If the head does come down with its occiput posterior, it is best delivered by forceps, either with rotation to an anterior position if possible or by sweeping the occiput, sinciput and then the face over the perineum with a marked upward direction of traction. This obviously greatly endangers the integrity of the pelvic floor, which is commonly seriously lacerated. Failing forceps, the fingers should be inserted into the vagina to discover whether the mouth can be entered under the symphysis. If this proves practicable, the head may be rotated in the cavity of the pelvis, an outside, abdominal hand aiding greatly in the rotation, while the body is held by an assistant.

Should the mouth be out of reach, Van Hoorn's maneuver may succeed. In this the fingers are hooked over the child's clavicles from behind, and the back is swept upward toward the symphysis, an abdominal hand meanwhile making firm pressure from above to push the occiput over the perineum.

It must be remembered that in all breech extractions there is a limited time after the birth of the umbilicus in which the delivery must be completed, if the child is to live.

Eight minutes is about the maximum for safety, for, while children do survive for a longer time after the placental circulation is cut off, late complications may carry them off, as pneumonia, atelectasis, etc.

In the mother, deep and extensive lacerations are to be apprehended especially if the delivery is a difficult one and the obstetrician loses finesse in his effort to conserve time.

Statistics have been adduced which show that the fetal mortality of breech presentations *per se*, without any complications of pregnancy or labor, is 6.5 per cent. If to this be added the tendency to prolapse of the cord, separation of the placenta, placenta praevia, etc., the danger to the child of this abnormal position will be readily understood.

CHAPTER XLIV

VERSION

By version is meant the reversal of the polarity of the fetus in relation to the mother, and hence there may be cephalic version, when a caudal presentation is converted into a cephalic one, or podalic version when a cephalic presentation is turned into a breech.

Version may be external, *i. e.*, performed entirely by abdominal taxis. Internal, when managed via the vagina, and combined, when both methods are utilized in conjunction.

External version has as its object the conversion of a breech or a transverse presentation into a cephalic one during pregnancy and always before labor has begun. The procedure is approved in many clinics, its object being to abolish the increased fetal mortality due to breech labor.

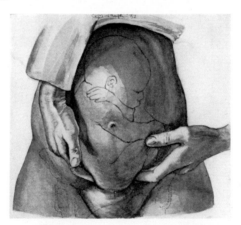

Fig. 460.—Gently mobilize the child, carefully dislodging the breech from the inlet. Listen to the fetal heart tones frequently. If the placenta is palpable on the anterior wall make only the gentlest motions. (M. E. Davis.)

External version may never be done, if labor pains have begun, nor if the breech be engaged. The optimum time for success is between the thirty-fourth and the thirty-sixth weeks of gestation.

The technic is simple.

In the ideal case, there should be no pelvic disproportion, the abdominal wall must be thin, the uterus relaxed, and there must be a sufficiency of liquor amnii (Figs. 460, 461, 462, 463).

The patient, undressed and draped, lies upon a table, the fetal heart tones are auscultated and the diagnosis of position confirmed.

699

The breech is then gently pushed upward and to one side with one hand, while the other manipulates the head downward on the opposite side of the abdomen. Should the uterus contract, the movements are

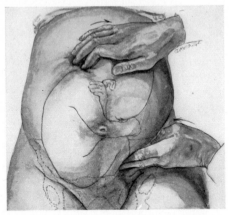

Fig. 461.—With one hand draw the breech out of the inlet into one iliac fossa, at the same time pressing the head toward the opposite flank with the other hand. (M. E. Davis.)

suspended until relaxation returns. When the head has been brought to the brim of the pelvis it is gently but firmly pressed into the inlet and held there for five or six minutes in the hope that fixation will take place.

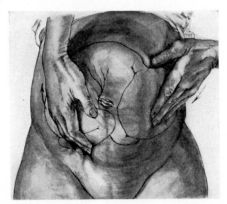

Fig. 462.—Listen to the fetal heart tones frequently for any change in rate or rhythm, which may signify interference with the fetal circulation. Turn the baby in the direction which maintains an attitude of complete flexion. If this fails, you may try to turn the child in the opposite direction. (M. E. Davis.)

Binders and pads along the sides of the uterus are of no value in maintaining the new position. Should recurrence occur, the maneuver may be repeated in a week. If a second attempt is unsuccessful, one should desist from efforts at external version. The fetal heart must be frequently auscultated during the procedure, any irregularity or marked alteration of rate constituting a danger sign.

Vaginal bleeding, strong uterine contractions and rupture of the membranes are contraindications to further manipulations. In my own clinics external version is rarely performed.

Cephalic version during labor is rarely done.

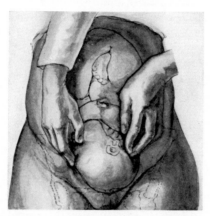

Fig. 463.—Hold the fetus in its new position, gently pressing the head down into the pelvic brim. If it engages easily, the new position will probably be retained. (M. E. Davis.)

Internal version is usually podalic in type.

The indications for its employment are:

Transverse lie of the fetus, usually shoulder.
Prolapse of the umbilical cord.
Errors in rotation and flexion of the head.
Parietal bone presentations.
Placenta praevia.
Any condition of mother or child demanding prompt delivery.
Slight pelvic contractions.

All of the foregoing indications are clear, with the exception of the last, which in the opinion of the writer exists only in unusual cases, expectancy followed by forceps being much safer for mother and child.

Conditions Necessary for Version:

The bladder and rectum must be empty.
The patient must be aseptically prepared.
The membranes must be intact or very recently ruptured.
The cervix must be fully dilated and effaced or very easily
    dilatable (except in Braxton Hicks' version, q. v.).
Surgical anesthesia is required.

The Contraindications to Version are:

Marked disproportion.

Tetanic contraction of the uterus, with a high contraction ring.

If the presenting part has passed through the external os.

Undilated cervix.

TECHNIC—COMBINED INTERNAL AND EXTERNAL PODALIC VERSION

The patient, being prepared and anesthetized, is placed on a table as for forceps extraction. The perineum is ironed out, and a preliminary episiotomy performed if this be deemed necessary.

The obstetrician should wear a short-sleeved gown and long version gloves which reach the elbow. A gown sleeve bunched at the wrist into the ordinary short glove makes an unwieldy and dangerous foreign body to introduce into the uterus.

The operator then introduces his most skilled hand into the vagina, without regard to the position of the child's back. If the cervix is not completely dilated this may be completed by manual stretching, but it is advised that version be postponed if possible until dilatation and effacement are complete.

When the membranes are unruptured, they should be preserved until the fingers have passed the level of the internal os, when they may be ruptured with the finger tips, the liquor amnii being retained in the uterus by the wrist which acts as a plug. The hand then passes up into the uterus, inside the membranes, and as the arms are reached, they are palpated, and if extended, are flexed on the child's chest.

The knee is then usually felt, and if the foot is difficult to reach the leg may be flexed by Pinard's maneuver, and the foot brought down. It is much better to endeavor to grasp both feet, since the full breech makes a better dilator for the birth canal and lessens the tendency to dystocia from an impacted after-coming head (Fig. 464).

Sometimes a tyro experiences difficulty in differentiating a hand from a foot, a knee from an elbow.

The knee is rounded, and usually its apex points toward the head. The elbow is sharp and usually points away from the head. The foot possesses the characteristic malleoli and the great toe cannot be abducted to any extent. The hand presents nothing comparable to the malleoli and the thumb may be separated widely from the fingers.

When both feet cannot be grasped, it is best to attempt to bring down the posterior one which tends to rotate the back forward so that the buttocks of the child may rest in the hollow of the sacrum.

In practice, however, it is wise to bring down that foot which is first grasped, provided both cannot be seized.

With the feet firmly held, traction is made upon them, while with the other hand, abdominal pressure is made upon the head pushing it upward and outward. A firm but gentle and sustained pull accompanied by a steady pushing upward of the head will generally bring about the desired reversal of polarity in a few minutes. Attempts at version should be discontinued during a uterine contraction, after which they may be resumed. When the knees appear at the vulva and the head is in the fundus, the version has been completed, and the delivery as a footling may be left to nature's efforts (not good practice) or extraction may follow in the manner before described.

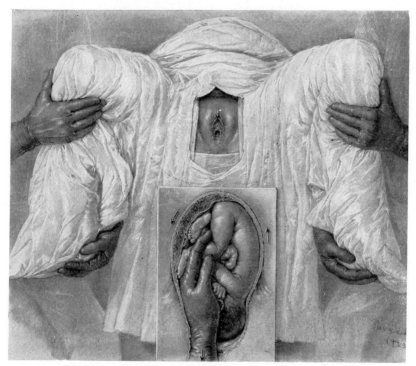

Fig. 464.—Patient in position for internal podalic version. Inset shows hand in uterus grasping the feet. (Williams, "Obstetrics," D. Appleton-Century Co., Publishers.)

Version in transverse presentation does not differ materially from podalic version, except that the feet are nearer the cervix, and there is a considerable probability of a prolapsed arm. In the latter case, a fillet should be placed around the wrist, and lightly held by an assistant in order to keep the arm lying alongside the chest, thus preventing extension of it over the head (Figs. 465, 466).

Braxton Hicks' Version.—This is a combined podalic version done often before the cervix is fully dilated and effaced. Its purpose is to bring down the buttocks of the child that they may press upon a placenta praevia and so reduce the bleeding from it.

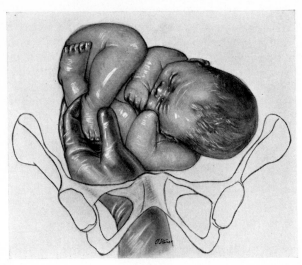

Fig. 465.—Version in transverse presentation seizing the anterior foot.

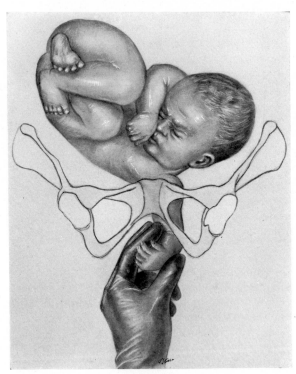

Fig. 466.—Version in transverse position. Replacing the prolapsed arm after it has been cleansed.

If the placenta is marginally or laterally placed, the membranes are ruptured beside it, and two fingers are inserted into the uterus. Only one foot is sought and when found it is brought down, the head being helped upward as before until the knee appears at the vulva. The breech is now in contact with the low-lying placenta, and spontaneous delivery is awaited, with a full knowledge that the child is in great danger from asphyxia by, as it were, sitting on its own blood supply. This operation, however, is always undertaken primarily in the interests of the mother, who lies in grave peril from hemorrhage. If the placenta praevia is central, the fingers must perforate this organ in order to reach the foot, a procedure generally attended by sharp bleeding which is only checked by the prompt pulling down of the breech to act as a tampon.

THE DANGERS OF VERSION

For the child the dangers are those of breech extraction: intracranial injury, asphyxiation, and fracture of limbs.

For the mother, the complications to be feared are rupture of the uterus, premature detachment of the placenta, laceration of the cervix and subsequent infection.

Rupture of the uterus is a too frequent sequel to version. When the operation is attempted long after the membranes have ruptured, and the uterus is closely molded to the contours of the child's body, with a high contraction ring, the introduction of the hand is often sufficiently traumatic to provoke a tear of the uterus. It is accordingly good practice to explore the uterus manually after every difficult version and extraction to determine whether or not such accident has occurred.

Premature detachment of the placenta may happen at any time during version. A sudden gush of blood will apprise the attendant of the accident, in which case the delivery should be completed as rapidly as may be and the uterus subsequently packed with sterile gauze.

Lacerations of the cervix are common when version is attempted before dilatation and effacement are complete. The manual dilatation which must precede the operation in such instances is traumatic and frequently results in extensive tears, even up to the broad ligament. It is this complication which renders routine version without indication such a dangerous practice, not only from the standpoint of mortality, but from the serious and permanent damage to the cervix which so often follows.

45

CHAPTER XLV

CESAREAN SECTION

CESAREAN section consists in the abdominal extraction of the child from an incision in the uterus, made after laparotomy. The history of this operation is an epitome of medical progress and the reader is referred to the memoirs of Pickerell and Schilling upon this interesting subject:

Indications.—The indications for cesarean section may be grossly divided into absolute and relative ones. Pelves with a true conjugate of 6 to 6½ cm. will not permit the vaginal delivery of a full-sized child, even though it be mutilated by embryotomy, and hence abdominal delivery is imperative and the indication is said to be absolute.

Relative indications for section are any others than the above and therefore vary widely under the influence of different schools of thought.

Cesarean section may be further divided into the *section of election,* when the procedure is determined prior to the onset of labor, and as a deliberate choice between abdominal and vaginal delivery, and the *section of necessity,* when dystocia or some accident of labor renders its performance indispensable.

The indications for the elective cesarean section are:

Contracted pelvis.

Placenta praevia.

Abruptio placentae.

Tumors of the pelvis obstructing labor.

Advanced systemic diseases, as cardiopathy, tuberculosis, etc.

Certain cases of eclampsia and preeclampsia.

Previous cesarean section with weak scars.

Dystocia from previous pelvic operations, as antefixation of the uterus.

Certain cases of malpresentation, especially if associated with minor degrees of pelvic contraction.

Rarely obstruction from rigidity or stenosis of cervix or vagina.

Sometimes in elderly primiparae, in the presence of fetal distress.

As may be inferred from the multiplicity of indications, delivery by cesarean section may be chosen in the presence of almost any of the complications of pregnancy or labor, and it is this fact which has led to its wholesale abuse, and the unsavory reputation which this invaluable procedure has acquired in many quarters.

It is true that anyone acquainted with the rudiments of abdominal surgery can perform an abdominal hysterotomy, and hence its employment by those untrained in the niceties of vaginal delivery.

The indications in detail have been fully discussed in the chapters devoted to these several subjects and hence need no repetition here.

A question which continually arises is whether cesarean section once performed requires a repetition of the operation in subsequent pregnancies. "Once a cesarean, always a cesarean," is an old dictum which still holds good in many instances, but not routinely so.

Statistics show that 3 per cent of cesarean scars rupture during succeeding labors, with a high maternal and fetal mortality, but like other statistics, these figures are subject to much correction. Who

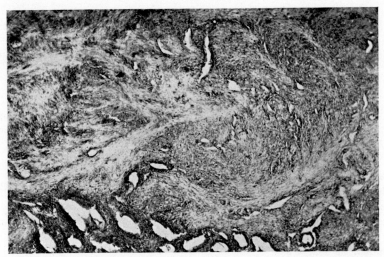

Fig. 467.—Uterine scar after two classical cesarean sections showing firm fibrous union.

did the section? Why? Under what conditions? All of these factors are of such paramount importance that they must be closely scrutinized if the truth is to prevail (Fig. 467).

When the operation has been done by skilled obstetricians, under correct conditions, the scar will not rupture subsequently in more than ½ of 1 per cent of all cases. On the other hand, if the uterine wound has not been properly coapted or if infection followed, the ratio of ruptures will be high. Sometimes even though the previous operation has been well done the placental site in the next pregnancy will lie over the scar, and this fact does tend to weaken it and so predispose to rupture during labor, although the complication is uncommon.

Obviously, if the indication for the first hysterotomy was a correctly diagnosed contracted pelvis, the same conditions demand repeated section. If the original procedure was inspired by placenta praevia, toxemia, etc., it may not at all be necessary to repeat it.

My own practice is as follows:

All cases in which pelvic disproportion once indicated cesarean, continue to indicate it, and the operation is routinely performed. When conditions other than pelvic contraction were responsible for the original operation, the patient must be delivered of later children in hospital, and upon the onset of labor, the operating room is set up in order that immediate laparotomy may be performed, should evidences of impending or actual rupture appear.

Types.—These are the varieties of cesarean section in common use:

The classical (Sanger) operation.

The low cervical (laparotrachelotomy).

Cesarean section with hysterectomy (miscalled the Porro operation).

Two other modifications for use in frankly infected cases are now being fairly widely used.

The Latzko extraperitoneal operation.

The Gottschalk-Portes operation.

Choice of which of these procedures offers the best hope of an optimum result depends upon the type of case and the skill and experience of the operator.

In recent statistics the low cervical operation is shown to be much safer for the mother than the classical one, but here again the figures are open to considerable criticism if it be remembered that the laparotrachelotomy type demands training and skill and is therefore done in the main, by obstetric specialists, whereas the classical operation is the one chosen by the occasional operator and the surgeon untrained in obstetrics.

In potentially infected cases the low operation is superior in that, should infection occur, its spread is more or less limited to the tissues under the bladder reflection and therefore it tends to remain extraperitoneal and become a parametritis or pelvic cellulitis a far safer variety of sepsis than that involving the general peritoneum.

Cesarean with hysterectomy, or the Latzko and Gottschalk-Portes procedures are reserved for frankly infected cases, although the first is utilized in instances of rupture of the uterus and certain types of abruptio placentae.

Choice of Anesthetic.—Local anesthesia by simple infiltration with ½ per cent novocain is the method of choice in all elective sections, and the writer has not had occasion to use any other variety in elective section during the past fifteen years.

If the patient be in active labor, nitrous oxide and oxygen, ethylene or ether where skilled anesthetists are lacking are used. Spinal anesthesia has many advocates but this is rarely used in my clinic.

Elective Cesarean Section.—If upon a fitting indication, elective section is selected as the type of delivery to be undertaken, the operation should be performed before the onset of labor if possible, the last two weeks of pregnancy being the most favorable time. Previous studies determine whether the child is living and in good condition since a dead or deformed child constitutes a major contraindication to section unless in the latter case the monster be of some type which is not amenable to vaginal delivery.

The patient herself should be prepared for the ordeal by a few days' rest and any appropriate medication. For elective section the classical operation is by far the best in my opinion. It is more easily and rapidly performed than any other, lends itself admirably to local anesthesia and if properly done carries no mortality or morbidity risk other than that of any intra-abdominal procedure.

Technic of Operation.—To obtain the optimum results from the elective section under local anesthesia, close attention to a number of small details is absolutely necessary. The patient is admitted to the hospital twenty-four hours before the contemplated operation and is subjected to the usual laboratory tests and a careful physical investigation. A vaginal examination, with estimation of the relation between fetal and pelvic size determines the correctness or error of the previous findings. The diet is light, with an abundance of fluids. The colon is emptied by a soapsuds enema. Three hours before operation, sodium luminal is administered by mouth, the dose varying from 3 to 5 grains, depending upon the physique of the patient. At this time her relatives are excluded from the darkened room and the woman usually rapidly falls asleep. Forty-five minutes before operation she is gently and quietly taken to the anesthesia or some other room adjacent to the operating room and is placed upon the operating table. A hypodermic injection of $\frac{1}{6}$ grain of morphine sulphate and $\frac{1}{150}$ grain of scopolamine hydrobromide is then given and absolute quiet maintained. At the appointed time, when all arrangements for operation have been completed, the operator and assistants scrubbed and ready, the patient, her eyes lightly covered, is wheeled into the operating room in which silence is maintained. The abdomen is gently swabbed with iodine followed by alcohol and then draped. Preoperative catheterization is not necessary. A line of incision 12 cm. long, extending from 3 cm. above the umbilicus to 9 cm. below it and about 2 cm. to the right of this point is then anesthetized with $\frac{1}{2}$ per cent novocain containing 10 minims of adrenalin to the ounce of solution. The skin, fascia, muscles, and peritoneum are in turn injected, slowly and painstakingly. The abdominal parietes are then incised, sponging being by gentle, quiet pressure, no wiping or rubbing being permitted. Bleeding is controlled by clamp and ligature and the peritoneum further injected with the anesthetic solution if the patient exhibits any evidence of pain. The fundus uteri now presses upward into the incision and a suture of No. 2 chromic catgut on a medium-sized curved needle is passed through the fascia, muscle and peritoneum at the extreme upper angle of the incision. The needle now pierces the uterine wall, a little to the right of the incision, thus correcting the normal dextroversion of that organ. Peritoneum, muscle and fascia on the opposite side of the incision are now transfixed and the sutures tied firmly, the ends left long and held by a hemostat. The

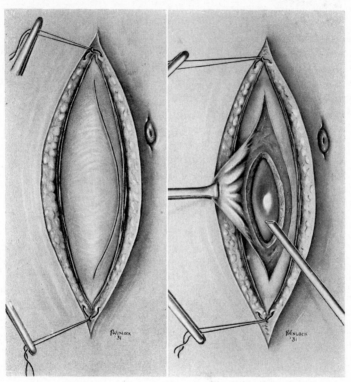

Fig. 468. Fig. 469.

Fig. 468.—Classical cesarean section. Author's technic. The abdominal incision and the uterus sutured to its angle to avoid intestinal protrusion and spill of liquor amnii. Semilunar incision of the uterine peritoneum.

Fig. 469.—The peritoneal flap retracted, the uterus incised and the membranes bulging through. Trocar to drain away liquor amnii. (Figures 468 and 469 from author's article in Amer. Jour. of Obstet. and Gynec., Feb., 1932, C. V. Mosby Co., Publishers.)

same maneuver is carried out at the extreme lower angle of the incision and when both sutures are tied and the hemostats attached to them are firmly held tight by an assistant, the anterior uterine wall is seen to be in intimate contact with the spread-open parietal peritoneum (Fig. 468). No further infiltration is necessary, the uterine wall being insensitive to pain.

A semilunar incision just through the uterine serosa is now made extending from one of the stay sutures to the other. The center of the flap so begun is grasped by an Allis clamp and with a few snips of the scissors the flap is dissected well back beyond the proposed line of incision in the uterine wall. The musculature under the flap is now carefully incised until a pouch of membranes bulges up into the wound (Fig. 469). The liquor amnii is then aspirated with a trocar, the fluid draining into a basin and so preventing spill and the soiling of the drapes. The uterine incision is then lengthened by cutting and tearing with the finger until it is approximately 11 cm. in length, and the fetus is grasped by the feet and extracted in the usual manner, except that owing to the shortness of the wound, the shoulders and head must be delivered slowly and carefully, the head being maintained in flexion by a finger inserted into the mouth.

A hypodermic injection of 1 cc. of pituitrin (obstetric) and 1 cc. of ergot is now administered and the placenta and membranes carefully withdrawn. The uterus is closed by tier suture, an inner layer

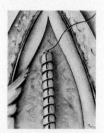

Fig. 470.—Closure of the uterine incision. (Author's article in Amer. Jour. of Obstet. and Gynec., Feb., 1932, C. V. Mosby Co., Publishers.)

of No. 0 chromic gut, a wide middle layer of No. 2 chromic gut, and the serosal flap is fastened back in place by a No. 0 gut suture, entirely covering the uterine muscle incision (Fig. 470).

If the uterine muscle is very thick, or if bleeding is troublesome mattress sutures of catgut may be required. At no time during the operation is the uterus eventrated, and the stay sutures are always held taut. No packing or walling-off is necessary nor is the abdominal cavity sponged at any time. The stay sutures are now cut away, the uterus sinks into the abdomen, and the abdominal incision is closed by tier suture, an intracutaneous skin stitch, or skin clips being utilized. A firm occlusive dressing of adhesive plaster is applied to complete the procedure. The uterus is not packed except in cases of placenta praevia when packing is always inserted.

Patients so treated usually take light diet on the evening of the operation and are subsequently managed as ordinary puerpera, out of bed on the tenth day and discharged on the fourteenth. Two minor points should never be neglected. If the operation has consumed some time, it will probably be necessary to reinfiltrate the parietal peritoneum and the skin with novocain to prevent a painful closure. Second, the moment it is observed that the patient does not respond well to local anesthesia and begins to complain or to move, this method should be abandoned at once and nitrous oxide inhalation be commenced. An anesthetist with gas apparatus should always be in attendance for this purpose. It is infinitely better surgery to admit the failure of local anesthesia early, than to prolong its use in a suffering, complaining patient.

Laparotrachelotomy is the low cervical section, devised by Frank, modified by Sellheim and perfected and popularized in America by Beck and DeLee.

This operation contemplates the separation of the bladder from the lower uterine segment, and the turning back a flap of peritoneum

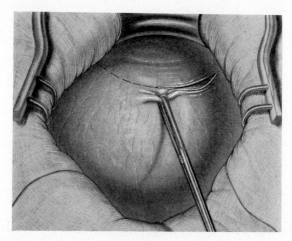

Fig. 471.—Low or cervical cesarean section. Incising the peritoneal reflection of the bladder.

on the anterior surface of the uterus, just above the bladder reflection. In the area of lower segment and cervix exposed by the retraction of these two flaps the uterus is incised, the child and placenta extracted, the former usually with forceps and the uterine wound closed, the peritoneal flaps being allowed to cover it and being sutured in position to complete the work. The operation is far easier of performance when the patient has been in active labor for several hours, since the stretching of the lower uterine segment gives more room, and draws the cervix away from the bladder. Its advantages are that infection, if it occurs, is less liable to become generalized, but rather tends to remain localized within the pelvis; there is less likelihood of peritoneal adhesion; the scar in the uterus is stronger and hence rupture in subsequent pregnancies is minimized; a true test of labor is possible, as uterine contractions rather aid the performance of this operation and also some women may deliver by the vaginal route after test of labor, who would otherwise have been subjected to section.

Technic.—A midline incision is made in the lower abdomen, entirely below the umbilicus.

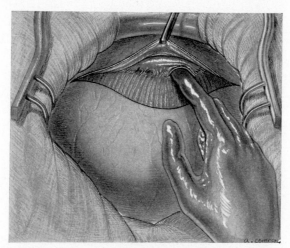

Fig. 472.—Low or cervical cesarean section. Separating the bladder.

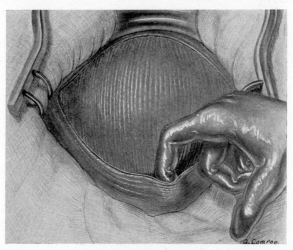

Fig. 473.—Low or cervical cesarean section. Separating and retracting the upper peritoneal flap.

The bladder reflection of the peritoneum is incised laterally for about 8 cm. and the bladder is separated either by blunt or sharp dissection and retracted downward (Figs. 471, 472, 473).

By means of scissors passed under it and then widely opened, an upper peritoneal flap is separated from the anterior surface of the uterus, and retracted upward. In the space thus obtained, the uterus is opened by a longitudinal incision, after traction sutures have been inserted at the upper and lower margins of the divided uterine sur-

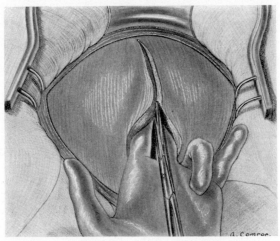

Fig. 474.—Low or cervical cesarean section. Incising the uterus.

face. (Some operators prefer a transverse incision in the uterus.) Intestinal forceps may be applied to the edges of the uterine wound to minimize bleeding (Fig. 474).

With a finger in the mouth, the face of the child is rotated anteriorly, and delivery is accomplished by forceps (Fig. 475), or the hand

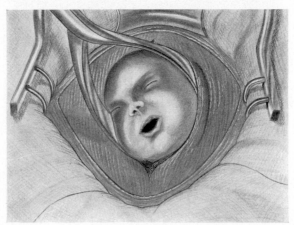

Fig. 475.—Low or cervical cesarean section. Extracting the child with forceps.

may be slipped under the head forcing it upward into the wound, while pressure on the fundus uteri from above pushes the head out of the opening. In the event of a breech presentation the infant is de-

livered by the feet. Pituitrin and ergot are administered hypodermically, and after the expulsion of the placenta, the uterine wound is

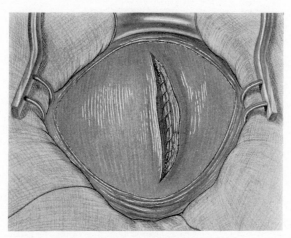

Fig. 476.—Low or cervical cesarean section. The first layer of sutures in the
uterine wall.

closed by interrupted sutures of catgut, silk, or whatever material is
preferred by the individual operator (Fig. 476).

A second layer of either interrupted or continuous sutures (Fig.
477) is now introduced and finally the peritoneal flaps are permitted

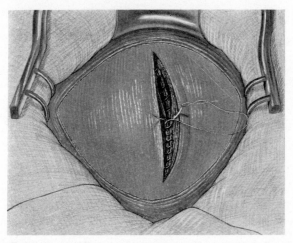

Fig. 477.—Low or cervical cesarean section. The second layer of sutures.

to cover the divided area of the uterus and are held in position by a
running suture of fine catgut (Fig. 478). The uterus may or may not
be packed with sterile gauze before closure, as desired (Fig. 479).

Packing is not generally used except in cases of placenta praevia when its employment should be universal.

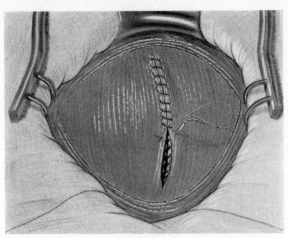

Fig. 478.—Low or cervical cesarean section. The superficial suture layer.

Cesarean Section with Hysterectomy.—This operation was devised by Porro of Pavia who fastened the cervical stump in the lower angle of the incision by a strong clamp, which held the crushed and avascular stump, outside the abodminal cavity. It has since been modified,

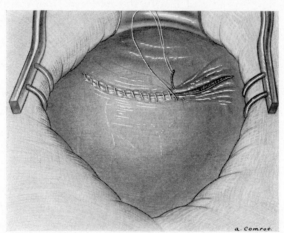

Fig. 479.—Low or cervical cesarean section. The bladder and upper peritoneal fold united. Completion of the operation.

and has become the usual type of supravaginal hysterectomy, with dropped stump.

The procedure is indicated in frankly infected cases, in rupture of the uterus, in presence of multiple or single large fibromata, and in abruptio placentae where the uterine muscle is infused with blood, which appears as petechiae under the serosal surface.

Technic.—The usual midline incision is followed by opening the uterus, withdrawing the child (taking care to avoid spill by detailed packing off the uterus from the other abdominal viscera), then closing the uterine incision by one or two deep sutures, the placenta and cord remaining within the cavity. The contracting uterus is then drawn out of the abdomen, and the intestines walled off by fresh abdominal pads.

A curved Kelly forceps is placed upon each broad ligament close to the uterine wall, the forceps including in their grasp, the fallopian tube, the ovarian ligament and the round ligament. These forceps prevent regurgitant bleeding from the uterus, and facilitate handling this organ.

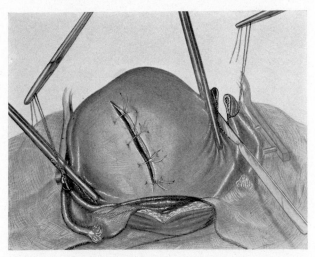

Fig. 480.—Cesarean section with hysterectomy. The incision in the uterine wall is held together by a few through-and-through sutures. The right broad ligament and ovarian artery are ligated.

The tubes and ovaries are usually to be conserved and accordingly a suture ligature of No. 2 chromic catgut is placed around the top of the broad ligament, about 1 inch distant to the uterus. This ligature controls the ovarian artery and the fallopian tube. The ends of the ligature are left long and held by a hemostat. Another suture ligature is placed on the round ligament, and cut short (Fig. 480).

The procedure is repeated on the opposite side, and both broad ligaments and the round ligaments cut, leaving sufficient stump to prevent slipping of the ligatures.

The bladder reflection of the peritoneum is now nicked and incised laterally to the sides of the uterus and the bladder is pushed down-ward with gauze, aided by occasional snips of the scissors if this be required (Fig. 481).

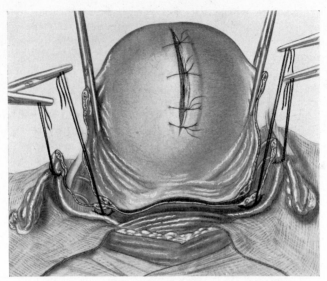

Fig. 481.—Both broad ligaments are divided. The bladder reflection is separated and the bladder pushed down.

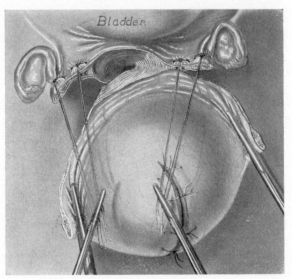

Fig. 482.—Both uterine arteries have been ligated and the fundus uteri amputated at the internal os.

The uterine arteries, running along the sides of the cervix and lower uterine segment may now be palpated, and tied with suture ligature, the needle being passed at right angles to the long axis of the uterus, just within the muscle, to surround the arteries. These ligatures are left long, and the uterus is then amputated with a scalpel, coning out the cervix a little in the process (Fig. 482). If the case is frankly infected the cervix may be amputated with the cautery, a sponge being placed in the cul-de-sac to absorb spill if any. As the anterior cervical wall is cut through, the stump is seized and held in forceps to prevent its dropping into the cul-de-sac. The cervix is

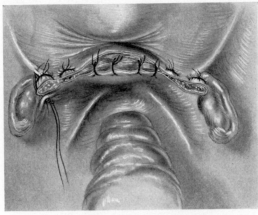

Fig. 483.—The cervical stump has been closed by interrupted sutures. Peritonealization begun.

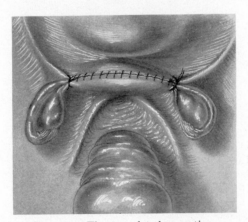

Fig. 484.—The completed operation.

then closed with interrupted sutures, the center one being placed first and its long ends used as a traction rod. The stumps of the broad ligaments are now surrounded with a second reinforcing ligature, and their cut ends sewn lightly to the cervical stump, as are the round ligaments. The bladder reflection is then pulled over the cervical stump and sutured in place with a continuous suture of No. 0 chromic gut and the operation is completed (Figs. 483, 484).

The above technic is simple, and by its use no clamps are placed upon tissues which are to remain, and these are therefore spared the traumatism of being crushed by the clamps. The abdominal incision is closed in the usual manner, without drainage.

The Latzko Operation.—This is a truly extraperitoneal operation, involving the dislocation of the bladder from its position on the anterior uterine wall, extracting the child through an incision in the area thus exposed, closing the wound, and allowing the bladder to resume its normal position. The peritoneal cavity is not invaded, and the operation offers excellent results in infected cases, its main disadvantage being its technical difficulty.

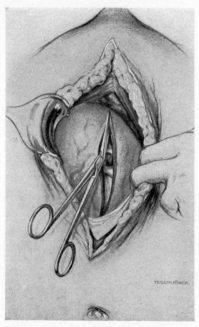

Fig. 485.—Latzko extraperitoneal cesarean section. Guided by the fingers, the thin lower uterine segment is incised. Avoid sharp retractors and too violent lateral pulling. (DeLee.)

The indications are the necessity for abdominal delivery in a frankly infected patient, with a living child.

Technic.—The bladder, after being emptied is filled with **200 cc.** of boric acid solution, introduced through an indwelling catheter, which is then clamped and fastened to the thigh.

The patient is placed in a high Trendelenburg position, the abdomen prepared, and a midline incision is made from the symphysis to the upper edge of the distended bladder. The incision is carried down to the fascia, and the anterior sheath of the rectus is divided a little to the left of the midline and the muscle dislocated and pulled

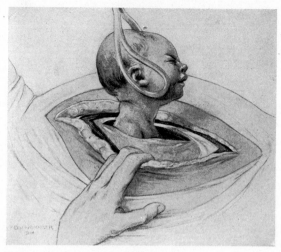

Fig. 486.—Latzko extraperitoneal cesarean section. Table horizontal. The head is pulled into position for forceps either by means of a finger in the mouth and the child delivered as in face presentation, or a vulsellum is fastened to the occiput and thus the head steadied for the application of the blades. Deliver slowly. If necessary to enlarge the uterine incision, do it under the eye. A tear would extend toward the side where are the ureter, large veins, and the uterine artery. The placenta may be removed manually or expressed by Credé. If needed, an injection of pituitrin may be given into the uterine muscle. (DeLee.)

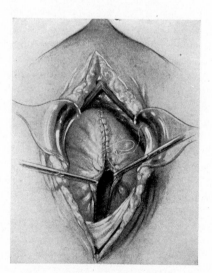

Fig. 487.—Latzko extraperitoneal cesarean section. Uterine suture, three rows. Now draw the peritoneum down, bring the bladder into position, and fasten it with a few sutures. Leave a rubber drain in the lowest corner of wound. Abdominal closure. (DeLee.)

46

to the left (Fig. 485). The posterior sheath of the rectus is then carefully incised, care being taken not to penetrate the bladder or peritoneum. The bladder is then separated from the posterior sheath of the rectus by blunt dissection, using the finger: this dissection aided by scissors is continued until the bladder is entirely free from the rectus fascia—up to the peritoneal reflection. The left side of the bladder is then separated from the uterus and the whole organ is gently worked off its uterine attachment toward the right. The vesico-uterine fold of peritoneum is then freed from the lower uterine segment, care being taken not to enter the peritoneal cavity at this point. The bladder is then emptied; and a longitudinal incision made in the lower uterine segment, and delivery effected by forceps as in laparotrachelotomy (Fig. 486). Pituitrin is administered and the placenta and membranes extracted. The uterine incision is then closed, by two layers of interrupted sutures or, the upper layer may be continuous, after which the bladder is allowed to drop back into place and so held by a few interrupted sutures. A small rubber dam drain is left in the retrovesical space, and the abdominal wound closed (Fig. 487).

The advantages of the Latzko operation are that the peritoneal cavity is not opened and hence the factor of sepsis is greatly minimized, and the operation is well fitted for use in infected patients.

Hemorrhage is not marked and postoperative shock is unusual.

The disadvantages are the technical difficulty of the procedure, which, however, can be overcome by familiarity with its details, the danger of opening the peritoneum, and the possibility of injury to the bladder. Any untoward effect of either of these accidents can be obviated by immediate repair of any wound made in either tissue.

The Gottschalk-Portes Operation.—This is a two-stage operation, designed for the treatment of frankly infected cases and has not yet enjoyed a widespread popularity. From personal experience I am inclined to believe it offers great hope of successful management of neglected cases, and may practically eliminate any necessity for the mutilation of the living child.

The procedure is as follows:

The first stage consists in making a midline incision long enough to permit eventration of the unopened uterus. This being delivered, is held forward in anteversion while the abdominal wound is closed to the posterior aspect of the cervix. The wound is then covered with a protective dressing, and the uterus is opened by a high fundal incision, the child, placenta and membranes are extracted. The uterine wound may then be closed, or if desired left open for drainage, although the latter method rather predicates an imperfectly healed uterine scar. The uterus is covered with dressings kept soft and moist with sterile albolene. This procedure can be easily carried out under local anesthesia and produces but little shock (Fig. 488).

The second stage may be conducted in one of two ways, depending upon the late developments. If the infection subsides, and the uterus involutes normally, it may be replaced within the abdomen

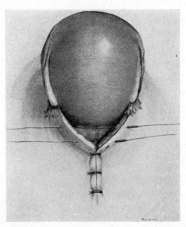

Fig. 488.—Portes operation. Median abdominal incision from symphysis to near xiphoid cartilage. The pregnant uterus is placed in marked anteversion to permit the rapid suturing of the abdominal wall. The sutured abdominal wall is covered with sterile towels; the uterus is dropped on it; gauze wicks are placed around the lower segment and an incision is made on the anterior wall, encroaching on the fundus. The fetus, placenta, and membranes are extracted and the uterine incision is closed in two layers with No. 2 chromic catgut. The uterus is covered with a moist sterile dressing and a tight abdominal binder is applied. (Phaneuf in Surg., Gynec., and Obstet., vol. 44, June, 1927.)

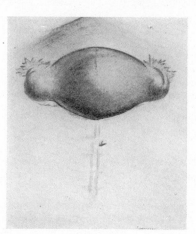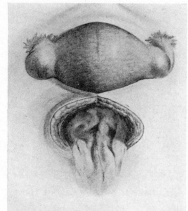

Fig. 489. Fig. 490.

Figs. 489 and 490.—Portes operation. The abdominal incision is reopened; the intestines are protected with gauze. Intestinal adhesions are exceptional. (Phaneuf in Surg., Gynec., and Obstet., vol. 44, June, 1927.)

when the wound in its anterior surface has firmly healed (Figs. 489, 490).

The uterus is carefully cleansed with tincture of green soap, followed by alcohol, the abdominal incision is reopened, the cervix freed from its adhesion to the lower angle of the wound, and dropped back into its normal position. A drain is laid in the cul-de-sac, and the abdominal incision again closed, about the drain (Figs. 491, 492).

If the infection grows worse, the uterus may be removed at any time postpartum, by the Porro technic and without other than local infiltration anesthesia in the broad ligaments. The ovaries may be retained, and subsequently dropped back into the abdomen, as described above.

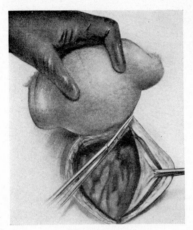 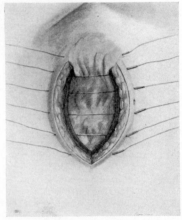

Fig. 491.   Fig. 492.

Fig. 491.—Portes operation. The adhesions to the uterovaginal pedicle are, at first, separated with scissors and then with the finger until the pedicle is free from the abdominal wall. The uterus and the adnexa are dropped in the pelvic cavity, where they assume their normal positions.

Fig. 492.—Portes operation. Through-and-through sutures of silkworm gut booted with fine rubber tubing are introduced. A cigaret drain is placed in the cul-de-sac of Douglas and comes out behind the uterus. The gauze is withdrawn, the omentum is brought down, and the sutures are tied. (Figs. 491 and 492 from Phaneuf in Surg., Gynec., and Obstet., vol. 44, June, 1927.)

The mortality of this operation as reported is 11 per cent, a very low incidence considering the desperate condition of many of the patients upon whom it was performed.

At least four women, in the reported series, have carried later pregnancies to term and have been successfully delivered by classical cesarean section, done electively.

THE AFTER-CARE OF CESAREAN SECTION PATIENTS

The usual postoperative care prescribed for laparotomies in general is used after cesarean section. When inhalation anesthesia has been employed, liquid diet for two days, an enema on the third and, when the bowels have moved, light diet is the ordinary routine. Morphine is given freely for pain, and laxatives are avoided until after the third postoperative day. If the patient is enfeebled or has been vomiting, glucose solution 10 per cent is administered intravenously in 500 to 1000 cc. amounts, every day or two for the first three days. The baby should nurse as usual, and the patient, if all goes well, may sit out of bed on the tenth postoperative day and leave the hospital on the fourteenth. Catheterization is generally necessary for a day or two, and after voluntary voiding has been established, it is well to catheterize the patient once or twice to be certain that residual urine does not remain in the bladder. If this is found to be the case the catheterization should be continued until the bladder has regained its tone and is able to empty itself completely.

THE COMPLICATIONS AND DANGERS OF CESAREAN SECTION

The two complications of importance which may follow cesarean section are peritonitis and hemorrhage.

The former is an ever-present peril, not threatening when the case is a purely elective one, done before the onset of labor and without vaginal manipulation, but becomes more and more perilous, as preoperative infection is more definitely present.

The rupture of the membranes implies potential infection and it has been shown abundantly that the danger of sepsis increases in almost direct ratio to the time intervening between such rupture and operation. This danger is immensurably increased after vaginal manipulation and attempt at forceps delivery or, worse still, version.

If the patient have an elevation of temperature or a foul vaginal discharge, prior to operation, the outlook is serious indeed.

The average gross maternal mortality following this operation in the United States is somewhere about 10 per cent. Inasmuch as this includes all cases, the correctly performed ones done on true indications, as well as those which, unfortunately, have been performed by unskilled operators, untrained in the selection of the proper operation to meet the needs of the individual case, the figures do not represent an entirely accurate estimate of the dangers of this procedure *in trained hands*. In the great clinics of the country, the mortality will range between 2 and 4 per cent, this also including neglected cases, admitted in extremis, as well as those done solely in the interests of the child as in moribund eclamptics, etc.

The real facts are, that elective cesarean section, done before the onset of labor, or immediately following it, in a well organized hospital will carry a mortality of considerably under 1 per cent. In the section of necessity, in neglected cases, this figure will rise to 6 or 7 per cent but no higher.

The crux of the matter lies in the selection of the patient to be operated upon, the training of the operator and the type of operation chosen.

In elective cesarean section, excellent results are obtained following the classical operation, under local anesthesia, since this may be done in a minimum of time, with a minimum of trauma and shock.

When rupture of the membranes, vaginal examination of doubtful asepsis, long hours of labor and so on render infection probable, laparotrachelotomy is the procedure of choice, and should be done to the exclusion of the classical type.

In frankly infected cases, bad surgical risks, etc., section with hysterectomy, the Latzko or the Portes operations offer the best hope.

When the child is dead, embryotomy should be given the preference over section whenever this is possible.

THE CLINICAL COURSE OF INFECTION FOLLOWING CESAREAN SECTION

When sepsis follows the classical operation, it usually takes the form of a generalized peritonitis, with distention, paralytic ileus, vomiting, septic temperature and death within a few days.

In the event that the infection develops after laparotrachelotomy, while general peritonitis may occur, there is more apt to be a parametritis and pelvic cellulitis with its characteristic signs (*q. v.*) and with a much less grave prognosis. This is also the case with the Latzko operation.

Untoward results after hysterectomy usually take the form of general peritonitis.

Hemorrhage.—The danger of bleeding during the operation has been greatly reduced since the introduction of local anesthesia and the technic of administering pituitrin immediately before the making of the uterine incision.

Nevertheless, sometimes, when the placenta lies under the wound and must be penetrated or detached in order to reach the child, bleeding is active and even alarming. Intestinal forceps may be used on the wound edges to control the uterine sinuses, and controlled speed in completing the extraction of the child and placenta, will obviate the danger in great measure. Speed in closing the uterine wound is essential.

Bleeding from the vagina after the completion of the operation sometimes arises, but may usually be controlled by the exhibition of pituitrin and ergot.

In patients suffering from placenta praevia the uterus should be firmly packed through the abdominal wound before it is sutured.

Donors for blood transfusion should always be in readiness, they having been typed and matched with the patient prior to the operation.

It is important for one to realize that there is rarely any urgency in operating upon women in labor, except in case of hemorrhage from placenta praevia, or abruptio placentae. All too often an exhausted, dehydrated woman is rushed from the admission office to the operating room which has hastily been set up, when a few hours' rest by the aid of morphine, with adrenalin if necessary to relax a Bandl's contraction ring which threatens uterine rupture, control of dehydration by the use of glucose intravenously, blood transfusion if indicated, and the administration of nourishing and refreshing liquids, will render a slightly delayed section infinitely safer for both patients.

Morbidity.—Moderate elevation of temperature for two or three postoperative days is common in cesarean section, except in the purely elective form when this should be no greater than after any clean laparotomy. In the slightly infected cases the fever may persist during the first week, after which it generally subsides.

Tympanitis and distention are common because liquor amnii is an irritant to the peritoneum. However if the patient be free from infection this distressing complication usually disappears after the second day. Should it continue, the usual management of lavage, intermittent or continuous, the withholding of food by mouth, enemata, morphine and pituitrin will ordinarily control the symptoms.

Repeated Cesarean Section.—This matter has been touched upon previously. If the indication for the first operation was a properly diagnosed pelvic disproportion, subsequent gestation should always be terminated by the same means.

The important point in repeated section is the nature of the uterine scar, and it seems true that if the original approximation of the wound edges was well done and no postoperative infection supervened the scar will be strong, and even though much fibrous tissue is intermingled with the muscle bundles, there is sufficient elasticity to withstand stretching and the contractions of labor.

In one patient upon whom the writer performed five classical cesarean sections in eight years, there was never any gross evidence of a previous uterine wound found, and this has been the case in many second and third sections.

The scar following low cervical section is said by its advocates to be more firm than that in the upper segment, but this requires further study of material before the statement can be substantiated.

Cesarean Section on the Dead and Dying.—Postmortem section when the child is living has been practiced through the ages, but the children who have survived are few indeed. If the woman has died from a disease of long duration, or when the vital processes have been at a low ebb, the prognosis for the child is almost hopeless, but when death comes suddenly to a woman whose circulation has been active, there is a slightly better outlook. Unfortunately, sudden death does not often occur where immediate operation can be done, and since the child perishes in from five to ten minutes after the death of the mother, the opportunity to perform section under these conditions does not often offer itself.

Section on the dying, while permissible, is extremely repugnant to most persons and is but rarely done.

Sterilization in Connection with Cesarean Section.—The question of sterilization often arises when a woman is to undergo abdominal hysterotomy. It seems reasonable that a person who has once been put in the peril of an abdominal section in order to produce a child, should have the privilege of refusing to undergo the ordeal a second time. Therefore, if sterilization is demanded by the wife and husband in writing, the obstetrician is entirely justified in acceding to their request.

If the operation is performed upon the indication of grave systemic disease, sterilization should be advised by the attending physician.

If the section be done for contracted pelvis, it is wise to point out to the patient and her husband, the safety of the operation, and the desirability of having a family of at least two children.

At a second section, every woman has a right to be sterilized if she so desires. The religious aspect should be given due weight and no procedure is permissible which is in opposition to the tenets of the patient's religious creed.

Technic.—The Bellevue technic, based upon the procedure of Madlener is satisfactory. Each fallopian tube is grasped at about its middle point by forceps, and after crushing a loop of the tube, a suture ligature is passed through the mesosalpinx and strongly tied about the ends of the loop, the intervening portion being then cut off.

If the section is an elective one, under local anesthesia, with the technic as described above, sterilization may be accomplished by cutting the lower fixation suture, which attaches the uterus to the abdominal wall, rotating the uterus on the upper stitch, which is still in place, injecting the mesosalpinx and tube with $\frac{1}{2}$ per cent novocain, through a long needle, and then tying off and excising a loop of tube as before.

By retaining the upper suture, the intestines and omentum are kept out of the incision and no packing off is required.

CHAPTER XLVI

MUTILATING OPERATIONS ON THE CHILD

THESE are procedures designed to reduce the size of the infant, in order that its body, either entire or dismembered, may be drawn through the birth canal, in cases when this is impossible unless the bulk of the fetus be lessened.

CRANIOTOMY

Craniotomy is the name given to the process of perforating the skull of the child and evacuating the brain after which the head is crushed and extracted.

Indications.—Craniotomy should be performed when the child is dead, and pelvic disproportion exists to a degree incompatible with a safe forceps delivery.

The procedure is not often enough used for this indication, many obstetricians either fearing its danger or disliking its brutality, and hence exposing the mother to extensive laceration only to deliver a dead baby.

When the child is living, the decision as to craniotomy is a momentous one. As DeLee well says: "the obstetrician is judge, jury and perhaps executioner of an innocent baby and he can hardly be blamed if he shrinks from the painful task." If the question be considered from its medical and sociological side alone, religious views being set aside, certain facts become self-evident.

In isolated districts, where skilled hands for the performance of extraperitoneal cesarean section are not available, when labor is absolutely obstructed, and both mother and child are doomed unless the latter is sacrificed, surely the operator is justified.

In hospital practice, when the primiparous mother is in such grave condition that only a hysterecomy may possibly save her, it would seem wise to destroy the already injured baby, and permit the woman to again become pregnant under happier auspices, than to doom her to subsequent childlessness.

The religious tenets of the family must be scrupulously respected, and craniotomy on the living child may never be performed without the knowledge and consent of both parents.

Happily the steady increase of hospital facilities and the development of extraperitoneal methods of cesarean section render this decision more and more unnecessary, as life-saving methods for both mother and infant become more generally applicable.

Advanced hydrocephalus constitutes a strong indication for craniotomy.

Conditions Necessary for Craniotomy.—The true conjugate must not be less than 6 cm. in length, for even a child with crushed skull cannot be extracted through so small a canal. Here abdominal delivery is an absolute necessity.

The cervix must be dilated, or easily dilatable.

The patient must be anesthetized.

Bladder and rectum must be empty.

Technic.—The patient being draped and prepared, in the lithotomy position, the head is grasped with a volsellum forceps and steadied. The hand is then introduced into the vagina and under its guidance a perforator, Smellie's scissors, or Naegele's perforator (Fig. 493), is thrust into the skull, preferably into a suture or fontanel.

The perforator is widely opened in several directions, cutting an irregular and jagged wound in the cranium. It is then thrust into the brain and moved about, tearing and cutting the cerebrum and the cerebellum. The bits of brain may be flushed out by the use of a metal catheter or cannula, and a stream of mild antiseptic solution.

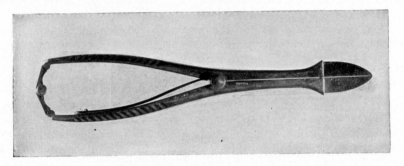

Fig. 493.—Naegele's perforator. (DeLee.)

The head may now be crushed and extracted with the cephalotribe, cranioclast, or basiotribe.

The cephalotribe is an instrument constructed like the obstetric forceps with a very small cephalic cavity, and a powerful screw lock. The blades are applied as are the obstetric forceps, the head crushed and extraction follows.

A more powerful instrument is Tarnier's basiotribe. This is a three-bladed instrument which is at once perforator, crusher and extractor. The middle, spear-pointed blade is a perforator and is introduced either through the opening previously made or is used without any previous perforation and forced to the base of the skull.

The shorter of the forceps-like blades is then passed to the left side of the fetal head and the two blades are joined by the compression screw and locked, being held in contact with a hasp fitted to the handle. The compression screw is then released, the third and longer blade applied to the right side of the head and the compression screw again tightened until the head is crushed, after which the child is extracted, its course through the birth canal being guided by the vaginal hand.

The cranioclast is another instrument available for craniotomy. It consists of two blades, an inner solid one and an outer one fenestrated to fit over the inner one. In use, the solid blade is thrust into the fetal skull, through the perforation previously made, and the outer blade is placed on the outside of the head. The blades are locked, the compression screw tightened, and the head extracted, while a vaginal hand protects the soft parts from damage (Fig. 496).

Sometimes a portion of the bone tears away, in which case, the cranioclast must be reapplied to a firmer portion of the skull.

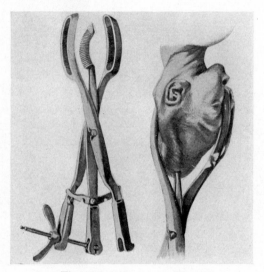

Fig. 494.   Fig. 495.

Figs. 494 and 495.—Auvard's three-bladed cranioclast and its use. (Bumm.)

Craniotomy is not a simple procedure and in the presence of an impacted head may occasion great difficulty. The chief dangers are perforation of the uterus or deep cutting injuries of the vaginal walls by sharp and jagged ends of bone, and infection of the mother from a time-consuming and traumatic procedure. Both of these contingencies can be avoided by care and watchfulness while operating (Fig. 497).

Embryotomy is a term used to describe the evisceration of the child through an opening made in the abdomen or thorax, or, as it is more generally employed, the decapitation of the fetus.

In certain cases of transverse presentation with the thorax or abdomen anterior, and in such conditions as general edema of the fetus, evisceration is a valuable aid to delivery.

Technic.—With the body of the child steadied by suprapubic pressure, an opening is made in the abdomen or thorax with scissors. Through this opening the viscera are slowly torn from their attachments and drawn out, after which the body of the child is doubled up and delivered, or this may be effected by version and extraction.

Decapitation or beheading is usually done because of neglected shoulder presentation, sometimes in locked twins, the child being dead and version impracticable.

Technic.—The prolapsed arm, if present, is firmly drawn down and held by an assistant. The operator inserts the whole hand into the

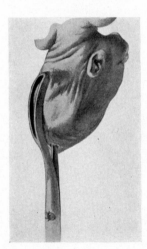

Fig. 496.—The head extracted by the cranioclast. (Bumm.)

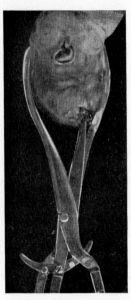

Fig. 497.—Showing the perforation through the posterior fontanel in case of extreme flexion of the head. It will be observed that the blade placed over the face does not reach further than the forehead. (Kerr.)

vagina, the finger acting as a guide for the decapitating instrument which is either Braun's blunt hook, or the sickle knife of Ransbotham. The hook is carefully introduced around the neck of the child, and the tip is covered by a finger to prevent injury to the maternal tissues.

Strong traction is then made upon the handle with an oscillating to-and-fro movement, which disarticulates the cervical vertebrae. When this is accomplished the soft tissues of the neck are severed with scissors, and the body of the child extracted either by traction upon the prolapsed arm or by version.

The head is expressed in a manner similar to simple expression of the placenta and if this does not serve, the finger is inserted into the mouth and delivery concluded by combined traction from below and suprapubic pressure.

Occasionally it may be necessary to crush the head with one of the craniotomy instruments before extraction.

Cleidotomy.—The shoulders may be too broad for delivery, in which case, the clavicles may be severed by cutting them with heavy blunt-pointed scissors, under the guidance of the hand.

BIBLIOGRAPHY

In writing this work the standard textbooks and systems of obstetrics have been consulted and freely quoted. To avoid repetition, detailed reference to these various works has not been made.

CHAPTER I

ANATOMY OF THE FEMALE REPRODUCTIVE ORGANS

Anson, B. J.: Curtis' Obstetrics and Gynecology, Philadelphia, W. B. Saunders Co., 1933, vol. I, pp. 195 on.

Arey, L. B.: Developmental Anatomy, Philadelphia, W. B. Saunders Co., 1934.

Frankel, O.: Physiology and Pathology of the Isthmus Uteri, Jour. Obstet. and Gynæc. Brit. Emp., 40: 397, 1933.

Halban and Seitz: Biologie u. Pathologie des Weibes, Urban und Schwarzenberg, 1921.

O'Leary, J. L., and Culbertson, C.: The Form Changes in the Human Uterine Gland During the Menstrual Cycle, Surg., Gynec., and Obstet., 227, 1928.

Polano, O.: Geburtshilfliche-gynäkologische Propedeutik, Leipzig, C. Kabitsch, 1920.

Sobotta and McMurrich: Atlas and Text-Book of Human Anatomy, New York, G. E. Steckert, 1930.

Tandler, J.: Lehrbuch der Systematische Anatomie, Leipzig, F. C. W. Vogel, 1929.

Thoma: Lehrbuch der Anatomie, Stuttgart, Enke, 1894.

CHAPTER II

PHYSIOLOGY OF THE REPRODUCTIVE ORGANS

Anderson, Dorothy: The Rate of the Passage of the Mammalian Ovum Through Various Portions of the Fallopian Tube, Amer. Jour. Physiol., 82: 557, 1927.

Arey, L. B.: Developmental Anatomy (q. v.).

Corner, G. W., and Allen, W. M.: Amer. Jour. Physiol., 88: 326, 1929.

Fraenkel, L.: Arch. f. Gynäk., 91: 705, 1910.

———: Deutsch. med. Wchnschr., 53: 2154, 1927.

Frank, R. T.: The Female Sex Hormone, Springfield, Ill., Charles C. Thomas, 1929.

Hitschmann and Adler: Monatschr. f. Geburtsh. u. Gynäk., 27: 1, 1908.

Loeb, L.: The Cyclic Changes in the Ovum of the Guinea Pig, Jour. Morphol., 22: 37, 1911.

Norris, C. C.: The Menopause, Amer. Jour. Obstet., 61: 2030, 1910.

Novak, E.: Menstruation and Its Disorders, New York, D. Appleton and Co., 1931.

Papanicolaou, G. N.: Jour. Amer. Med. Assoc., 86: 1422, 1926.

Schäffer: Arch. f. Gynäk., 84: 657, 1909.

Schröder, R.: Arch. f. Gynäk., 101: 1, 1913.

———: Arch. f. Gynäk., 104: 27, 1915.

Smith, P. E., and Engel, E. T.: Amer. Jour. Anat., 40: 159, 1927.

Snyder, F. F.: Changes in the Human Oviduct During the Menstrual Cycle and Pregnancy, Bull. Johns Hopkins Hosp., 35: 141, 1924 (Literature).

Zondek, B.: Hypophysenvorderlappen und Ovarium, Berlin, 1931.

CHAPTERS III, IV, V, AND VI

FERTILIZATION OF OVUM—FETAL MEMBRANES—GROWTH OF FETUS—PHYSIOLOGY OF FETUS

Adair, F. L., and Schumann, E. A.: Curtis' Obstetrics and Gynecology, Philadelphia, W. B. Saunders Co., 1933, vol. 1.

Bryce, T. H., and Teacher, J. H.: Contribution to the Study of the Early Development and Embedding of the Human Ovum, Glasgow, Maclehose and Sons, 1908.

Greenhill, J. P.: A Young Human Ovum in Situ, Amer. Jour. Anat., 40: 315, 1927.

Grosser, O.: Frühentwicklung, Eihautbildung und Placentation des Menschen und der Säugetiere, München, Bergmann, 1927.

Mall, F. P.: On the Age of Human Embryos, Amer. Jour. Anat., 23: 397, 1918.

Peters, H.: Über die Einbettung des Menschlichen Eies, Leipzig, Deuticke, 1899.

Preyer: Specielle Physiologie des Embryo, Leipzig, 1885.

Slemons, J. M.: Nutrition of the Fetus, New Haven, Yale University Press, 1919.

Young: Study of an Early Human Ovum, Tr. Edinburgh Obstet. Soc., 46: 113, 1926.

CHAPTER VII

THE PHYSIOLOGY OF PREGNANCY

Heart and Circulatory System

Frey: Herz und Schwangerschaft, Leipzig, 1923.

Gammeltoft, R.: Surg., Gynec., and Obstet., 46: 382, 1928.

Grollman, A.: Amer. Jour. Physiol., 86: 117, 1928.

Hinselmann, H.: Monatschr. f. Geburtsh. u. Gynäk., 42: 1923.

Stander, H. J., and Cadden, J. F.: The Cardiac Output in Pregnant Women, Amer. Jour. Obstet. and Gynec., 20: 13, 1932.

Blood

Arneth, J.: Arch. f. Gynäk., 74: 145, 1904.

Bland, P. B.; First, A., and Goldstein, L.: The Blood Platelets in Pregnancy and in the Puerperium, Amer. Jour. Obstet. and Gynec., 20: 165, 1930.

Bland, P. B., and Goldstein, L.: Coagulability of the Blood in Pregnancy, Amer. Jour. Obstet. and Gynec., 23: 815, 1932.

Bland, P. B.; Goldstein, L., and First, A.: The Physiological Anemia of Pregnancy, Surg., Gynec., and Obstet., 50: 954, 1930.

Caldwell, Wm. E., and Lyle, Wm. G.: Blood Chemistry in Normal and Abnormal Pregnancies, Amer. Jour. Obstet. and Gynec., 2: 1, 1921.

Dietrich: Studien über Blutveränderungen bei Schwangeren, u. s. w., Arch. f. Gynäk., 94: 383, 1911.

Griffin, R. J.: The Sedimentation Rate and Schilling Index in Pregnancy, Amer. Jour. Obstet. and Gynec., 28: 532, 1934.

Hofbauer, J.: Für die placentare Theorie du Eklampsie-Aetiologie, Zentralbl. f. Gynäk., 32: 1469, 1908.

Kühnel: Untersuchungen über die Physiol. Schwangerschaftsanamie, Zeitschr. f. Geburtsh. u. Gynäk., Stuttgart, 90: 511, 1927.

Lyon, E. C.: Anemia in Late Pregnancy, Jour. Amer. Med. Assoc., 90: 11, 1929.

Miller, Keith and Rowntree: Plasma and Blood Volume in Pregnancy, Jour Amer. Med. Assoc., 65: 779, 1915.

Rucker, M. P. A.: Study of the Hemoglobin After Childbirth with Special Reference to the Resumption of Menstruation, Amer. Jour. Obstet. and Gynec., 1: 964, 1921.

Respiratory System

Hofbauer, J.: Monatschr. f. Geburtsh. u. Gynäk., **28:** 45, 1908.
Klaften: Zentralbl. f. Gynäk., 931, April, 1925.
Zuntz: Arch. f. Gynäk., **90:** 452, 1910.

Weight Changes

Kerwin, Wm.: Weight Estimation During Pregnancy, Amer. Jour. Obstet. and Gynec., **11:** 1926.
Randall, L. M.: The Weight Factor in Pregnancy, Amer. Jour. Obstet. and Gynec., **9:** 529, 1925.
Zangemeister, W.: Über das Körpergewicht Schwangerer nebst Bemerkungen über des Hydrops Gravidarum, Zeitschr. f. Geburtsh. u. Gynäk., **78:** 325, 1916.

Alimentary Tract

D'Amato, G., and Gmelin, E.: The Effect of Pregnancy and Puerperium upon the Gall Tract, Zentralbl. f. Gynäk., **51:** 1031, 1928.
Freiheit, J. M.: The Bromsulphalein Test for Liver Function in Toxemias of Pregnancy, Amer. Jour. Obstet. and Gynec., **23:** 797, 1932.
Potter, M. G.: Observations on the Gall Bladder and Bile During Pregnancy at Term, Jour. Amer. Med. Assoc., **106:** 1073, 1936.
Schmidt, H. R., and Jonen: Zentralbl. f. Gynäk., **91:** 527, 1924.

Pelvic Articulations

Abramson, D.; Roberts, S. M., and Wilson, P. D.: Relaxation of the Pelvic Joints in Pregnancy, Surg., Gynec., and Obstet., **58:** 595, 1934.
Chamberlain, W. E.: Symphysis Pubis in the Roentgenological Examination of the Sacroiliac Joint, Amer. Jour. Roentgenol., **24:** 806, 1930.
Duncan, M.: Researches in Obstetrics, Edinburgh, 1868.
Litzenberg, J. C.: Sacroiliac Joints in Obstetrics and Gynecology, Jour. Amer. Med. Assoc., **59:** 1759, 1917.
Lynch, W. W.: The Pelvic Articulation During Pregnancy, Labor and the Puerperium, Surg., Gynec., and Obstet., **575,** 1920.

Endocrines and Metabolism

Baer, Joseph L.: Amer. Jour. Obstet. and Gynec., **2:** 249, 1921.
Bar, Paul: Leçons de Pathologie Obstetricale, vol. 11, Paris, 1907.
Hinton, J. W.: Hyperthyroidism Associated with Pregnancy, Amer. Jour. Obstet. and Gynec., **20:** 183, 1930.
Marshall, F. H. A.: The Physiology of Reproduction, New York, Longmans, Green and Co., 1922.
Murlin: Energy Metabolism of the Pregnant Dog, Amer. Jour. Physiol., **26:** 1910.
Schwarz, O. H., and Drabkin, C.: Basal Metabolic Rates in Late Pregnancy and the Puerperium, Amer. Jour. Obstet. and Gynec., **22:** 571, 1931.
Trumper, Max: Fundamental Biochemical Factors in Pregnancy, Amer. Jour. Obstet. and Gynec., **20:** 209, 1930.

Urinary Tract

Hofbauer, J. I.: Curtis' Obstetrics and Gynecology, Philadelphia, W. B. Saunders Co., 1933, vol. I.
Hundley, J. M., Jr. et al: Physiologic Changes Occurring in the Urinary Tract During Pregnancy, Amer. Jour. Obstet. and Gynec., **30:** 625, 1935.
Strumpf, I. J.: Changes in the Urinary Tract During Pregnancy, Amer. Jour. Obstet. and Gynec., **26:** 857, 1933.

CHAPTER VIII

THE DIAGNOSIS OF PREGNANCY

Ahlfeld, F.: Beobachtungen über die Dauer der Schwangerschaft, Monatschr. f. Geburtsh. u. Gynäk., 34: 180, 1869.

Aschheim, C., and Zondek, B.: Klin. Wchnschr., 7: 8, 1928.

Baer, J. L.: Amer. Jour. Obstet. and Gynec., 2: 249, 1921.

Bouchacourt: L'Obstetrique, 5: 20, 1900.

Case, J. J.: Curtis' Obstetrics and Gynecology, Philadelphia, W. B. Saunders Co., 1933, vol. III, p. 762.

Chadwick, J. R.: The Value of the Bluish Discoloration of the Vaginal Entrance as a Sign of Pregnancy, Jour. Amer. Gynec. Soc., 11: 399, 1886.

Edling: Text a. d. Geb. a Röntgenstrahlen, 17: 3457, 1911.

Frank, R. T.: Jour. Lab. and Clin. Med., 17: 61, 1931.

Friedman, M. H.: Amer. Jour. Physiol., 89: 438, 1929.

————: Amer. Jour. Physiol., 90: 617, 1929.

Friedman, M. D., and Lapham, M. E.: Amer. Jour. Obstet. and Gynec., 21: 405, 1931.

Hicks, J. Braxton: On the Contraction of the Uterus Throughout Pregnancy, Jour. Obstet. Soc., London, 13: 216, 1872.

Jarcho, J.: Amer. Jour. Surg., XII, 3: 417, 1931.

Liese, G., and Auer, E. S.: Amer. Jour. Obstet. and Gynec., 20: 667, 1930.

MacDonald, Ellice: The Diagnosis of Early Pregnancy, Amer. Jour. Obstet., 57: 323, 1908.

Mathieu, A.; Palmer, A., and Holman, A.: Northwest Medicine, Seattle, 31: 215, 1932.

Mazer, Charles H., and Goldstein, L.: Clinical Endocrinology in the Female, Philadelphia, W. B. Saunders Co., 1932, p. 390.

McDonald, E.: Jour. Amer. Med. Assoc., 47: 1979, 1906.

Montgomery, W. F.: An Exposition of the Signs and Symptoms of Pregnancy, London, 1856, p. 82.

Rakhmanoff: Vratch, p. 1456: 1901: quoted by Metchnikoff, The Nature of Man.

Schatz-Klein: Beiträge zum Physiologie der Schwangerschaft, Leipzig, 1910.

Schneider, P. H.: Surg., Gynec., and Obstet., 52: 56, 1931.

Schnitker, M. A.; Hodges, P. C., and Whitacre, F. E.: Roentgenologic Evidence of Fetal Death, Amer. Jour. Roentgenol. and Radium Therap., 28: September, 1932.

CHAPTER IX

THE MANAGEMENT OF PREGNANCY

Adair, F. L., and Maland, E. O.: Results Gained in Maternity Cases in Which Prenatal Care Has Been Given, Jour. Amer. Med. Assoc., 81: 992, 1923.

Baer, J. L.: Basal Metabolism in Pregnancy and the Puerperium, Amer. Jour. Obstet. and Gynec., 2: 249, 1921.

Danforth, W. C.: Management of Normal Pregnancy, Curtis' Obstetrics and Gynecology, Philadelphia, W. B. Saunders Co., 1933, vol. I, Chap. XXI.

McCord, J. R.: Prenatal Care, South. Med. Jour., 25: 166, 1932.

Standards of Prenatal Care. Prepared by the Joint Committee of American Gynecological Society, American Association of Obstetricians, Gynecologists and Abdominal Surgeons and American Child Health Association, Amer. Jour. Obstet. and Gynec., 12: 754, 1926.

Urner, J. A.: Vitamins in Pregnancy, Curtis' Obstetrics and Gynecology, Philadelphia, W. B. Saunders Co., 1933, vol. I., Chap. XXI.

CHAPTER X

THE FETUS IN UTERO—POSITION AND PRESENTATION

Barnum, J.: The Effect of Gravitation on the Presentation and Position of the Fetus, Jour. Amer. Med. Assoc., **64:** 458, 1915.

Duncan, J. M.: Researches in Obstetrics, Edinburgh, 1886.

Hillis, D. S.: Presentation and Position of the Fetus, Curtis' Obstetrics and Gynecology, Philadelphia, W. B. Saunders Co., 1933, vol. I., Chap. XVIII.

Leff, M. A.: Fetal Heart Stethoscope, Amer. Jour. Obstet. and Gynec., **20:** 158, 1930.

Schatz, F.: Zentralbl. f. Gynäk., **40:** 1033, 1900.

CHAPTER XI

THE ANATOMY AND PHYSIOLOGY OF LABOR

Calkins, L. S.; Irvine, J. R., and Horsley, G. W.: Variation in the Length of Labor, Amer. Jour. Obstet. and Gynec., **19:** 294, 1930.

Dickinson, R. L.: Studies on the Levator Ani Muscle, Amer. Jour. Obstet., **22:** 897, 1889.

Dodek, S. M.: A New Method for Graphically Recording the Contractions of the Parturient Human Uterus, Surg., Gynec., and Obstet., **55:** 45, 1932.

Gibbons, R. A.: Causes of the Onset of Labor, Brit. Med. Jour., **34:** 739, 1927.

Schatz, F.: Beiträge zur Physiologischen Geburtskunde, Arch. f. Gynäk., **3:** 58, 1872.

Thoms, H.: Variations in the Female Pelvis in Relation to Labor, Surg., Gynec., and Obstet., **60:** 680, 1935.

Whitehouse and Featherstone: Certain Observations on the Innervation of the Uterus, Jour. Obstet. and Gynæc. Brit. Emp., **30:** 565, 1923.

Williams, J. W.: Histological Study of Fifty Uteri Removed at Cesarean Section, Bull. Johns Hopkins Hosp., **28:** 335, 1917.

Zweifel, P.: Über das Untere Uterinsegment, Zentralbl. f. Gynäk., **38:** 1376, 1914.

CHAPTER XII

THE MECHANISM OF LABOR

Caldwell, W. E.; Moloy, H. C., and D'Esopo, D. A.: A Roentgenologic Study of the Mechanism of the Engagement of the Fetal Head, Amer. Jour. Obstet. and Gynec., **28:** 824, 1934.

———: Further Studies in the Mechanism of Labor, Amer. Jour. Obstet. and Gynec., **30:** 763, 1935.

Garnett, A. Y. P., and Jacobs, J. B.: Pelvic Inclination, Amer. Jour. Obstet. and Gynec., **31:** 388, 1936.

Goodall, J. R.: The Caput Succedaneum: A Hindrance to Labor, Jour. Obstet. and Gynæc. Brit. Emp., **40:** 1021, 1933.

Paramore: A Critical Inquiry into the Causes of Internal Rotation of the Fetal Head, Jour. Obstet. and Gynæc. Brit. Emp., October, 1909.

Rudolph, R., and Ivy, A. C.: Internal Rotation of the Fetal Head from the Viewpoint of Comparative Obstetrics, Amer. Jour. Obstet. and Gynec., **25:** 74, 1933.

Rydberg, E.: Jour. Obstet. and Gynæc. Brit. Emp., **42:** 797, 1935.

Sellheim: Die Beziehungen des Geburtskanales u. des Geburtsobjektes zur Geburtsmechanik, Leipzig, 1906.

Stude, W. C.: Factors Influencing the Variety and Position of Occipital Presentation, Surg., Gynec., and Obstet., **59:** 913, 1934.

Zweifel, P.: Erfahrungen an den letzten 10,000 Geburten, u. s. w., Arch. f. Gynäk., **101:** 643, 1914.

CHAPTERS XIII AND XIV

THE CLINICAL COURSE OF LABOR—THE CONDUCT OF LABOR

Aldridge, A. H., and Watson, P.: Analysis of End Results of Labor in Primiparas After Spontaneous versus Prophylactic Methods of Delivery, Amer. Jour. Obstet. and Gynec., **30**: 1554, 1935.

Calkins, L. A.; Litzenberg, J. C., and Plass, E. D.: Management of the Third Stage of Labor with Special Reference to Blood Loss, Amer. Jour. Obstet. and Gynec., **21**: 175, 1931.

Mayes, H. W.: Vaginal vs. Rectal Examination, etc., Surg., Gynec., and Obstet., **45**: 771, 1932.

Pomeroy, R.: Shall We Cut and Reconstruct the Perineum for Every Primipara, Amer. Jour. Obstet., **78**: 211, 1918.

Williams, P. F. (Chairman): Maternal Mortality in Philadelphia. Report of the Committee on Maternal Welfare, Philadelphia County Medical Society, 1934.

CHAPTER XV

ANALGESIA AND ANESTHESIA IN OBSTETRICS

Bourne, W.: Vinal Ether Obstetric Anesthesia for General Practice, Jour. Amer. Med. Assoc., **105**: 2047, 1935.

Colvin, E. D., and Bartholomew, R. A.: The Advantages of Paraldehyde as a Basic Amnesic Agent in Obstetrics, Jour. Amer. Med. Assoc., **104**: 362, 1935.

Gwathmey, J. J., and McCormick, C. O.: Ether-Oil Rectal Analgesia in Obstetrics, Jour. Amer. Med. Assoc., **105**: 2044, 1935.

Irving, F. C.; Berman, S., and Nelson, H. B.: The Barbiturates and Other Hypnotics in Labor, Surg., Gynec., and Obstet., **58**: 1, 1934.

McIlroy, L., and Rodney, H. E.: The Alleviation of Pain in 560 Cases of Spontaneous Labor, Jour. Obstet. and Gynæc. Brit. Emp., **40**: 1175, 1933.

CHAPTER XVI

THE PUERPERIUM

Adair, F. L.: The Influence of Diet on Lactation, Amer. Jour. Obstet. and Gynec., **9**: 56, 1925.

Döderlein: Das Scheidensekret, Leipzig, 1892.

Frommel, Rich.: Zeitschr. f. Geburtsh. u. Gynäk., **7**: 305, 1882.

Harding, V. J.; Murphy, H., and Downs, C. E.: Observations on Blood Sugar and Serum Calcium in Relation to Lactation in Women, etc., Amer. Jour. Obstet. and Gynec., **16**: 765, 1928.

Jacquet, Rich.: Über Atrophia Uteri, Berlin. Beitr. zum Geburtsh. u. Gynäk., **2**: 1–11, 1873.

Sharp, E. A.: Amer. Jour. Obstet. and Gynec., **30**: 411, 1935.

Williams, J. W.: Regeneration of the Uterine Mucosa After Delivery; with Especial Reference to the Placental Site, Amer. Jour. Obstet. and Gynec., **22**: 664, 1931.

CHAPTER XVII

THE TOXEMIAS OF PREGNANCY

Anselmino, K. J., and Hoffman, F.: Die Übereinstimmungen in den Klinischen Symptomen der Nephropathie und Eklampsie der Schwangeren mit den Wirkungen des Hypophysenhinterlappenhormons, Arch. f. Gynäk., **147**: 597, 1931.

Arnold, J. O.: Med. Clin. N. A., July, 1934.

Bell, E. T.: Renal Lesions in the Toxemias of Pregnancy, Amer. Jour. Path., **8**: 1, 1932.

Bissell, Dougal: Amer. Jour. Obstet. and Gynec., **9**: 118, 1925.

Bode, O.: Polyneuritis und Eklampsie, Arch. f. Gynäk., **146**: 118, 1931.

Cantarow, A.; Montgomery, T. L., and Bolton, W. A.: The Calcium Partition in Pregnancy, Parturition, and the Toxemias, Surg., Gynec., and Obstet., **51**: 469, 1930.

Clifford, S. H.: Jour. Amer. Med. Assoc., **103**: 1117, 1934.

Cushing: Secretion of Urine, 2nd ed., London, 1926.

Davis, A. B., and Harrar, J. A.: Toxemia of Pregnancy. 875 Cases with Convulsions at the New York Lying-in Hospital, Bull. N. Y. Lying-in Hospital, **13**: 135, 1927.

Dieckman, W. J.: The Hepatic Lesion in Eclampsia, Amer. Jour. Obstet. and Gynec., **17**: 454, 1929.

Duncan, J. W., and Harding, W. J.: A Report on the Effect of High Carbohydrate Feeding on the Nausea and Vomiting of Pregnancy, Canadian Med. Assoc. Jour., **8**: 1057, 1918.

Fahr, T.: Die Eklampsie, Bonn, 1924.

Fieux: Ann. de gynec. et d'obstet., **60**: 718, 1912.

Greenhill, J. P.: Eclampsia at the Chicago Lying-in Hospital. Immediate and Late Results, Jour. Amer. Med. Assoc., **87**: 228, 1926.

Günter and Schultze: Eclampsie und Kalzium, Zentralbl. f. Gynäk., **50**: 57, 1926.

Harding, W. J., and Van Wyck, H. B.: Serum Protein in Nausea and Vomiting of Pregnancy, Jour. Obstet. and Gynec., **15**: 511, 1928.

Harrar, J. A.: Bull. Lying-in-Hosp., New York, **2**: 72, 1905.

Hinselmann, H.: Die Eklampsie, Bonn, 1924.

Irving, F. C.: The Vascular Aspect of Eclampsia, Amer. Jour. Obstet. and Gynec., **31**: 466, 1936.

Keutmann, E. H., and McCann, W. S.: Dietary Protein in Hemorrhagic Bright's Disease; Effects Upon Course of Disease with Special Reference to Hematuria and Renal Function, Jour. Clin. Investigation, **11**: 973, 1932.

King, A G.: Eclampsia Without Convulsions Terminating in Cerebral Apoplexy, Jour. Amer. Med. Assoc., **100**: 15, 1933.

King, E. L.: Liver Function Tests in Toxemias of Pregnancy, South. Med. Jour., **23**: 285, 1930.

Lazard, E. M.; Irwin, J. C., and Vruwink, J.: The Intravenous Magnesium Sulphate Treatment of Eclampsia, Amer. Jour. Obstet. and Gynec., **12**: 1926.

Levy-Solal, M.: L'eclampsie-syndrome, Paris méd., **1**: 600, 1927.

Levy-Solal and Le Loup: Paris méd., **13**: 217, 1923.

MacGregor, L.: Histological Changes in the Renal Glomerulus in Essential (primary) Hypertension, Arch. Path., **6**: 347, 1930.

McPherson, quoted by Kosmak: The Toxemias of Pregnancy, New York, D. Appleton and Co., 1922, p. 24.

Missett, J. V.: The Relationship between the Early and Late Toxemias of Pregnancy, Amer. Jour. Obstet. and Gynec., **27**: 697, 1934.

Mussey, R. D.: Recurring Preeclamptic Toxemia. Its Clinical Significance, Minnesota Med., **14**: 889, October, 1931.

Oppenheimer, W.: Arch. f. Gynäk., Berlin, July, 1924, p. 158.

Peckham, C. H., and Stout, M. L.: A Study of the Late Effects of the Toxemias of Pregnancy, Bull. Johns Hopkins Hosp., **49**: 225, 1931.

Peters and Van Slyke: Quantitative Clinical Chemistry, Baltimore, Williams and Wilkins. Toxemias of Pregnancy, vol. 1, p. 983. Pregnancy and Pregnancy Toxemias, vol. 1, p. 784.

Schumann, E. A.: Amer. Jour. Obstet. and Gynec., **21**: 381, 1931.

Stander, H. J.: The Treatment of Eclampsia by the Stroganoff Method, Amer. Jour. Obstet. and Gynec., **9**: 327, 1925.

Stander, H. J.; Ashton, P., and Cadden, J. F.: The Value of Various Kidney Function Tests in the Differentiation of Toxemias of Pregnancy, Amer. Jour. Obstet. and Gynec., **23**: 461, 1932.

Stander, H. J., and Cadden, J. F.: Blood Chemistry in Preeclampsia and Eclampsia, Amer. Jour. Obstet. and Gynec., 28: 856, 1934.

Stander, H. J., and Peckham, C. H.: A Classification of the Toxemias of the Latter Half of Pregnancy, Amer. Jour. Obstet. and Gynec., 11: 583, 1926.

Stander, H. J., and Peckham, C. H.: Basal Metabolism in Toxemias of Pregnancy, Bull. Johns Hopkins Hosp., 38: 227, 1926.

Thalheimer, Wm.: Insulin Treatment of the Toxemic Vomiting of Pregnancy, Surg., Gynec., and Obstet., 39: 237, 1924.

Theobald, G. W.: Two Cases of Eclampsia Developing without Albuminuria, and One Fatal Case of Hydatidiform Mole without Albuminuria, Jour. Obstet. and Gynæc. Brit. Emp., 36: 803, 1929.

Titus, P., and Givens, M. H.: Intravenous Injection of Glucose in Toxemia of Pregnancy, Jour. Amer. Med. Assoc., 78: 92, 1922.

Titus, Paul et al.: Amer. Jour. Obstet. and Gynec., 18: 29, 1929.

Weill, A., and Laudat, P.: Bull. Soc. d'Obst. et de Gynec. de Paris, 13: 348, 1924.

Zangemeister, W.: Der Hydrops Gravidarum, sein Verlauf und seine Beziehungen Zum Nephropathie und Eklampsie, Zeitschr. f. Geburtsh. u. Gynäk., 81: 491, 1919.

CHAPTER XVIII

ABORTION AND PREMATURE LABOR

Clifford, S. H.: Reduction of Premature Infant Mortality Through Determination of Fetal Size in Utero, Jour. Amer. Med. Assoc., 103: 1117, 1934.

————: A Consideration of the Obstetrical Management of Premature Labor, New England Med. Jour., 210: 570, 1934.

Huntington, J. L.: A Review of the Pathology of Miscarriage, Amer. Jour. Obstet. and Gynec., 17: 32, 1929.

Litzenberg, J. C.: Missed Abortion, Amer. Jour. Obstet. and Gynec., 1: 475, 1920.

Taussig, F. J.: Abortion, Spontaneous and Induced, St. Louis, C. V. Mosby Co., 1935.

CHAPTER XIX

DISPLACEMENTS OF THE UTERUS

Polak, J. O.: The Influence of Fibroids in Pregnancy and Labor, Surg., Gynec., and Obstet., 46: 71, 1928.

Reis, R. A., and Chaloupka, A. J.: Jour. Amer. Med. Assoc., 94: 255, 1930.

Robinson, A. L., and Duvall, A. M.: Torsion of the Pregnant Uterus, Jour. Obstet. and Gynæc. Brit. Emp., 38: 55, 1931.

Schumann, E. A.: Observations Upon the Coexistence of Carcinoma Fundus Uteri and Pregnancy, Amer. Jour. Obstet. and Gynec., 14: 573, 1927.

CHAPTER XX

EXTRA-UTERINE PREGNANCY

Beck, A. C.: Treatment of Extra-Uterine Pregnancy After the Fifth Month, Jour. Amer. Med. Assoc., 73: 962, 1919.

Berkeley and Bonney: Tubal Gestation, A Pathological Study, Jour. Obstet. and Gynæc. Brit. Emp., 7: 77, 1905.

Caturani, M.: To What Extent Must We Depend Upon the Microscopical Examination to Support the Clinical Diagnosis of Ectopic Pregnancy? Amer. Jour. Obstet., 79: 716, 1919.

Clement, F.: Death of Fetus After Tubal Pregnancy of Six Months, Unruptured, Bull. et mém. Soc. de Paris, 24: 203, 1932.

Frank, R. T.: Amer. Jour. Obstet., 65: 466, 1912.

Gagnon, F.: Tubal Pregnancy at Term, Bull. Soc. méd. d'hôp. Universitaires de Quebec, December, 1934, p. 422.

Heinz, H.: Case of Sixth Month Unruptured Isthmial Pregnancy, Amer. Jour. Obstet. and Gynec., 24: 757, 1932.

Hellman, A. M., and Simon, H. J.: Full Term Abdominal Pregnancy, Amer. Jour. Surg., 29: 403, 1935.

Hull, E. T.: Unruptured Utero-Interstitial Pregnancy at Term, Amer. Jour. Obstet. and Gynec., 28: 452, 1934.

Kline, B. S.: The Decidual Reaction in Extrauterine Pregnancy, Amer. Jour. Obstet. and Gynec., 17: 42, 1929.

Litzenberg, J. C.: Microscopic Studies of Tubal Pregnancy, Amer. Jour. Obstet. and Gynec., 1: 223, 1920.

Mall, F. P.: The Fate of the Human Embryo in Tubal Pregnancy, Carnegie Inst. Pub. No. 221.

Mall and Cullen: An Ovarian Pregnancy Located in the Graafian Follicle, Surg., Gynec., and Obstet., 17: 698, 1913.

Norris, C. C.: Primary Ovarian Pregnancy, Surg., Gynec., and Obstet., 9: 123, 1909.

Novak, E: Combined Intrauterine and Extrauterine Pregnancy with a Report of 276 Cases, Surg., Gynec., and Obstet., 34: 26, 1926.

Pelkonen, E.: Full Term Ampulla Pregnancy at Duodecim, 50: 723, 1934.

Polak, J. O.: Observations in 227 Cases of Ectopic Pregnancy, Amer. Jour. Obstet., 71: 946, 1915.

Schumann, E. A.: Amer. Jour. Obstet., 69: 127, 1914.

———: Extrauterine Pregnancy, New York, D. Appleton and Co., 1921.

Siddall, R. S.: The Occurrence and Significance of Decidual Changes in the Endometrium in Extrauterine Pregnancy, Amer. Jour. Obstet. and Gynec., 31: 420, 1936.

Sittner, A.: Arch. f. Gynäk., 64: 526, 1901.

———: Zentralbl. f. Gynäk., 27: 33, 1903.

———: Deutsch. med. Wchnschr., 29: 743, 1903.

———: Die Kinderheilkunde, 12: 201, 1908.

Smith, R. R.: Ectopic Pregnancy and Repeated Ectopic Pregnancies, Surg., Gynec., and Obstet., 18: 684, 1914.

Tait, R. L.: Lectures on Ectopic Pregnancy and Pelvic Hematocele, Birmingham, 1888.

Webster, J. C.: Ectopic Pregnancy, Edinburgh, 1895, p. 76.

Weinbrenner: Über Interstitielle Schwangerschaft, Zeitschr. f. Geburtsh. u. Gynäk., 51: 57, 1904.

Williams, C. D.: Etiology of Ectopic Gestation, Surg., Gynec., and Obstet., 7: 519, 1908.

Wynne, H. M. N.: Bull. Johns Hopkins Hosp., 30: 15, 1919.

CHAPTER XXI

DISEASES OF THE EMBRYO AND APPENDAGES

Bell, W. Blair: Prolonged Retention of Hydatidiform Moles, etc., Jour. Obstet. and Gynæc. Brit. Emp., 31: 278, 1924.

Benthin: Monatschr. f. Geburtsh. u. Gynäk., 39: 1914.

Gardiner, J. P.: Surg., Gynec., and Obstet., 34: 252, 1922.

Gerhartz: Deutsch. med. Wchnschr., 43: 74, 1917.

Lull, C. B.: Chorionepithelioma Following Full Term Pregnancy, Amer. Jour. Obstet. and Gynec., 30: 730, 1935.

Mathieu, A., and Palmer, A.: The Early Diagnosis of Chorioepithelioma, Surg., Gynec., and Obstet., 61: 336, 1935.

Novak, E., and Koff, A. K.: Chorioepithelioma, Amer. Jour. Obstet. and Gynec., 20: 153, 1930.

Schiller, W., and Toll, R. M.: An Inquiry into the Cause of Oligohydramnios, Amer. Jour. Obstet. and Gynec., 13: 689, 1927.

Schumann, E. A.: Observations upon Hydatidiform Mole, Amer. Jour. Obstet. and Gynec., **4:** 386, 1922.

———: Further Observations on Hydatidiform Mole, Amer. Jour. Obstet. and Gynec., **18:** 768, 1929.

———: Curtis' Obstetrics and Gynecology, Philadelphia, W. B. Saunders Co., 1933. (Full literature.)

Wilson, R. A.: Placenta Accreta, Amer. Jour. Obstet. and Gynec., **17:** 58, 1929.

CHAPTER XXII

PLACENTA PRAEVIA

Greenhill, J. P.: The Present Day Treatment of Placenta Praevia, Surg., Gynec., and Obstet., **50:** 113, 1930.

Kellogg, F. S.: Treatment of Placenta Praevia Based on a Study of 303 Consecutive Cases at the Boston Lying-in Hospital, Amer. Jour. Obstet. and Gynec., **11:** 112, 1926.

Stein, I. F., and Leventhal, M. L.: Surg., Gynec., and Obstet., **45:** 798, 1927.

Strassman, P.: Placenta Praevia, Arch. f. Gynäk., **21:** 112, 1902.

Ude, W. H., and Urner, J. A.: Roentgenological Diagnosis of Placenta Praevia, Amer. Jour. Obstet. and Gynec., **29:** 667, 1935.

CHAPTER XXIII

ABRUPTIO PLACENTAE

Browne, F. J.: Further Experimental Observations of Etiology, Accidental Hemorrhage and Placental Infarct, Jour. Obstet. and Gynæc. Brit. Emp., 1928.

Davis, M. E.: Abruptio Placentae, Surg., Gynec., and Obstet., **53:** 768, 1931.

Essen-Moeller: L'hemorrhage Retroplacentaire, Arch. mens. d'obst. et de gynéc., Paris, **4:** 145, 1913.

Fitzgibbon, G.: Revised Conception of Antepartum Accidental Hemorrhage, Jour. Obstet. and Gynæc. Brit. Emp., **33:** 2, 1926.

Holmes, R. W.: Uteroplacental Apoplexy and Ablatic Placentae, Amer. Jour. Obstet. and Gynec., **6:** 517, 1923; Amer. Jour. Obstet., **44:** 753, 1901; Jour. Amer. Med. Assoc., **56:** 1845, 1908.

Kraul, L.: Premature Separation of the Placenta, 27 Cases, Wien. med. Wchnschr., **77:** 509, 1927.

McGlinn, J. A., and Harer, W. B.: The Treatment of Abruptio Placentae, Amer. Jour. Obstet. and Gynec., **30:** 226, 1935.

Rigby: An Essay on Uterine Hemorrhage, 6th ed., 1776.

Scott, R. A.: Premature Separation of Normally Implanted Placenta. Review literature, Surg., Gynec., and Obstet., **38:** 450, 460, 1924.

CHAPTER XXIV

THE LOCAL DISEASES ACCIDENTAL TO PREGNANCY

Davis, C. H., and Colwell, C.: Trichomonas Vaginalis (Donné), Preliminary Report on Experimental and Clinical Study, Jour. Amer. Med. Assoc., **92:** 306, 1929.

Livermore, G. R., and Schumann, E. A.: Gonorrhea and Kindred Affections in the Male and Female, New York, D. Appleton and Co., 1929.

Noeggerath, E.: Die Latente Gonorrhoe im Weiblichen Geschlecht, Bonn, 1872.

Schumann, E. A.: The Relation of Venereal Diseases to Childbirth, Amer. Jour. Obstet. and Gynec., **8:** 257, 1924.

CHAPTER XXV

MALFORMATION OF UTERUS AND VAGINA

Baldwin, J. F.: Artificial Vagina by Intestinal Transplantation, Jour. Amer. Med. Assoc., 54: 1362, 1915.

Ballantyne, J. A.: Eden and Lockyer's Gynecology, New York, The Macmillan Co., 1917, vol. 1, p. 215.

Crossen, H. S.: Operative Gynecology, St. Louis, C. V. Mosby Co., ed. 3, 1925.

Findley, P.: Pregnancy in Uterus Didelphys, Amer. Jour. Obstet. and Gynec., 12: 318, 1926.

Frank, R. J.: Gynecological and Obstetrical Pathology, New York, D. Appleton and Co., 1922.

Gellhorn, G.: Unilateral Defect of Tube and Ovary, Amer. Jour. Obstet., 76: 877, 1917.

Huffman, O. V.: Ectopic Pregnancy Associated with Anomalous Fallopian Tubes, Surg., Gynec., and Obstet., 16: 548, 1913.

Humpstone, O. P.: Pregnancy in Rudimentary Horn of Uterus, Surg., Gynec., and Obstet., 31: 501, 1920.

Kaufmann, E.: Lehrbuch der Speziellen Pathologischen Anatomie, Berlin, G. Reimer, 1911, vol. 2, p. 908.

Kerwin, W.: Uterus Septus with Special Reference to Operative Technic, Amer. Jour. Obstet. and Gynec., 9: 369, 1925.

Miller, N. F.: Uterus Didelphys, Amer. Jour. Obstet. and Gynec., 4: 398, 1922.

Moench, G. L.: Uterus Duplex Bicollis, Vagina Simplex and Superfetation, Amer. Jour. Obstet. and Gynec., 13: 60, 1927.

Rockey, A. E.: Double Uterus and Vagina, Ann. Surg., 63: 615, 1916.

Schubert, G.: The Formation of a New Vagina in the Case of Congenital Vaginal Malformation, Surg., Gynec., and Obstet., 19: 376, 1914.

Schumann, E. A.: Observations on the Comparative Anatomy of the Female Genitalia, Amer. Jour. Obstet., 64: 626, 1911.

Schwarz, E.: Uterus Bicornis, Amer. Jour. Obstet., 77: 583, 1918.

Smith, F. R.: The Significance of Incomplete Fusion of the Müllerian Ducts in Pregnancy and Parturition, Amer. Jour. Obstet. and Gynec., 22: 714, 1931.

Wardlow, Y., and Smith, W. P.: Uterus Duplex Bicornis, Surg., Gynec., and Obstet., 35: 497, 1922.

CHAPTER XXVI

MULTIPLE PREGNANCY

Adair, F. L.: Fetal Malformations in Multiple Pregnancy, Amer. Jour. Obstet. and Gynec., 20: 539, 1930.

Badouin: La Grossesse Sextuple, Gaz. de méd. de Paris, 157, 1909.

Newman, H. H.: The Biology of Twins, University of Chicago Press, 1917.

Stockard, C. R.: An Experimental Study of Twins, Double Monsters and Single Deformities, Amer. Jour. Anat., 28: 115, 1921.

Streeter: Formation of Single Ovum Twins, Bull. Johns Hopkins Hosp., 30: 235, 1919.

Williams, J. W.: Note on Placentations in Quadruplet and Triplet Pregnancy, Bull. Johns Hopkins Hosp., 39: 271, 1926.

CHAPTER XXVII

MATERNAL ILLNESSES ACCIDENTAL TO PREGNANCY

Pregnancy and Tuberculosis

Adair, F. L., and Whitacre, F. E.: Tuberculosis and Reproduction, Jour. Mich. State Med. Soc., January, 1932.

Barnes, H. L., and Barnes, S. R. P.: Pregnancy and Tuberculosis, Amer. Jour
Obstet. and Gynec., 19: 490, 1930.
Hill, Alice M.: A Statistical Study of the Relationship Between Pregnancy and
Tuberculosis, Amer. Rev. Tuberc., 17: 113, 1928.
Matthew, H. B., and Bryant, L. S.: Jour. Amer. Med. Assoc., 95: 1707, 1930.

Syphilis

Cole, H. N. *et al.:* Jour. Amer. Med. Assoc., 106: 464, 1936.
Gellhorn, G.: Syphilis in Women, Nelson's Loose-Leaf Surgery, 1928.
————: Syphilis in Women, Curtis' Obstetrics and Gynecology, Philadelphia, W.
B. Saunders Co., 1933 (complete literature).
Ingraham, N. R., and Kahler, J. E.: The Diagnosis and Treatment of Syphilis
Complicating Pregnancy (complete review of literature), Amer. Jour. Obstet.
and Gynec., 27: 134, 1934.
McCord, J. R.: Syphilis and Pregnancy, Jour. Amer. Med. Assoc., 105: 89, 1935.
McKelvey, J. L., and Turner, J. B.: Syphilis and Pregnancy, Jour. Amer. Med.
Assoc., 102: 503, 1934.

Cardiovascular

Carr, B. F., and Hamilton, B. E.: Amer. Jour. Obstet. and Gynec., 26: 824, 1933.
Clifford, S. H.: Jour. Amer. Med. Assoc., 103: 1117, 1934.
Gilchrist, A. R.: Tr. Edinburgh Obstet. Soc., 90: 121, 1931.
Hamilton, B. E., and Kellog, F. S.: Amer. Jour. Obstet. and Gynec., 13: 535, 1927.
McIlroy, L., and Rendel, O.: The Problem of the Damaged Heart in Obstetrical
Practice, Jour. Obstet. and Gynæc. Brit. Emp., 38: 7, 1931.
Newell, F. S.: Boston Med. and Surg. Jour., 197: 757, 1927.
Reis, R. A., and Frankenthal, L. E.: Amer. Jour. Obstet. and Gynec., 29: 44, 1935.
Teel, Harold M.: Fetal Mortality in Patients with Organic Heart Disease, Amer.
Jour. Obstet. and Gynec., 30: 53, 1935.

Anemias

Mosher, G. C.: The Complication of Purpura with Gestation, Surg., Gynec., and
Obstet., 36: 502, 1923.
Mussey, R. D. *et al.:* Observations on Secondary Anemia During Pregnancy,
Amer. Jour. Obstet. and Gynec., 24: 179, 1932.
Osler, W.: The Severe Anemias of Pregnancy and the Postpartum State, Brit.
Med. Jour., 1: 1919.
Pepper, O. H. P.: A Review of Our Knowledge of the Anemias of Pregnancy,
Med. Clin. N. A., 12: 925, 1929.
Ridder: Chronische Myeloidische Leukämie und Schwangerschaft, Münch. med.
Wchnschr., 77: 2057, 1930.

Respiratory System

Johnson, R. A., and Morgan, H. J.: Acute Lobar Pneumonia and Hematogenous
Puerperal Infection, Bull. Johns Hopkins Hosp., 33: 106, 1922.
Levy: Über Intrauterine Infektion mit Pneumonia Crouposa, Arch. f. Exp.
Path., 26: 595, 1896.

Digestive System

Baer, J. L.; Reis, R. A., and Arens, R. A.: Appendicitis in Pregnancy with
Changes in Position and Axis of the Normal Appendix in Pregnancy, Jour.
Amer. Med. Assoc., 98: 1359, 1932.
Jefferson, J. C.: Intestinal Obstruction Complicating Pregnancy, Lancet, 2: 855,
1924.
Mull, J. W., Bill, A. H., and Kinney, F. M.: Variations of Serum Calcium and
Phosphorus During Pregnancy, The Effects on the Occurrence of Dental
Caries, Amer. Jour. Obstet. and Gynec., 27: 679, 1934.

Peterson, R.: Gallstones During Pregnancy and the Puerperium, Surg., Gynec., and Obstet., **11**: 1, 1910.

Royston, G. D., and Fisher, A. O.: Appendicitis in Pregnancy, Amer. Jour. Obstet. and Gynec., **11**: 184, 1926.

Wilson, R. A.: Acute Appendicitis Complicating Pregnancy, Labor and the Puerperium, Surg., Gynec., and Obstet., **47**: 620, 1927.

Ziskin, D. E.; Blackberg, S. N., and Stout, A. P.: The Gingivas During Pregnancy, Surg., Gynec., and Obstet., **57**: 719, 1933.

Urinary System

Dodds, G. H.: Immediate and Remote Prognosis of Pyelitis of Pregnancy and and the Puerperium, Jour. Obstet. and Gynæc. Brit. Emp., **39**: 46, 1932.

Hofbauer, J. I.: Contributions to the Etiology of Pyelitis in Pregnancy, Bull. Johns Hopkins Hosp., **42**: 118, 1928.

Klein, P.: Pyelitis Gravidarum, und Schwangerschaftsunterbrechung, Arch. f. Gynäk., **137**: 1047, 1929.

Matthews, H. B.: Pregnancy After Nephrectomy, Jour. Amer. Med. Assoc., **77**: 1634, 1921.

Williams, J. T.: Pyelographic Findings in Pyelitis Complicating Pregnancy (Stoeckel, W.), Münch. med. Wchnschr., **71**: 257, 1924.

Nervous Systemic Diseases

Campbell, A. M.: Chorea Gravidarum, Amer. Jour. Obstet. and Gynec., **16**: 88, 1928.

Plass, E. D., and Woods, E. B.: Hemorrhagic Encephalitis (neoarsphenamine) in Obstetric Patients, Amer. Jour. Obstet. and Gynec., **29**: 509, 1935.

Schumann, E. A., and Fist, H. S.: Organic Diseases of Nervous System Complicating Pregnancy, Amer. Jour. Obstet. and Gynec., **4**: 67, 1922.

Wilson, K. M., and Garvey, Paul: Polyneuritis Gravidarum, Amer. Jour. Obstet. and Gynec., **23**: 775, 1932.

Infectious Diseases

Blacklock, D. B., and Gordon, R. M.: Malaria Infection as It Occurs in Late Pregnancy, etc., Amer. Jour. Trop. Med. and Parasit., **19**: 327, 1925.

Bland, P. B.: Influenza in Its Relation to Pregnancy and Labor, Amer. Jour. Obstet., **79**: 184, 1919.

Harris, J. W.: Influenza Occurring in Pregnant Women, Jour. Amer. Med. Assoc., **72**: 978, 1919.

Hicks, H. F., and French, E.: Typhoid Fever and Pregnancy with Special Reference to Fetal Infection, Lancet, **1**: 1491, 1905.

Posch, W.: Über Scharlach im Wochenbett, Zeitschr. f. Geburtsh. u. Gynäk., **90**: 609, 1926.

Simpson, W. M., and Frazier, E.: Undulant Fever, Jour. Amer. Med. Assoc., **93**: 1958, 1929.

Endocrine System

Bokelmann, O., and Scheringer, W.: Beiträge zur Kenntniss der Schilddrüsenfunktions und des Stoffwechsels in der Gestation, Arch. f. Gynäk., **143**: 512, 1931.

Carlson, A. J., and Ginsburg, H.: The Influence of Pregnancy on the Hyperglycemia of Pancreatic Diabetes, Amer. Jour. Physiol., **36**: 217, 1915.

Davis, C. H.: Thyroid Hypertrophy and Pregnancy, Jour. Amer. Med. Assoc., **87**: 1004, 1926.

Hartley, E. C.: The Tetanoid Syndrome in Obstetrics, Amer. Jour. Obstet. and Gynec., **19**: 54, 1930.

Liebmann, S.: Über den Verlauf der mit Diabetes Komplizierten Schwangerschaften und Geburten, Monatschr. f. Geburtsh. u. Gynäk., **91**: 398, 1932.

Litzenberg, J. C., and Carey, J. B.: Relation of Basal Metabolism to Gestation, Amer. Jour. Obstet. and Gynec., 17: 550, 1929.

McCruden, F. H., and Fales, H.: Studies in Bone Metabolism, etc., Arch. Int. Med., 5: 596, 1910.

Meinert, E.: Tetanie in der Schwangerschaft, Arch. f. Gynäk., 30: 444, 1887.

Rowntree, L. G., and Snell, A. M.: A Clinical Study of Addison's Disease, Philadelphia, W. B. Saunders Co., 1931.

CHAPTER XXVIII

ANOMALIES OF THE FORCES OF EXPULSION

Bourne, A., and Bell, A. C.: Uterine Inertia, Jour. Obstet. and Gynæc. Brit. Emp., 40: 423, 1933.

Brown, R. C.: Prolonged First Stage of Labor, Jour. Obstet. and Gynæc. Brit. Emp., 40: 240, 1933.

Goodall, J. R.: The Inertia Syndrome, Jour. Obstet. and Gynæc. Brit. Emp., 41: 256, 1934.

Rucker, M. P.: The Treatment of Contraction Ring Dystocia with Adrenalin, Amer. Jour. Obstet. and Gynec., 14: 609, 1927.

White, C.: On Contraction and Retraction Rings, Amer. Jour. Obstet. and Gynec., 11: 364, 1926.

CHAPTER XXIX

ANOMALIES IN FORCES OF RESISTANCE

Bell, T. Floyd: Occiput Posterior Position, West. Jour. Surg., Gynec., and Obstet., October, 1933.

Brooklyn Gynecological Society Analysis of 3301 Breech Deliveries in the Hospitals of Brooklyn, Amer. Jour. Obstet. and Gynec., 28: 40, 1934.

Caldwell, Wm. E., and Studdiford, W. E.: Review of Breech Deliveries at Sloane Hospital for Women, Amer. Jour. Obstet. and Gynec., 18: 623, 1929.

Cannell, D. E., and Dodek, S. M.: Amer. Jour. Obstet. and Gynec., 27: 517, 1934.

Essen-Möller, E.: Acta Obstet. et Gynaec. Scandinav., 8: 103, 1929.

King, E. L., and Gladden, A. H., Jr.: Amer. Jour. Obstet. and Gynec., 17: 78, 1929.

Morton, D. G.: Amer. Jour. Obstet. and Gynec., 24: 853, 1932.

Nathanson, J. N.: Amer. Jour. Obstet. and Gynec., 30: 159, 1935.

Quigley, J. K.: Amer. Jour. Obstet. and Gynec., 21: 234, 1931.

Reed, C. B.: Persistent Mento-Posterior Positions, Amer. Jour. Obstet., 51: 615, 1905.

Schulze, Margaret: Labor in the Elderly Primipara, Jour. Amer. Med. Assoc., 93: 824, 1929.

Thoms, H.: Occipito-Posterior Position and the Transversely Contracted Pelvis, Amer. Jour. Obstet. and Gynec., 24: 50, 1932.

Thorn, W.: Zur Manuellen Umwandlung der Gesichtslagen in Hinterhauptslagen, Zeitschr. f. Geburtsh. u. Gynäk., 13: 186, 1886.

CHAPTER XXX

CONTRACTED PELVIS

Caldwell, W. E., and Moloy, H. C.: Anatomical Variations in the Female Pelvis and Their Effect in Labor with a Suggested Classification, Amer. Jour. Obstet. and Gynec., 24: 479, 1933.

Clifford, S. H.: The X-ray Measurement of the Fetal Head in Utero, Surg., Gynec., and Obstet., 58: 727, 1934.

Friedman, L. J.; Michels, L. M., and Rossitter, A. F.: Practical Roentgen Pelvimetry, Surg., Gynec., and Obstet., 61: 735, 1935.

Hanson, S.: X-ray Cephalometry, Amer. Jour. Obstet. and Gynec., **27:** 691, 1934.

Hillis, D. S.: Diagnosis of Contracted Pelvis by Impression Method, Surg., Gynec., and Obstet., **51:** 852, 1930.

Jarcho, J.: Roentgenographic Measurement of Pelvic and Cephalic Measurements, Amer. Jour. Surg., **14:** 419, 1931.

————: The Value of the Walcher Position in Contracted Pelvis, Surg., Gynec., Obstet., 854, 1929.

Pride, W. T.: Pelvic Measurements in the White and Colored Female and Their Significance in Childbirth, Amer. Jour. Obstet. and Gynec., **31:** 495, 1936.

Stone, E. L.: (Literature of Osteomalacia.) Surg., Gynec., and Obstet., **39:** 599, 1924.

Thoms, H.: The Inadequacy of External Pelvimetry, Amer. Jour. Obstet. and Gynec., **27:** 270, 1934.

————: Fetal Cephalometry in Utero, Jour. Amer. Med. Assoc., **95:** 21, 1930.

————: Shortening of the Transverse Diameter of the Superior Strait, Amer. Jour. Obstet. and Gynec., **19:** 539, 1930.

————: Roentgen Pelvimetry, Radiology, **21:** 125, 1933.

————: Variations of the Female Pelvis in Relation to Labor, Surg., Gynec., and Obstet., **60:** 680, 1935.

————: The Diagnosis of Disproportion, Surg., Gynec., and Obstet., **52:** 963, 1931.

————: What is a Normal Pelvis? Jour. Amer. Med. Assoc., **102:** 2075, 1934.

Williams, N. H.: A Comparison of Clinical and X-ray Pelvimetry, West. Jour. Obstet. and Gynec., February, 1935.

CHAPTER XXXI

DYSTOCIA DUE TO ANOMALIES OF THE BIRTH CANAL

Barley, H.: Trial Labor in 477 Cases of Contracted Pelvis, Amer. Jour. Obstet. and Gynec., **12:** 550, 1926.

Barris, J. D.: Induction of Labor for Disproportion, Jour. Obstet. and Gynæc. Brit. Emp., **36:** 287, 1925.

Michaelis: Das Enge Becken, Leipzig, 1851.

Skutsch: Die Beckenmessung, Jena, 1886.

Williams, J. W.: Frequency, Etiology and Practical Significance of Contraction of the Pelvic Outlet, Surg., Gynec., and Obstet., **8:** 619, 1909.

Zangemeister: Beiträge zur Lehre vom Engen Becken, Zentralbl. f. Gynäk., 1395, 1922.

CHAPTER XXXII

DYSTOCIA DUE TO ABNORMALITIES OF THE FETUS

Ballantyne, J. W.: The Diseases of the Fetus, Edinburgh, 1892.

Ballard: Jour. de méd. de Bordeaux, **91:** 159, 1920.

Falls, F. H.: The Diagnosis of Fetal Deformities in Utero, Amer. Jour. Obstet. and Gynec., **16:** 803, 1928.

Freund, H.: Deutsch. med. Wchnschr., **31:** 667, 1905.

Gustafson, G. W.: Intra-Uterine Diagnosis of Monstrosities, Surg., Gynec., and Obstet., **59:** 223, 1934.

Schumann, E. A.: A Study of Hydrops Universalis Fetus, Amer. Jour. Obstet., **72:** 590, 1915.

————: Observations Upon the Formation of Teratomata, Amer. Jour. Obstet., **57:** 608, 1913.

————: Some General Observations Upon Antenatal Pathology, Amer. Jour. Obstet., **75:** 592, 1917.

Spangler, D.: Amer. Jour. Roentgenol., **11:** 238, 1924.

Zangemeister and Lehn: Die Geburtshilfliche Bedeutung Übergrosses Fruchtentwicklung, Arch. f. Gynäk., **109:** 500, 1918.

CHAPTER XXXIII

RUPTURE OF THE UTERUS

Bell, W. Blair: Manual Rupture of the Puerperal Uterus, Jour. Obstet. and Gynæc. Brit. Emp., **31:** 430, 1924.

Mandelstamm, A.: Zur Frage des Geburtsshockes und des Plötzlichen Todes Nach der Geburt, Arch. f. Gynäk., **38:** 543, 1929.

Riddel: Rupture of the Uterus During Pregnancy, Jour. Obstet. and Gynæc. Brit. Emp., **33:** 1, 1926.

Sachs, S.: Über Uterus Rupturen in den Geburt, Zentralbl. f. Gynäk., **54:** 1180, 1930.

CHAPTER XXXIV

INJURIES OF THE BIRTH CANAL

Goff, B. H.: Prophylaxis in Gynecology with Especial Reference to the Immediate Care of the Postpartum Cervix, Trans, Amer. Gynec. Soc., **60:** 167, 1935.

Olshausen: Über Dammverletzung und Dammschutz, Samml. klin. Vortr., Leipzig, No. 44, 1872.

CHAPTER XXXV

POSTPARTUM HEMORRHAGE

Labhardt: Beiträge zur Kenntniss der Anatomischen Grundlagen der Postpartum Blutungen, Zeitschr. f. Geburtsh. u. Gynäk., **66:** 374, 1910.

Momberg: Blutelehre der Unteren Körperhälfte, Zentralbl. f. Gynäk., 716, 1909.

Peckham, C. K., and Kuder, K.: Some Statistics of Postpartum Hemorrhage, Amer. Jour. Obstet. and Gynec., **26:** 361, 1933.

Polak, J. O.: Postpartum Hemorrhage, N. Y. State Jour. Med., **26:** 1030, 1930.

Stoeckel: Pathologie u. Therapie der Nachgeburtsblutungen, Arch. f. Gynäk., **125:** 1, 1925.

Williams, J. W.: The Tolerance of Freshly Delivered Women to Excessive Loss of Blood, Amer. Jour. Obstet., **80:** 1, 1919.

CHAPTER XXXVI

INVERSION OF UTERUS AND PROLAPSE OF CORD

Fritsch, J.: Zur Aetiologie der Puerperalen Uterusinversion, Zentralbl. f. Gynäk., **31:** 427, 1907.

Huntington, J. L.; Irving, F. C., and Kellog, F. S.: Amer. Jour. Obstet. and Gynec., **15:** 34, 1928.

McCullough, W. McK. H.: Inversion of the Uterus: A Report of Three Cases and an Analysis of 230 Recently Recorded, Jour. Obstet. and Gynæc. Brit. Emp., **32:** 280, 1925.

Miller, N. F.: Pregnancy Following Inversion of the Uterus, Amer. Jour. Obstet. and Gynec., **13:** 307, 1927.

Phaneuf, L. E.: Amer. Jour. Obstet. and Gynec., **11:** 116, 1926.

Schiller, W.: Über Nabelschnurvorfall, Monatschr. f. Geburtsh. u. Gynäk., **88:** 52, 1931.

Spinelli, P. G.: Della Inversione Uterina, Riv. di ginec. contemp., **1:** 1, 1897.

Vogel, G.: Beiträge zur Lehre von der Inversio Uteri, Zeitschr. f. Geburtsh. u. Gynäk., **42:** 490, 1900.

CHAPTERS XXXVII AND XXXVIII

PUERPERAL SEPSIS

Adair, F. L., and Tiber, J. L.: Amer. Jour. Obstet. and Gynec., 17: 559, 1929.

Bernstine, J. B.: Further Studies in the Treatment of Puerperal Septicemia and Other Blood Stream Infections with Metaphen, Amer. Jour. Obstet. and Gynec., 25: 849, 1933.

Crocker, W. J.; Valentine, E. H., and Brody, W.: Hemography-Controlled Nonspecific Immunotransfusion in Treatment of Sepsis, Jour. Lab. and Clin. Med., 20: 482, 1935.

Findley, P.: The Biologic Defense in Puerperal Infection, Amer. Jour. Obstet. and Gynec., 13: 514, 1927.

Goodall, J. R.: Puerperal Infection, Montreal, 1932.

Halban and Kohler: Die Pathologische Anatomie des Puerperal Prozesses, Braumüller, Leipzig, 1919.

Hofbauer: Cellular Defense in the Parametrium. Function of Hofbauer Cells, Amer. Jour. Obstet. and Gynec., 10: 1–14, July, 1925.

Holmes, O. W.: Puerperal Fever as a Private Pestilence, Boston, 1855.

Lea, Arnold W.: Puerperal Sepsis, Oxford University Press, 1910.

Little, H. M.: Bacteriology of the Puerperal Uterus, Amer. Jour. Obstet., 52: 815–847, October, 1905.

Logan, W. R.: The Relation of the Vaginal Reaction and Flora During Pregnancy to Puerperal Sepsis, Jour. Obstet. and Gynæc. Brit. Emp., 38: 788, 1931.

Miller, C. J.: The Therapy of Puerperal Infection, Surg., Gynec., and Obstet., 51: 557, 1930.

Polak, J. O.: Pelvic Inflammation in Women, New York, D. Appleton and Co., 1921.

——: Further Studies in Puerperal Sepsis, Amer. Jour. Obstet. and Gynec., 10: 521–527, 1925.

Prevost, A. R.: Les streptocoques anaerobiques, Ann. de l'inst. Pasteur, Paris, 39: 417–447, 1925, Thèse de Paris, 1924.

Pyrah, L. N., and Oldfield, C.: Puerperal General Peritonitis, Jour. Obstet. and Gynæc. Brit. Emp., 40: 3, 1933.

Schottmüller: Zur Bedeutung Einiger Anaeroben in der Pathol. Inbesondern bei Puerperalen Erkrankungen, Mitt. a. d. Grenzgeb. d. Med. u. Chir., 1910, vol. XXI. Zur Aetiologie des Febris Puerperalis, Münch. med. Wchnschr., 2011, 1911.

Schwarz, O. H., and Brown, J. K.: Puerperal Infection Due to Anaerobic Streptococci, Amer. Jour. Obstet. and Gynec., 31: 379, 1936.

Semmelweis, I.: Die Aetiologie der Begriff u. der Prophylaxis des Kindbettfiebers, Pest, Vienna and Leipzig, 1861.

Stetson, R. E.: The Therapeutic Value of Blood Transfusions with Report of 68 Cases of Sepsis, Amer. Jour. Med. Sci., 168: 534, No. 4, October, 1924.

Stolz, M.: Beiträge z. Geburtsh. u. Gynäk., 7: 406, 1903.

Watson, B. P.: Puerperal Infection, Amer. Jour. Obstet. and Gynec., 16: 157–179, August, 1928. Postpartum Pelvic Infections, ibid., 16: 536–546, October, 1928.

White, Chas.: A Treatise on the Management of Pregnant and Lying-in Women, London, 1773.

CHAPTER XXXIX

PUERPERAL DISEASES AND ANOMALIES OF THE BREASTS

Bumm, E.: Zur Aetiologie der Puerperalen Mastitis, Arch. f. Gynäk., 27: 460, 1886.

Klein, M. D.: A Clinical Study of Effect of Camphor in Oil on Lactation, Amer. Jour. Obstet. and Gynec., 31: 894, 1936.

Schumann, E. A.: A Study of Carcinoma Mastitoides, Ann. Surg., 53: 69, 1911.
Storrs: Checking the Secretion of the Lactating Breast, Surg., Gynec., and Obstet., 9: 401, 1909.

CHAPTER XL

INJURIES AND ACCIDENTS OF THE INFANT

Ballantyne, J. W.: Antenatal Pathology and Hygiene, Edinburgh, 1904.
Ehrenfest, H.: Birth Injuries of the Child, New York, D. Appleton and Co., 1922.
Henderson, Y.: The Prevention and Treatment of Asphyxia in the Newborn, Jour. Amer. Med. Assoc., 90: 583, 1928.
McGrath, M. D., and Kuder, K.: Resuscitation of the Newborn, Jour. Amer. Med. Assoc., 106: 885, 1936.
Plass, E. D., and Jeans, P. C.: Intracranial Hemorrhage in the Newborn, Early and Late Manifestations, Jour. Iowa State Med. Soc., September, 1932.
Schultze: Zur Behandlung des Scheintodes Neugeborenen, Zeitschr. f. Geburtsh. u. Gynäk., 68: 591, 1911.
Schwartz, P., and Fink, L.: Morphologie und Entstehung der Geburtstraumatischen Blutungen in Gehirn und Schädel des Neugeborenen, Zeitschr. f. Kinderh., 40: 427, 1926.
Seitz: Die Fötalen Herztöne Während den Geburt, Munich, 1903 (literature).
Sharpe, Wm.: Intracranial Hemorrhage in the Newborn, Jour. Amer. Med. Assoc., 81: 620, 1923.

CHAPTER XLI

OPERATIVE OBSTETRICS

Champetier de Ribes: De l'accouchement provoqué, Ann. de gynéc. et d'obstét., Paris, 30: 401, 1888.
Denman: An Introduction to the Practise of Midwifery, London, (7th ed.), p. 318, 1823.
Dührssen: Über den Werth der Tiefen Cervix und Scheiden-Damm Einschnitte in der Geburtshilfe, Arch. f. Gynäk., Berlin, 37: 27, 1890.
Hofbauer and Hoerner: The Nasal Application of Pituitary Extract for the Induction of Labor, Amer. Jour. Obstet. and Gynec., 14: 137, 1927.
Morton, D. G.: Induction of Labor by Means of Artificial Rupture of the Membranes, etc., Amer. Jour. Obstet. and Gynec., 26: 323, 1933.
Slemons, J. M.: Induction of Labor at Term, Amer. Jour. Obstet. and Gynec., 26: 494, 1932.
Williamson: The Induction of Premature Labor, Jour. Obstet. and Gynæc. Brit. Emp., 8: 252, 1905.

CHAPTER XLII

THE OBSTETRICAL FORCEPS

Aveling: The Chamberlens and the Midwifery Forceps, London, 1882.
Baer, J. L.: The Use of Forceps, Illinois Med. Jour., 56: 379, 1929.
Barton, L. G., Caldwell and Studdiford, W. E.: A New Obstetric Forceps, Amer. Jour. Obstet. and Gynec., 15: 16, 1928.
Bill, A. H.: The Modified Scanzoni Maneuver in the Treatment of Vertex-Occipito-Posterior Positions, Amer. Jour. Obstet. and Gynec., 9: 342, 1925.
Das, K.: The Obstetric Forceps, Its History and Evolution, St. Louis, C. V. Mosby Co., 1929.
DeLee, J. B.: The Prophylactic Forceps Operation, Jour. Amer. Med. Assoc., 75: 145, 1920.
Jarcho, J.: The Kielland Obstetric Forceps and Its Application, Amer. Jour. Obstet. and Gynec., 10: 35, 1925.

Kielland: Über die Anlegung der Zange am nicht Rotierten Kopf mit Beschreibung Eines Neuen Zangemodelles, Monatschr. f. Geburtsh. u. Gynäk., Berlin, 43: 47, 1916.
Piper, E. B.: Prevention of Fetal Injuries in Breech Delivery, Jour. Amer. Med. Assoc., 92: 217, 1929.
Scanzoni: Lehrbuch der Geburtshilfe, 2nd ed., 1853.
Tarnier: Description de deux nouveaux forceps, Paris, 1877.

CHAPTER XLIII

BREECH EXTRACTION

Litzmann: Der Mauriceau-Levret-sche Handgriffe, Arch. f. Gynäk., Berlin, 31: 102, 1887.
Mauriceau, F.: Traité des Maladies des Femmes Grosses, 6th ed., p. 280, 1721.
Piper, E. B.: Curtis' Obstetrics and Gynecology, Philadelphia, W. B. Saunders Co., 1933, vol. II, Chap. XXXVI.
Smellie, Wm.: Treatise on the Theory and Practise of Midwifery (8th ed.), 1774, p. 195.
Veit, G.: Über die Beste Methode zur Extraktion des nachfolgenden Kindeskopfes, Greifswald med. Beiträge, vol. 2, No. 1, 1863.
Wiegand: Über Wendung durch Äussere Handgriffe, Hamburg med. Mag., 1: 52, 1807

CHAPTER XLIV

VERSION

Baer, J. L.; Reis, R. A., and Lutz, J. J.: The Present Position of Version and Extraction, etc., Amer. Jour. Obstet. and Gynec., 24: 599, 1932.
Bartholomew, R. H.: Prophylactic External Version, Amer. Jour. Obstet. and Gynec., 14: 648, 1927.
Hicks, J. Braxton: On Combined External and Internal Version, London, 1864.
Holland, E.: Cranial Stress in the Fetus During Labor, Jour. Obstet. and Gynæc. Brit. Emp., 29: 551, 1922.
Paré, A.: Edition Malgaigne, 1840, vol. 2, 623.
Pinard, A.: De la Version par les Manoeuvres Externes Traité du Palper Abdominal, Paris, 1889.
Potter, I.: The Place of Version in Obstetrics, St. Louis, C. V. Mosby Co., 1922.

CHAPTER XLV

CESAREAN SECTION

Beck, A. C.: The Advantages and Disadvantages of the Two-flap Low Incision Cesarean Section, etc., Amer. Jour. Obstet. and Gynec., 1: 586, 1921.
Burns, H. T.: Study of 79 Patients Delivered by the Latzko Extraperitoneal Cesarean Section, Amer. Jour. Obstet. and Gynec., 28: 556, 1934.
———: The Latzko Extraperitoneal Cesarean Section, Amer. Jour. Obstet. and Gynec., 19: 759, 1930.
DeLee, J. B.: Low or Cervical Cesarean Section, Jour. Amer. Med. Assoc., 84: 791, 1925.
Dührssen, A.: Der Vaginale Kaiserschnitt, 1896.
Gordon, C. A.: A Survey of Cesarean Sections in Brooklyn, Amer. Jour. Obstet. and Gynec., 16: 307, 1928.
Greenhill, J. P.: Histologic Study of Uterine Scars After Cervical Cesarean Section, Jour. Amer. Med. Assoc., 21: 92, 1929.
King, E. L.: The End Results of Abdominal Cesarean Section, Jour. Amer. Med. Assoc., 79: 112, 1922.

48

Latzko: Über den Extraperitonealen Kaiserschnitt, Zentralbl. f. Gynäk., p. 275, 1909.

Lull, C. B.: A Survey of Cesarean Sections Performed in Philadelphia During 1931, Amer. Jour. Obstet. and Gynec., 25: 426, 1933.

Maxwell, Alice F.: A Review of Cesarean Section, West. Jour. Surg., Gynec., and Obstet., 42: 14, 1934.

Nicholson, Wm. R.: Rupture of the Cesarean Scar in Succeeding Pregnancy, Amer. Jour. Obstet. and Gynec., 26: 387, 1933.

Phaneuf, L.: Cesarean Section Followed by Temporary Exteriorization of the Uterus, Surg., Gynec., and Obstet., 44: 788, 1927.

————: Some Historical Notes on the Technic of Cesarean Section, Surg., Gynec., and Obstet., 47: 857, 1928.

Pickrell, K. L.: An Inquiry into the History of Cesarean Sections, Bull. Soc. Med. Hosp. of Chicago, 4: 414, 1935.

Porro: Della Amputazione Utero-ovarica, Milan, 1876.

Portes: La césarienne suivive d'exteriorisation de l'uterus, Gynéc. et obstét., 10: 225, 1924.

Sänger: Der Kaiserschnitt bei Uterusmyomen, Leipzig, 1882.

Schumann, E. A.: The Elective Cesarean Section as a Prophylactic Measure Against Obstetric Mortality and Morbidity, Amer. Jour. Obstet. and Gynec., 23: 248, 1932.

Sellheim: Der Extraperitoneale Uterusschnitt, Zentralbl. f. Gynäk., p. 133, 1908.

CHAPTER XLVI

MUTILATING OPERATIONS ON THE CHILD

Davis, E. P.: Operative Obstetrics, Philadelphia, W. B. Saunders Co., 1911.

Mendenhall, A. M.: Amer. Jour. Obstet. and Gynec., 5: 372, 1923.

Simpson, J. Y.: Cranioclast, Med. News and Gazette, 1860, vol. 1.

Tarnier, A.: Le Basiotribe, Ann. de gynéc. et d'obstét., 21: 74, 1884.

INDEX

755